£80.00 WL410 HAN

KT-150-243

WL410 HAN
Hankey Graeme J.

Stroke treatment and prevention: an
evidence based approach

£80.00   25/04/2006

STAFF LIBRARY
WILLOW HOUSE
WATFORD GENERAL HOSPITAL
VICARAGE ROAD
WATFORD WD18 0HB

DEMCO

Stroke Treatment and Prevention

Stroke is the third most common cause of death in the world, and a major source of a disability. This invaluable reference will provide clinicians caring for stroke patients with ready access to the optimal evidence for best practice in acute stroke treatment and secondary prevention. The author, who is a Member of the Editorial Board of the Cochrane Stroke Review Group, describes all available treatments for acute stroke and secondary prevention, the rationale for using them, and, where available, the highest-level evidence (level 1) for their safety and effectiveness.

Where level 1 evidence is not available, he offers advice on reasonable practice and information about current research. The evidence for each treatment is followed by the author's interpretations, and the implications of the evidence in the care of stroke patients.

This is therefore an essential resource for clinicians, translating into practice advances that have been made in the treatment and prevention of stroke, and suggesting the most appropriate interventions.

MEDICAL LIBRARY
HEMEL HEMPSTEAD HOSPITAL
HILLFIELD ROAD
HEMEL HEMPSTEAD
HERTS   HP2 4AD

Stroke Treatment and Prevention

An Evidence-Based Approach

Graeme J. Hankey MBBS, MD, FRCP, FRCPEdin, FRACP

Neurologist
Stroke Unit
Department of Neurology
Royal Perth Hospital
Perth, Australia

Clinical Professor
School of Medicine and Pharmacology
The University of Western Australia
Australia

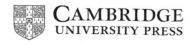
CAMBRIDGE
UNIVERSITY PRESS

CAMBRIDGE UNIVERSITY PRESS
Cambridge, New York, Melbourne, Madrid, Cape Town, Singapore, São Paulo

CAMBRIDGE UNIVERSITY PRESS
The Edinburgh Building, Cambridge CB2 2RU, UK
Published in the United States of America by Cambridge University Press, New York

www.cambridge.org
Information on this title: www.cambridge.org/9780521827195

© Cambridge University Press 2005

This book is in copyright. Subject to statutory exception and
to the provisions of relevant collective licensing agreements,
no reproduction of any part may take place without the
written permission of Cambridge University Press.

First published 2005

Printed in the United Kingdom at the University Press, Cambridge

A catalogue record for this book is available from the British Library

Library of Congress Cataloguing in Publication data

ISBN-13 978-0-521-82719-5 hardback
ISBN-10 0-521-82719-1 hardback

Cambridge University Press has no responsibility for the
persistence or accuracy of URLs for external or third-party
Internet web sites referred to in this book, and does not
guarantee that any content on such web sites is, or will
remain, accurate or appropriate.

Every effort has been made in preparing this book to provide accurate and
up-to-date information which is in accord with accepted standards and practice
at the time of publication. Although case histories are drawn from actual cases,
every effort has been made to disguise the identities of the individuals involved.
Nevertheless, the authors, editors and publishers can make no warranties that the
information contained herein is totally free from error, not least because clinical
standards are constantly changing through research and regulation. The authors,
editors and publishers therefore disclaim all liability for direct or consequential
damages resulting from the use of material contained in this book. Readers are
strongly advised to pay careful attention to information provided by the
manufacturer of any drugs or equipment that they plan to use.

This book is dedicated to my wonderful and
loving parents (Jean and John)
and
daughters (Genevieve and Michelle)

Contents

Preface

Stroke is an enormous public health problem. It is the third most common cause of death (causing 4.4 million deaths worldwide in 1990) and the most important cause of disability among adults (with an estimated prevalence of 0.6% population) in the world. It also imposes an enormous cost on the community, accounting for about 5% of all health service costs.

During the past decade, several promising treatments for stroke have been evaluated by means of the most reliable methods – the randomised-controlled trial (RCT) and the systematic review and meta-analysis of RCTs – providing a reasonably reliable body of evidence for the efficacy and safety of several treatments for stroke. In order for these advances to make an important difference to patient outcome and the health of nations, they need to be translated into practice. One way to facilitate this is by increasing the access to best evidence for stroke care practitioners and consumers. At present, these data are available at several sites including the *Cochrane Library*, MEDLINE, and Evidence-Based Medicine publications and web sites such as Clinical Evidence http://www.clinicalevidence.org/, EBM Guidelines http://www.ebm-guidelines.com/ and the Scottish Intercollegiate Guidelines Network http://www.sign.ac.uk/guidelines/index.html. Furthermore, they are regularly updated to incorporate new evidence as it arises. However, none are dedicated in a single corpus specifically for clinicians who manage stroke patients and their families.

The aim of this book is to provide stroke clinicians (and their patients and families), with ready access to the optimal evidence to guide best practice in acute stroke treatment and (secondary) prevention of recurrent serious vascular events. Where available, I have quoted the highest level of evidence (level 1) to guide practice – RCTs and systematic reviews and meta-analyses of RCTs – and have predominantly sourced the *Cochrane Library*, to whom I am grateful for allowing me to reproduce their work. Of course, by the time you read this book, there will have been further updates in the *Cochrane Library* every quarter, with new reviews and updated earlier reviews, which I would encourage you to 'visit'. After each section describing the evidence, I have made a comment about my interpretation of the evidence, and the implications of the evidence for clinical practice and research. As level 1 evidence is not (yet) available for many areas of stroke management, I have tried to define which areas are 'evidence-poor' and even 'evidence-free', what might be reasonable practice under these circumstances (acknowledging that absence of evidence of effectiveness does not necessarily mean evidence of absence of effectiveness (Alderson, 2004)), and what research is ongoing and needed.

Ultimately, in order to translate evidence into practice, clinicians must be aware of, and prescribe, the most appropriate interventions for their patients based on effectiveness, safety, affordability and patient preferences. And patients must be adequately informed and consent to comply with the prescription. Since most strokes are first-ever strokes and sudden in onset, it is commonly a shock for previously healthy people with a first-ever stroke or transient ischaemic attack (TIA) to be suddenly impaired neurologically, to be asked to consider sometimes risky and costly investigations and treatments (e.g. catheter angiography, thrombolysis, decompressive neurosurgery, carotid surgery or stenting), and prescribed at least three drugs (e.g. antithrombotic, statin and antihypertensive) for life. Consequently, all the options must be presented sensitively, simply and repeatedly by clinicians who know the risks (large and small) and benefits (large and small) of the treatments. And this must be done quickly, on the day of presentation or as soon as possible thereafter, because of the high risk of early recurrent stroke. Perhaps the drugs should be introduced one at a time so that any early adverse effects can be correctly attributed. Stroke medicine therefore remains an art as well as a science. It cannot be undertaken solely by 'robots' according to a 'cook-book' or protocol; the results of RCTs and meta-analyses have to be interpreted accurately, and coupled with clinical experience, acumen and common sense, in order to be applied optimally to individual patients (Warlow *et al.*, 2003).

I am grateful to Professors Charles Warlow and Peter Sandercock (Edinburgh, Scotland) and Jan van Gijn (Utrecht, The Netherlands) for introducing me to evidence-based stroke medicine, and to John Wiley and Sons Limited for granting me permission to reproduce many of the figures in this book from the *Cochrane Library*.

Graeme Hankey

The size of the problem of stroke

Stroke is an enormous and serious public health problem. It is the third most common cause of death in the world, after ischaemic heart disease and all types of cancer combined. Stroke caused 4.4 million deaths in 1990, and two thirds of these occurred in less developed countries (Murray and Lopez, 1996, 1997). Stroke is also the most important cause of disability among adults. The estimated prevalence of stroke-related disability is more than 0.6% of the population of the world, which represented 3% of the world's disability burden in 1990 (Murray and Lopez, 1996, 1997; Lopez and Murray, 1998).

In the USA in 1994, stroke was the second most common cause of death, the fourth greatest cause of disability-adjusted life years, the fifth highest consumer of days in hospital, the fifth most prevalent major disorder and the eighth most commonly occurring disorder (incidence) (Gross et al., 1999).

Stroke is therefore costly (and becoming increasingly costly) to health care systems. It is estimated that stroke accounts for 4–6% of health care budgets, excluding the costs of social services and carers. Stroke accounts for almost 6% of total health care costs in Finland, 5% in the UK and over 3% in the Netherlands (Isaard and Forbes, 1992; Taylor et al., 1996; Evers et al., 1997; Dewey et al., 2001; Payne et al., 2002; Levy et al., 2003; Evers et al., 2004; Martinez-Vila and Irimia, 2004). However, stroke attracts far less research funding than heart disease or cancer (Rothwell, 2001; Pendlebury et al., 2004).

Incidence

The incidence of new cases of first-ever stroke, standardised for age and sex, is about 200 per 100,000 per year (i.e. 0.2% of the population (and 0.4% of people aged <45 years)) in the few white populations studied in Europe, the USA and Australia, and non-white populations in development countries (Fig. 1.1) (Sudlow and Warlow, 1997; Feigin et al., 2003; Warlow et al., 2003; Feigin, 2005, Lavados et al., 2005). However, the incidence of stroke may be higher, and up to twice as common in Siberia, Eastern Europe and China, and lower in some parts of France, such as Dijon, which has the lowest incidence.

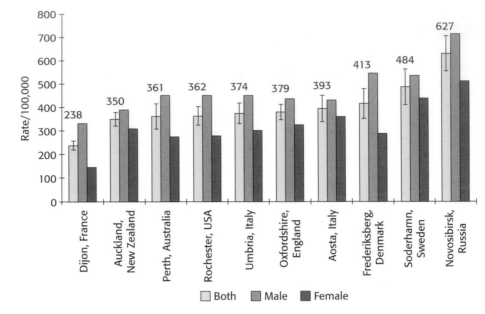

Figure 1.1   Incidence of stroke (ischaemic and haemorrhagic combined) amongst 10 different communities according to age groups 45 years and older. Reproduced from Sudlow and Warlow (1997), with permission form the authors and Lippincott Williams & Wilkins.

The incidence of stroke, in white populations at least, is roughly equal in men and women, and rises steeply with age; about a quarter occur below the age of 65 years and about a half below the age of 75 years. Consequently, the absolute number of stroke patients is likely to increase in the future, because of the ageing of most populations, despite uncertainty over whether stroke incidence is rising, falling or remaining static (see below).

Among incidence studies with the highest rates of brain imaging, the distribution of the pathological types of stroke among populations is similar (about 80% ischaemic, 15% primary intracerebral haemorrhage and 5% subarachnoid haemorrhage) (Warlow et al., 2003). The proportion of stroke due to primary intracerebral haemorrhage is reported be higher in Africa and Asia but this claim remains to be confirmed by well-conducted population-based studies.

Prevalence

The prevalence of stroke is probably somewhere between 5 and 12 per 1000 population (i.e. 1% of the population) but this estimate depends on the age and sex structure of the population (Bonita et al., 1997). In women and men aged 65–74 years, the prevalence of stroke is 25 and 50 per 1000, respectively (Wyller et al., 1994;

Table 1.1. Age-standardised stroke mortality (per 100,000 population) between 40 and 69 years of age in 27 countries in 1985 (Bonita *et al.*, 1990).

	Men		Women	
Country	Rank	Rate	Rank	Rate
Bulgaria	1	249	1	156
Hungary	2	229	2	130
Czechoslovakia	3	177	4	103
Romania	4	172	3	129
Yugoslavia	5	145	5	101
Singapore	6	136	6	92
Japan	7	107	11	60
Scotland	8	99	7	77
Finland	9	98	13	57
Poland	10	96	10	62
Hong Kong	11	94	9	64
Austria	12	90	16	48
Northern Ireland	13	84	8	67
Ireland	14	72	12	59
England and Wales	15	71	14	54
Germany	16	68	19	39
Belgium	17	64	18	41
New Zealand	18	62	15	50
France	19	60	26	28
Australia	20	60	17	45
Denmark	21	55	20	38
Norway	22	55	22	35
Sweden	23	48	24	30
The Netherlands	24	47	23	31
USA	25	45	21	35
Canada	26	39	25	28
Switzerland	27	38	27	21

Bots *et al.*, 1996; Geddes *et al.*, 1996). Stroke prevalence also depends on incidence and survival.

Mortality

The mortality rates of stroke vary widely among countries for which routine death-certificate data are available, from about 20 to 250 per 100,000 population per year (Sarti *et al.*, 2000) (Table 1.1).

Table 1.2. Factors influencing stroke mortality rates.

- The incidence of stroke and its pathological and aetiological subtypes
- The severity and case fatality of stroke
- The age and gender of the population affected by stroke
- The accuracy of death certificates

Stroke mortality varies because of many factors (Table 1.2). For example, pathological stroke subtypes with a very low case fatality (e.g. lacunar infarction) contribute little to mortality statistics whereas pathological and aetiological subtypes with a high case fatality (e.g. primary intracerebral haemorrhage, total anterior circulation infarction) do. As stroke mortality rises rapidly with age, any assessment of mortality must account for age, and any comparisons in mortality must be age standardised or, perhaps better, restricted to certain age groups where the diagnosis of stroke is most likely to be correct (age 55–64 years) or where the number of strokes is largest (age 65–74 years). However, even after adjusting for age, the age-standardised death rate attributed to stroke varies 6-fold among developed countries (Table 1.1) (Bonita *et al.*, 1990; Sarti *et al.*, 2000). In the early 1990s, stroke mortality was lowest in western Europe, the USA, Japan and Australia, and highest in Eastern Europe and countries of the former Soviet Union (Sarti *et al.*, 2000).

Very little is known about stroke mortality in the developing world, nor about the relative distribution of stroke subtype mortality among different countries anywhere in the world.

Case fatality, recurrent stroke and functional outcome

The case fatality rates after a first-ever stroke (all types combined) are about 12% at 7 days, 20% at 30 days, 30% at 1 year, 60% at 5 years and 80% at 10 years (Dennis *et al.*, 1993; Hankey *et al.*, 2000; Hardie *et al.*, 2003). The relative risk of death in stroke survivors is about twice the risk of people in the general population, and the risk persists for several years.

Death within a few hours to days after stroke is usually due to the direct effects of the brain lesion itself (usually intracerebral or subarachnoid haemorrhage, and less commonly massive brainstem infarction) or its complications (e.g. brain oedema) causing brain herniation. Later, the complications of immobility (e.g. bronchopneumonia, venous thromboembolism) and recurrent vascular events of the brain and heart are the common causes of death (Fig. 1.2).

The risk of a recurrent stroke among survivors of stroke in the community is up to about 10% within 7 days, and about 18% within the first 3 months (Fig. 1.3) (Coull *et al.*, 2004; Hill *et al.*, 2004; Hankey *et al.*, 2005). The risk is 3-fold higher if the transient ischaemic attack (TIA) or ischaemic stroke is caused by large artery disease,

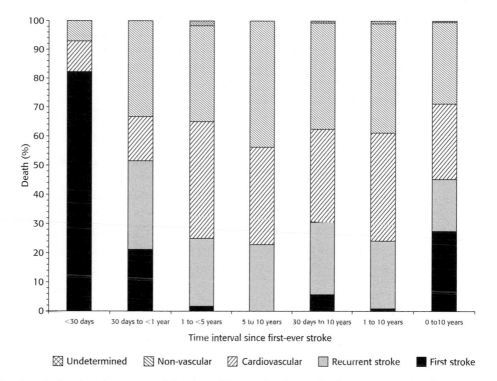

Figure 1.2   Graph showing the causes of death at different time intervals after stroke. Each column represents deaths within a defined period after stroke, and the bars within each column indicate the proportion of deaths during each period due to particular causes. Note how most deaths in the first 30 days after stroke are due to the direct effects of the stroke, whereas most deaths in subsequent years are due to cardiovascular disease and recurrent stroke. Reproduced from Hardie *et al.* (2003), with permission from the authors and Lippincott Williams & Wilkins.

and 5-fold lower if the cause is small artery disease (Lovett *et al.*, 2004). Thereafter, the risk falls to a nadir of 3 to 4% per year at 3 years, after which it gradually increases to about 7 to 8% per year at 10 years (Hankey *et al.*, 1998; Hardie *et al.*, 2004; van Wijk *et al.*, 2005). But the absolute risk varies depending on the prevalence and level of other vascular risk factors (Dippel *et al.*, 2004; van Wijk *et al.*, 2005; Rothwell *et al.*, 2005).

Among stroke survivors, neurological function begins to improve within the first few days due to resolution of the ischaemic penumbra, cerebral oedema and comordities (e.g. infection) that exacerbate the functional effects of the stroke. Thereafter, neurological and functional recovery continues, and is most rapid in the first 3 months due to neural plasticity (by which neurons adopt new functions), the acquisition of new skills through training (physiotherapy and occupational therapy) and modification of the patient's environment. Recovery continues

Table 1.3. Predictors of survival free of dependency after stroke.

- The pathological type of stroke (haemorrhage or infarction)
- The clinical syndrome and aetiological subtype of ischaemic stroke
- Age at the time of stroke
- Living alone (nobody permanently living with the patient before the stroke)
- Independent in activities of daily living before the stroke (Oxford Handicap score ≤2 before stroke)
- Normal verbal Glasgow Coma Scale score (=5)
- Arm strength: can lift both arms to horizontal
- Able to walk without the help of another person (can use stick/Zimmer frame)

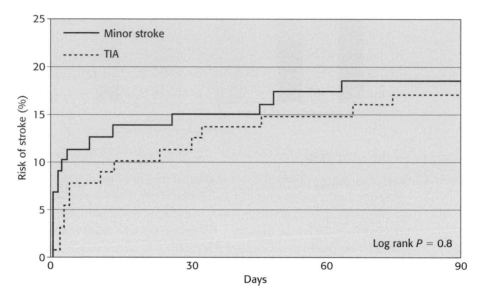

Figure 1.3   Cumulative risk of stroke in the first 90 days after a TIA or minor stroke in the Oxford Vascular Study. Reproduced with permission from the *British Medical Journal* Publishing Group and Coull *et al. BMJ* 2004; 328: 326–8.

more slowly over the next 6–12 months, with some gains still being realised 1–2 years after stroke (not all of which are functional adaptations).

The risk of being physically or cognitively dependent at 1 year after a stroke is about 20–30%. At 12 months after first-ever stroke, about one-third of all stroke patients have died, about 20–30% are dependent on another person for everyday activities (e.g. washing, dressing, mobilising) and 40–50% are independent (Hankey *et al.*, 2000, 2002; Warlow *et al.*, 2003; Hardie *et al.*, 2004).

The major clinical factors at the time of stroke or soon after a stroke which are predictive of being alive and independent at 6 months after a stroke are shown in Table 1.3 (Counsell *et al.*, 2002).

These factors seem to be equally predictive whether they are assessed within 48 h of stroke onset or later, whether the stroke is ischaemic or haemorrhagic in type, and whether the patient has had a previous stroke or not (Counsell *et al.*, 2002).

Trends in stroke mortality over time

Stroke mortality rates are declining in most places where it has been measured, with the exception of eastern Europe. Indeed, the decline in stroke mortality in some countries is even more rapid than in coronary heart disease mortality. However, in other countries, such as Australia, there has been a deceleration in the decline in stroke mortality (Feigin *et al.*, 2003).

The reason for the decline in stroke mortality is less clear; it may reflect a decline in the incidence of stroke (all types of stroke, or just those which are more likely to be fatal, such as haemorrhagic stroke), an improvement in case fatality (survival) after stroke (perhaps due to better medical care or reduced stroke severity) or an improvement in the accuracy of classifying stroke as a cause of death (e.g. less misclassification of sudden deaths as stroke) (Hankey, 1999).

Trends in stroke incidence over time

Recent data from the Oxford Vascular Study indicate that in Oxfordshire, UK, the incidence of stroke has declined over the past 20 years, particularly for ischaemic stroke and intracerebral haemorrhage (Rothwell *et al.*, 2004). There has also been a significant reduction in stroke mortality, but not case fatality. Similar results have been reported in Perth, Australia (Jamrozik *et al.*, 1999) but this finding is not consistent in other areas (Feigin *et al.*, 2003; Warlow *et al.*, 2003).

The Oxford Vascular Study suggests that the reduction in stroke incidence may be attributable to improved recognition and treatment of modifiable causal risk factors (such as high blood pressure, high blood cholesterol) and the increased use of other effective stroke prevention strategies (such as antiplatelet therapy) in appropriate individuals (Rothwell *et al.*, 2004). These data suggest that stroke is preventable.

Future trends in burden of stroke

The burden of stroke is likely to remain substantial for the foreseeable future, if not increase. If the incidence of stroke does not fall by at least 2% per year, every year, then the absolute number of incident stroke cases is likely to increase, given the ageing of the population (Bonita *et al.*, 2004). In developed countries, any increasing burden is likely to fall more on the acute hospital services than on rehabilitation facilities, because strokes are more likely to be fatal in very elderly and disabled people than in younger and fitter patients (Malmgren *et al.*, 1989).

Strategies to reduce the future burden of stroke

There are two main strategies to reduce the burden of stroke:

1 Prevention of first-ever and recurrent stroke by means of the population (mass) and high-risk approaches (Rose, 1992).

2 Treatment of acute stroke to optimise survival free of complications of stroke, recurrent stroke (and coronary events – the major cause of death in long-term survivors of stroke) and handicap.

This book focuses on the second strategy.

Understanding evidence

One of the challenges in finding effective treatments for stroke is that stroke is not a single entity. Stroke has a broad spectrum of clinical features, pathologies, aetiologies and prognoses. Consequently, there is wide variation in the types of treatments for stroke and in the response of patients to effective treatments. This means that there is a low likelihood that there will ever be a single 'magic bullet' to treat all types of stroke. A similar analogy can be seen with infectious diseases and cancers. They also have a broad spectrum of clinical features, pathologies, causes and outcomes. As a result, there are a range of antibiotic and antineoplastic treatments targeting different aetiologies and mechanisms of cellular injury and, even in targeted patients, their effectiveness is variable. This is because the response of patients is also determined by other genetic and acquired factors.

Given that there are likely to be different treatments for different causes and sequelae of stroke, and different responses in different patients, stroke researchers need to ideally aim to evaluate the effects of treatments for particular pathological and aetiological subtypes and sequelae of stroke, and stroke clinicians need to ideally strive to target effective treatments to appropriate patients who are likely to respond favourably.

Stroke clinicians therefore need to know which treatments for patients with particular types and sequelae of stroke are effective (and ineffective), and their respective risks and costs. Theory alone is insufficient for guiding practice; treatments should have been tested appropriately and thoroughly in clinical practice (Doust and Del Mar, 2004). Although appropriate evaluation usually requires enormous efforts and resources, this is several-fold less than the costs of misplaced enthusiasm which leads to the introduction of, and perseverence with, ineffective and dangerous treatments. Indeed, if the extracranial–intracranial bypass trial had not been undertaken and reported (showing no overall effectiveness), this costly and risky procedure would still be practised widely today as a plausible, relatively safe and effective procedure (EC–IC Bypass Study Group, 1985). It can only be hoped that the future will not judge us as irresponsible when we choose to not evaluate

Table 2.1. Common treatments used in neuroscience today which are (sadly) lacking evidence of effectiveness and safety from RCTs.

- Thrombolysis for thrombosis of the basilar artery
- Anticoagulants for intracranial venous thrombosis
- Early surgery for ruptured intracranial aneurysms
- Surgery for intracerebral haemorrhage
- Surgery for cervical spondylotic myelopathy
- Surgery for syringomyelia
- Thymectomy for myasthenia gravis
- Radiation therapy for glioma
- Dopamine agonists for Parkinson's disease (different preparations, timing)

Table 2.2. Reasons for using ineffective or harmful treatments.

- Lack of reliable evidence of safety and effectiveness
- Over-reliance on surrogate outcomes
- Anecdotal clinical experience (i.e. historical controls)
- Theoretical benefit (e.g. love of the pathophysiological model, which is incorrect)
- Natural history of the disease (e.g. poor prognosis)
- Patients' expectations (real or assumed)
- A desire to 'do something'
- Ritual
- No questions asked

established procedures in the same way, on the (in my opinion undefensible) grounds that it is 'unethical' (Table 2.1) (van Gijn, 2004, 2005).

Indeed, a primary reason for the wide variation in stroke management among different clinics, cities, regions and countries, and use of ineffective and harmful treatments, is continuing uncertainty about the safety and effectiveness of many of the available treatments due to the lack of reliable evidence of efficacy and safety (Table 2.2) (Chalmers, 2004; Doust and Del Mar, 2004).

In the presence of uncertainty about the relative intrinsic merits of different treatments, clinicians cannot be certain about those merits in any given use of one of them – as in treating an individual patient. Therefore, it seems irrational and unethical to insist one way or another before the completion of a suitable evaluation/trial of the different treatments. So, the best treatment for the patient is to participate in a relevant trial. Although this is experimentation, it is simply choice under uncertainty, coupled with data collection. The choice is random, and constructive doubt is its practical counterpart, but this should not matter as there is no better mechanism for choice under uncertainty (Ashcroft, 2000). Indeed, the entry criteria into clinical trials can be simplified by using the 'uncertainty principle' which states that a patient can be entered if, and only if, the responsible clinician is substantially uncertain which of the trial treatments would be most appropriate for that particular patient. A patient should not be entered if the responsible clinician or the patient is, for medical or non-medical reasons, reasonably certain that one of the treatments that might be allocated would be inappropriate for this particular patient (in comparison with either no treatment or some other treatment that could be offered to the patient in- or outside the trial) (Peto and Baigent, 1998).

In order to assess the effects of a treatment on outcome after stroke, the treatment must be evaluated in patients, and it must be compared with patients who have not been exposed to the treatment, but who are ideally identical in all other ways such as in prevalence and level of prognostic factors that influence outcome (i.e. a control group). A control group is needed because the outcome after stroke is neither uniformly poor or good (i.e. it is variable), and because it is difficult to accurately predict the outcome of any individual patient (see Chapter 1).

As stroke commonly causes substantial loss of brain function within minutes to hours, and there are many possible treatable causes of stroke, it is most unlikely that any single treatment for stroke will have a dramatically favourable or unfavourable effect on patient outcome after stroke. If there is such a treatment, it will either substantially improve outcome among a group of patients with a poor prognosis or substantially harm outcome among a group of patients with a good prognosis. Such large treatment effects can be identified reliably from observational studies of the outcome of treated patients compared with untreated historical, literature or concurrent controls; without the need for large randomised trials. This is because any possible modest effects of systematic error or random error, even if in the opposite direction to the treatment effect (i.e. reducing the true treatment effect), are not likely to be large enough to disguise the dramatic effect of the treatment (Table 2.3). For example, the striking effectiveness of drugs such as penicillin were realised from observational studies of treated patients with hitherto uniformly fatal or disabling diseases such as pneucoccal meningitis, who subsequently recovered dramatically after penicillin. Randomised-controlled trials (RCTs) were not required.

However, most (if not all) treatments for stroke are likely to have *modest* effects at the best. Yet, these may be clinically worthwhile, particularly if the treatment is safe, inexpensive and widely applicable, and if the disease (e.g. stroke) is common, disabling and expensive (Warlow, 2004).

In order to reliably identify such modest, yet important, treatment effects, it is necessary to ensure that they are not underestimated or even nullified (and therefore missed) by modest systematic or random errors (false negative, or type II error)

Table 2.3. Common sources of error in studies of interventions for stroke.

Systematic errors (biases) in the assessment of treatment effects
- Selection bias (systematic pretreatment differences in comparison groups)
- Performance bias (systematic differences in the care provided apart from the intervention being evaluated)
- Attrition bias (systematic differences in withdrawals from the trials)
- Recording/detection bias (systematic differences in outcome assessment)

Random errors in the assessment of treatment effects
- Relate to the impact of the play of chance on comparisons of the outcome between those exposed and not exposed to the treatment of interest
- Are determined by the number of relevant outcome events in the study
- The potential error can be quantified by means of a confidence interval (CI) which indicates the range of effects statistically compatible with the observed result
- Can prevent real effects of treatment being detected or their size being estimated reliably

Table 2.4. Strategies to minimise systematic and random errors.

Minimisation of systematic error
- Proper randomisation
- Analysis by allocated treatment (including all randomised patients: intention to treat)
- Outcome evaluation blind to the allocated treatment
- Chief emphasis on overall results (without undue data-dependent emphasis on particular subgroups)
- Systematic review of all relevant studies (without undue data-dependent emphasis on particular studies)

Minimisation of random error
- Large numbers of major outcomes (with streamlined study methods to facilitate recruitment)
- Systematic review of all relevant studies (yielding the largest possible number of major outcome events)

(Table 2.3) (Collins and MacMahon, 2001). Similarly, for treatments with no effect, it is necessary that modest systematic and random errors are minimised, and not sufficiently large to produce an erroneous conclusion that the treatment is effective or harmful (false positive, or type I error).

Strategies to minimise systematic and random errors

Reliable and accurate identification of modest, but important, treatment effects requires simultaneous minimisation of systematic errors (bias) and random errors (Table 2.4).

Table 2.5. Hierarchy of study types.

- Systematic reviews and meta-analyses of RCTs
- Randomised-controlled trials (RCTs)
- Non-randomised controlled intervention studies
- Controlled observational studies
- Case series
- Expert opinion

Table 2.6. Levels of evidence about health care interventions.

E1, Level I: Evidence obtained from a systematic review of all relevant RCTs

E2, Level II: Evidence obtained from at least one properly designed RCT

E3$_1$, Level III-1:   Evidence obtained from well-designed pseudo-RCTs (alternate allocation or some other method)

E3$_2$, Level III-2:   Evidence obtained from comparative studies with concurrent controls and allocation not randomised (cohort studies), case–control studies, or interrupted time series without a parallel control group

E3$_3$, Level III-3:   Evidence obtained from comparative studies with historical controls, two or more single-arm studies, or interrupted time series without a parallel control group

E4, Level IV: Evidence obtained from case series, either post test or pre- and post-test

Source: National Health and Medical Research Council (1999).

Randomisation is the most efficient method of minimising systematic bias in treatment allocation, *blinded outcome evaluation* is the most efficient method of minimising observer or recording/detection bias, and registering and analysing *large numbers of primary outcome measures* (and therefore randomising large numbers of patients) is the main method of minimising random error (Sackett *et al.*, 2000; Collins and MacMahon, 2001).

Of these, random error is arguably the most important to minimise. Surprisingly large numbers of patients (often thousands or even tens of thousands) must be included in randomised trials of stroke treatments to provide really reliable estimates of effect. Trials of such size are rare in stroke medicine.

Therefore, the best evidence about the effects of a treatment with potentially modest, mild or no treatment effect comes from large RCTs in which there are large numbers of outcome events, and in which outcome evaluation is undertaken by observers who are blinded to the treatment allocation.

The hierarchy of study types adopted by the Agency for Health Care Policy and Research is widely accepted as reliable in this regard and is given in Table 2.5 (Harbour *et al.*, 2001).

Levels of evidence about health care interventions have been developed from this hierarchy (Table 2.6).

Table 2.7. Revised grading system for recommendations in evidence-based guidelines (Harbour *et al.*, 2001).

Levels of evidence

1++	High quality meta-analyses, systematic reviews of RCTs, or RCTs with a very low risk of bias
1+	Well-conducted meta-analyses, systematic reviews of RCTs, or RCTs with a low risk of bias
1−	Meta-analyses, systematic reviews or RCTs, or RCTs with a high risk of bias
2++	High-quality systematic reviews of case-control or cohort studies *or* High-quality case-control or cohort studies with a very low risk of confounding, bias or chance and a high probability that the relationship is causal
2+	Well-conducted case-control or cohort studies with a low risk of confounding, bias, or chance and a moderate probability that the relationship is causal
2−	Case-control or cohort studies with a high risk of confounding, bias, or chance and a significant risk that the relationship is not causal
3	Non-analytic studies (e.g. case reports, case series)
4	Expert opinion

Grades of recommendations

A	At least one meta-analysis, systematic review, or RCT rated as 1++ and directly applicable to the target population *or* A systematic review of RCTs or a body of evidence consisting principally of studies rated as 1+ directly applicable to the target population and demonstrating overall consistency of results
B	A body of evidence including studies rated as 2++ directly applicable to the target population and demonstrating overall consistency of results *or* Extrapolated evidence from studies rated as 1++ or 1+
C	A body of evidence including studies rated as 2+ directly applicable to the target population and demonstrating overall consistency of results *or* Extrapolated evidence from studies rated as 2++
D	Evidence level 3 or 4 *or* Extrapolated evidence from studies rated as 2+

Grading system for recommendations in evidence-based guidelines

A revised grading system (Table 2.7) has been proposed to strike an appropriate balance between incorporating the complexity of type and quality of the evidence and maintaining clarity for guideline users (Harbour *et al.*, 2001). The key changes from the Agency for Health Care Policy and Research system are that the study type and quality rating are combined in the evidence level; the grading of recommendations extrapolated from the available evidence is clarified; and the grades of recommendation are extended from three to four categories, effectively by splitting the previous grade B which was seen as covering too broad a range of evidence type and quality.

Key elements to the design of a clinical trial of a treatment for stroke

All clinical trials *should* be designed and reported using the CONSORT guidelines (Moher *et al.*, 2001; Altman *et al.*, 2001). However, not all trials are reported in this way, and not all journals insist on it. Thus some trials may have been carried out adequately but reported inadequately, and others may have been designed and carried out inadequately. When reviewing a study, the following points should be considered (Altman *et al.*, 2001; Lees *et al.*, 2003; Lewis and Warlow, 2004; Lader *et al.*, 2004; Rothwell, 2005a,b; Rothwell *et al.*, 2005c). For further details of what to look for in a report of a RCT, I would recommend Lewis and Warlow (2004), Rothwell (2005a, b), and Rothwell *et al.* (2005).

Hypothesis and aim
- Are the study hypothesis and aim clearly stated?
- Did the study hypothesis pre-specify any proposed subgroup analyses (*a priori*)?

Design
- What is the study design?
- Is it a randomised trial?
- Is the method of randomisation described and was it an appropriate method? Was the decision to enter each patient made irreversibly in ignorance of which trial treatment that each patient would be allocated? If not (e.g. if 'randomisation' was based on date of birth, date of admission or alternation (e.g. an odd or even day of the week)), foreknowledge of the next treatment allocation could affect the decision to enter the patient, and those allocated one treatment might then differ systematically from those allocated another.
  Were adequate measures undertaken to conceal allocations, such as central randomisation; serially numbered, opaque, sealed envelopes; or other descriptions with convincing concealment?

Patients
- Were explicit and clearly operational inclusion and exclusion criteria employed?

Follow-up
- Were all patients followed up prospectively at pre-specified, regular intervals?
- Was patient follow-up complete?
  If not, this can lead to attrition bias (systematic differences in withdrawals from trials) because patients who are withdrawn from, or stop participating in, a trial tend to differ from those who remain in the study (e.g. they may have a higher rate of complications or adverse effects from the disease or treatment respectively). This type of bias can be minimised by performing an 'intention-to-treat analysis'

where the analysis of results at the end of the study includes every patient who was assigned to the intervention or control group, regardless of whether they received the assigned treatment or subsequently dropped out of the trial (see below).

Outcome measures

Is the primary measure of outcome:
- relevant to the patient (e.g. death, functional dependency, serious vascular event)?
- relevant to the intervention (i.e. potentially modifiable)?
- valid (measures what it is supposed to measure)?
- reliable (reproducible)?
- simple?
- communicable?

Avoid surrogate outcomes in phase III studies:
- Surrogate outcomes may reflect only one part of the disease process and their treatment may not produce worthwhile improvements in survival and functional outcome. Deciding if a treatment is safe and effective just on the basis of its effects on a physiological measurement, an imaging test or some complex scale may be misleading.
- Treating surrogate outcomes may be hazardous. Cardiac dysrhythmias are associated with a poor prognosis and antidysrhythmic drugs can markedly reduce their frequency. However, various antidysrhythmic drugs, although they reduce the surrogate outcome (dysrhythmias), they actually increase mortality.

Outcome evaluation

- Were the outcome events recorded in such a way to reduce the risk of bias (i.e. blind to the assigned treatment)?

Statistical analysis

- Is the primary analysis by intention-to-treat (i.e. is the final analysis based on the groups to which all randomised patients were originally allocated)?

  Even in a properly randomised trial, bias can be inadvertently introduced by the post-randomisation exclusion of certain patients (e.g. those who are non-compliant with treatment), particularly if the outcome of those excluded from one treatment group differs from that of those excluded from another. 'On-treatment' comparisons, among only those who were compliant, are therefore potentially biased. However, because there is always some non-compliance with allocated treatments in clinical trials, an intention-to-treat analysis tends to underestimate the effects produced by full compliance with study treatments. In order to estimate the treatment effect with full compliance, it is more appropriate to avoid using potentially biased 'on-treatment' comparisons, and to apply the approximate estimate of level of compliance seen in the trial (e.g. 80%) to the estimate of the treatment effected provided by the intention-to-treat comparison (e.g. 30% relative risk reduction (with 80% compliance)). Doing this reveals a less-biased estimate of therapeutic effect with full compliance (e.g. 35–40% relative risk reduction with 100% compliance).

- Was the treatment effect given with its confidence interval (CI)?
  It is important that the results are expressed with a CI, not just as 'significant' or 'not significant' (e.g. 25% reduction, 95% CI: 22–28%). Trials should give a precise estimate of treatment effect and therefore have narrow CIs.

- Was the result clinically significant as well as statistically significant?
  Large relative treatment effects look impressive (e.g. '50% reduction'), but if event rates are low, the absolute benefit is small and may be clinically insignificant.

- Are there any subgroup analyses, and if so, are they appropriate and *a priori* (Rothwell, 2005b)?
  As individual patients differ from each other, there is an understandable temptation to examine treatment effects in subgroups of interest, particularly if the overall trial result is negative. However, the more subgroups that are examined the more likely that an effect will be identified due to chance (e.g. analysing 20 subgroups will lead to one being statistically significant at the $P = 0.05$ level (1 out of 20) just due to the play of chance) (Cook *et al.*, 2004). *Post hoc* subgroup analyses cannot, therefore, be regarded as anything more than hypothesis generating. Any apparent treatment effect must be confirmed in a further trial in which there is an *a priori* hypothesis that a particular subgroup of patients will benefit while other subgroups will not. The most reliable estimate of a treatment effect, even in a subgroup, is that obtained in the whole sample of randomised patients. It can be assumed that subgroups will differ *quantitatively* in their response to treatment to some extent, but it cannot be assumed that there will be an unexpected *qualitative* difference in the direction of the treatment effect, such that treatment is harmful for one subgroup of patients but beneficial for another. A subgroup analysis may be appropriate when the overall treatment effect is substantial, and highly significant. This is measured by the z-value, the size of the treatment effect divided by its standard deviation. For reliable subgroup analyses z should be 10 or greater, as seen in the Antithrombotic Trialists' Collaboration (2002) where the estimate of effectiveness of antiplatelet therapy vs control in preventing serious vascular events was an odds ratio (OR) of 22% and the standard deviation was only 2. The z-value was therefore more than 10, and so there was sufficient statistical power to conduct a reliable subgroup analysis of the effectiveness of antiplatelet therapy in subgroups, such as patients with previous myocardial infarction, previous stroke, and other high risk groups. Very few trials achieve this sort of power.

- Are they any additional ('on-treatment') analyses, and are they appropriate? An 'on-treatment' analysis may be of value in describing the frequency of specific adverse effects among only those who actually received the treatment; strictly randomised comparisons may not be needed to assess extreme relative risks.

Conclusion

It can never be absolutely correct to claim that treatments have no effect or that there is no difference in the effects of treatments, because it is impossible to prove a negative or that two treatments have an identical effect. There is always some uncertainty surrounding estimates of treatment effects, and a small difference can never be excluded (Altman and Bland, 1995; Alderson and Chalmers, 2003). Claims of no effect or no difference may mean that patients continue to be denied or exposed to interventions with important (beneficial or harmful) effects. They may also suggest that further research is unnecessary, which may delay reliable estimates of treatment effects. The impossibility of proving no effect or no difference should be distinguished from the concept used for equivalence trials, where limits are set on the differences that are considered clinically significant.

Trial sponsorship and competing interests

The development of new interventions requires funding, and elements of a market economy are indispensable. However, capitalism should be subject to restraining forces to ensure an appropriate balance, as with any other endeavour in society. Sponsors of trials of interventions have a right to evaluate their intervention as they would like to, but they also have a responsibility to the future users and recipients of the intervention to include clinicians in the design, management and reporting of the studies (van Gijn, 2004, 2005).

Due to the potential for the best interests of patients and society to be compromised by the financial interests of the sponsors and prescribing clinicians, it is essential that the highest form of honesty and integrity prevails (Shaw, 1908).

'*Good Clinical Practice Guidelines*' have been developed as preliminary regulations of drug trials. However, they focus on an abundance of minor details, such as those pertaining to the relations between the clinical investigator and both the patient and the sponsor, how often every value in the trial records of individual patients should be checked against their hospital records, and which disciplines should be represented in the institutional review boards. The major issues, however, are not addressed. There are no rules governing the trial design, or the integrity of the data storage, management and analysis; and therefore no rules that a trial should be run by a steering committee of clinicians who are independent from the sponsor (Donnan *et al.*, 2003; van Gijn, 2004).

There is evidence that research funded by pharmaceutical companies is more likely to have outcomes favouring the sponsor than research funded from other sources (Bekelman *et al.*, 2003; Lexchin *et al.*, 2003). This is not because the research by pharmaceutical companies is of different quality, but because of publication bias; the companies may have a tendency to not publish unfavourable results.

It is crucial that trial sponsorship and all potential competing interests are presented in any report of a study.

Limitations of RCTs

Sample size (random error and imprecise estimates of treatment effects)

Although RCTs provide the least biased and hence most reliable evaluation of whether a treatment is effective and safe, they are commonly limited by suboptimal sample size. As a result there is potential for some random error and therefore imprecision in the estimate of the treatment effect.

Generalisability/external validity

Another weakness of RCTs is limited generalisability. The results of trials conducted in a single centre, region or country, and in a single racial or ethnic group, or type of patients, cannot necessarily be generalised (applied) to other centres, regions or countries, and other racial or ethnic groups, or patients respectively. Even well-executed trials with sound internal validity may not necessarily inform us about the effect of a treatment among patients who were not entered into the trial (i.e. its external validity) (Rothwell, 2005a).

One of the solutions to the above limitations of RCTs is to conduct multicentre trials in multiple countries, but the disadvantages include practical difficulties, time and cost. Another solution, particularly if large multicentre RCTs are impractical, is a systematic review, or meta-analysis, of all trials.

Systematic reviews and meta-analyses of RCTs

A systematic review and meta-analysis seeks to reduce systematic error (bias) and random error by applying scientific methods to the review of all of the published and unpublished research evidence; in this case RCTs.

Systematic reviews

The scientific methods or strategies of a systematic review include:
- Defining the *research question* to ensure the review will be relevant and reliable, and guide the development of the review protocol. Most reviews define a broad

question (e.g. does thrombolysis in acute ischaemic stroke improve outcome) which includes several pre-specified subquestions (e.g. does thrombolysis with tissue plasminogen activator (tPA) within 3 h reduce death and dependency at 6 months after stroke).

- Developing a *review protocol* based on the research question. The protocol contains specific, explicit and reproducible inclusion and exclusion criteria for selecting trials for the review in order to minimise bias in trial selection. The protocol also contains explicit methods of data extraction and synthesis to minimise bias during data collection and the analysis of results.
- Undertaking a systematic and *comprehensive search* for all potentially relevant trials.
- Applying the pre-specified eligibility criteria to *select relevant trials.*
- Performing a *critical appraisal* of the methodological quality (research designs and characteristics) of the trials to ensure that most emphasis is given to the most methodologically sound trials.
- *Extracting and analysing data* using pre-defined, explicit methods. The statistical synthesis or analysis of the results is called a meta-analysis (see page 21).
- *Interpreting* the results, and drawing conclusions based on the totality of the available evidence (not a biased subset).

Therefore, a *systematic review* provides a method of reviewing the available evidence using explicit scientific strategies to reduce any bias (e.g. in trial selection and data extraction) in the estimate of the direction of the treatment effect from using only selected trials, and to increase the precision of the estimate of the treatment effect by examining a larger amount of data and thereby reducing random error (Collins *et al.*, 1987; Peto, 1987).

Sources of bias in systematic reviews

There are three main sources of bias in systematic reviews: publication bias, study quality bias and outcome recording bias.

Publication bias

Systematic reviews aim to identify and include all trials that are relevant to the research question. However, some studies are difficult to find, and these may tend to differ from trials which are easy to find. For example, studies which have concluded a 'positive' or interesting results are more likely to be published, and therefore easier to locate, than studies which have produced 'negative' or neutral results (see Chapter 7, Fig. 7.12) (Easterbrook, 1991). The conduct of a systematic review therefore needs to engage multiple overlapping sources of study ascertainment. The search should cover electronic databases (which are unfortunately restricted to only certain journals in certain languages (e.g. Embase, Medline)), hand searching of journals, and active searching of conference abstracts, theses and unpublished trials (Alderson, 2004).

Study quality bias

There is sound empirical evidence that more methodologically robust trials tend to indicate that new treatments are less effective than do less reliable trials (Shultz, 1994). It is therefore important that the conduct of a systematic review includes a measure of the methodological quality of the trials included, and if possible a sensitivity analysis of the results according to the methodological quality of the trials (Glasziou *et al.*, 2004).

Outcome recording bias

Most clinical trials measure and analyse several outcomes. There is a tendency for some trials to publish the results of their most impressive outcomes and to not report their least impressive results. If a systematic review then combines all of the published results, there is likely to be a bias towards only the most impressive results. Such outcome recording bias is minimised by defining, in advance, the outcomes which are to be used in the systematic review and then collecting the relevant data consistently from each study. Thereby the relevant outcomes for the research question should be recorded in a similar manner among the different trials.

Meta-analyses

A *meta-analysis* is a statistical process for combining data from different trials.

The type of technique to analyse the data depends on the type of outcome event to be analysed. Most trials of stroke treatment and prevention have recorded dichotomous outcomes for patients, which are split into two groups (e.g. dead or alive, dependent or independent, survival free of recurrent stroke or not). However, some trials have reported the mean and standard deviation of results such as a disability score or length of stay in hospital.

If the control and treatment groups contain the same number of patients followed up in the same way for the same time, the most simple analysis of dichotomous outcomes (e.g. dead or alive) is to compare the combined total of the outcome events in the control group of each trial (e.g. c, Table 2.8), with the combined total of outcome events in the intervention group of each trial (e.g. a, Table 2.8). However, this is rarely the case, and other types of analyses are needed (O'Connell *et al.*, 2004) (Table 2.8).

Table 2.8. Risks and odds.

- The *risk* of an event is the number of people with an outcome event of interest divided by the total number of observations (e.g. a/(a + b), or (a + c)/(a + b + c + d)).
- The *odds* of an event is the number of people with an outcome events of interest divided by the number of people who do not have an outcome event (e.g. a/b, or (a + c)/(b + d)).
- The *risk ratio* (relative risk) is the risk of an event among patients assigned the intervention divided by the risk among patients assigned no intervention ([a/(a + b)]/[c/(c + d)]). An example is the statement: 'for stroke patients being treated with intervention "y", the risk of an event at 6 months after stroke was 80% of the risk for patients who are not treated. In other words, treatment reduced the risk of an event by 20%'. A risk ratio of 1.0 (or 100%) indicates no effect of the intervention.
- The *odds ratio* is the odds of an event among patients assigned the intervention divided by the odds among patients assigned no intervention ((a/b)/(c/d)). An example is the statement: 'for stroke patients being treated with intervention "y", the odds of an event at 6 months after stroke was 80% of the odds for patients who are not treated. In other words, treatment reduced the odds of an event by 20%'. An OR of 1.0 indicates no effect of the intervention.
- The (absolute) *risk difference* is the risk of an event among patients assigned the intervention (a/(a + b)) minus the risk of an event among patients assigned no intervention (c/(c + d)). An absolute risk difference of 0 indicates no effect of the intervention. The risk difference is the easiest to interpret (e.g. 'if all patients are treated with the intervention, about 20% would have a good outcome').

		Outcome		
		Yes	No	Total
	Yes	a	b	a + b
Intervention				
	No	c	d	c + d
	Total	a + c	b + d	a + b + c + d

Example of the calculation of different measures of effect of a treatment in a controlled trial.

	Control group (*n* = 1000)	Treatment group (*n* = 1000)
Number of outcome events	**100**	**60**
Absolute risk	100/1000 = **10%**	60/1000 = **6%**
Absolute risk difference	10% − 6% = **4%**	
95% CI for risk difference	**1.6%–6.4%**	
P-value for risk difference	2*P* < **0.001**	
Number needed to treat (NNT)	1/0.04 (4%) = **25**	
95% CI for NNT	1/0.064–1/0.016 = 15.6–62.5	
Relative risk (or risk ratio) (treatment vs control)	6%/10% = **0.6**	

Table 2.8. (*Cont.*)

	Control group (*n* = 1000)	Treatment group (*n* = 1000)
Relative risk reduction (absolute risk difference/absolute risk in control group)	4%/10% = 40%	
Odds of an event	100/900 = **11.1%**	60/940 = **6.4%**
Odds ratio	6.4%/11.1% = **0.57**	
95% CI of OR	**0.41–0.80**	
P-value for OR	2*P* = **0.001**	

Odds ratio

An OR is the ratio of the odds (chance) of an outcome occurring amongst patients allocated the intervention compared with the corresponding odds (chance) of that outcome occurring amongst patients allocated control (Sandercock, 1989) (Table 2.8). An OR = 1 (unity) indicates identical odds (1:1) of an outcome occurring amongst patients allocated the intervention and control, whereas an OR <1 indicates lower odds (chance) of an outcome occurring amongst patients allocated the intervention compared with control.

For example, if we consider a 'trial' in which two coins are tossed, the odds (chance) of a 'heads' as the outcome using coin A (the 'intervention' group) should be equal to the odds (chance) of a 'heads' as the outcome using coin B (the 'control' group). However, due to the play of chance (random error), this does not always occur. For example, if each coin is tossed 5 times, it is possible that coin A appears as 'heads' 4 times and 'tails' 1 time (odds 4:1), and coin B appears as 'heads' 2 times and 'tails' 3 times (odds 2:3). In this case, the OR of achieving a 'heads' with coin A, compared to coin B, is 4/1 divided by 2/3, which is 6.0 (i.e. 6.0:1).

Any calculated OR is an imperfect, and therefore imprecise, estimate of the 'true' result. The degree of imprecision can be demonstrated by means of a CI. This is the range of estimates of the OR that would be obtained if the 'trial' was repeated several times. For example, if the trial of coin tossing were repeated 100 times, the 95% CI represents the range of estimates of the OR that would be obtained 95% of the time (i.e. in 95 of the 100 trials); the results of the other five trials (per 100) would be more extreme, and outside those 95% confidence limits (Gardner and Altman, 1986). As the estimates (e.g. of the OR) will follow a normal distribution due to chance, the estimate obtained in any one trial is more likely to lie in the middle of the CI (or range) than at the extremes.

So, in the example above, a simple calculation of the 95% CI of the OR of 6.0 indicates that the 'true' result could possibly lie in range from an OR of

0.35–101.57 (i.e. there is a 95% chance that the true result (an OR of 1.0 in this case of coin tossing) lies within this range) (Gardner and Altman, 1989), and it is more likely to be in the middle of the range than at the extremes.

There are several methods of calculating odds ratios and their CIs (Der Simonian and Laird, 1986; Peto, 1987; Gardner and Altman, 1989). The 'fixed effects model' is a standard approach but it may be unreliable when the results of individual trials differ substantially from one another (i.e. there is heterogeneity among the trials; see below). The 'random effects model' is more appropriate if there is heterogeneity, but it tends to over-emphasise the effects of small trials.

If the 'trial' of coin tossing above were to be repeated, it is likely that a different result would occur, due to the play of chance (random error). And, if there were more tosses of the coin, it is likely that there would be less random error, and a more precise result. For example, if each coin is now tossed 10 times, it is possible that coin A appears as 'heads' 6 times and 'tails' 4 times (odds 6:4), and coin B appears as 'heads' 3 times and 'tails' 7 times (odds 3:7). In this case, the OR of achieving a 'heads' with coin A, compared to coin B, is 6/4 divided by 3/7, which is 3.50 (95% CI: 0.55–22.30).

And, if each coin is now tossed 100 times, it is possible that coin A appears as 'heads' 53 times and 'tails' 47 times (OR 53:47), and coin B appears as 'heads' 45 times and 'tails' 55 times (OR 45:55). In this case, the OR of achieving a 'heads' with coin A, compared to coin B, is 53/47 divided by 45/55, which is 1.38 (95% CI: 0.79–2.40). As can be seen, the larger the number of coin tosses, the larger the number of outcomes ('heads' or 'tails'), the lower the random error, the more precise the estimate of the odds ratio, and the more precise (i.e. smaller) the range of the 95% CI.

If the 95% CI of the OR does not include (i.e. does not overlap with) an OR of 1.0 (unity), the result is statistically significant at the $P = 0.05$ level. The larger the number of outcome events in the trial or meta-analysis, the greater the statistical power, the more precise the result, the narrower the 95% CIs, and the smaller the treatment effect that can be statistically significant. This can be seen in Fig. 2.1.

Presentation of results of systematic reviews and meta-analyses

The results of systematic reviews and meta-analyses are conventionally presented in the format of a graph, called a forest plot (Fig. 2.1). For a designated outcome, the result of each trial is allocated a row, and the name of the study is in the first column. The second column describes the results for patients randomly allocated to the experimental treatment; 'n' represents the number of patients in the treatment group who registered the outcome of interest, and 'N' is the total number of patients in the treatment group. The third column describes the results for patients

Review: Calcium antagonists for acute ischemic stroke
Comparison: 01 Calcium antagonists vs control in acute "ischaemic" stroke.
Outcome: 01 Poor outcome at end of follow up

Study	Treatment n/N	Control n/N	Peto Odds Ratio 95% CI	Weight (%)	Peto Odds Ratio 95% CI
01 Nimodipine vs control					
Bogousslavsky 1990	2 / 30	3 / 30		0.3	0.65 [0.11, 4.00]
Bridgers 1991	103 / 138	43 / 66		2.5	1.59 [0.83, 3.04]
Canwin 1993	39 / 96	42 / 93		3.1	0.83 [0.47, 1.48]
Gelmers 1984	2 / 29	12 / 31		0.7	0.17 [0.05, 0.57]
Gelmers 1988	24 / 93	34 / 93		2.7	0.61 [0.33, 1.13]
German-Austrian 1994	60 / 239	63 / 243		6.2	0.96 [0.64, 1.44]
Heiss 1990	5 / 14	4 / 13		0.4	1.24 [0.26, 5.96]
INWEST 1990	133 / 195	54 / 100		4.1	1.84 [1.12, 3.03]
Kaste 1994	44 / 176	31 / 174		4.0	1.53 [0.92, 2.55]
Lowe 1989	34 / 56	23 / 56		1.9	2.18 [1.04, 4.56]
Martinez-Vila 1990	18 / 81	22 / 83		2.0	0.79 [0.39, 1.62]
Mohr 1992	475 / 800	155 / 264		12.9	1.03 [0.77, 1.38]
NEST 1993	197 / 437	211 / 443		14.7	0.90 [0.69, 1.18]
NIMPAS 1999	11 / 25	10 / 25		0.8	1.17 [0.39, 3.57]
Paci 1989	2 / 19	5 / 22		0.4	0.43 [0.09, 2.16]
TRUST 1990	275 / 607	257 / 608		20.1	1.13 [0.90, 1.42]
VENUS 1999	71 / 225	62 / 229		6.3	1.24 [0.83, 1.86]
Wimalaratna 1994	57 / 146	28 / 69		3.0	0.94 [0.52, 1.69]
Yordanov 1984	70 / 121	62 / 117		4.0	1.22 [0.73, 2.03]
Subtotal (95% CI)	1022 / 3527	1121 / 2759		90.3	1.07 [0.96, 1.19]

Test for heterogeneity chi-square=29.75 df=18 p=0.04
Test for overall effect=1.20 p=0.2

02 Flunarizine vs control					
FIST 1990	93 / 166	83 / 165		5.6	1.26 [0.82, 1.94]
Limburg 1990	3 / 12	8 / 14		0.4	0.28 [0.06, 1.30]
Subtotal (95% CI)	96 / 178	91 / 179		6.0	1.13 [0.74, 1.71]

Test for heterogeneity chi-square=3.40 df=1 p=0.0653
Test for overall effect=0.56 p=0.6

03 Isradipine vs control					
ASCLEPIOS 1990	47 / 120	44 / 114		3.8	1.02 [0.61, 1.73]
Subtotal (95% CI)	47 / 120	44 / 114		3.8	1.02 [0.61, 1.73]

Test for heterogeneity chi-square=0.00 df=0
Test for overall effect=0.09 p=0.9

Total (95% CI)	1765 / 3825	1256 / 3052		100.0	1.07 [0.97, 1.18]

Test for heterogeneity chi-square=33.23 df=21 p=0.0437
Test for overall effect=1.30 p=0.19

.1   .2   1   5   10

Figure 2.1   Forest plot showing the effects of calcium antagonists compared with control in patients with acute ischaemic stroke on poor outcome (death or dependency) at the end of the scheduled follow-up period among individual trials (each line), and pooled (summary at the bottom). The OR of a poor outcome in the calcium antagonists group compared with that in the control group is plotted for each trial (black square), along with its 95% CI (horizontal line). Meta-analysis of the pooled results of all trials is represented by a black diamond showing the OR, and the 95% CI of the OR. Reproduced from Horn and Limburg (2000), with permission from the authors and John Wiley & Sons Limited. Copyright Cochrane Library, reproduced with permission.

randomly allocated to the control intervention; 'n' represents the number of patients in the control group who registered the outcome of interest, and 'N' is the total number of patients in the control group. The fourth column contains a black square and a horizontal line. The black square represents the OR calculated for that individual trial and the horizontal line depicts the 95% CI. The fifth column, on the right-hand side of the figure, displays the OR and its 95% CI numerically. The summary result for the group of trials is shown in the bottom row as a diamond where the centre of the diamond indicates the summary OR and the breadth of the diamond indicates the 95% CI of that OR.

If the meta-analysis does not show a statistically significant effect of an intervention it does not necessarily mean that the intervention and the control group are equivalent. An intervention is only considered equivalent to control if equivalence limits have been pre-specified and if the 95% CIs of the OR lie completely within the pre-specified equivalence limits. The equivalence limits encompass a modest treatment difference that would not matter to clinicians or patients (i.e. it would not be of clinical significance).

Clinical significance depends on whether the results are important for clinicians or patients.

Consistency and heterogeneity

Since systematic reviews bring together studies that are diverse clinically (e.g. differences in dose and duration of follow-up) and methodologically (e.g. differences in study quality and inclusion criteria), it is expected that the results will be heterogeneous quantitatively but not qualitatively. The magnitude of the treatment effect is likely to differ (quantitatively), but the direction (positive or negative) of the treatment effects is likely to be the same (i.e. all positive or all negative) qualitatively compared with control.

The value of systematic reviews and meta-analyses is greatest when the results of the studies they include show clinically important effects of similar direction and magnitude. However, the conclusions are less clear when the included studies have differing results. In an attempt to establish objectively whether studies in the meta-analysis are consistent, a statistical test of heterogeneity is usually presented. This test seeks to determine whether there are genuine differences underlying the results of the studies (heterogeneity), or whether there is consistency of the effects across the studies, with any variation in findings among the studies being compatible with chance alone (homogeneity). Unless we know how consistent the results are we cannot determine the generalisability of the results of the meta-analysis. Indeed, several hierarchical systems for grading evidence state that the results of the studies must be consistent or homogeneous to obtain the highest grading (Harbour *et al.*, 2001).

A test for heterogeneity examines the null hypothesis that all studies are evaluating the same effect. The usual test statistic (Cochran's Q) is computed by summing the squared divisions of each study's estimate from the overall estimate of the meta-analysis, weighting each study's contribution in the same manner as in the meta-analysis (Cochran, 1954). *P*-values are obtained by comparing the statistic with a Chi-square distribution with $k - 1$ degrees of freedom (where k is the number of studies). The test is therefore susceptible to the number of trials included in the meta-analysis. As meta-analyses of stroke trials often include small numbers of studies the power of the test is low, and the test is poor at detecting true heterogeneity among studies as significant. In these circumstances, a non-significant result cannot be taken as evidence of homogeneity.

Rather than simply testing for homogeneity, and ascertaining whether it is significant or not statistically, Higgins *et al.* (2003) propose that it is more important and preferable to determine the extent to which heterogeneity affects the conclusions of the meta-analysis. They have developed a new quantity I^2, which ranges from 0% to 100%, and which measures the degree of consistency across studies in the meta-analysis (Higgins *et al.*, 2003). I^2 can be compared directly between meta-analyses with different numbers of studies and different types of outcome data.

Where to find clinical trials and systematic reviews

Source of information about clinical trials and systematic reviews are given in Table 2.9.

Table 2.9. Sources of information about clinical trials and systematic reviews.

• Cochrane Library contents (www.cochrane.org; http://www3.interscience.wiley.com/cgi-bin/mrwhome/106568753/home)		
Cochrane Database of Systematic Reviews	3925	Reviews
Database of Abstracts of Reviews of Effects	5205	Abstracts
Cochrane Central Register of Controlled Trials	446,156	Reports of trials
Cochrane Database of Methodology Reviews	19	Reviews
Health Technology Assessment database	4548	Reports
Health Economic evaluation database	15496	Assessments
• MEDLINE (http://medline.cos.com) (fails to detect many trials)		
• Evidence-Based Medicine websites		
Clinical Evidence http://www.clinicalevidence.com/		
EBM Guidelines http://www.ebm-guidelines.com/		
• Guideline websites		
Scottish Intercollegiate Guidelines Network http://www.sign.ac.uk/guidelines/index.html		

What if there is no robust evidence from systematic reviews of RCTs?

When robust evidence from RCTs in patients is not available, the various examples and the corresponding actions are listed out in Table 2.10.

Table 2.10. When robust evidence from RCTs in your patients is not available.

No RCTs exist at all

Reasons

- RCT not feasible because the condition is so rare and patients are so few.
- RCT not undertaken due to lack of burning question, or resources.
- The intervention is new, and has not had time to be evaluated.

Examples

- Steroids and cyclophosphamide for cerebral angiitis.
- Drainage of acute hydrocephalus after subarachnoid haemorrhage.
- Intra-arterial thrombolysis for basilar artery occlusion.

Action

- Use reasoning from experience with individual patients but beware of the potential fallacies.
- Plan or join (as a collaborator) a RCT, if feasible.
- Obtain experience with any new operative intervention before evaluating it by means of RCTs.

Only a single RCT exists

Examples

- Folic acid-based multivitamin therapy for patients with ischaemic stroke (Toole *et al.*, 2004).
- Hemicraniectomy plus duraplasty for cerebral oedema following extensive cerebral hemispheric infarction.
- Extended-release dipyridamole plus aspirin vs aspirin for patients with ischaemic stroke (Diener *et al.*, 1996).

Actions

- Have faith in the results, but only partially (could they be a false positive result or false negative result?). If we had relied on the results of the first trial of aspirin in patients with transient ischaemic attack (TIA) and ischaemic stroke (The Canadian Cooperative Study Group, 1978) women would have been denied aspirin therapy which was later shown to be equally effective for them in a meta-analysis (Antithrombotic Trialists' Collaboration, 2002). If we had relied on the results of an early single trial showing that nimodipine decreased case fatality after ischaemic stroke (Gelmers *et al.*, 1998) we would not have later retreated when a meta-analysis proved this to be a false positive (Fig. 2.1) (Horn and Limburg, 2000).
- Plan a new RCT or join a RCT to determine the consistency of the result in another population of patients, and improve the precision of the estimate of the overall treatment effect.

Several RCTs exist but a systematic review reveals non-significant or equivocal results

Example

- Anticoagulation for cerebral venous sinus thrombosis (de Bruijn and Stam, 1999).

Table 2.10. (*cont.*)

Actions
- Review the 95% CIs of the overall estimate of the result and the statistical test for heterogeneity, and consider the possibility of a modest, but clinically important treatment effect being missed (e.g. a false negative result).
- Plan or join (as a collaborator) a RCT if a potentially important treatment effect may have been misinterpreted as false negative result because of inadequate statistical power.
- In the meantime, reasoning is required, but beware of the potential fallacies of reasoning.

RCTs exist but certain types of patients were not included in the trials
Examples
- Elderly patients with atrial fibrillation;
- Patients with basilar artery aneurysm who were not included in the International Subarachnoid Aneurysm Trial (ISAT) because these aneurysms are difficult to clip surgically and easier to coil angiographically (International Subarachnoid Aneurysm Trial (ISAT) Collaborative Group, 2002).

Action
- Use reasoning when extrapolating the results of RCTs to other patients, but beware of the potential fallacies.

Source: van Gijn (2004, 2005).

SUMMARY

1 *Stroke treatments with large benefits are rare* It is rare for treatments for neurological diseases to have really large benefits. When they do, it is usually obvious in studies with weak designs (observational studies with historical controls, or concurrent non-randomised controls), particularly if the untreated condition is associated with a very bad outcome. Randomised trials were not needed to show that penicillin was effective for bacterial meningitis or that intravenous (i.v.) glucose was lifesaving in hypoglycaemic coma.

2 *Most stroke treatments have modest benefits* So be sceptical about trials designed in the expectation that the treatments they are testing will have large effects. If uncertainty exists about the effect of a treatment for a neurological disease, it is likely that the treatment effect is in fact modest. However, even a modest treatment effect can be clinically worthwhile for the patient.

3 *To detect modest treatment benefits, trials must avoid bias and random error* The common sources of error in studies of interventions are systematic error (bias) and random error.

4 *'Ingredients' for a good trial*
   Evidence from a randomised trial is likely to be more reliable if there is:
   - proper randomisation *and* concealment of allocation (i.e. clinician cannot have foreknowledge of next treatment allocation);

- outcome evaluation blind to the allocated treatment;
- analysis by allocated treatment (including all randomised patients: intention to treat);
- large numbers of major outcomes and correspondingly narrow CIs;
- chief emphasis on overall results (without undue data-dependent emphasis on particular subgroups).

5 *Advantages of systematic reviews (over traditional reviews)*
- Use explicit, well-developed methods to reduce bias.
- Summarise large amounts of data explicitly.
- Provide all available data.
- Increase statistical power and precision.
- Look for consistencies/inconsistencies.
- Improve generalisability.

6 *Cochrane Reviews*
- Generally higher quality than other systematic reviews.
- Periodically updated.
- Available over internet/on CDROM.
- Abstracts available free of charge at: www.cochrane.org; www.update-software.com/clibng/cliglogon.htm.
- Reprints of full Cochrane Reviews also available for a small fee.

Organised acute stroke care

The principles of management of patients with a suspected acute stroke are to:
- make an accurate diagnosis of stroke, its pathological type (i.e. infarct or haemorrhage) and aetiological subtype (cause of the infarct of haemorrhage);
- accurately assess the patient's impairments, disabilities and handicaps, and compare with previous impairments, disabilities and handicaps;
- estimate the prognosis for survival, recurrent stroke, other serious vascular events and future handicap;
- discuss the prognosis with the patient and family (if possible), and set shared, common short- and long-term goals;
- consider which services are required to meet the shared common goals and how to access and deliver them;
- optimise survival free of handicap by immediate brain reperfusion strategies in appropriate patients with ischaemic stroke, optimise physiological homoeostasis, anticipate and prevent complications of stroke, prevent recurrence of stroke and other major vascular events, begin rehabilitation immediately, and continue longer-term rehabilitation and support.

The management of stroke patients (and their carers and families) requires an integrated, comprehensive and coordinated stroke service which meets the needs (and wishes) of patients and carers in an effective, efficient and equitable manner.

The major components of an organised stroke service are as follows:
1. *A fast-track outpatient clinic*: To provide rapid assessment, diagnosis and secondary prevention measures for patients with suspected transient ischaemic attack (TIA) and non-disabling stroke.
2. *A comprehensive stroke unit*: To provide rapid assessment, diagnosis and intervention by a specialist multidisciplinary team.
3. *Early supported discharge*: To facilitate earlier discharge from hospital with enhanced support and rehabilitation input in the home setting.
4. *Longer-term support and rehabilitation*: To review continued progress, and new and ongoing needs, and maintain rehabilitation and support (Langhorne, 2002).

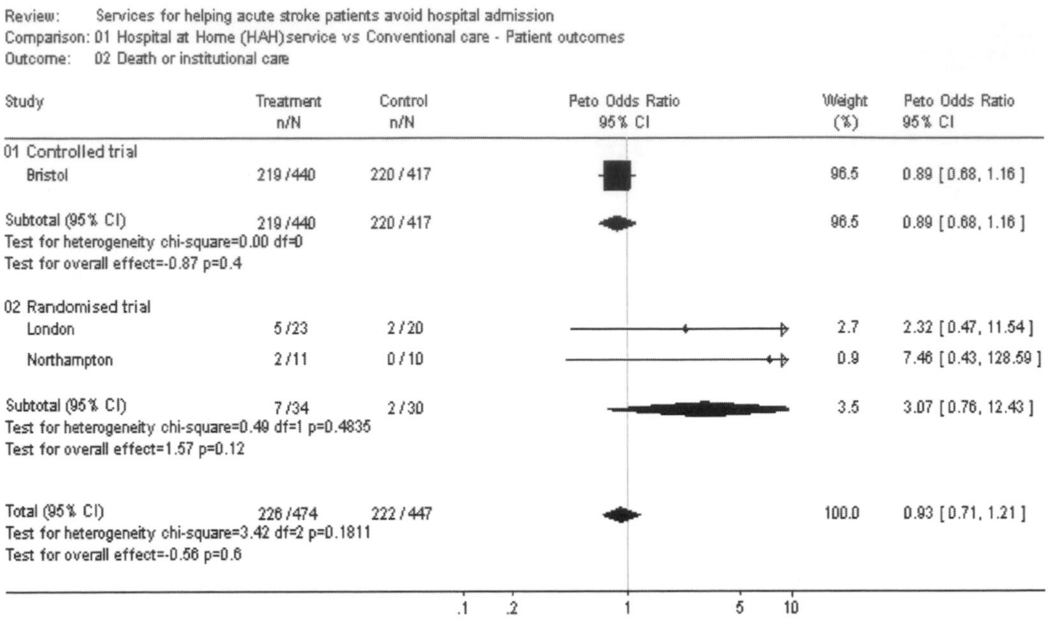

Review: Services for helping acute stroke patients avoid hospital admission
Comparison: 01 Hospital at Home (HAH) service vs Conventional care - Patient outcomes
Outcome: 02 Death or institutional care

Study	Treatment n/N	Control n/N	Peto Odds Ratio 95% CI	Weight (%)	Peto Odds Ratio 95% CI
01 Controlled trial					
Bristol	219 /440	220 / 417		96.5	0.89 [0.68, 1.16]
Subtotal (95% CI)	219 /440	220 / 417		96.5	0.89 [0.68, 1.16]
Test for heterogeneity chi-square=0.00 df=0					
Test for overall effect=-0.87 p=0.4					
02 Randomised trial					
London	5 /23	2 / 20		2.7	2.32 [0.47, 11.54]
Northampton	2 /11	0 / 10		0.9	7.46 [0.43, 128.59]
Subtotal (95% CI)	7 /34	2 / 30		3.5	3.07 [0.76, 12.43]
Test for heterogeneity chi-square=0.49 df=1 p=0.4835					
Test for overall effect=1.57 p=0.12					
Total (95% CI)	226 /474	222 / 447		100.0	0.93 [0.71, 1.21]
Test for heterogeneity chi-square=3.42 df=2 p=0.1811					
Test for overall effect=-0.56 p=0.6					

.1   .2   1   5   10

Figure 3.1   Forest plot showing the proportional effects (OR and its 95% CI) of home-based stroke services compared with conventional hospital-based stroke services on death or institutionalisation at the end of the scheduled follow-up period for each individual trial (each single line), and as a pooled summary estimate of the results of all trials at the bottom (black diamond). Reproduced from Langhorne *et al.* (1999), with permission from the authors and John Wiley & Sons Limited. Copyright Cochrane Library, reproduced with permission.

Management of stroke patients at home (vs in hospital)

Evidence

Three controlled clinical trials have compared the effect of routine processes of caring for stroke patients (often involving admission to hospital) with the effect of caring for stroke patients by means of a multidisciplinary domiciliary team aiming to provide care in the home (Langhorne *et al.*, 1999). The trials used a range of services to serve as their control (or comparison) group, such as care in a general medical ward (GMW), by a mobile stroke team in the hospital, and in a stroke ward. Overall, there was no significant difference in the proportion of patients who had died or were in institutional care at 1 year after stroke onset among the home-based care group compared with the conventional hospital-based care group (odds ratio (OR): 0.93, 95% confidence interval (CI): 0.71–1.21) (Fig. 3.1) (Langhorne *et al.*, 1999).

Among elderly medical patients there was also no difference in mortality (OR: 1.00, 95% CI: 0.70–1.44) (Fig. 3.2) (Shepperd and Iliffe, 2001).

Review: Hospital at home versus in-patient hospital care
Comparison: 01 Hospital at home versus in-patient care
Outcome: 07 mortality - elderly medical

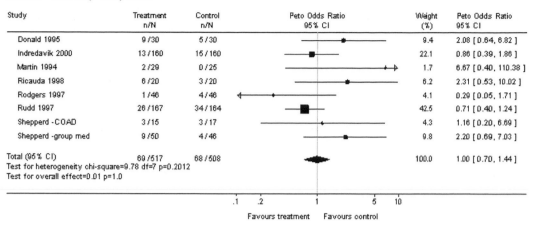

Study	Treatment n/N	Control n/N	Peto Odds Ratio 95% CI	Weight (%)	Peto Odds Ratio 95% CI
Donald 1995	9/30	5/30		9.4	2.08 [0.64, 6.82]
Indredavik 2000	13/160	15/160		22.1	0.86 [0.39, 1.86]
Martin 1994	2/29	0/25		1.7	6.67 [0.40, 110.38]
Ricauda 1998	6/20	3/20		6.2	2.31 [0.53, 10.02]
Rodgers 1997	1/46	4/46		4.1	0.29 [0.05, 1.71]
Rudd 1997	26/167	34/164		42.5	0.71 [0.40, 1.24]
Shepperd -COAD	3/15	3/17		4.3	1.16 [0.20, 6.69]
Shepperd -group med	9/50	4/46		9.8	2.20 [0.69, 7.03]
Total (95% CI)	69/517	68/508		100.0	1.00 [0.70, 1.44]

Test for heterogeneity chi-square=9.78 df=7 p=0.2012
Test for overall effect=0.01 p=1.0

.1   .2   1   5   10

Favours treatment   Favours control

Figure 3.2   Forest plot showing the proportional effects of home-based services compared with conventional hospital inpatient care on death at the end of the scheduled follow-up period among elderly medical patients. Reproduced from Shepperd and Iliffe (2001), with permission from the authors and John Wiley & Sons Limited. Copyright Cochrane Library, reproduced with permission.

These trials were besieged with practical problems. In some of the trials, the actual number of hospital bed days used by the patients randomised to care at home was as great as the patients randomised to care in hospital. In other words, many of the patients ended up going to hospital, and so the home-based care plan was far more expensive than the hospital plan. In subsequent trials, patients allocated at random to care at home had to be eventually admitted to the stroke unit (Hacke, 2000; Kalra et al., 2000). Understandably, there was a trend for greater resource consumption among those randomised to home-based care.

Comment

Interpretation of the evidence

The debate about hospital vs home care has mainly been an issue in the UK. The above data provide no evidence to support a radical change in policy from hospital- to home-based acute stroke care.

Implications for practice

All stroke patients should have immediate and equitable access to appropriate assessment and management, and most should be admitted to hospital.

However, hospital admission is also dependent on other factors (Table 3.1).

Table 3.1. Factors influencing hospital admission rates.

- The patient's functional state, prognosis, area of residence and expectations
- The clinician's plan for investigations and management
- The level of organisation of the primary care and hospital-based care
- Local custom and practice

Table 3.2. The type of stroke patients who should be managed in hospital.

- Patients who may benefit from organised care by a multidisciplinary team in a stroke unit; or from appropriate and effective acute medical and surgical therapies, besides aspirin, such as i.v. thrombolysis (ischaemic stroke within 3 h of onset) and suboccipital craniectomy (*cf.* cerebellar infarction and oedema)
- Patients who are at risk of life threatening, preventable or treatable complications such as airway obstruction and respiratory failure; swallowing problems causing aspiration, dehydration and malnutrition; epileptic seizures; venous thromboembolism; and infections
- Patients who are disabled and require nursing care

Table 3.3. The type of stroke patients who may be managed at home.

- Patients who are not disabled, or were previously disabled and well cared for (e.g. in a nursing home)
- Patients who can be diagnosed accurately (including stroke pathology, aetiology and prognosis) as an outpatient
- Patients who can be cared for at home, including appropriate secondary stroke prevention and, where appropriate, domiciliary rehabilitation

The type of patients who should probably be managed in hospital are listed in Table 3.2.

The type of patients who can probably be managed at home are listed in Table 3.3.

Implications for research

The debate about hospital vs home care has largely been superseded by the compelling evidence of the superior effectiveness of organised care in a stroke unit in optimising survival and functional outcome after stroke (see below). However, there is increasing evidence that the home does have an important role in post-hospital care, and in facilitating accelerated discharge from hospital to home. Early supported home-based rehabilitation has been shown to reduce length of hospital stay, and in selected patients it may reduce disability and institutional care (Early Supported Discharge Trialists, 2001; Indredavik *et al.*, 2000; Fjaertoft *et al.*, 2003; Langhorne, 2003; Langhorne *et al.*, 2005; Meijer and van Limbeek *et al.*, 2005) (see below).

Table 3.4. The three main models of organised stroke care.

- Care in a *geographically dedicated stroke ward (stroke unit)* by a multidisciplinary team. Within the geographically dedicated stroke ward there are three models:
  (i) Acute (intensive care) stroke unit: provides stroke unit care in the first few days after stroke. Patients are admitted directly to the unit for acute assessment, investigation and intervention.
  (ii) Rehabilitation stroke unit: admits patients 1–2 weeks after stroke and continues rehabilitation for several weeks to months as required.
  (iii) Comprehensive stroke unit: combines both acute care and rehabilitation.
- Care in a several wards by a *mobile stroke team.*
- Care in a *mixed assessment/rehabilitation unit*: a generic disability unit which specialises in the management of disabled patients, irrespective of the cause.

Hospital-based care

Terminology

The term 'stroke unit' encompasses the provision and coordination of multidisciplinary stroke care in a geographically defined area, such as a stroke ward (Langhorne and Dennis, 1998). The core disciplines involved are usually medical, nursing, speech and swallowing therapy/pathology, physiotherapy, occupational therapy, social work and dietetics. Information regarding patient assessment, goals, interventions, progress and discharge planning are coordinated by regular (at least weekly) multidisciplinary meetings.

Types of organised (stroke unit) care

The three main models of organised stroke care are listed in Table 3.4.

Evidence

Death

A systematic review of 23 randomised-controlled trials (RCTs) involving almost 5000 patients in eight countries showed that, compared with alternative conventional services usually provided in a GMW, organised multidisciplinary care in a stroke unit was associated with a statistically significant reduction in the odds of death recorded at final follow-up (median 1 year, ranges from 6 weeks to 12 months) by about 18% (OR: 0.82, 95% CI: 0.71–0.94, $P = 0.005$) from 25% (596/2396) to 21% (522/2525) (Fig. 3.3) (Stroke Unit Trialists' Collaboration, 2001). This is an absolute risk reduction of 4% (25% − 21%), indicating that for every 100 patients assigned to organised care in a stroke unit, there were four fewer deaths at final follow-up compared to care in a GMW.

Review: Organised inpatient (stroke unit) care for stroke
Comparison: 01 Organised stroke unit care vs Alternative service
Outcome: 01 Death by the end of scheduled follow up

Study	Treatment n/N	Control n/N	Peto Odds Ratio 95% CI	Weight (%)	Peto Odds Ratio 95% CI
01 Stroke ward vs General medical ward					
Akershus	61 /271	70 /279		12.5	0.87 [0.59, 1.28]
Dover	34 /98	35 /89		5.5	0.82 [0.45, 1.48]
Edinburgh	48 /155	55 /156		8.7	0.82 [0.51, 1.32]
Goteborg-Ostra	16 /215	12 /202		3.3	1.27 [0.59, 2.73]
Goteborg-Sahlgren	45 /166	19 /83		5.3	1.25 [0.68, 2.27]
Nottingham	14 /98	10 /76		2.6	1.10 [0.46, 2.61]
Orpington-1993	3 /53	6 /48		1.0	0.43 [0.11, 1.70]
Orpington-1995	7 /36	17 /37		2.0	0.31 [0.12, 0.81]
Perth	4 /29	6 /30		1.1	0.65 [0.17, 2.50]
Stockholm	49 /269	46 /225		9.5	0.89 [0.57, 1.40]
Svendborg	14 /31	12 /34		2.0	1.50 [0.56, 4.02]
Trondheim	27 /110	36 /110		5.7	0.67 [0.37, 1.20]
Umea	43 /110	75 /183		8.3	0.92 [0.57, 1.50]
Subtotal (95% CI)	365 /1641	398 /1552		67.3	0.87 [0.74, 1.03]
Test for heterogeneity chi-square=10.31 df=12 p=0.5885					
Test for overall effect=-1.60 p=0.11					
02 Mixed rehabilitation ward vs General medical ward					
Birmingham	4 /29	2 /23		0.7	1.63 [0.30, 8.90]
Helsinki	26 /121	27 /122		5.2	0.96 [0.52, 1.77]
x Illinois	0 /56	0 /35		0.0	Not estimable
Kuopio	8 /50	10 /45		1.8	0.67 [0.24, 1.86]
x New York	0 /42	0 /40		0.0	Not estimable
Newcastle	11 /34	12 /33		1.9	0.84 [0.31, 2.28]
Subtotal (95% CI)	49 /332	51 /298		9.6	0.91 [0.58, 1.42]
Test for heterogeneity chi-square=0.86 df=3 p=0.8352					
Test for overall effect=-0.43 p=0.7					
03 Mobile stroke team vs General medical ward					
Montreal	16 /65	21 /65		3.3	0.69 [0.32, 1.47]
Uppsala	27 /60	26 /52		3.5	0.82 [0.39, 1.72]
Subtotal (95% CI)	43 /125	47 /117		6.8	0.75 [0.44, 1.28]
Test for heterogeneity chi-square=0.11 df=1 p=0.7448					
Test for overall effect=-1.05 p=0.3					
04 Stroke ward vs Mixed rehabilitation ward					
Dover	5 /18	11 /28		1.3	0.61 [0.18, 2.08]
Nottingham	11 /78	16 /63		2.7	0.48 [0.21, 1.12]
Orpington-1993	6 /71	12 /73		2.0	0.48 [0.18, 1.30]
Tampere	30 /98	27 /113		5.2	1.40 [0.76, 2.58]
Subtotal (95% CI)	52 /265	66 /277		11.2	0.82 [0.54, 1.24]
Test for heterogeneity chi-square=5.83 df=3 p=0.1201					
Test for overall effect=-0.96 p=0.3					
05 Stroke ward vs Mobile stroke team					
Orpington-2000	13 /152	34 /152		5.0	0.35 [0.19, 0.65]
Subtotal (95% CI)	13 /152	34 /152		5.0	0.35 [0.19, 0.65]
Test for heterogeneity chi-square=0.00 df=0					
Test for overall effect=-3.33 p=0.0009					
Total (95% CI)	522 /2515	596 /2396		100.0	0.82 [0.71, 0.94]
Test for heterogeneity chi-square=25.19 df=23 p=0.3406					
Test for overall effect=-2.78 p=0.005					

.1   .2   1   5   10

Favours treatment   Favours control

Figure 3.3   Forest plot showing the proportional effects of organised stroke unit care compared with alternative services on *death* at the end of the scheduled follow-up

Death or institutionalisation

Random allocation to organised multidisciplinary care in a stroke unit was associated with a statistically significant reduction in the odds of the combined outcome of death or institutionalisation at final follow-up by about 20% (OR: 0.80, 95% CI: 0.71–0.90, $P = 0.0002$) from 45% (1077/2373) to 40% (944/2486) (Fig. 3.4), indicating that for every 100 patients assigned to organised care in a stroke unit, there were five fewer patients who died or were institutionalised at final follow-up compared to care in a GMW (Stroke Unit Trialists' Collaboration, 2001).

Death or dependency

Random allocation to organised care in a stroke unit was associated with a statistically significant reduction in the odds of the combined outcome of death or dependency by 22% (OR: 0.78, 95% CI: 0.68–0.89, $P = 0.0003$), from 61% (1171/1935) to 56% (1117/2000), indicating that for every 100 patients assigned to organised care in a stroke unit, there were five fewer patients who died or dependent at final follow-up compared to care in a GMW (Fig. 3.5) (Stroke Unit Trialists' Collaboration, 2001).

Absolute effects of organised care on death, institutional care and dependency

Overall, for every 100 stroke patients randomly allocated organised (stroke unit) care, four additional patients survived (21% (stroke unit) vs 25% (GMW)), two avoided long-term care in an institution (19% (stroke unit) vs 21% (GMW)) and an additional six returned home, of whom one was physically or cognitively dependent (16% (stroke unit) vs 15% (GMW)) and five were independent (44% (stroke unit) vs 39% (GMW)) (Stroke Unit Trialists' Collaboration, 2001).

On average, the number of patients needed to treat with organised (stroke unit) care to prevent one death was 33 (95% CI: 20–100), to prevent one patient being unable to live at home was 20 (95% CI: 12–50) and to prevent one patient failing to regain independence was 20 (95% CI: 12–50). However, there could be a wide range of results as the 95% CI of these estimates and the absolute outcome rates varied considerably (Stroke Unit Trialists' Collaboration, 2001).

Caption for fig. 3.3 (*cont.*)
period among individual trials (each line) and pooled (summary at the bottom). The OR for death in the organised stroke unit care group compared with that in the alternative services group is plotted for each trial (black square), along with its 95% CI (horizontal line). Meta-analysis of the pooled results of all trials is represented by a black diamond showing the OR, and the 95% CI of the OR. Reproduced from the Stroke Unit Trialists' Collaboration (2001), with permission from the authors and John Wiley & Sons Limited. Copyright Cochrane Library, reproduced with permission.

Review: Organised inpatient (stroke unit) care for stroke
Comparison: 01 Organised stroke unit care vs Alternative service
Outcome: 02 Death or institutional care by the end of scheduled follow up

Study	Treatment n/N	Control n/N	Peto Odds Ratio 95% CI	Weight (%)	Peto Odds Ratio 95% CI
01 Stroke ward vs General medical ward					
Akershus	101 / 271	113 / 279		12.1	0.87 [0.62, 1.23]
Dover	50 / 98	48 / 89		4.3	0.89 [0.50, 1.58]
Edinburgh	66 / 155	78 / 156		7.2	0.74 [0.48, 1.16]
Goteborg-Ostra	49 / 215	43 / 202		6.6	1.09 [0.69, 1.73]
Goteborg-Sahlgren	64 / 166	34 / 83		4.9	0.90 [0.53, 1.55]
Nottingham	28 / 98	21 / 76		3.2	1.05 [0.54, 2.03]
Orpington-1993	9 / 53	12 / 48		1.5	0.62 [0.24, 1.61]
Orpington-1995	18 / 36	30 / 37		1.5	0.26 [0.10, 0.67]
Perth	6 / 29	14 / 30		1.2	0.32 [0.11, 0.93]
Stockholm	150 / 269	117 / 225		11.2	1.16 [0.82, 1.66]
Svendborg	18 / 31	20 / 34		1.5	0.97 [0.36, 2.58]
Trondheim	41 / 110	61 / 110		5.1	0.48 [0.28, 0.82]
Umea	51 / 110	105 / 183		6.3	0.64 [0.40, 1.03]
Subtotal (95% CI)	651 / 1641	696 / 1552		66.7	0.82 [0.71, 0.95]

Test for heterogeneity chi-square=20.16 df=12 p=0.0642
Test for overall effect=-2.64 p=0.008

02 Mixed rehabilitation ward vs General medical ward					
Helsinki	36 / 121	46 / 122		5.0	0.70 [0.41, 1.19]
Illinois	22 / 56	17 / 35		2.0	0.69 [0.29, 1.61]
Kuopio	22 / 50	23 / 45		2.2	0.75 [0.34, 1.68]
New York	15 / 42	17 / 40		1.8	0.75 [0.31, 1.82]
Newcastle	18 / 34	21 / 33		1.5	0.65 [0.25, 1.70]
Subtotal (95% CI)	113 / 303	124 / 275		12.5	0.71 [0.51, 0.99]

Test for heterogeneity chi-square=0.08 df=4 p=0.9992
Test for overall effect=-2.01 p=0.04

03 Mobile stroke team vs General medical ward					
Montreal	57 / 65	52 / 65		1.6	1.76 [0.69, 4.46]
Uppsala	40 / 60	35 / 52		2.3	0.97 [0.44, 2.13]
Subtotal (95% CI)	97 / 125	87 / 117		3.9	1.24 [0.68, 2.27]

Test for heterogeneity chi-square=0.91 df=1 p=0.3406
Test for overall effect=0.71 p=0.5

04 Stroke ward vs Mixed rehabilitation ward					
Dover	11 / 18	18 / 28		1.0	0.88 [0.26, 2.94]
Nottingham	34 / 78	32 / 63		3.2	0.75 [0.39, 1.46]
Orpington-1993	24 / 71	33 / 73		3.2	0.62 [0.32, 1.21]
Tampere	43 / 98	42 / 113		4.7	1.32 [0.76, 2.29]
Subtotal (95% CI)	112 / 265	125 / 277		12.1	0.90 [0.64, 1.27]

Test for heterogeneity chi-square=3.33 df=3 p=0.344
Test for overall effect=-0.60 p=0.5

05 Stroke ward vs Mobile stroke team					
Orpington-2000	21 / 152	45 / 152		4.8	0.40 [0.23, 0.68]
Subtotal (95% CI)	21 / 152	45 / 152		4.8	0.40 [0.23, 0.68]

Test for heterogeneity chi-square=0.00 df=0
Test for overall effect=-3.33 p=0.0009

Total (95% CI)	994 / 2486	1077 / 2373		100.0	0.80 [0.71, 0.90]

Test for heterogeneity chi-square=34.03 df=24 p=0.0842
Test for overall effect=-3.67 p=0.0002

```
        .1   .2        1        5   10
         Favours treatment   Favours control
```

Figure 3.4   Forest plot showing the proportional effects of organised stroke unit care compared with alternative services on *death or institutionalisation* at the end of the scheduled follow-up

Length of stay

Length of stay data were available for 17 individual trials which compared organised inpatient (stroke unit) care with an alternative service. Mean (or median) length of stay ranged from 13 to 162 days in the stroke unit groups and from 14 to 137 days in controls. The calculation of a summary result for length of stay was subject to major methodological limitations; length of stay was calculated in different ways (e.g. acute hospital stay, total stay in hospital or institution), two trials recorded median rather than mean length of stay, and in two trials the standard deviation had to be inferred from the P-value or from the results of similar trials. Overall, using a random effects model, there was a modest reduction in the length of stay in the stroke unit group (standardised mean difference: -0.17, 95% CI: -0.33 to -0.01, $P = 0.03$) which is approximately equivalent to a reduction of 6 (2–10) days (Fig. 3.6) (Stroke Unit Trialists' Collaboration, 2001). The summary estimates were complicated by considerable heterogeneity which limits the extent to which more general conclusions can be inferred.

Longer-term outcomes up to 5 years after stroke

Two trials (Nottingham, Trondheim) carried out supplementary studies extending patient follow-up to 5 years post-stroke. Care in a stroke unit was associated with a 37% reduction in odds of death (OR: 0.63, 95% CI: 0.45–0.89, $P < 0.01$), 38% reduction in odds of death or institutional care (OR: 0.62, 95% CI: 0.43–0.89, $P < 0.01$) (Fig. 3.7) and 41% reduction in odds of death or dependency (OR: 0.59, 95% CI: 0.38–0.92, $P < 0.05$). One trial (Trondheim) extended follow up to 10 years post-stroke and found a similar pattern of results: a 54% reduction in the odds of death (OR: 0.46, 95% CI: 0.23–0.91), a 60% reduction in odds of death or institutional care (OR: 0.40, 95% CI: 0.18–0.86) and 38% reduction in odds of death or dependency (OR: 0.62, 95% CI: 0.26–1.46) (Stroke Unit Trialists' Collaboration, 2001).

Patient satisfaction and quality of life

Only two trials (Nottingham, Trondheim) recorded outcome measures related to patient quality of life (Nottingham Health Profile). In both cases there was significantly improved quality of life among survivors of care in a stroke unit. There was no systematically gathered information on patient preferences (Stroke Unit Trialists' Collaboration, 2001).

Caption for fig. 3.4 (*cont.*)
period among individual trials (each line) and pooled (summary at the bottom). Reproduced from the Stroke Unit Trialists' Collaboration (2001) and with permission from the authors and John Wiley & Sons Limited. Copyright Cochrane Library, reproduced with permission.

Review: Organised inpatient (stroke unit) care for stroke
Comparison: 01 Organised stroke unit care vs Alternative service
Outcome: 03 Death or dependency by the end of scheduled follow up

Study	Treatment n/N	Control n/N	Peto Odds Ratio 95% CI	Weight (%)	Peto Odds Ratio 95% CI
01 Stroke ward vs General medical ward					
Akershus	103 /271	110 /279		15.4	0.94 [0.67, 1.33]
Dover	54 /98	50 /89		5.5	0.96 [0.54, 1.70]
Edinburgh	93 /155	94 /156		8.8	0.99 [0.63, 1.56]
Goteborg-Sahlgren	108 /166	54 /83		6.0	1.00 [0.58, 1.74]
Nottingham	63 /98	52 /76		4.6	0.83 [0.44, 1.56]
Orpington-1993	38 /53	39 /48		2.2	0.59 [0.24, 1.48]
x Orpington-1995	36 /36	37 /37		0.0	Not estimable
Perth	10 /29	14 /30		1.7	0.61 [0.22, 1.71]
Trondheim	54 /110	81 /110		6.2	0.36 [0.21, 0.61]
Umea	52 /110	102 /183		8.1	0.71 [0.44, 1.14]
Subtotal (95% CI)	611 /1126	633 /1091		58.5	0.80 [0.67, 0.95]
Test for heterogeneity chi-square=12.18 df=8 p=0.1432					
Test for overall effect=-2.51 p=0.01					
02 Mixed rehabilitation ward vs General medical ward					
Birmingham	8 /29	9 /23		1.4	0.60 [0.19, 1.90]
Helsinki	47 /121	65 /122		7.2	0.56 [0.34, 0.93]
Illinois	20 /56	17 /35		2.5	0.59 [0.25, 1.39]
Kuopio	31 /50	31 /46		2.6	0.74 [0.32, 1.72]
New York	23 /42	23 /40		2.4	0.90 [0.38, 2.13]
Newcastle	26 /34	28 /33		1.3	0.59 [0.18, 1.96]
Subtotal (95% CI)	155 /332	173 /298		17.2	0.63 [0.46, 0.88]
Test for heterogeneity chi-square=1.02 df=5 p=0.9609					
Test for overall effect=-2.75 p=0.006					
03 Mobile stroke team vs General medical ward					
Montreal	58 /65	60 /65		1.3	0.69 [0.21, 2.27]
Uppsala	45 /60	41 /52		2.4	0.81 [0.34, 1.94]
Subtotal (95% CI)	103 /125	101 /117		3.7	0.77 [0.38, 1.55]
Test for heterogeneity chi-square=0.04 df=1 p=0.8411					
Test for overall effect=-0.74 p=0.5					
04 Stroke ward vs Mixed rehabilitation ward					
Dover	11 /18	19 /28		1.2	0.75 [0.22, 2.56]
Nottingham	60 /78	48 /63		3.0	1.04 [0.48, 2.27]
Orpington-1993	63 /71	69 /73		1.3	0.47 [0.15, 1.53]
Tampere	53 /98	55 /113		6.2	1.24 [0.72, 2.13]
Subtotal (95% CI)	187 /265	191 /277		11.7	1.01 [0.68, 1.50]
Test for heterogeneity chi-square=2.40 df=3 p=0.4933					
Test for overall effect=0.05 p=1.0					
05 Stroke ward vs Mobile stroke team					
Orpington-2000	61 /152	73 /152		8.9	0.73 [0.46, 1.14]
Subtotal (95% CI)	61 /152	73 /152		8.9	0.73 [0.46, 1.14]
Test for heterogeneity chi-square=0.00 df=0					
Test for overall effect=-1.38 p=0.17					
Total (95% CI)	1117 /2000	1171 /1935		100.0	0.78 [0.68, 0.89]
Test for heterogeneity chi-square=19.04 df=21 p=0.5827					
Test for overall effect=-3.60 p=0.0003					

.1   .2   1   5   10

Favours treatment   Favours control

Figure 3.5   Forest plot showing the proportional effects of organised stroke unit care compared with alternative services on *death or dependency* at the end of the scheduled follow-up period among individual trials (each line) and pooled (summary at the bottom). Reproduced from the Stroke Unit Trialists' Collaboration (2001), with permission from the authors and John Wiley & Sons Limited. Copyright Cochrane Library, reproduced with permission.

Review: Organised inpatient (stroke unit) care for stroke
Comparison: 01 Organised stroke unit care vs Alternative service
Outcome: 04 Length of stay (days) in a hospital and/or institution

Study	Treatment N	Mean (SD)	Control N	Mean (SD)	Standardised Mean Difference (Random) 95% CI	Weight (%)	Standardised Mean Difference (Random) 95% CI
01 Stroke ward							
Akershus	271	8.00 (8.00)	279	10.00 (7.00)		6.9	-0.31 [-0.47, -0.14]
Dover	112	116.00 (99.00)	117	113.00 (96.00)		6.2	0.03 [-0.23, 0.29]
Edinburgh	155	55.00 (47.00)	156	75.00 (64.00)		6.5	-0.36 [-0.58, -0.13]
Goteborg-Ostra	215	16.00 (15.00)	202	14.00 (15.00)		6.7	0.13 [-0.06, 0.33]
Goteborg-Sahlgren	166	28.00 (17.00)	83	36.00 (17.00)		6.2	-0.47 [-0.74, -0.20]
Orpington-1993	124	55.00 (30.00)	121	98.00 (50.00)		6.2	-1.04 [-1.31, -0.78]
Orpington-2000	152	32.00 (30.00)	149	30.00 (40.00)		6.5	0.06 [-0.17, 0.28]
Perth	29	24.00 (30.00)	30	27.00 (30.00)		4.2	-0.10 [-0.61, 0.41]
Stockholm	269	21.00 (20.00)	225	20.00 (20.00)		6.8	0.05 [-0.13, 0.23]
Svendborg	31	12.00 (22.00)	34	23.00 (34.00)		4.4	-0.38 [-0.87, 0.12]
Tampere	98	13.00 (30.00)	113	15.00 (38.00)		6.1	-0.06 [-0.33, 0.21]
Trondheim	110	75.00 (84.00)	110	123.00 (105.00)		6.2	-0.55 [-0.82, -0.28]
Umea	110	21.00 (16.00)	183	31.00 (27.00)		6.4	-0.42 [-0.66, -0.19]

Subtotal (95% CI)   1842   1802   87.7   -0.26 [-0.44, -0.08]
Test for heterogeneity chi-square=83.97 df=12 p<0.00001
Test for overall effect=-2.80 p=0.005

02 Mixed rehabilitation ward							
Helsinki	121	24.00 (39.00)	122	31.00 (71.00)		6.3	-0.12 [-0.37, 0.13]
Kuopio	42	162.00 (125.00)	35	129.00 (119.00)		4.7	0.27 [-0.18, 0.72]
Newcastle	34	52.00 (46.00)	33	41.00 (34.00)		4.4	0.27 [-0.21, 0.75]

Subtotal (95% CI)   197   190   9.6   0.08 [-0.21, 0.37]
Test for heterogeneity chi-square=0.42 df=2 p=0.1904
Test for overall effect=0.54 p=0.6

03 Mobile stroke team							
Uppsala	60	30.00 (27.00)	52	23.00 (20.00)		5.3	0.29 [-0.08, 0.66]

Subtotal (95% CI)   60   52   2.7   0.29 [-0.08, 0.66]
Test for heterogeneity chi-square=0.00 df=0
Test for overall effect=1.52 p=0.13

Total (95% CI)   2099   2044   100.0   -0.17 [-0.33, -0.01]
Test for heterogeneity chi-square=98.70 df=16 p<0.00001
Test for overall effect=-2.11 p=0.03

       -4   -2   0   2   4
Favours treatment   Favours control

Figure 3.6   Forest plot showing the effects of organised stroke unit care compared with alternative services on *length of hospital stay (days, mean)* at the end of the scheduled follow-up period among individual trials (each line) and pooled (summary at the bottom). Reproduced from the Stroke Unit Trialists' Collaboration (2001), with permission from the authors and John Wiley & Sons Limited. Copyright Cochrane Library, reproduced with permission.

Subgroup analyses by trial characteristics

In view of the variety of trial methodologies, a subgroup analysis was undertaken based only on those trials with a low risk of bias: (a) secure randomisation procedures, (b) unequivocally blinded outcome assessment and (c) a fixed 1 year period of follow-up. Among the five trials (Goteborg-Sahlgren; Helsinki; Kuopio; Nottingham; Orpington-2000) that met all of these criteria, stroke unit care was associated with significant reductions in the odds of death (OR: 0.74, 95% CI: 0.55–0.99, $P < 0.05$), death or institutional care (OR: 0.71, 95% CI: 0.55–0.90,

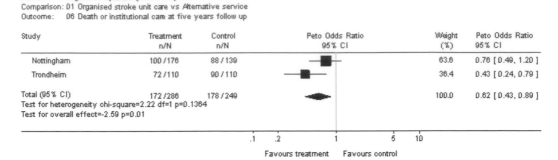

Review: Organised inpatient (stroke unit) care for stroke
Comparison: 01 Organised stroke unit care vs Alternative service
Outcome: 06 Death or institutional care at five years follow up

Study	Treatment n/N	Control n/N	Peto Odds Ratio 95% CI	Weight (%)	Peto Odds Ratio 95% CI
Nottingham	100 / 176	88 / 139		63.6	0.76 [0.49, 1.20]
Trondheim	72 / 110	90 / 110		36.4	0.43 [0.24, 0.79]
Total (95% CI)	172 / 286	178 / 249		100.0	0.62 [0.43, 0.89]

Test for heterogeneity chi-square=2.22 df=1 p=0.1364
Test for overall effect=-2.59 p=0.01

.1   .2   1   5   10

Favours treatment   Favours control

Figure 3.7   Forest plot showing the proportional effects of organised stroke unit care compared with alternative services on *death or institutionalisation at 5 years follow-up* among individual trials (each line) and pooled (summary at the bottom). Reproduced from the Stroke Unit Trialists' Collaboration (2001), with permission from the authors and John Wiley & Sons Limited. Copyright Cochrane Library, reproduced with permission.

$P < 0.001$) and death or dependency (OR: 0.70, 95% CI: 0.55–0.89, $P < 0.001$) (Stroke Unit Trialists' Collaboration, 2001).

Subgroup analyses by patient characteristics

Pre-defined subgroup analysis including data from the majority of trials (at least 2500 patients randomised) were carried out based on the patients' age, sex and initial stroke severity. The results are summarised in Table 3.5.

Subsequent studies have supported the benefits of stroke unit care among patients with severe stroke (Jorgensen *et al.*, 2000) and suggested that the benefits of stroke unit management may also vary according to stroke subtype. A *post hoc* analysis of one RCT suggests that stroke unit care improved the outcome of patients with large vessel infarcts, but not those with lacunar syndromes (Evans *et al.*, 2002).

These subgroup analyses should be interpreted with caution, however, as they are based on a small number of outcome events and are, therefore, imprecise and not statistically robust. Also the results may vary according to the outcome measure chosen. For example, patients with stroke of mild severity did not appear to benefit from stroke unit care in terms of a reduced risk of death (OR: 0.96, 95% CI: 0.58–1.60) or death or institutional care (OR: 0.95, 95% CI: 0.66–1.36), but they had a significantly reduced risk of survival with dependency (OR: 0.51, 95% CI: 0.33–0.79, $P < 0.001$) (Stroke Unit Trialists' Collaboration, 2001).

Organised (stroke unit) care vs general medical wards

Three different models of organised stroke unit care (comprehensive stroke ward, rehabilitation stroke ward and mixed assessment/rehabilitation ward) tended to be

Table 3.5. OR (95% CI) for Death or Institutional Care among patients randomly assigned to care in a stroke unit, compared with a general ward, according to the patients age, sex and stroke severity at the time of randomisation.

Patient characteristics	OR (95% CI)
Age up to 75 years	0.77 (0.63–0.94)
Age more than 75 years	0.69 (0.56–0.85)
Male	0.66 (0.51–0.85)
Female	0.77 (0.60–0.98)
Mild stroke	0.95 (0.66–1.36)
Moderate stroke	0.70 (0.58–0.84)
Severe stroke	0.55 (0.38–0.81)

more effective than GMW care. There were insufficient data to draw conclusions on the comparison of mobile team care (peripatetic service) vs GMWs. The apparent benefits of stroke unit care were seen in units with both an acute admission policy and a delayed admission policy.

Different types of organised stroke unit care: direct comparisons (Fig. 3.8)

Three different types of organised (stroke unit) care could be compared; that is care:

1 in a ward dedicated only to stroke care (dedicated stroke ward),
2 by a mobile stroke team, or
3 by a generic disability service (mixed rehabilitation unit) which specialises in the management of disabling illness including stroke.

Acute stroke ward vs mixed assessment/rehabilitation ward

One trial (Tampere) compared an acute stroke unit with a mixed assessment/ rehabilitation ward and there was no statistically significant difference in the odds of death (OR: 1.4, 95% CI: 0.76–2.58), death or institutional care (OR: 1.32, 95% CI: 0.76–2.29) (Fig. 3.8), or death or dependency (OR: 1.24, 95% CI: 0.72–2.13). However, there were insufficient data to draw firm conclusions.

Rehabilitation stroke ward vs mixed assessment/rehabilitation ward

Three trials (Dover, Orpington-1993, Nottingham) incorporated designs in which patients could be randomised either to a stroke rehabilitation ward or to conventional care in either a GMW or mixed assessment/rehabilitation ward within a department of geriatric medicine.

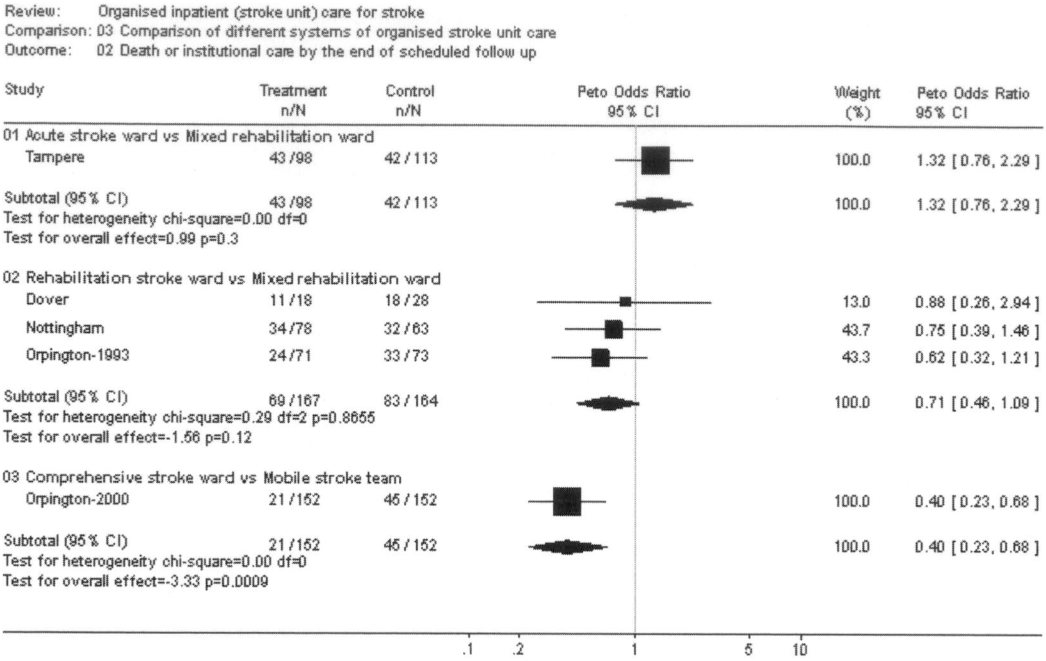

Review: Organised inpatient (stroke unit) care for stroke
Comparison: 03 Comparison of different systems of organised stroke unit care
Outcome: 02 Death or institutional care by the end of scheduled follow up

Study	Treatment n/N	Control n/N	Peto Odds Ratio 95% CI	Weight (%)	Peto Odds Ratio 95% CI
01 Acute stroke ward vs Mixed rehabilitation ward					
Tampere	43 /98	42 / 113		100.0	1.32 [0.76, 2.29]
Subtotal (95% CI)	43 /98	42 / 113		100.0	1.32 [0.76, 2.29]
Test for heterogeneity chi-square=0.00 df=0					
Test for overall effect=0.99 p=0.3					
02 Rehabilitation stroke ward vs Mixed rehabilitation ward					
Dover	11 /18	18 / 28		13.0	0.88 [0.26, 2.94]
Nottingham	34 /78	32 / 63		43.7	0.75 [0.39, 1.46]
Orpington-1993	24 /71	33 / 73		43.3	0.62 [0.32, 1.21]
Subtotal (95% CI)	69 /167	83 / 164		100.0	0.71 [0.46, 1.09]
Test for heterogeneity chi-square=0.29 df=2 p=0.8655					
Test for overall effect=-1.56 p=0.12					
03 Comprehensive stroke ward vs Mobile stroke team					
Orpington-2000	21 /152	45 / 152		100.0	0.40 [0.23, 0.68]
Subtotal (95% CI)	21 /152	45 / 152		100.0	0.40 [0.23, 0.68]
Test for heterogeneity chi-square=0.00 df=0					
Test for overall effect=-3.33 p=0.0009					

.1   .2   1   5   10

Figure 3.8   Forest plot showing a comparison of the effects of different systems of organised stroke unit care on *death or institutionalisation* at the end of the scheduled follow-up period among individual trials (each line) and pooled (summary at the bottom). Reproduced from the Stroke Unit Trialists' Collaboration (2001), with permission from the authors and John Wiley & Sons Limited. Copyright Cochrane Library, reproduced with permission.

Patients randomly assigned to care in the stroke rehabilitation ward had significantly fewer deaths (OR: 0.51, 95% CI: 0.29–0.90), and a non-significant trend towards fewer patients with the composite end point of death or requiring institutional care (OR: 0.71, 95% CI: 0.46–1.09) (Fig. 3.8), and death or dependency (OR: 0.8, 95% CI: 0.45–1.42). However, the numbers were small and no definite conclusions can be drawn.

Comprehensive stroke unit vs mobile stroke team

One trial (Orpington-2000) compared a comprehensive stroke ward (providing acute care and rehabilitation) with admission to general wards where care was provided by a mobile stroke team. Among patients randomly allocated to care in comprehensive stroke ward, there was a significant reduction in death (OR: 0.35, 95% CI: 0.19–0.65), and the combined outcome of death or institutional care compared with patients cared for by a mobile stroke team (OR: 0.40, 95% CI: 0.23–0.68) (Fig. 3.8), and a non-significant trend to a reduction in death or dependency (OR: 0.73, 95% CI: 0.46–1.14) at the end of follow-up.

Another trial also found that, compared with care in a GMW, patients who were randomised to comprehensive (acute and rehabilitation) care in a *stroke ward* had the greatest reduction in death and dependency at 1 year ($P = 0.008$), followed by patients randomised to care in a *rehabilitation ward* ($P = 0.04$), followed by patients cared for by a *mobile stroke team* (Kalra *et al.*, 2000; Stroke Unit Trialists' Collaboration, 2001).

Different processes of care: indirect comparisons

The improved functional outcome at the time of discharge, and shorter length of stay in hospital, of patients cared for in a stroke ward compared to a GMW or a mobile stroke team was associated with fewer systemic complications, which may be attributable to different processes of care (Evans *et al.*, 2001; Fuentes *et al.*, 2001). Patients in stroke wards were monitored more frequently and more patients received oxygen, antipyretics, measures to reduce aspiration, and early nutrition, than those in general wards (Evans *et al.*, 2001).

The characteristic processes of care in a stroke unit are listed in Table 3.6 (Indredavik *et al.*, 1999; Langhorne and Pollock, 2002; Langhorne and Dennis, 2004).

A recent pilot randomised trial tested the conventional stroke unit (featuring systemic early assessment of problems, provision of intravenous (i.v.) fluids, team rehabilitation and weekly multidisciplinary team meetings) with a stroke-care monitoring unit (same model of care but also providing continuous monitoring of oxygen saturation, electrocardiogram, temperature, blood pressure and glucose level with intervention for abnormalities) (Sulter *et al.*, 2003). Early case fatality was reduced with stroke-care monitoring but the magnitude was imprecise (wide CIs). These findings require confirmation in other studies but are an important development in the further exploration of why stroke units may be effective.

Care pathways

A care pathway (or clinical pathway, or critical pathway) can be defined as a plan of care that is developed and used by a multidisciplinary team, and is applicable to more than one aspect of care (Kwan and Sandercock, 2004, 2005). It can be a printed document or an electronic program, and it usually forms all or part of the patient's case record. Care pathways are often used in conjunction with other strategies of care such as case management, and are intended to assist healthcare professionals in clinical decision-making (Hydo, 1995; Lanska, 1998). Despite their popularity, the evidence to support their use is weak.

Evidence

A systematic review identified three RCTs (total of 340 patients) and 12 non-randomised studies (total of 4081 patients) which compared the effects of care

Table 3.6. Features of stroke units studied in randomised trials.

Assessment and monitoring	
Medical	Systematic clinical history and examination
	Routine investigations
	CT brain scan
	Blood tests: haematology and serum biochemistry
	Electrocardiogram
	Investigations in selected patients
	Carotid ultrasound
	Echocardiogram
	Magnetic resonance imaging
Nursing	
	General care needs
	Vital signs
	Swallow assessment
	Fluid balance
	Pressure-area risks
	Neurological monitoring
Therapy	
	Assessment of impairments and function
Early management	
Physiological management	Careful management of food and fluids (often i.v. saline over the first 12–24 h)
	Monitoring and treatment of infection, pyrexia, hypoxia and hyperglycaemia
Early mobilisation	Early measures to get patient sitting up, standing and walking
Nursing care	Careful positioning and handling, and pressure-area care
	Management of swallowing problems
	Avoidance of urinary catheters if possible
Multidisciplinary team rehabilitation	
Rehabilitation process	Formal multidisciplinary meetings once a week (plus informal meetings)
	Early rehabilitation, goal setting and involvement of carers
	Close linking of nursing with other multidisciplinary care
	Provision of information on stroke, recovery and services
Discharge planning	Early assessment of discharge needs
	Discharge plan involving patient and carers

Source: Langhorne and Pollock (2002) and Langhorne and Dennis (2004).

pathways with standard medical care among patients admitted to hospital with acute stroke (Kwan and Sandercock, 2004, 2005). There was no significant difference between care pathway and control groups in terms of death, or discharge destination. However, patients managed with a care pathway were more dependent at discharge ($P = 0.04$). More reliable data, from RCTs, are required.

Implications for clinical practice
There is currently insufficient evidence to justify routine implementation of care pathways for acute stroke management or stroke rehabilitation in hospital.

Implications for research
Further research by means of well conducted randomised and non-randomised studies and qualitative research are needed, particularly addressing the effects of care pathways on processes of care, implementation of evidence-based practice, functional outcomes, quality of life, patient and carer satisfaction, and hospital cost.

Comment

Interpretation of the evidence

These data indicate that patients who receive organised inpatient (stroke unit) care are more likely to survive, regain independence and return home than those receiving a less organised service. The benefit for stroke unit patients appears to be sustained for up to 5 or 10 years.

The apparent benefits were consistent among men and women, those aged above and below 75 years, and those with mild and severe strokes. Patients with more severe stroke symptoms are at greater risk of death or requiring institutional care and hence stand to gain more from treatment, whereas patients with mild stroke appeared to benefit from stroke unit care in terms of reduction in death or dependency rather than a reduction in death or the composite outcome of death or institutional care.

The benefits were observed in all types of stroke unit which were able to provide a period of care lasting several weeks if necessary (i.e. comprehensive stroke units and rehabilitation stroke units), and were most apparent in units based in a dedicated ward (rather than a mobile stroke team). Effective units were operational in a variety of departments including neurology, geriatric medicine, general/internal medicine and rehabilitation medicine. What they had in common was similar processes of care (Table 3.6, see below).

The *specific* processes of care in the stroke units to which their effectiveness in saving lives (mainly between 1 and 4 weeks after stroke) and reducing dependency after stroke are not clear (Langhorne and Pollock, 2002). The stroke units included in the systematic review did not regularly use thrombolytic agents or other acute specific treatments, and they did not provide intensive monitoring of physiological variables. Other features of care must be important, by reducing the risks of complications and by identifying and treating complications early. The number of potential post-stroke physiological abnormalities, neurological and general complications that need to be expected, prevented, detected and effectively treated to optimise the outcome for the patient is likely to be very extensive, but much of the benefit may be attributable to:

1 coordinated care by a multidisciplinary team;
2 awareness, anticipation and preventions of complications of stroke in high risk individuals (e.g. aspiration pneumonia, pulmonary embolism, pressure sores);
3 maintenance of physiological homoeostasis (Stroke Unit Trialists' Collaboration, 2001; Evans *et al.*, 2001; Langhorne and Pollock, 2002).

There is also evidence that some of the beneficial effect of care in a stroke unit may be attributable to patients in a stroke ward receiving greater amounts of therapy (Kalra *et al.*, 2000). Augmented exercise therapy has a small but favourable effect on activities of daily living (ADL), particularly if implemented within the first few months after stroke (Kwakkel *et al.*, 2004).

The crucial ingredients, therefore, appear to be coordinated multidisciplinary assessment, intervention, and optimisation of physiological homoeostasis; measures to risk stratify, record and prevent complications; active rehabilitation; education and training in stroke care; and specialisation of all staff in the team. It is uncertain whether more intensive medical monitoring is beneficial.

As the major direct health care costs of acute stroke management are from nursing care and hospital overheads, length of hospital stay is an important determinant of initial costs. In the longer term, direct costs are more determined by residual disability, and the care of dependent individuals in hospitals and nursing homes. If stroke unit care really does reduce long-term disability without increasing the mean length of stay in a hospital or institution, and without increasing the cost of inpatient care then it is likely to be cost-effective compared with conventional care. Preliminary economic analyses suggest that stroke unit care is likely to be associated with a modest increase in cost but it improves outcomes and saves resources (Major and Walker, 1998; Patel *et al.*, 2004).

Implications for practice

Generalisability

Evidence from prospective observational studies of more than 14,000 patients admitted to 80 Swedish hospitals, and of 7352 patients admitted to 240 hospitals in England, Wales and Northern Ireland, indicate that the results of the systematic review of randomised trials outlined above may be reproducible in, and generalisable to, routine clinical settings. Although biases are inherent in such observational data, patients admitted to a stroke unit in Sweden had reduced dependence at 3 months (relative risk reduction (RRR) 6%, 95% CI: 1–11%) (Stegmayr *et al.*, 1999; Glader *et al.*, 2001) and patients admitted to a stroke unit in England, Wales and

North Ireland had a 25% (95% CI: 10–40%) lower case fatality, irrespective of case mix (Rudd *et al.*, 2005).

The absolute benefits of organised inpatient (stroke unit) care appear to be sufficiently large (numbers needed to treat to ensure one extra 'good' outcome are 33 for survival, 20 to regain independence and 20 to return home) to justify the organisation of stroke services.

Structure of the stroke unit

Stroke ward or mobile team?   Acute stroke patients should be offered organised inpatient (stroke unit) care which is typically provided by a coordinated multidisciplinary team operating within a discrete stroke ward, which can offer a substantial period of rehabilitation if required (Kalra *et al.*, 2000; Fuentes *et al.*, 2001).

However, if a geographically dedicated stroke unit is not feasible, it is nevertheless important to establish a multidisciplinary stroke team that meets regularly and follows the principles of regular patient assessment, goal setting, intervention, re-assessment and re-intervention. Indeed, the rural general practitioner (GP) can provide an excellent stroke service if he/she is *interested* in TIA/stroke patients, enthusiastic to teach and coordinate nurses and any available allied health professionals, and motivated to lobby for essential resources such as a computed tomographical (CT) scan.

Telemedicine also has great potential to facilitate organised stroke care in rural and remote areas, through links with more specialised urban units.

Acute stroke ward or rehabilitation ward?   The benefits of admitting all patients immediately to an acute stroke unit are that it facilitates the early implementation of a uniform and standardised approach to assessment, goal setting, intervention (including rehabilitation), discharge planning and research. Transfer to a rehabilitation stroke ward (which is ideally linked with the acute stroke ward) is then seamless, continuous and consistent.

Stroke unit size   The size of the stroke unit will vary according to the incidence of stroke in the catchment population of the service and the activity of the hospital. A stroke unit should generally be large enough to be flexible to accommodate fluctuating demands; the number, gender ratio, severity and length of stay of patients will not be constant throughout the year.

Stroke unit staffing

Stroke units require a multidisciplinary team, which is made up of one or more doctors (e.g. stroke consultant, registrar and resident), nurses (including specialist stroke liason nurse), physiotherapists, occupational therapists, a speech and language therapist, and social worker as a basic minimum. A number of other health professionals also have an important role in the management of some stroke patients, such as a dietician, pharmacist, clinical neuropsychologist, specialist in orthotics/prosthetics, neuroradiologist, neurosurgeon and vascular surgeon.

The core features of these staff are that they are interested in stroke and have been trained in stroke management. Therefore, they have the necessary knowledge and enthusiasm.

The stream of basic training of doctors (i.e. neurology, geriatric, general medical) is not as important as the interest of the doctors and the comprehensiveness of their subsequent training in stroke medicine. Consequently, stroke units are managed effectively by neurologists, geriatricians, general physicians and rehabilitation specialists around the world, all who have been well trained in stroke medicine (Caplan, 2003; Lees, 2003; Donnan and Davis, 2003).

Patient selection criteria

There are no firm grounds for restricting access according to a patient's age, sex or stroke severity. Organised stroke care should be accessible to a wide range of patients extending to those of all ages and degrees of disability, according to their needs. Local conditions often dictate whether a geriatric service is a better option for the very elderly, particularly those with pre-existent handicap and multiple comorbidities.

However, when demand for beds exceeds supply, there are two options. The ideal is to re-configure the beds and training staff to allow care of all stroke patients in a stroke unit (Intercollegiate Stroke Working Party, 2002; Stone, 2002). This requires flexibility which may not be practical or possible. The other alternative is to prioritise patients according to different needs and services. In this case, it is important to establish local agreement about appropriate triage.

Duration of stay

A defined maximum length of stay should not be needed if the unit:
- is of sufficient size for the population needs,
- works flexibly,
- is efficient in discharging patients.

Ideally, an appropriately sized stroke unit should be allowed flexibility with its operating procedures and have the facility to provide care until discharge from hospital to home, an ongoing rehabilitation facility, or to placement in appropriate alternative care. Wherever the patient is discharged or transferred, it is important to ensure a seamless/continuous transition of care.

The only rationale for having a maximum length of stay is to prevent 'bed blocking' and to ensure that resources are appropriately utilised and managed. If a maximum length of stay is established, facilities and staff must be able to deliver appropriate continuing/ongoing care.

General processes of care in the stroke unit (care pathways)
Stroke units should aim to replicate those core service characteristics identified in
the randomised trials (Table 3.6).

Assessment   Patients are assessed as soon as possible by all core and relevant
members of the stroke unit.

The medical assessment comprises a relevant and targeted clinical history and
examination, documenting the nature of the symptoms and physical impairments,
the timing of the onset, any precipitating factors, and the subsequent course. In
addition, relevant aetiological (e.g. vascular risk factors), social, vocational and
emotional factors are recorded. Initial investigations include brain imaging by cranial CT scan or MRI, full blood count, erythrocyte sedimentation rate (ESR), creatinine, electrolytes, glucose, electrocardiography (ECG) and urine analysis. The
assessment is directed to answering each of the following questions:

  (i) **Is it a stroke** (*clinical diagnosis*)?
 (ii) **Where is the stroke** (*anatomical diagnosis*: which part of the brain is affected
      and what vascular territory)?
(iii) **What is the cause of the stroke** (*ischaemic or haemorrhagic*, and causes of the
      ischaemia or haemorrhage)?
 (iv) **What are the patient's impairments, disabilities and handicaps?**
  (v) **What is the patient's prognosis and goals?**
 (vi) **How should the patient be treated** (to minimise brain damage, prevent
      recurrent stroke and complications, optimise physiological homeostasis, and
      rehabilitation)?

The nursing assessment includes the patient's neurological status, impairments,
disabilities and function; swallowing function, bladder and bowel function, skin
status, psychosocial status and risk of complications (e.g. aspiration pneumonia,
venous thromboembolism, urinary tract infection and skin pressure sores), followed by a plan of general care needs of the patient.

The speech and swallowing therapist (speech pathologist) assesses communication,
receptive and expressive language skills, articulation, swallowing function, and risk of
aspiration by means of clinical skills, sometimes supplemented by videofluoroscopy.

The physiotherapist assesses the patient's respiratory function, muscle tone,
movement and mobility. This includes an assessment of the recovery level of the
arm(s), trunk and leg(s) and the assistance required with bed mobility and to sit up
from lying. Sitting balance is evaluated with the patient sitting on the edge of the
bed. If the patient is medically stable and not drowsy then standing balance, ability
to transfer (e.g. to commode and chair) and ambulation is evaluated if appropriate.

The occupational therapist assesses the patient's functional impairments, disabilities and handicaps, and abilities to perform ADL, work and leisure activities.

The social worker assesses the patients' social situation, support from family and friends, accommodation and financial status, occupational status and goals, and access to community resources (e.g. home help, meals on wheels).

The dietician assesses the dietary habits and nutritional needs of the patient and, together with the swallowing therapist, recommends an appropriate diet.

Goal setting (including discharge planning)   In every stroke patient, intermediate- and long-term goals should be agreed and described so that progress towards them can be measured. Moreover, everyone will feel a sense of achievement when the goals are met.

Where a patient is failing to achieve his or her goals (or milestones) then it is crucial to identify the cause and, if possible, do something about it. The reasons for failure to achieve goals are many. They may be medical (e.g. a recurrent stroke or other serious vascular event has occurred, or a medical complication has developed (e.g. pneumonia, pulmonary embolism, or the patient has become depressed and lost interest and motivation) or may reflect an inaccuracy in the teams' understanding of the patient's pathology and likely clinical course (e.g. being over optimistic about progress).

Goal setting may sometimes involve just an individual professional but more often needs to involve the rest of the team, the patient and sometimes the patient's family.

It is important to know the home and social circumstances of a stroke patient for early decision-making (such as the desirability of emergency operation) and for later rehabilitation and discharge from hospital.

Goals should be meaningful, and challenging but achievable.

Communication   A distinctive finding of the systematic review by the Stroke Unit Trialists' Collaboration is that stroke units were uniformly characterised by a multidisciplinary team which was coordinated/chaired by a leader (usually the senior doctor or other senior member of staff), and meets at least once a week to discuss all of the patients. Although the team is multidisciplinary, the interaction is interdisciplinary. The meeting is structured such that a doctor summarises the key features of the patient (age, date of stroke, clinical syndrome, pathology, aetiology, key treatments, major problems and goals), and then a brief (1–2 min) report on the progress of each patient in the preceding few days or week is given by the nurse, speech and swallowing therapist, physiotherapist, occupational therapist, and social worker. If relevant the dietician and pharmacist also report.

The patient's progress is matched with the original short- and long-term goals. If progress is not as good as expected, reasons are sought for failure to achieve goals, such as recurrent stroke, intercurrent medical problems, depression, incorrect original diagnosis, inaccurate team assessment, etc. Goals are reset and a future management plan detailed.

Besides a formal weekly meeting, which normally lasts about 60–90 min for 15 patients, team members communicate directly on the ward (or through the written medical record) with each other during the week about the patient. Many units also hold less formal meetings on other occasions to ensure effective multidisciplinary operation and involvement of family and carers. Key decisions are not made without widespread team consultation and approval.

Another key feature of stroke unit care is the early involvement of carers in the assessment and rehabilitation process, including the provision of appropriate information regarding the nature and cause of the stroke, and its management.

Intervention   Rehabilitation begins on day 1, following initial assessments. It is essential that rehabilitation techniques being taught in the therapy areas are carried over into every day practice on the ward (and at home) by the nurses and carers. Carers are therefore encouraged to attend therapy sessions, and nurses are encouraged to reinforce these behaviours in the everyday handling of the patient.

Discharge planning and post-discharge support   After a short period in hospital, during which the patient's status and progress have been documented, it is possible to re-assess goals, re-assess future management, and plan for early supported discharge home (Early Supported Discharge Trialists, 2001), another stroke rehabilitation facility, or to longer-term care.

Implications for research

Future trials should focus on direct comparisons of different models of organised stroke unit care, examining the potentially important components of stroke unit care, such as intensive monitoring of physiological abnormalities, very early mobilisation, novel strategies to detect and prevent complications, acute supportive therapies, and systems of rehabilitation (Langhorne and Dennis, 2004).

Outcome measures should not only include the outcomes of death, dependency and institutionalisation, but also domains of patient satisfaction, quality of life and cost.

Pre-planned collaboration between comparable trials could alleviate some of the problems of retrospective systematic reviews.

Early supported discharge

Evidence

There have been 11 RCTs randomising stroke a total of 1597 patients in hospital to either conventional care or any early supported discharge (ESD) service intervention

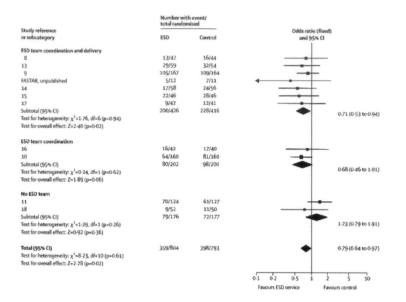

Figure 3.9   Forest plot showing a comparison of the effects of an early supported discharge service vs conventional care (control) on *death* or *dependency* in Activities of Daily Living (ADL) at the end of scheduled follow-up. Reproduced from Langhorne *et al.* (2005), with permission from the authors and Elsevier Limited, Publishers of the Lancet.

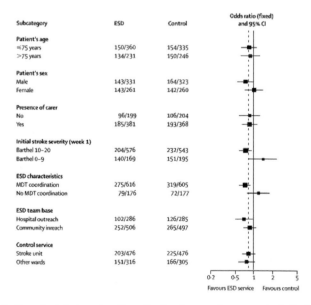

Figure 3.10   Forest plot showing the effects of an early supported discharge service vs conventional care in various subgroups of patients and services on *death or dependency* at the end of scheduled follow-up. Reproduced from Langhorne *et al.* (2005), with permission from the authors and Elsevier Limited, Publishers of the Lancet.

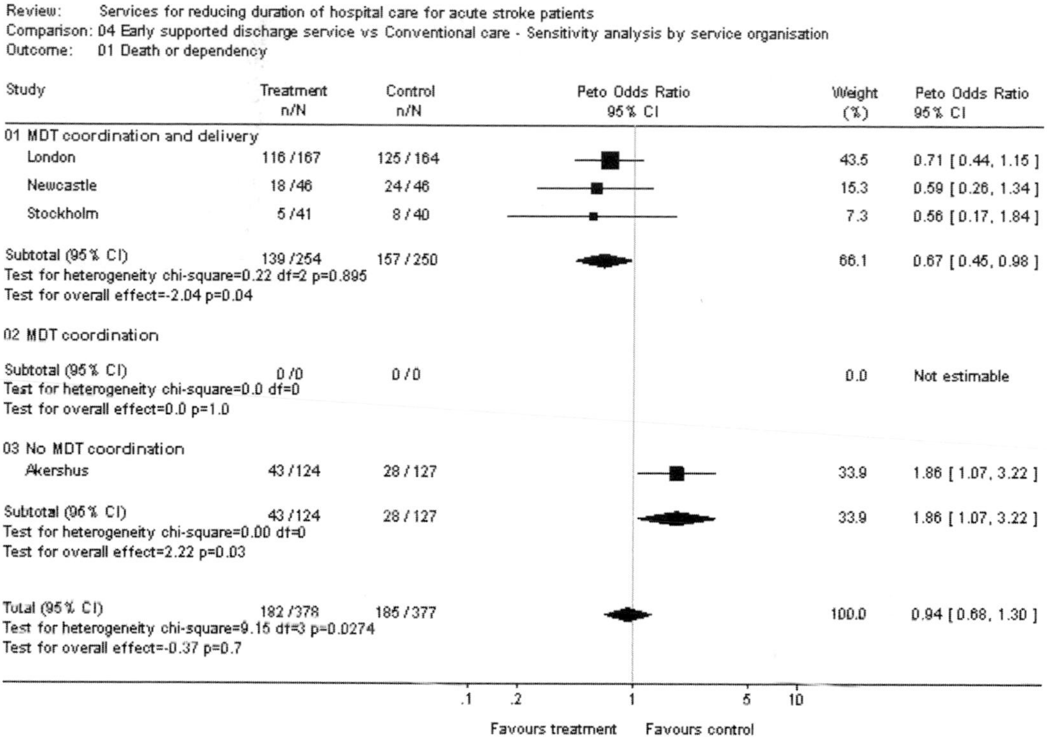

Review: Services for reducing duration of hospital care for acute stroke patients
Comparison: 04 Early supported discharge service vs Conventional care - Sensitivity analysis by service organisation
Outcome: 01 Death or dependency

Study	Treatment n/N	Control n/N	Peto Odds Ratio 95% CI	Weight (%)	Peto Odds Ratio 95% CI
01 MDT coordination and delivery					
London	116 / 167	125 / 164		43.5	0.71 [0.44, 1.15]
Newcastle	18 / 46	24 / 46		15.3	0.59 [0.26, 1.34]
Stockholm	5 / 41	8 / 40		7.3	0.56 [0.17, 1.84]
Subtotal (95 % CI)	139 / 254	157 / 250		66.1	0.67 [0.45, 0.98]
Test for heterogeneity chi-square=0.22 df=2 p=0.895					
Test for overall effect=-2.04 p=0.04					
02 MDT coordination					
Subtotal (95 % CI)	0 / 0	0 / 0		0.0	Not estimable
Test for heterogeneity chi-square=0.0 df=0					
Test for overall effect=0.0 p=1.0					
03 No MDT coordination					
Akershus	43 / 124	28 / 127		33.9	1.86 [1.07, 3.22]
Subtotal (95% CI)	43 / 124	28 / 127		33.9	1.86 [1.07, 3.22]
Test for heterogeneity chi-square=0.00 df=0					
Test for overall effect=2.22 p=0.03					
Total (95% CI)	182 / 378	185 / 377		100.0	0.94 [0.68, 1.30]
Test for heterogeneity chi-square=9.15 df=3 p=0.0274					
Test for overall effect=-0.37 p=0.7					

.1   .2   1   5   10

Favours treatment   Favours control

Figure 3.11   Forest plot showing a comparison of the effects of early supported discharge vs conventional care on *death or dependency* at the end of the scheduled follow-up period. From the Early Supported Discharge Trialists (2001), with permission from the authors and John Wiley & Sons Limited. Copyright Cochrane Library, reproduced with permission.

providing rehabilitation and support in a community setting with an aim of reducing the duration of hospital care (Langhorne *et al.*, 2005). Overall, the ORs (95% CI) were 0.90 (0.64–1.27) for death, 0.74 (0.56–0.96) for death or institutionalisation, and 0.79 (0.64–0.97) for death or dependency (Figs 3.9–3.10) (Early Supported Discharge Trialists, 2001; Fjaertoft *et al.*, 2003; Langhorne *et al.*, 2005; Meijer and van Limbeek, 2005). Apparent benefits were more evident in the trials evaluating a coordinated multidisciplinary early supported discharge (ESD) team (Fig 3.11) and in stroke patients with mild to moderate disability. The ESD group showed significant reductions ($P < 0.001$) in the length of hospital stay equivalent to approximately 8 days.

Comment

These data suggest that appropriately resourced ESD services provided for a selected group of stroke patients can reduce the length of hospital stay and improve functional outcomes in the longer term with lower rates of dependency and admission to institutional care (Indredavik *et al.*, 2000; Early Supported Discharge Trialists, 2001; Langhorne, 2003; Langhorne *et al.*, 2005).

Therapy-based rehabilitation for stroke patients living at home

Evidence

A systematic review of 14 RCTs of therapy-based rehabilitation services (defined as input from physiotherapy, occupational therapy or a multidisciplinary team) targeted to a total of 1617 stroke patients living at home revealed that patients allocated therapy-based rehabilitation services were less likely to deteriorate in ability to perform ADL (OR: 0.72, 95% CI: 0.57–0.92, $P = 0.009$; absolute risk reduction: 7%) and more likely to be able to perform personal ADL (standardised mean difference: 0.14, 95% CI: 0.02–0.25, $P = 0.02$) (Legg and Langhorne, 2004).

Comment

Further research is needed to define the most effective interventions, their functional and economic benefit, and the most appropriate level and means of service delivery.

SUMMARY

Most patients with suspected stroke should not be managed at home, but should be transported without delay to a hospital, which has access to the required diagnostic tests 24 h/day and 7 days/week.

Once admitted, patients should be managed in a stroke unit rather than a GMW.

Geographically defined stroke units, dedicated to organised stroke care, appear to be more effective than stroke care on general wards with input from a mobile stroke team. There appears to be no systematic increase in length of hospital stay associated with organised (stroke unit) care.

In order to meet the needs of the local stroke population (which are likely to increase), and the anticipated increasing role of acute diagnostic techniques and interventions, it is crucial that future plans anticipate the requirements for trained staff and an adequate numbers of stroke unit beds for acute stroke.

Processes of care on a stroke unit should mirror those found to be effective in RCTs. Stroke care should be specialised, organised and multidisciplinary (i.e. provided by medical, nursing, physiotherapy, occupational therapy, speech therapy and social work staff who are interested and trained in stroke care). The multidisciplinary stroke team should meet at least once weekly to discuss patient assessments, goals, progress and management, and discharge plans.

The other beneficial components of organised stroke care are likely to be many, but it remains uncertain which are the most effective. Future research should be directed at identifying the crucial ingredients in this 'black box' so that they can be the focus of future care and optimise judicious use of resources.

Early discharge from the stroke unit with support from a domiciliary rehabilitation team (coordinated by the stroke unit) promises to reduce hospital length of stay (and thus increase turnover in the stroke unit) and improve rehabilitation in the home and patient outcome.

General supportive acute stroke care

As discussed in Chapter 3, there is some preliminary evidence that part of the effectiveness of organised care in a stroke unit can be attributed to general supportive stroke care, which includes optimisation of physiological homoeostasis (i.e. keeping physiological variables within 'normal' limits), and early anticipation and prevention of complications of stroke (Langhorne *et al.*, 2000; Evans *et al.*, 2001). Associations between abnormal measurements of physiological parameters (e.g. blood pressure (BP), temperature, blood glucose) in the setting of acute stroke and poor outcomes have been reported in epidemiological studies, but it remains unknown whether interventions which aim to return the physiological measurement to normal will improve patient outcome. This is because physiological measures are only potential surrogate measures of outcome. An abnormal physiological measurement may simply indicate that the patient has developed a complication, such as fever as a result of aspiration pneumonia or venous thromboembolism (VTE), and this may not (or may) correlate with outcome. Hence, an intervention that simply aims to normalise the abnormality may not be very effective unless the underlying cause is identified and treated. Although it can be argued that large randomised-controlled trials (RCTs) are not required to establish the effectiveness of close monitoring of patients with acute stroke, a more compelling argument can be made that any invasive monitoring, or intervention aimed at preventing complications or normalising physiological measurements should be evaluated by RCTs if the intervention could have adverse effects or is costly, to establish the balance between benefit and risk. Few RCTs have been completed, but several are in progress.

This chapter discusses the rationale for specific aspects of supportive stroke care. An important preface is that because there have been very few RCTs evaluating these aspects of stroke care, many of the following comments and recommendations are based on reasoning (which can be flawed (see Chapter 2)) and not reliable evidence from RCTs.

Preserving vital functions and optimising physiological homoeostasis

Interventions which aim to preserve vital functions and optimise physiological homoeostasis include the use of oxygen (O_2) therapy to correct hypoxia, administration of fluids by means of nasogastric tube (NGT) or intravenous (i.v.) drip in those who cannot swallow safely to maintain hydration (i.e. to optimise fluid balance and prevent or treat dehydration), use of antipyretics and antibiotics to maintain a normal body temperature, and the use of insulin therapy in patients with hyperglycaemia to maintain a normal blood glucose (Indredavik *et al.*, 1999).

Airway and oxygenation

Maintenance of a patent airway and adequate oxygenation are fundamental to good stroke care and preservation of neurones in the ischaemic penumbra. Abnormal patterns of respiration, such as hyperventilation and periodic breathing, are common after stroke, particularly severe stroke (Nachtmann *et al.*, 1995), but if present in a stroke patient with depressed consciousness, it is important to ensure that the patient does not have an intermittently obstructed airway.

Monitoring

Monitoring of respiratory function and pulse oximetry is being used increasingly in the acute phase of stroke to alert the stroke team to significant oxygen desaturation. This may occur as a result of extensive brainstem or hemispheric infarction, large brain haemorrhage, sustained seizure activity, or to complications such as severe pneumonia, particularly in patients at risk of aspiration, heart failure, pulmonary embolism (PE), or exacerbation of chronic obstructive pulmonary disease.

Supplemental oxygen

Supplemental oxygen should not be required if patients are breathing normally and maintaining good oxygenation on room air. Despite the fact that there is no convincing evidence that oxygen supplementation at low or high flow rates is effective in acute ischaemic stroke (Ronning and Guldvog, 1999; Singhal *et al.*, 2005), if hypoxia is present, it should probably be corrected with supplemental oxygen 2–4 l/min via a nasal tube, and all possible causes of the hypoxia sought and treated (e.g. pulmonary oedema, embolism or infection).

Hyperbaric oxygen therapy

Despite theoretical benefits of hyperbaric oxygen therapy (HBO) (increased oxygen delivery, maintenance of blood–brain barrier integrity and decreased cerebral oedema) a randomised, double-blind, sham-controlled trial of 60 min in a monoplace hyperbaric chamber pressurised with 100% oxygen to 2.5-atmospheric pressure absolute (ATA) in the HBO group, or 1.14 ATA in the sham group, among 33 patients with acute ischaemic stroke showed that at 3 months, a larger percentage of sham patients had a good outcome compared with the HBO group (National Institutes of Health Stroke Scale (NIHSS) 80% vs 31.3%; $P = 0.04$; modified Rankin Scale 82% vs 31%; $P = 0.02$) (Rusymiak *et al.*, 2003).

Intubation

Early intubation may be necessary in the presence of a severely compromised respiratory pattern, severe hypoxaemia or hypercarbia, and in unconscious patients (Glasgow Coma Scale (GCS) $\leqslant 8$) at high risk for aspiration.

Comment (all grade D recommendations based on level IV evidence)

- Monitoring of oxygenation by means of pulse oximetry is recommended in acute ischaemic stroke.
- Supplemental oxygen is recommended for patients with hypoxaemia (O_2 saturation <92% by pulse oximetry and to aim for O_2 saturation $\geqslant 95\%$).
- Airway support and ventilatory assistance is recommended for patients with depressed levels of consciousness or a compromised airway; or potentially reversible respiratory insufficiency.

Cardiac care

Cardiac output

Cardiac output should be optimised by maintaining a normal heart rate and a high normal BP in the setting of an acute ischaemic stroke. An adequate intravascular volume is necessary for the latter, and so re-hydration with i.v. fluids is often necessary in patients who cannot swallow safely. The central venous pressure should be maintained at approximately 8–10 cmH$_2$O, but its monitoring is not usually necessary unless early warning of a volume deficiency or volume overload is required.

Low cardiac output

Stroke may be complicated by low cardiac output due to dehydration, heart failure, acute myocardial infarction (acute MI), and cardiac dysrhythmias, particularly atrial fibrillation (Broderick *et al.*, 1992; Vingerhoets *et al.*, 1993), and particularly with cerebral infarcts involving the insular cortex (Oppenheimer *et al.*, 1996).

The cause of low cardiac output should be ascertained and treated. If necessary, restoration of normal cardiac rhythm using drugs, cardioversion, or pacemaker support should be performed in co-operation with internists or cardiologists. If ino-tropic agents are required, dobutamine has the advantage of increasing cardiac output without substantially affecting either heart rate or BP. Dopamine may be particularly useful in patients with arterial hypotension or renal insufficiency.

Electrocardiography monitoring

Every stroke patient should have an initial electrocardiography (ECG), but continuous ECG monitoring is not usually necessary unless the patient has, or is prone to, low cardiac output (see below). Significant ECG alterations in the ST segments and the T waves and QT prolongation mimicking myocardial ischaemia may appear in the acute phase.

Comment (all grade D recommendations based on level IV evidence)

Continuous cardiac monitoring should be considered in the first 48 h of stroke onset in patients with:

- previous known cardiac disease,
- history of dysrhythmias,
- unstable BP,
- clinical signs/symptoms of heart failure,
- abnormal baseline ECG,
- stroke involving the insular cortex.

Fluid and electrolytes

Dehydration

Dehydration to some degree is common after stroke and, by compromising brain perfusion and renal function, may be related to bad outcome (Bhalla *et al.*, 2000).

In patients with brain oedema, a slightly negative fluid balance is recommended, and hypotonic solutions (NaCl 0.45% or glucose 5%) are contraindicated.

Otherwise, fluid balance should be restored in all acute stroke patients. Most patients, particularly those who cannot swallow safely, require i.v. fluid replacement. Unless the blood glucose is known, no glucose solution should be given to a stroke patient due to the potential detrimental effects of hyperglycaemia (see page 63). Fluid should be replaced in the form of normal saline.

Peripheral venous access is usually sufficient for initial fluid management, while a central venous catheter is required in case of infusion of larger volumes of fluids (or hyperosmolar) solutions. Uncontrolled volume replacement may precipitate cardiac failure and pulmonary oedema.

Electrolyte imbalance

Serious electrolyte abnormalities are uncommon in patients with ischaemic stroke, unless precipitated by the stroke (e.g. hyponatraemia due to syndrome of inappropriate antidiuretic hormone (SIADH)) or treatments (e.g. hypokalaemia due to diuretics) (Diringer, 1992). The cause should be treated, and the electrolytes replaced if necessary.

Serum electrolytes should be assessed at baseline, and subsequently if the patient deteriorates.

Nutrition

Under-nutrition is common in stroke survivors; estimates vary from 8% (Unosson *et al.*, 1994) to 34% (Choi-Kwon *et al.*, 1998).

Under-nutrition is associated with increased case fatality and poor functional status at 6 months after stroke, even after adjusting for other prognostic factors (The FOOD Trial Collaboration, 2003).

It is unclear if and how patients should be fed after acute stroke.

Food supplementation

Evidence

A systematic review of RCTs for the Cochrane Library identified one RCT of nutritional supplementation in a total of 42 patients (Bath *et al.*, 1999). Since there were only a total of nine outcome events (case fatality), the trial was underpowered statistically, and reported very imprecise estimates of the effects of supplementation on case fatality (odds ratio (OR): 0.25, 95% confidence interval (CI): 0.06 to 1.08) (Fig. 4.1).

Since this review, the Feed Or Ordinary Diet (FOOD) trial recruited 4023 patients with recent stroke (median 5 days, IQR 3–9 days) who were able to swallow

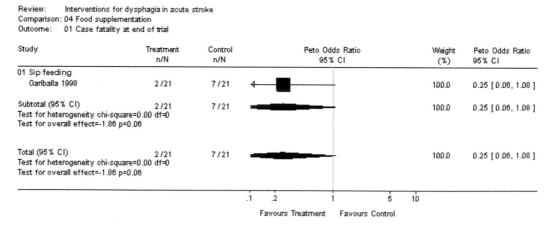

Figure 4.1   Forest plot showing the effects of *food supplementation* compared with no food supplementation on *case fatality* at the end of the scheduled follow-up period among individual trials (each line), and pooled (summary at the bottom). Reproduced from Bath *et al.* (1999), with permission from the authors and John Wiley & Sons Limited. Copyright Cochrane Library, reproduced with permission.

safely and who were admitted to 125 hospitals in 15 countries between 1996 and 2003 (The FOOD Trial Collaboration, 2005a).

A total of 2007 patients were randomised to carry on with their normal hospital diet until discharge from hospital whereas 2016 patients were randomised to their normal hospital diet plus oral nutritional (protein-energy) supplements, equivalent to 360 ml of 6.27kJ/ml and 62.5 g/l in protein per day, until hospital discharge.

Random assignment to a supplemented diet was associated with no significant change in the odds of death (OR: 0.94, 95% CI: 0.78 to 1.13) or the composite end-point of death or poor outcome (OR: 1.03, 95% CI: 0.91 to 1.17) at 6 months after randomisation. The supplemented diet was associated with a non-significant absolute reduction in the risk of death of 0.7% (95% CI: −1.4% to +2.7%) and an absolute increase in risk of death or poor outcome of 0.7% (−2.3% to +3.8%).

An updated systematic review RCTs of the effects of nutritional supplementation in stroke patients, comprising the results of the trial by Gariballa *et al.* (1998) and The FOOD Trial Collaboration (2005a), reveal that nutritional supplementation is associated with no significant reduction in odds of death (OR: 0.92, 95% CI: 0.76 to 1.11).

Comment

The available evidence does not support a policy of routine oral nutritional supplementation after stroke.

Blood glucose

Hypoglycaemia

Hypoglycaemia is an important treatable state which must be excluded immediately in any patient with suspected transient ischaemic attack (TIA) or stroke because it may be the underlying cause of the focal neurological symptoms and signs (e.g. hemiparesis), and thus mimic a TIA or stroke (Huff, 2002). If not corrected promptly, permanent disability and death may ensue. Appropriate treatment comprises i.v. dextrose bolus or infusion of 10–20% glucose, preferably via a central venous line.

Hyperglycaemia

Hyperglycaemia is far more common than hypoglycaemia after stroke, and may be due to diabetes (known or occult) or an acute stress response. Whatever its cause, hyperglycaemia after stroke is associated with a poor outcome (Capes *et al.*, 2001; Parsons *et al.*, 2002; Lindsberg & Roine, 2004). Experimental data from animal models suggests that the association may be causal, but further research is required to determine whether the association between hyperglycaemia and a poor outcome is confounded by hyperglycaemia simply being a marker of the severity of the stroke or underlying vascular disease.

In light of this uncertainty, it is presently not known how aggressively hyperglycaemia should be corrected. The United Kingdom Glucose Insulin in Stroke Trial (GIST-UK) is a multicentre RCT comparing an i.v. infusion of glucose (10% dextrose) + potassium chloride (20 mmol) + insulin (variable-dose soluble human Actrapid insulin, initial insulin 16 U) (GKI) with an i.v. infusion of 0.9% normal saline (154 mmol/l sodium), both administered at 100 ml/h for 24 h, in acute stroke patients with mild to moderate hyperglycaemia (admission plasma glucose 6.0–17 mmol/l) (GIST-UK Protocol, 2004. http://www.gist-uk.org). An interim analysis of the capillary Boehringer–Mannheim (BM) glycemia test-strip monitor and plasma glucose concentrations in the two treatment groups showed that the mean plasma glucose levels decline spontaneously with time, and the GIST-GKI regimen rapidly achieves euglycaemia at significantly lower levels than with saline hydration alone, and with a low risk of hypoglycaemia. However, long-term clinical benefits of routine management of hyperglycaemia in acute stroke remains to be determined from the ongoing RCTs (Scott *et al.*, 1998, 1999; Gray *et al.*, 2004). In the meantime, an empirical recommendation is to try to maintain the blood glucose within normal limits, and to actively correct blood glucose levels above at least 15 mmol/l, and probably above 10 mmol/l, with an infusion of insulin, glucose and potassium (and even lower levels of hyperglycaemia if there are adequate facilities for closely monitoring blood glucose to minimise any risk of hypoglycaemia).

Comment (all grade D recommendations based on level IV evidence)

- Unless the blood glucose is known, no glucose solution should be given to a stroke patient due to the potential detrimental effects of hyperglycaemia.
- Rapidly correct low blood glucose concentrations with i.v. dextrose bolus or infusion of 10–20% glucose, and avoid hypotonic solutions (NaCl 0.45% or glucose 5%) to minimise brain oedema and the probable detrimental effects of hyperglycaemia associated with glucose infusions.
- Monitor serum glucose levels in diabetic patients.
- Gradually lower raised blood glucose concentrations with normal saline and insulin titration. The European Stroke Initiative (EUSI) recommends to lower blood glucose to about 10 mmol/l (European Stroke Initiative, 2003, 2004) whereas the American Stroke Association (ASA) recommends to aim for blood glucose <16.63 mmol/l (Adams *et al.*, 2003).
- Rapidly correct low blood glucose concentrations with i.v. dextrose bolus or infusion of 10–20% glucose, and avoid hypotonic solutions (NaCl 0.45% or glucose 5%) to minimise brain oedema and the probable detrimental effects of hyperglycaemia associated with glucose infusions.

Body temperature

Pyrexia is common in the first 48 h after stroke (Corbett *et al.*, 2000) and may be due to:

- preceding infection (e.g. encephalitis, infective endocarditis), which may be a risk factor for, or cause of, the stroke (Grau *et al.*, 1999, 2004; Lindsberg and Grau, 2003);
- the effects of the stroke itself or
- a complication of the stroke such as chest or urinary infection or VTE.

The underlying cause must be identified and treated. In the meantime the temperature can be lowered by simple measures (e.g. antipyretic drugs) in order to make the patient feel more comfortable and perhaps improve patient outcome.

Paracetamol, given in a dose of 1000 mg 4 hourly (6000 mg/day) has been shown in a RCT to lower body temperature by 0.4°C (95% CI: 0.1 to 0.7°C), even in normothermic and subfebrile patients (Dippel *et al.*, 2001). A more recent observational study in 63 patients with acute ischaemic stroke and a body temperature >37.5°C showed that an acetaminophen suppository 1000 mg produced significantly more reductions in body temperature (60%), and normothermia (20%), at 1 h after treatment than acetylsalicyclic acid 500 mg i.v. (37% and 5%, respectively) (Sulter *et al.*, 2004). At 3 h after treatment, both interventions had similar effects, with normothermia only being achieved in 37–38% of patients. Fever (>38°C) and evidence of an infection were related to unresponsiveness to treatment. The authors concluded that in most patients with acute ischaemic stroke, an acetaminophen suppository of 1000 mg and acetylsalicyclic acid 500 mg i.v. are insufficient to reduce an elevated body temperature to a state of normothermia.

A systematic review of observational studies suggests that raised temperatures after stroke are associated with poor outcomes (Reith *et al.*, 1996; Hajat *et al.*, 2000). Mechanisms for hyperthermia-induced ischaemic brain damage include increased metabolic demand in the penumbra, enhanced release of excitatory amino acids and free radical formation, and changes in the blood–brain barrier (Fukuda *et al.*, 1999).

However, it has not been proven that hyperthermia independently affects outcome adversely. This is because it has not been shown that lowering body temperature improves outcome (Kasner *et al.*, 2002; Dippel *et al.*, 2001; Sulter *et al.*, 2004). This remains the subject of ongoing research studies and clinical trials.

Comment

- Body temperature ≥37.5°C should be investigated (for the cause) and treated probably with antipyretic agents and, if appropriate, relevant antibiotics.
- Antibiotic, anti-mycotic and anti-viral prophylaxis is not recommended in immuno-competent patients.

Blood Pressure (BP)

Normally, within a mean BP range of 60–150 mmHg, blood flow to the brain is maintained at a constant level by cerebral autoregulation; cerebral blood vessels dilate in response to a fall in BP and constrict in response to a rise in BP. However, after a stroke, cerebral autoregulation is disturbed in the region of focal brain infarction or haemorrhage such that cerebral blood flow (CBF) is no longer maintained and is directly dependent on systemic BP (i.e. CBF is pressure dependent) (Meyer *et al.*, 1973). Hence, if the systemic BP falls, so does the blood flow to the affected part of the brain because flow in the ischaemic penumbra becomes passively dependent on mean arterial pressure (Eames *et al.*, 2002). It therefore seems prudent to avoid abrupt systemic hypotension in acute stroke patients.

BP and stroke outcome

There is a U-shaped relationship between BP in acute stroke and outcome (Fig. 4.2). Early death and a poor long-term outcome are more frequent in patients with BP in the highest and lowest quartiles of systolic BP (Leonardi-Be *et al.*, 2002; Aslanyan *et al.*, 2003; Vemmos *et al.*, 2003, 2004a, b; Boysen, 2004; Castillo *et al.*, 2004; Willmot *et al.*, 2004). The higher mortality in patient with low admission BP values

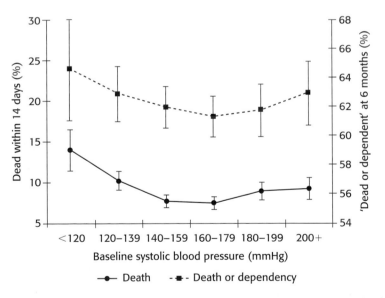

Figure 4.2   Proportion of patients who died within 14 days (solid lines) or were dead or dependent at 6 months (dashed lines) after stroke by baseline systolic BP (SBP). Circles and squares indicate the mean percentage of patients who had died within 14 days and patients who had died or were dependent at 6 months, respectively, within each BP subgroup; 95% CIs are represented by T bars. Reproduced from Leonardi-Be *et al.* (2002), with permission from the authors and Lippincott, Williams and Wilkins.

is likely to reflect the association with heart failure (particularly in patients with cardioembolic ischaemic stroke) and coronary heart disease (particularly in patients with lacunar stroke) (Vemmos *et al.*, 2003, 2004b). The mechanisms by which high BP may adversely affect outcome are probably by increasing the risk of cerebral oedema (Vemmos *et al.*, 2003, 2004a; Boysen, 2004) and perhaps also by haemorrhagic transformation of brain infarction.

Hypotension

Low-normal BP (systolic BP <120 mmHg) is uncommon (about 5% of patients) after acute stroke. It is usually caused by hypovolaemia due to excessive fluid loss through sweating and by insufficient fluid intake by mouth or tube (i.e. dehydration). This can be ascertained by examining the patient and fluid balance chart. However, hypotension may also reflect underlying sepsis, coexistent heart disease (dysrhythmias, acute MI) or heart failure (Vemmos *et al.*, 2003; 2004b).

Hypotension should be recognised and corrected promptly by treating the underlying cause, raising the foot of the bed, and replacing fluids via a safe route with crystalloid (saline) or, occasionally, colloid, solutions. Low cardiac output may also need inotropic support.

Hypertension

Acute stroke, due to infarction or haemorrhage, is associated with high BP (>140/90 mmHg) in about 75% of patients, of whom 50% have a previous history of high BP and are taking antihypertensive therapy at the time of the stroke (Britton *et al.*, 1986; Oppenheimer *et al.*, 1992).

The BP falls spontaneously in most patients over the 1st week after acute stroke, although a third of patients remain hypertensive (Wallace & Levy, 1981; Britton *et al.*, 1986; Carlsson & Britton, 1993; Harper *et al.*, 1994).

The mechanisms underlying hypertension in stroke are complex but pre-existing hypertension, hospitalisation stress, and activation of the sympathetic, ACTH–cortisol and renin–angiotensin–aldosterone systems, and the Cushing reflex (hypertension secondary to raised intracranial pressure) all contribute (Myers, 1982; Carlberg *et al.*, 1991).

Treatment of BP after stroke

It is currently unclear how BP should be managed during the acute phase of ischaemic and haemorrhagic stroke (Bath & Bath, 1997; BP in Acute Stroke Collaboration, 2001; International Society of Hypertension Writing Group, 2003). In the Intravenous Nimodipine West European Stroke Trial (INWEST), the rapid hypotensive action of i.v. nimodipine was shown to increase the risk of neurological deterioration (Wahlgren *et al.*, 1994; Ahmed *et al.*, 2000). A recent small trial randomised 339 patients with acute ischaemic stroke and elevated BP (≥200 mmHg systolic and/or $\geqslant 110$ mmHg diastolic 6–24 h after admission or $\geqslant 180$ mmHg systolic and/or $\geqslant 105$ mmHg diastolic 24–36 h after admission) to placebo ($n = 166$ patients) or candesartan cilexetil (4 mg on day 1; 8 or 16 mg on day 2; $n = 173$ patients) for 7 days, with the aim of lowering BP by 10–15% within the first 24 h (Schrader *et al.*, 2003). After 7 days, patients assigned candesartan who were still hypertensive (mean daytime BP $>135/85$ mmHg) were treated with increased doses of candesartan or an additional antihypertensive drug, in addition to continuing candesartan for a year. Patients assigned placebo who were hypertensive were started on candesartan for a year and the dose was adjusted to lower BP to $<140/90$ mmHg (office) or $<135/85$ mmHg (mean daytime BP). Two patients assigned placebo were normotensive and did not receive antihypertensive medication. During the placebo-controlled phase in the first 7 days, and the subsequent 12 months of follow-up, BP levels were similar in both treatment groups. However, the cumulative 12-month mortality (placebo: 7.2% vs candesartan: 2.9%; $P = 0.07$) and number of vascular events (placebo: 18.7% vs candesartan: 19.8%; $P = 0.026$; OR: 0.474, 95% CI: 0.25 to 0.895) differed significantly in favour of candesartan (Schrader *et al.*, 2003). If these results can be confirmed in other RCTs, the uncertain mechanism by which early angiotensin type-1 receptor blockade may affect long-term cardiovascular morbidity and mortality remains to be elucidated.

Randomised trials of sufficient size are needed to determine the effect of lowering and increasing BP in acute stroke on functional outcome, and of continuing or temporarily stopping prior antihypertensive medication treatment. The Efficacy of Nitric Oxide in Stroke (ENOS) trial aims to address these issues in 5000 randomised patients (Bath, 2004). As of May 2005, a total of 345 patients have been randomised.

Meanwhile, guidelines recommend that BP should only be lowered actively within the first 72 h after stroke, and cautiously at that (by about 15% over 24 h), in the presence of hypertensive crises such as hypertensive encephalopathy, left ventricular failure, acute aortic dissection, or intracerebral bleeding, or if the BP is very high and poses a real risk of cerebral haemorrhage (Adams *et al.*, 2003, 2005; European Stroke Initiative, 2003, 2004). It is not known what level of BP is too high but the guidelines recommend treatment if:

Systolic BP	>200–220 mmHg (ischaemic stroke) or
	>180–200 (haemorrhagic stroke) or
Diastolic BP	>120–130 mmHg (ischaemic stroke) or
	>100–110 mmHg (haemorrhagic stroke)

However, the guidelines are based on theoretical arguments and individual case series (i.e. level IV evidence), and not on the results of systematic overviews of large intervention trials of BP manipulation in acute stroke on important clinical outcomes, which are not (yet) available (i.e. level I evidence).

However, there is a systematic review of data from 32 RCTs involving 5368 patients which indicates that i.v. calcium channel blockers (CCBs), oral CCBs and β-blockers significantly lowered BP during the first 3 days of treatment in acute stroke. Angiotensin converting enzyme inhibitors, nitric oxide donors and prostacyclin also appeared to lower BP as compared to the controls. In contrast, magnesium, naftidrofuryl and piracetam had no effect on BP (The Blood Pressure in Acute Stroke Collaboration, 2004).

It is recommended that nifedipine capsules and parenteral medications should be avoided because of the risk of abrupt reduction of BP (Grossman *et al.*, 1996), possible ischaemic steal (Adams *et al.*, 1994; Ahmed *et al.*, 2000) and overshoot hypertension. Oral Captopril (6.25–12.5 mg), may be used instead, but has a short duration of action and can have an abrupt effect. In North America, i.v. labetalol (10 mg) is frequently recommended. Intravenous urapidil is also increasingly used in this situation. Sodium nitroprusside is sometimes recommended despite possible major side-effects, such as reflex tachycardia and coronary artery ischaemia.

Comment (all grade D recommendations based on level IV evidence)

- Routine BP lowering is not recommended, except for extremely elevated values (>200–220 mmHg systolic BP or >120 mmHg diastolic BP for ischaemic stroke, >180/105 mmHg for haemorrhagic stroke) confirmed by repeated measurements.
- Immediate antihypertensive therapy for more moderate hypertension is recommended in case of stroke and heart failure, aortic dissection, acute MI, acute renal failure, thrombolysis or i.v. heparin but should be applied cautiously.
- Recommended target BP in patients:
  - as a general rule, lower BP by 10–15%;
    - with prior hypertension, 180/100–105 mmHg;
    - without prior hypertension, 160–180/90–100 mmHg;
    - considering thrombolysis, lower BP below 180/110 mmHg before commencing thrombolysis.
- Recommended drugs for BP treatment:
  - i.v. labetalol 10–20 mg over 1–2 min; may repeat or double every 10 min (max dose 300 mg);
  - i.v. nicardipine 5 mg/h i.v. infusion as initial dose; titrate to desired effect by increasing 2.5 mg/h every 5 min to maximum of 15 mg/h
  - i.v. urapidil,
  - i.v. sodium nitroprusside 0.5 μg/kg/min i.v. infusion as initial dose with continuous BP monitoring,
  - i.v. nitroglycerine or
  - oral captopril.
- Avoid sublingual nifedipine which is rapidly absorbed and may cause a precipitous fall in BP.

• Avoid hypotension, particularly in unstable patients, and treat by administering adequate amounts of fluids (see further on) and, when required, volume expanders and/or catecholamines (epinephrine 0.1–2 mg/h plus dobutamine 5–50 mg/h).

Prevention of medical complications

Within hours of a stroke, and in the days and weeks thereafter, various life threatening, preventable or treatable complications may occur such as airway obstruction and respiratory failure; swallowing problems causing aspiration, dehydration and malnutrition; epileptic seizures; VTE and infections (Davenport *et al.*, 1996; Langhorne *et al.*, 2000). Early assessment and anticipation coupled with appropriate intervention can minimise these and improve outcome.

Aspiration pneumonia, dehydration and malnutrition

Swallowing function is impaired in up to 50% of hospitalised stroke patients, precluding safe oral nutrition and hydration until swallowing function recovers and predisposing to complications (e.g. aspiration pneumonia) and a poor functional outcome (Smithard *et al.*, 1996; Mann *et al.*, 1999, 2000).

The management of patients with swallowing impairment aims to facilitate the recovery of swallowing function by standardised swallowing therapy and, in the meantime, to feed and hydrate the patients safely by means of tube feeding.

Swallowing therapy

Evidence

A Cochrane Review of two RCTs in a total of 85 patients found that formal swallowing therapy does not significantly reduce end-of-trial dysphagia rates (OR: 0.55, 95% CI: 0.18 to 1.66) (Bath *et al.*, 1999). One small trial of drug therapy with nifedipine for dysphagia in 17 patients found no effect on end-of-trial case fatality (Bath *et al.*, 1999; Fig. 4.3).

Tube feeding for patients with swallowing disability

Evidence

A Cochrane Review of two RCTs comparing percutaneous endoscopic gastrostomy (PEG) vs nasogastric tube (NGT) feeding reported that the overall OR for death was 0.28 (95% CI: 0.09 to 0.89) in favour of PEG feeding (Bath *et al.*, 1999; Fig. 4.4).

Since this Cochrane Review, the much larger FOOD trial (The FOOD Trial Collaboration, 2005b) was designed to answer two main questions:

1 Does early initiation of enteral tube feeding improve outcomes (early vs avoid)?
2 Does enteral tube feeding via a PEG, compared with a nasogastric (NG) tube improve outcomes (PEG vs NG)?

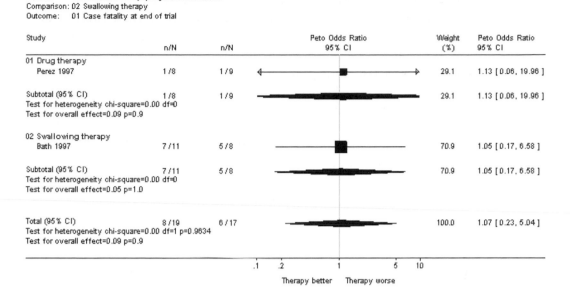

Figure 4.3   Forest plot showing the effects of *swallowing therapy* compared with *no swallowing therapy* on *case fatality* at the end of the scheduled follow-up period among individual trials (each line), and pooled (summary at the bottom). Reproduced from Bath *et al.* (1999), with permission from the authors and John Wiley & Sons Limited. Copyright Cochrane Library, reproduced with permission.

Review: Interventions for dysphagia in acute stroke
Comparison: 01 Feeding route
Outcome: 01 Case fatality at end of trial

Study	Treatment n/N	Control n/N	Peto Odds Ratio 95% CI	Weight (%)	Peto Odds Ratio 95% CI
01 PEG versus NGT					
Bath 1997	6/10	6/9		40.4	0.76 [0.12, 4.69]
Norton 1996	2/16	8/14		59.6	0.14 [0.03, 0.61]
Subtotal (95% CI)	8/26	14/23		100.0	0.20 [0.00, 0.89]
Test for heterogeneity chi-square=1.94 df=1 p=0.1642					
Test for overall effect=-2.15 p=0.03					
Total (95% CI)	8/26	14/23		100.0	0.28 [0.09, 0.89]
Test for heterogeneity chi-square=1.94 df=1 p=0.1642					
Test for overall effect=-2.15 p=0.03					

.1   .2   1   5   10

PEG better   NGT better

Figure 4.4   Forest plot showing the effects of *feeding by PEG tube* compared with *feeding by NGT* on *case fatality* at the end of the scheduled follow-up period. Reproduced from Bath *et al.* (1999), with permission from the authors and John Wiley & Sons Limited. Copyright Cochrane Library, reproduced with permission.

Early tube feeding vs avoid tube feeding for more than 7 days   In the 'early vs avoid' tube feeding FOOD trial, 859 patients who presented to 83 hospitals in 15 countries with dysphagia due to recent stroke (<30 days) were randomly assigned within seven days of admission to early enteral tube feeding ($n = 429$ (387 were fed by a NGT and 36 by a PEG tube)) and 430 to avoid tube feeding for more than 7 days (and maintain fluid input by giving parenteral fluids i.v. or subcutaneously (s.c.)).

Early tube feeding was associated with no significant change in odds of death at 6 months after randomisation, compared with avoid tube feeding (42.4% early tube, 48.3% avoid tube; OR: 0.79, 95% CI: 0.60 to 1.03), which is an absolute reduction in risk of death at 6 months of 5.8% (95% CI: -0.8 to $+12.5$%; $P = 0.09$).

Early tube feeding was also associated with no significant change in odds of death or a poor outcome at 6 months after randomisation, compared with avoid tube feeding (79.0% early tube, 80.2% avoid tube; OR: 0.93, 95% CI: 0.67 to 1.30), which is an absolute reduction in risk of death or poor outcome of 1.2% (95% CI: -4.2 to $+6.6$%; $P = 0.7$).

PEG vs NG tube   In the PEG vs NG FOOD trial, 321 patients with dysphagia due to recent stroke (<30 days) were enrolled by 47 hospitals in 11 countries and randomised within 7 days of admission to enteral feeding by PEG tube ($n = 162$ patients) or NGT ($n = 159$ patients) within 3 days of enrolment.

Enteral feeding by PEG was associated with no significant change in odds of death at 6 months after randomisation, compared with NGT (48.8% PEG, 47.8% NGT; OR: 1.04, 95% CI: 0.67 to 1.61), which is an absolute difference in death rates at 6 months of 1.0% (95% CI: -10.0 to $+11.9$%; $P = 0.9$).

Enteral feeding by PEG was associated with a borderline significant increase in odds of death or a poor outcome at 6 months after randomisation compared with NGT (88.9% PEG, 81.1% NGT; OR: 1.86, 95% CI: 0.99 to 3.50), which is an absolute increase in death or poor outcome at 6 months of 7.8% (95% CI: 0.0 to 15.5%; $P = 0.05$).

Comment

Early tube feeding via a NGT within the first few days of admission may reduce case fatality (compared with delayed or avoid tube feeding) in dysphagic stroke patients, but perhaps at the expense of increasing the proportion of patients surviving with a poor outcome (Finestone, 2000).

There is no evidence to support a policy of early initiation of PEG tube feeding in dysphagic stroke patients (unless the patient cannot tolerate an NGT).

PEG tube feeding is preferred for patients who are likely to require prolonged feeding by tube (i.e. for more than a few weeks).

Aspiration pneumonia after stroke may not be prevented by tube feeding but if present, should be treated with appropriate antibiotics.

Bladder function and risk of infection

Bladder dysfunction

The most common cause of bladder dysfunction after stroke is detrusor hyper-reflexia as a direct result of the stroke, which may be compounded by immobility (e.g. unable to sit or stand), urinary tract infection, and pre-stroke bladder outflow obstruction (e.g. prostatomegaly). Detrusor hyper-reflexia tends to cause urge incontinence and frequency of micturition.

Incontinence

Incontinence of urine is common in the first few days after stroke, and provokes considerable distress among patients and their carers. It is usually due to a combination of factors such as detrusor hyper-reflexia, impaired sphincter control, pre-existing bladder outflow obstruction (e.g. prostatomegaly, gynaecological problems), constipation, immobility, inability to communicate, inadequate response (e.g. inadequate nursing), confusion, impaired consciousness and urinary tract infection (Nakayama *et al.*, 1997).

Management of incontinence aims to identify and rectify the underlying cause (e.g. infection, outflow obstruction) and exacerbating factors (excessive fluids, uncontrolled hyperglycaemia or diuretics), and commence bladder 'retraining' where patients are prompted to void regularly. A bedside ultrasound machine can be used to exclude a postmicturition residual volume of 100 ml or more. If present, an anticholinergic drug (e.g. oxybutynin) can be used (if there are no contraindications such as closed angle glaucoma), coupled with regular (6 hourly) bladder emptying by intermittent catheterisation.

Indwelling catheters should be restricted to patients in whom the above measures are impractical, such as those in whom it is difficult to transfer and in whom pressure areas are a cause for concern. This is because the risks of an indwelling catheter include urinary tract trauma and infection. However, because incontinence of urine frequently resolves spontaneously during the first or second week after stroke, it is important to remove the catheter for a 'trial of voiding' and re-assessment of bladder function as soon as the patient's condition begins to improve.

For patients with persisting incontinence, cystoscopy and urodynamic investigations may be indicated to assess bladder contractility and outflow.

Retention

Urinary retention is common, especially in men with pre-existing bladder outflow obstruction, and must be systematically anticipated and excluded in patients with dribbling incontinence, agitation, confusion, impaired consciousness or communication difficulties, particularly if the have been exposed to precipitants such as drugs (tricyclic antidepressants which have antimuscarinic effects), immobility and constipation.

A urethral catheter provides prompt relief but in men with benign prostatic hypertrophy. α-blocking drugs (e.g. prazosin) or finasteride (which inhibits the metabolism of testosterone to dihydrotestosterone in the prostate) may enable the catheter to be removed without recurrence of retention.

Comment

Bladder function should be assessed soon after stroke onset. The patient's abdomen should be palpated for a distended bladder. After attempted voiding, a bladder ultrasound should be performed to assess the residual bladder volume of urine. If the residual urine volume is more than 100 ml, the bladder should be emptied regularly by attempted voiding followed by an 'in and out' urinary catheter, and the process repeated every 6–8 h until the residual urine volume is less than 100 ml.

An indwelling catheter should be avoided if possible because this makes resolution of urinary incontinence impossible to detect and may lead to a number of complications.

Risks of immobility

Immobile patients are at increased risk of:

- pneumonia (see above);
- decubitus ulcers (pressure sores);
- joint contractures;
- painful 'frozen' shoulder;
- deep venous thrombosis (DVT) and PE.

Pressure areas

Pressure sores or decubitus ulcers are avoidable, and if allowed to develop they cause the patient considerable pain and slow the patient's recovery (or are sometimes fatal). Prevention relies on an early and accurate assessment of the patient's risk of pressure sores, expert and interested nursing care, regular turning (e.g. every 2 h) and the judicious use of specialised cushions and mattresses (Nuffield Institute of Health, 1995).

Although not proven by RCTs, both the ASA and the EUSI state that early mobilisation is favoured to prevent numerous complications after stroke including aspiration pneumonia, VTE, decubital ulcers (pressure sores) and contractures (Indredavik et al., 1999; Adams et al., 2003; The European Stroke Initiative, 2003, 2004).

Painful 'frozen' shoulder and joint contractures

Shoulder pain after stroke is common, poorly understood, difficult to prevent and no proposed treatment is supported by reliable evidence.

Venous thromboembolism

About 5% of hospitalised stroke patients develop a clinically evident DVT (Warlow *et al.*, 1972; Warlow, 1978; Davenport *et al.*, 1996; Langhorne *et al.*, 2000) and about 2% a pulmonary embolus (Warlow, 1978; Kalra *et al.*, 1995; McClatchie, 1980). However, prospective studies that systematically screen stroke patients for DVT with compression Doppler ultrasound or magnetic resonance imaging identify DVT in up to half of patients (Kelly *et al.*, 2001).

Patients at greatest risk of developing a DVT and PE are those who are immobile (e.g. due to severe leg weakness) and obese, and who have a history of previous VTE or a prothrombotic state.

Strategies to prevent DVT and VTE include physical measures (e.g. re-hydration, early mobilisation (including regular passive and active joint movement) and compression stockings), and antithrombotic drug therapy (aspirin, heparin).

Compression stockings

Evidence   A meta-analysis of 17 small RCTs compression stockings in the peri-operative period suggest that stockings reduce the risk of post-operative VTE by about two-thirds (Wells *et al.*, 1994). Only two RCTs have tested physical methods such as graded elastic compression stockings and intermittent pneumatic compression in stroke patients and these were far too small to provide a reliable estimate of the effect (Muir *et al.*, 2000; Mazzone *et al.*, 2004; Grandi *et al.*, 2005).

Comment   It is not known if the results obtained with compression stockings that are applied before the onset of paralysis and for only a few days in the peri-operative period can be generalised to stroke patients in whom stockings are applied after (not before) the onset of limb paresis, and in whom immobilisation is frequently prolonged (rather than brief).

It is important to demonstrate the effectiveness of compression stockings in stroke patients because they are not without discomfort for the patients (particularly in hot environments), distressing in some patients (e.g. those with urinary incontinence), and potentially hazardous, causing skin necrosis and even gangrene, in patients with peripheral vascular disease and peripheral neuropathy, such as diabetics.

The Clots in Legs Or Teds after Stroke (CLOTS) trial is a family of two multicentre international RCTs which is currently evaluating whether full-length graduated compression stockings reduce the risk of DVT after stroke compared with no stockings, and whether full-length stockings are more effective than below-knee graduated compression stockings (www.clotstrial.com).

Whilst awaiting further evidence from the CLOTS trial, it is recommended that immobile stroke patients are mobilised as early as possible after stroke, and that compression stockings are reserved for patients at high risk of DVT (e.g. immobile or a history of previous DVT or prothrombotic state) and low risk of complications (e.g. no peripheral arterial disease or peripheral neuropathy).

Antiplatelet therapy

Evidence   Aspirin administered within 48 h of onset of acute ischaemic stroke reduces the odds of PE (OR: 0.71, 95% CI: 0.53 to 0.96) compared with control (Fig. 4.5), as it does in several other clinical scenarios (Antiplatelet Trialists' Collaboration, 1994). Although the absolute reduction is about one PE prevented per 1000 patients treated with aspirin (0.48% control, 0.34% aspirin), aspirin also significantly reduces the risk of long-term death and dependency (see Chapter 10) (Sandercock et al., 2003).

Comment   Aspirin is prescribed immediately in all patients with acute ischaemic stroke, unless contraindicated, because it reduces the absolute risk of early recurrent ischaemic stroke (by about 0.7%) and the risk of VTE (by about 0.1%) without causing an excess of haemorrhagic stroke (0.2%) that would nullify its beneficial effects. Consequently, there is a long-term net benefit from aspirin in reducing death and dependency (1.2%) (refer to Chapter 10) (Sandercock et al., 2003).

Anticoagulation

Evidence   Subcutaneous heparin significantly reduces the risk of DVT (OR: 0.21, 95% CI: 0.15 to 0.29) (Fig. 4.6) and PE (OR: 0.60, 95% CI: 0.44 to 0.81) (Fig. 4.7) (Gubitz et al., 2004). However, this favourable effect if offset by an excess risk of haemorrhagic transformation of the cerebral infarct (HTI) and extracranial haemorrhage, such that at 6 months post-stroke the risk of death and dependency is the same, whether the patient is treated early within the first 14 days of acute ischaemic stroke with s.c. heparin or not (see Chapter 9) (Gubitz et al., 2004). However, there are probably patients at particularly high risk of VTE (e.g. immobile and a history of previous VTE) and low risk of HTI (e.g. lacunar infarction) who may benefit if treated with s.c. heparin (e.g. standard unfractionated heparin (UFH) 5000 U bid).

As the risks of haemorrhagic complications of heparin are dose related, the risks of bleeding are less with low-dose heparins. Direct comparisons indicate that low-molecular-weight heparins (LMWHs) and heparinoids are more effective than

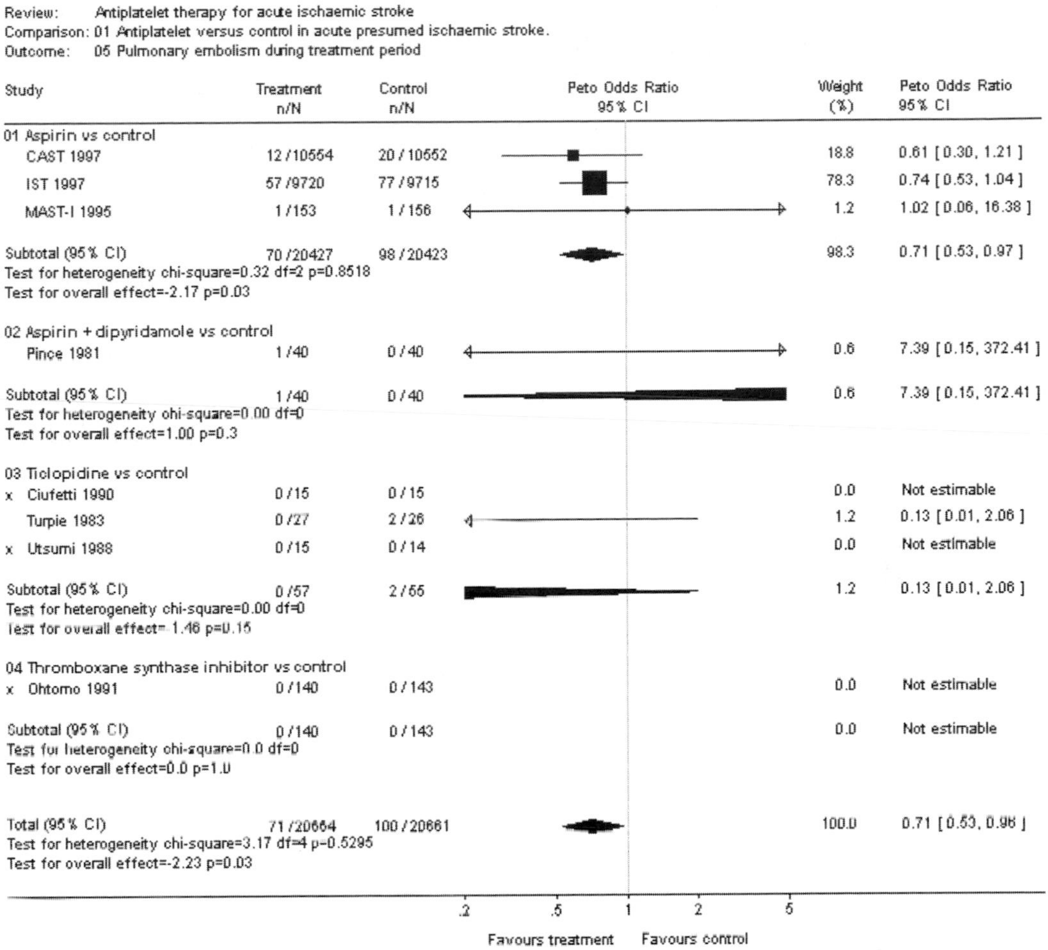

Review: Antiplatelet therapy for acute ischaemic stroke
Comparison: 01 Antiplatelet versus control in acute presumed ischaemic stroke.
Outcome: 05 Pulmonary embolism during treatment period

Study	Treatment n/N	Control n/N	Peto Odds Ratio 95% CI	Weight (%)	Peto Odds Ratio 95% CI
01 Aspirin vs control					
CAST 1997	12/10554	20/10552		18.8	0.61 [0.30, 1.21]
IST 1997	57/9720	77/9715		78.3	0.74 [0.53, 1.04]
MAST-I 1995	1/153	1/156		1.2	1.02 [0.06, 16.38]
Subtotal (95% CI)	70/20427	98/20423		98.3	0.71 [0.53, 0.97]
Test for heterogeneity chi-square=0.32 df=2 p=0.8518					
Test for overall effect=-2.17 p=0.03					
02 Aspirin + dipyridamole vs control					
Pince 1981	1/40	0/40		0.6	7.39 [0.15, 372.41]
Subtotal (95% CI)	1/40	0/40		0.6	7.39 [0.15, 372.41]
Test for heterogeneity chi-square=0.00 df=0					
Test for overall effect=1.00 p=0.3					
03 Ticlopidine vs control					
x Ciufetti 1990	0/15	0/15		0.0	Not estimable
Turpie 1983	0/27	2/26		1.2	0.13 [0.01, 2.06]
x Utsumi 1988	0/15	0/14		0.0	Not estimable
Subtotal (95% CI)	0/57	2/55		1.2	0.13 [0.01, 2.06]
Test for heterogeneity chi-square=0.00 df=0					
Test for overall effect=-1.46 p=0.15					
04 Thromboxane synthase inhibitor vs control					
x Ohtomo 1991	0/140	0/143		0.0	Not estimable
Subtotal (95% CI)	0/140	0/143		0.0	Not estimable
Test for heterogeneity chi-square=0.0 df=0					
Test for overall effect=0.0 p=1.0					
Total (95% CI)	71/20664	100/20661		100.0	0.71 [0.53, 0.96]
Test for heterogeneity chi-square=3.17 df=4 p=0.5295					
Test for overall effect=-2.23 p=0.03					

.2   .5   1   2   5

Favours treatment   Favours control

Figure 4.5   Forest plot showing the effects of *antiplatelet therapy* compared with *control* in patients with acute ischaemic stroke on *PE* at the end of the treatment period among individual trials (each line), and pooled (summary at the bottom). Reproduced from Sandercock *et al.* (2003), with permission from the authors and John Wiley & Sons Limited. Copyright Cochrane Collaboration, reproduced with permission.

standard UFH in preventing DVT in patients with acute ischaemic stroke (Fig. 4.8) (refer to Chapter 9) (Counsell and Sandercock, 2002; Sandercock *et al.*, 2005). In order to follow up on the promising results of a small trial (Hillbom *et al.*, 2002), a larger RCT is currently comparing s.c. LMWH (enoxaparin) with UFH. This is called the prevention of VTE after acute ischaemic stroke with the LMWH Enoxaparin (PREVAIL) trial. It is an open-label, randomised, parallel-group, trial evaluating the efficacy sand safety of enoxaparin 40 mg s.c. qid with UFH 5000 U s.c. q 12 h given for 10 ±4 days in the prevention of VTE as assessed by bilateral

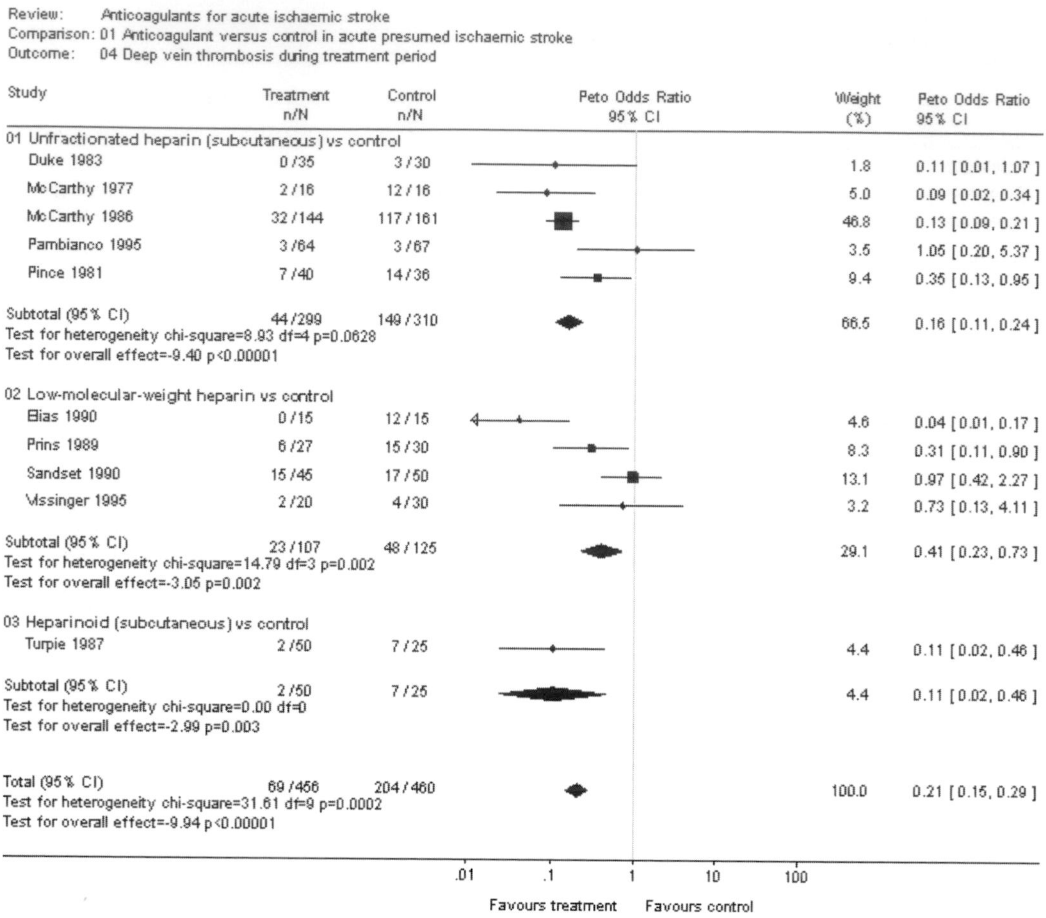

Review: Anticoagulants for acute ischaemic stroke
Comparison: 01 Anticoagulant versus control in acute presumed ischaemic stroke
Outcome: 04 Deep vein thrombosis during treatment period

Study	Treatment n/N	Control n/N	Peto Odds Ratio 95% CI	Weight (%)	Peto Odds Ratio 95% CI
01 Unfractionated heparin (subcutaneous) vs control					
Duke 1983	0 /35	3 /30		1.8	0.11 [0.01, 1.07]
McCarthy 1977	2 /16	12 /16		5.0	0.09 [0.02, 0.34]
McCarthy 1986	32 /144	117 /161		46.8	0.13 [0.09, 0.21]
Pambianco 1995	3 /64	3 /67		3.5	1.05 [0.20, 5.37]
Pince 1981	7 /40	14 /36		9.4	0.35 [0.13, 0.95]
Subtotal (95% CI)	44 /299	149 /310		66.5	0.16 [0.11, 0.24]
Test for heterogeneity chi-square=8.93 df=4 p=0.0628					
Test for overall effect=-9.40 p<0.00001					
02 Low-molecular-weight heparin vs control					
Elias 1990	0 /15	12 /15		4.6	0.04 [0.01, 0.17]
Prins 1989	6 /27	15 /30		8.3	0.31 [0.11, 0.90]
Sandset 1990	15 /45	17 /50		13.1	0.97 [0.42, 2.27]
Vissinger 1995	2 /20	4 /30		3.2	0.73 [0.13, 4.11]
Subtotal (95% CI)	23 /107	48 /125		29.1	0.41 [0.23, 0.73]
Test for heterogeneity chi-square=14.79 df=3 p=0.002					
Test for overall effect=-3.05 p=0.002					
03 Heparinoid (subcutaneous) vs control					
Turpie 1987	2 /50	7 /25		4.4	0.11 [0.02, 0.46]
Subtotal (95% CI)	2 /50	7 /25		4.4	0.11 [0.02, 0.46]
Test for heterogeneity chi-square=0.00 df=0					
Test for overall effect=-2.99 p=0.003					
Total (95% CI)	69 /456	204 /460		100.0	0.21 [0.15, 0.29]
Test for heterogeneity chi-square=31.61 df=9 p=0.0002					
Test for overall effect=-9.94 p<0.00001					

.01   .1   1   10   100

Favours treatment   Favours control

Figure 4.6   Forest plot showing the effects of *anticoagulant therapy* compared with *control* in patients with acute ischaemic stroke on *deep vein thrombosis* during the treatment period. Reproduced from Gubitz *et al.* (2004), with permission from the authors and John Wiley & Sons Limited. Copyright Cochrane Library, reproduced with permission.

contrast venography of the lower extremities at the end of the treatment period for asymptomatic patients, and an appropriate diagnostic procedure in patients with symptomatic DVT or PE. The study aims to include 1760 patients (880) per treatment group, and identify a reduction in odds of VTE by 35%, from 20% with UFH to 14% with enoxaparin.

Comment

Due to the lack of reliable evidence from RCTs, the optimal prophylactic management of VTE after acute stroke is controversial (Adams, 2004; Davis & Donnan, 2004; Dennis, 2004).

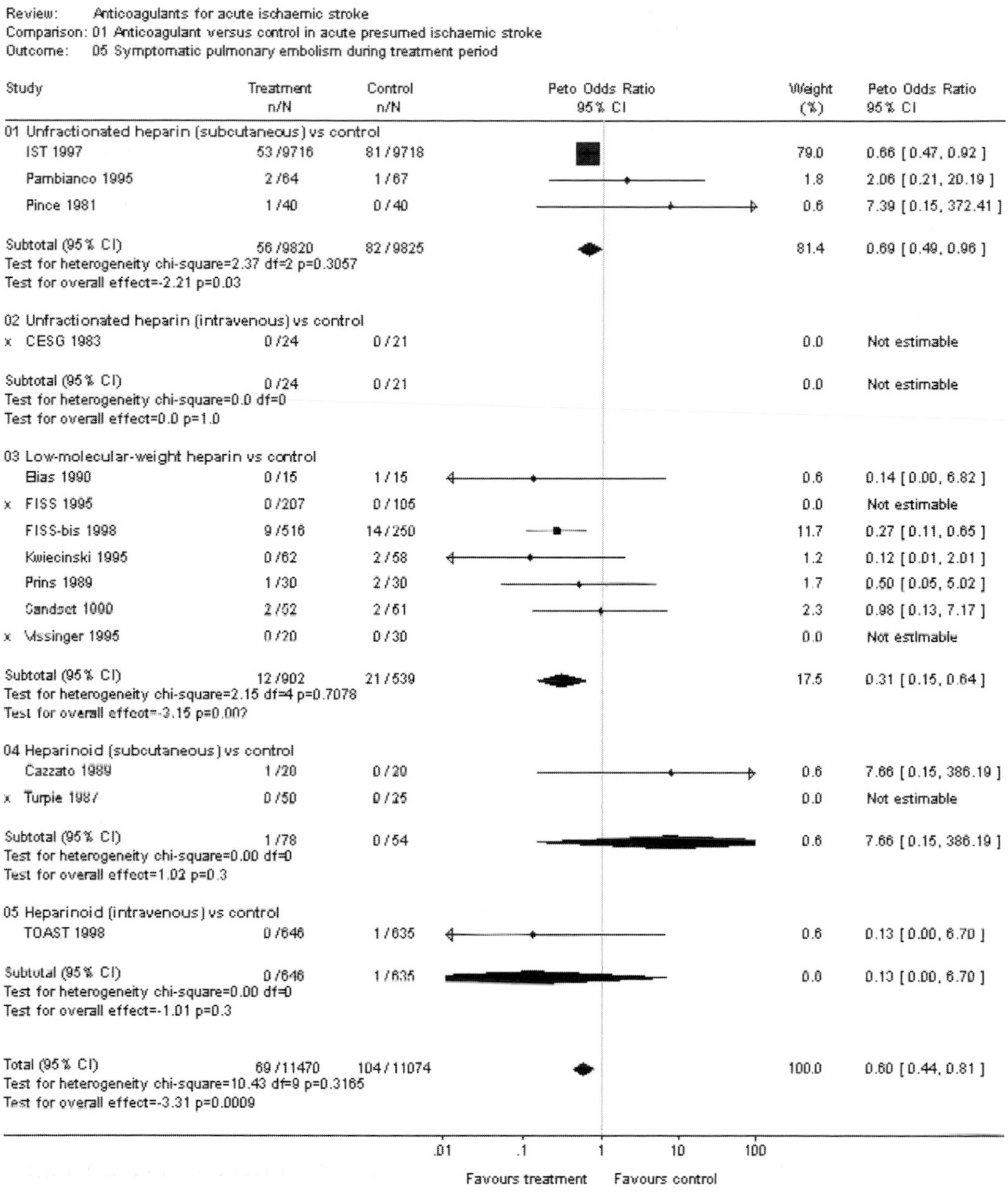

Review: Anticoagulants for acute ischaemic stroke
Comparison: 01 Anticoagulant versus control in acute presumed ischaemic stroke
Outcome: 05 Symptomatic pulmonary embolism during treatment period

Study	Treatment n/N	Control n/N	Peto Odds Ratio 95% CI	Weight (%)	Peto Odds Ratio 95% CI
01 Unfractionated heparin (subcutaneous) vs control					
IST 1997	53 /9716	81 /9718		79.0	0.66 [0.47, 0.92]
Pambianco 1995	2 /64	1 /67		1.8	2.06 [0.21, 20.19]
Pince 1981	1 /40	0 /40		0.6	7.39 [0.15, 372.41]
Subtotal (95% CI)	56 /9820	82 /9825		81.4	0.69 [0.49, 0.96]
Test for heterogeneity chi-square=2.37 df=2 p=0.3057					
Test for overall effect=-2.21 p=0.03					
02 Unfractionated heparin (intravenous) vs control					
x CESG 1983	0 /24	0 /21		0.0	Not estimable
Subtotal (95% CI)	0 /24	0 /21		0.0	Not estimable
Test for heterogeneity chi-square=0.0 df=0					
Test for overall effect=0.0 p=1.0					
03 Low-molecular-weight heparin vs control					
Elias 1990	0 /15	1 /15		0.6	0.14 [0.00, 6.82]
x FISS 1995	0 /207	0 /105		0.0	Not estimable
FISS-bis 1998	9 /516	14 /250		11.7	0.27 [0.11, 0.65]
Kwiecinski 1995	0 /62	2 /58		1.2	0.12 [0.01, 2.01]
Prins 1989	1 /30	2 /30		1.7	0.50 [0.05, 5.02]
Sandset 1990	2 /52	2 /61		2.3	0.98 [0.13, 7.17]
x Vissinger 1995	0 /20	0 /30		0.0	Not estimable
Subtotal (95% CI)	12 /902	21 /539		17.5	0.31 [0.15, 0.64]
Test for heterogeneity chi-square=2.15 df=4 p=0.7078					
Test for overall effect=-3.15 p=0.002					
04 Heparinoid (subcutaneous) vs control					
Cazzato 1989	1 /28	0 /20		0.6	7.66 [0.15, 386.19]
x Turpie 1987	0 /50	0 /25		0.0	Not estimable
Subtotal (95% CI)	1 /78	0 /54		0.6	7.66 [0.15, 386.19]
Test for heterogeneity chi-square=0.00 df=0					
Test for overall effect=1.02 p=0.3					
05 Heparinoid (intravenous) vs control					
TOAST 1998	0 /646	1 /635		0.6	0.13 [0.00, 6.70]
Subtotal (95% CI)	0 /646	1 /635		0.0	0.13 [0.00, 6.70]
Test for heterogeneity chi-square=0.00 df=0					
Test for overall effect=-1.01 p=0.3					
Total (95% CI)	69 /11470	104 /11074		100.0	0.60 [0.44, 0.81]
Test for heterogeneity chi-square=10.43 df=9 p=0.3165					
Test for overall effect=-3.31 p=0.0009					

.01   .1   1   10   100

Favours treatment   Favours control

Figure 4.7   Forest plot showing the effects of *anticoagulant therapy* compared with *control* in patients with acute ischaemic stroke on *symptomatic PE* during the treatment period. Reproduced from Gubitz *et al.* (2004), with permission from the authors and John Wiley & Sons Limited. Copyright Cochrane Library, reproduced with permission.

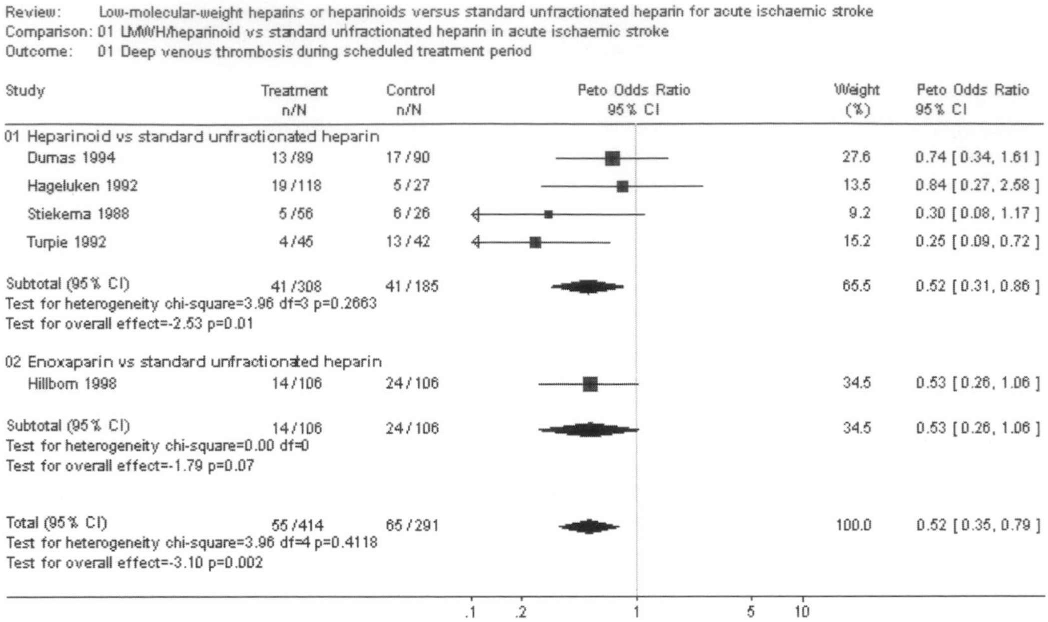

Review: Low-molecular-weight heparins or heparinoids versus standard unfractionated heparin for acute ischaemic stroke
Comparison: 01 LMWH/heparinoid vs standard unfractionated heparin in acute ischaemic stroke
Outcome: 01 Deep venous thrombosis during scheduled treatment period

Study	Treatment n/N	Control n/N	Peto Odds Ratio 95% CI	Weight (%)	Peto Odds Ratio 95% CI
01 Heparinoid vs standard unfractionated heparin					
Dumas 1994	13 /89	17 /90		27.6	0.74 [0.34, 1.61]
Hageluken 1992	19 /118	5 /27		13.5	0.84 [0.27, 2.58]
Stiekema 1988	5 /56	6 /26		9.2	0.30 [0.08, 1.17]
Turpie 1992	4 /45	13 /42		15.2	0.25 [0.09, 0.72]
Subtotal (95% CI)	41 /308	41 /185		65.5	0.52 [0.31, 0.86]
Test for heterogeneity chi-square=3.96 df=3 p=0.2663					
Test for overall effect=-2.53 p=0.01					
02 Enoxaparin vs standard unfractionated heparin					
Hillbom 1998	14 /106	24 /106		34.5	0.53 [0.26, 1.06]
Subtotal (95% CI)	14 /106	24 /106		34.5	0.53 [0.26, 1.06]
Test for heterogeneity chi-square=0.00 df=0					
Test for overall effect=-1.79 p=0.07					
Total (95% CI)	55 /414	65 /291		100.0	0.52 [0.35, 0.79]
Test for heterogeneity chi-square=3.96 df=4 p=0.4118					
Test for overall effect=-3.10 p=0.002					

.1   .2   1   5   10

Figure 4.8   Forest plot showing the effects of *low-molecular weight heparinoid* compared with *standard UFH* in patients with acute ischaemic stroke on *deep vein thrombosis* during the treatment period. Reproduced from Sandercock *et al.* (2005), with permission from the authors and John Wiley & Sons Limited. Copyright Cochrane Library, reproduced with permission.

The EUSI states that the incidence of VTE may be reduced by early re-hydration and mobilisation, and graded external compression stockings (level IV), and that low-dose s.c. heparin or LMWHs should only be considered for patients at high risk of VTE (level II) (European Stroke Initiative, 2004).

In contrast, the ASA recommends s.c. administration of anticoagulants to prevent VTE among all immobilised patients, or the use of intermittent external graduated compression stockings or aspirin for patients who cannot receive anticoagulants (Adams *et al.*, 2003).

For clinicians who are uncertain of the relative merits of graduated compression stockings compared with no stockings, or of below-knee compared with full-length stockings, patients can be randomised in the CLOTS trial.

For clinicians who are uncertain of the relative merits of unfractionated and low molecular weight heparin, patients can be randomised in the PREVAIL study.

Otherwise, there probably are patients at particularly high risk of VTE (e.g. immobile and a history of previous VTE) and low risk of HTI (e.g. small (lacunar) infarcts and perhaps no evidence of microhaemorrhages on graded echo magnetic resonance imaging of the brain) who are more likely to benefit if treated with prophylactic s.c. heparin (e.g. standard UFH 5000U bid, or enoxaparin) – and, in addition to aspirin (and stockings, re-hydration and passive limb movement), rather than instead of aspirin.

Seizures

Prophylactic administration of anticonvulsants to patients with recent stroke who have not had seizures is not recommended, whereas recurrent seizures should be treated as with any other acute neurological condition (Adams *et al.*, 2003; The European Stroke Initiative, 2004).

Monitoring of vital neurological functions in the stroke unit or in a normal ward

The intensity with which patients are monitored for physiological abnormalities and complications varies substantially between stroke units. At one extreme, stroke intensive-care units use one-to-one nursing, invasive monitoring of BP and intracranial pressure, and aggressive management of abnormal measurements. At the other extreme, patients may have only pulse, temperature, BP and GCS recorded. Although monitoring may seem innocuous enough, invasive monitoring has direct adverse effects (e.g. infection, bleeding) and any monitoring could lead to potentially harmful interventions (e.g. fluid overload, or excessive BP reduction). A small RCT has shown that a compromise with non-invasive monitoring, and protocols for treating abnormal physiological measurements, can reduce the frequency of early neurological deterioration (Davis *et al.*, 1999). Furthermore, the results of a small randomised pilot study suggest that admission of acute stroke patients to a Stroke Care Monitoring Unit, where oxygen saturation, body temperature, BP, blood glucose, and cardiac rhythm are monitored for the first 48 h, or longer until stable for 24 h (Table 4.1) may further optimise outcome (Sulter *et al.*, 2003).

In all stroke patients, the neurological status and vital functions (BP, pulse rate and temperature) should be continuously or regularly monitored. The neurological status is best monitored using validated neurological scales, such as the NIHSS, the Scandinavian Stroke Scale and the GCS.

In selected cases with past medical history of cardiac disease and/or dysrhythmias and in cases of unstable BP, on-line ECG monitoring is desirable. The electrodes for cardiac monitoring can also be used for respiratory monitoring, which is useful to detect respiration abnormalities during sleep. When instrumental monitoring is not feasible, repeat ECG, clinical checks of respiratory function and BP measurements with automatic inflatable sphygmomanometry can be performed. Pulse oximetry can also be useful for continuously monitoring the

Table 4.1. Monitoring protocol adopted by Sulter *et al.* (2003).

Parameter	Values	Interventions
BP (every 15 min)	Systolic BP ≤ 220 mmHg and mean BP < 130 mmHg	No intervention (unless lowering of BP is warranted – e.g., aortic dissection)
	Systolic BP > 220 mmHg or mean BP > 130 mmHg	10% reduction in BP: Labetalol 100–200 mg orally or 1 mg/min (maximum 200 mg) i.v. Enalapril 2.5–5.0 mg orally or 0.5–1 mg i.v.
	Mean BP < 80 mmHg	Volume expander (Gelofusine)
Oxygen saturation (pulse oximeter, continuous)	<95%	Oxygen via nasal prong or mask; start with 2–5 l/min
Body temperature (rectal thermometer, continuous)	>37.5°C	Acetylsalicylic acid (500 mg) or paracetamol suppository (1000 mg)
Blood glucose (every 6 h)	>10 mmol/l	Actrapid insulin via infusion pump
Cardiac rhythm (continuous 5-lead ECG for at least 48 h)	Dysrhythmia	Consult cardiologist

Mean BP = (systolic BP + 2 diastolic BP)/3.

patient's cardio-respiratory status. A central venous catheter, and occasionally central venous pressure monitoring, may be needed in severe stroke patients treated in specialised wards. A central venous catheter, provides indirect information on intravascular volume, cardiac function, and compliance within the venous system.

SUMMARY

Preserving vital functions and optimising physiological homoeostasis

Airway and oxygenation

- Monitoring of oxygenation by means of pulse oximetry is recommended in acute ischaemic stroke.
- Supplemental oxygen is recommended for patients with hypoxaemia (O_2 saturation <92% by pulse oximetry) and to aim for O_2 saturation ≥95%.
- Airway support and ventilatory assistance is recommended for patients with depressed levels of consciousness or a compromised airway; or potentially reversible respiratory insufficiency.

Cardiac care

Continuous cardiac monitoring should be considered in the first 48 h of stroke onset in patients with:
- previous known cardiac disease,
- history of dysrhythmias,
- unstable BP,
- clinical signs/symptoms of heart failure,
- abnormal baseline ECG,
- stroke involving the insular cortex.

Fluid and electrolytes

- Fluid balance should be restored (with normal saline, not dextrose) and maintained in all stroke patients.
- In patients with brain oedema, hypotonic solutions (NaCl 0.45% or glucose 5%) are contraindicated.
- Serum electrolytes should be assessed at baseline, and subsequently if the patient deteriorates.
- Electrolyte imbalances should be managed by treating the underlying cause and replacing the appropriate electrolytes if deficient.

Nutrition

- The available evidence does not support a policy of routine oral nutritional supplementation after stroke.

Blood glucose

- Unless the blood glucose is low, no glucose solution should be given to a stroke patient due to the potential detrimental effects of hyperglycaemia.
- Rapidly correct low blood glucose concentrations with i.v. dextrose bolus or infusion of 10–20% glucose, and avoid hypotonic solutions (NaCl 0.45% or glucose 5%) to minimise brain oedema.
- Monitor serum glucose levels in diabetic patients.
- Gradually lower raised blood glucose concentrations with normal saline and insulin titration.
- The EUSI recommends to lower raised blood glucose concentrations to about 10 mmol/l (European Stroke Initiative, 2004) whereas the ASA recommends to aim for blood glucose <16.63 mmol/l (Adams *et al.*, 2003).

Body temperature

- Body temperature ⩾37.5°C should be investigated (for the cause) and probably treated with antipyretic agents and, if appropriate, relevant antibiotics.
- Antibiotic, anti-mycotic and anti-viral prophylaxis is not recommended in immuno-competent patients.

BP

- Hypotension should be recognised and corrected promptly by treating the underlying cause, raising the foot of the bed, and replacing fluids via a safe route with crystalloid (saline) or, occasionally, colloid, solutions. Low cardiac output may also need inotropic support.
- Routine BP lowering is not recommended, except for extremely elevated values (>200–220 mmHg systolic BP or >120 mmHg diastolic BP for ischaemic stroke, >180/105 mmHg for haemorrhagic stroke) confirmed by repeated measurements.
- Immediate antihypertensive therapy for more moderate hypertension is recommended in cases of stroke with heart failure, aortic dissection, acute MI, acute renal failure, thrombolysis or i.v. heparin but should be applied cautiously.
- Recommended target BP in patients:
  - as a general rule, lower BP by 10–15%:
    with prior hypertension, 180/100–105 mmHg;
    without prior hypertension, 160–180/90–100 mmHg;
    considering thrombolysis, lower BP below 180/110 mmHg before commencing thrombolysis.
- Recommended drugs for BP treatment:
  - i.v. labetalol 10–20 mg over 1–2 min;
  - i.v. nicardipine 5 mg/h i.v. infusion at initial dose; titrate to desired effect by increasing 2.5 mg/h every 5 min to maximum of 15 mg/h;
  - i.v. urapidil;
  - i.v. sodium nitroprusside 0.5 μg/kg/min i.v. infusion as initial dose with continuous BP monitoring; or
  - i.v. nitroglycerine; or
  - oral captopril.
- Avoid sublingual nifedipine which is rapidly absorbed and may cause a precipitous fall in BP.
- Avoid and treat hypotension particularly in unstable patients by administering adequate amounts of fluids and, when required, volume expanders and/or catecholamines (epinephrine 0.1–2 mg/h plus dobutamine 5–50 mg/h).

PREVENTING MEDICAL COMPLICATIONS

Aspiration pneumonia, dehydration and malnutrition

Swallowing therapy

- This is very little evidence from RCTs of the effectiveness and safety of therapies to improve swallowing function.

Tube feeding

- Early tube feeding via a NGT within the first few days of admission may reduce case fatality (compared with delayed or avoid tube feeding) in dysphagic stroke patients, but perhaps at the expense of increasing the proportion of patients surviving with a poor outcome.
- There is no evidence to support a policy of early initiation of PEG tube feeding in dysphagic stroke patients (unless the patient cannot tolerate an NGT).
- PEG tube feeding is preferred for patients who are likely to require prolonged feeding by tube (i.e. for more than a few weeks).

Bladder dysfunction and infection

- Bladder function should be assessed soon after stroke onset. The patient's abdomen should be palpated for a distended bladder. After attempted voiding, a bladder ultrasound should be performed to assess the residual bladder volume of urine. If the residual urine volume is more than 100 ml, the bladder should be emptied regularly by attempted voiding followed by an 'in and out' urinary catheter, and the process repeated every 6–8 h until the residual urine volume is less than 100 ml.
- An indwelling catheter should be avoided if possible because this makes resolution of urinary incontinence impossible to detect and may lead to a number of complications.

Risks of immobility

Pressure sores

- Each patient's risk of pressure sores should be assessed and documented, and actions, appropriate to the level of risk, such as regular turning, should be taken to prevent sores developing.

Shoulder pain

- Shoulder pain after stroke is common, poorly understood, difficult to prevent and no proposed treatment is supported by reliable evidence.

Venous thromboembolism

- Immobile stroke patients should probably be treated with re-hydration, external graduated compression stockings, and aspirin in the acute phase, coupled with efforts to promote early mobilisation.
- If immobility persists for more than a few days, low-dose s.c. heparin or LMWHs should probably be added (as the risks of venous thrombosis increase, and the risks of HTI decrease).

Reperfusion of ischaemic brain by thrombolysis

Rationale

About 80% of all strokes are caused by occlusion of a cerebral artery, resulting in focal brain infarction (ischaemic stroke) (Warlow *et al.*, 2000). The cause is usually *in situ* atherothrombosis or an embolus from a proximal source such as the extracranial neck vessels, the aortic arch, the heart, and the leg and pelvic veins.

When a thrombus forms or is lodged in an artery, plasminogen, a precursor of plasmin, becomes trapped among the fibrin strands that constitute the bulk of the thrombus. Endogenous tissue plasminogen activator (t-PA), which is naturally made by endothelial cells, cleaves plasminogen on the surface of the thrombus, thereby releasing active plasmin. The plasmin, in turn, begins to degrade fibrin and thus expose more plasminogen. The process continues until the thrombus is lysed. Frequently, such spontaneous lysis of the thrombus, and recanalisation of the artery, do not occur until after the ischaemic brain has become infarcted.

Exogenous thrombolysis (or perhaps more correctly, fibrinolysis) aims to rapidly restore blood flow by lysing fresh thrombi (*in situ* or embolic) which underpin many, but not all, ischaemic strokes, before the ischaemic brain has become infarcted. However, although some emboli consist of fresh thrombus, which is lysable by thrombolysis, others are other non-lysable substances such as organised thrombus, calcium, bacteria, tumour and prosthetic material. Hence, not all ischaemic stroke is likely to respond to reperfusion by thrombolysis.

Thrombolysis has been used sporadically for more than 40 years in the treatment of acute ischaemic stroke (indeed, in the pre-computerised tomography (pre-CT) era, for the treatment of acute stroke of uncertain pathological type). However, evidence for its effectiveness and safety has only recently become available (Wardlaw *et al.*, 2003, 2004).

Evidence

Study designs and patients

A total of 18 randomised-controlled trials (RCTs) have compared thrombolytic treatment with placebo after onset of ischaemic stroke in 5727 highly selected patients (Wardlaw *et al.*, 2003, 2004). All patients underwent CT or magnetic resonance imaging (MRI) brain scan before randomisation to exclude non-stroke disorders and haemorrhagic stroke, and 4984 patients (15 trials) were treated within 6 h of onset of stroke. There are few data from patients aged over 80 years.

Much of the data comes from trials conducted in the first half of the 1990s when, in an effort to reduce delays to trial drug administration, on-site randomisation methods were used that, in consequence, limited the ability to stratify randomisation on key prognostic variables. Several trials, because of the biological effects of thrombolysis combined with the follow-up methods used, did not have complete blinding of outcome assessment.

Interventions

The thrombolytic agents tested were urokinase (UK), streptokinase (SK), recombinant tissue plasminogen activator (rt-PA) and recombinant pro-UK. About 50% of the data (patients and trials) come from trials testing intravenous (i.v.) rt-PA. Treatment allocation was double-blind in 16 of the 18 trials. Thrombolysis was administered by the i.v. route in 16 trials (98% of patients) and by intra-arterial (i.a.) route in two trials.

As different thrombolytic drugs were compared in only three trials, and with a very small number of patients ($n = 688$ patients) and outcome events, and no statistically significant difference was shown between the different agents (see below) (Mielke *et al.*, 2004), they are considered together in order to maximise statistical power.

Results for all patients and thrombolytic agents

Early death (within 10 days)

Overall, among patients treated up to 6 h after ischaemic stroke, random allocation to thrombolytic therapy was associated with a significant increase in early death, within the first 10 days of treatment compared with placebo (14.9% thrombolysis, 9.4% control; odds ratio (OR): 1.81; 95% confidence interval (CI): 1.46–2.24; $2P < 0.000001$) (Fig. 5.1) (Wardlaw *et al.*, 2003). This represents an excess of 59 (95% CI: 21–108) early deaths per 1000 patients treated with thrombolysis. There was borderline significant heterogeneity among the studies ($P = 0.048$), with a definite excess mortality in patients randomised to i.v. SK + aspirin compared with oral aspirin alone. The main cause of the increase in early deaths after thrombolysis was fatal sintracranial haemorrhage.

Data on early deaths were available for four trials using i.v. rt-PA, and showed a non-significant excess of early deaths (OR: 1.24, 95% CI: 0.85–1.81, $P = 0.3$) with no significant heterogeneity (Fig. 5.1). The absolute effect was 15 more (95% CI: 10 fewer to 50 more) deaths per 1000 patients treated. In the trials using SK, there was a statistically significant excess of early deaths (OR: 1.90, 95% CI: 1.37–2.63) (Fig. 5.1).

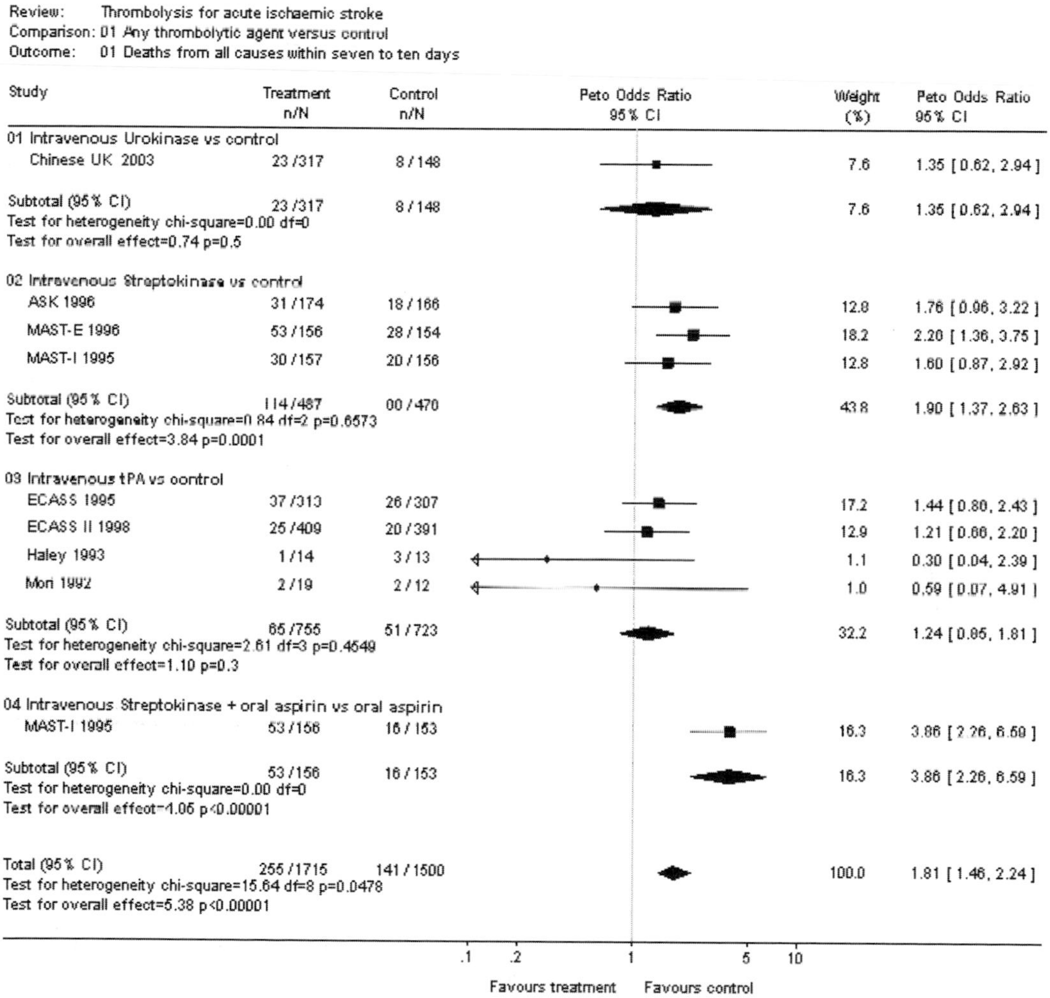

Review: Thrombolysis for acute ischaemic stroke
Comparison: 01 Any thrombolytic agent versus control
Outcome: 01 Deaths from all causes within seven to ten days

Study	Treatment n/N	Control n/N	Peto Odds Ratio 95% CI	Weight (%)	Peto Odds Ratio 95% CI
01 Intravenous Urokinase vs control					
Chinese UK 2003	23 /317	8 / 148		7.6	1.35 [0.62, 2.94]
Subtotal (95% CI)	23 /317	8 / 148		7.6	1.35 [0.62, 2.94]
Test for heterogeneity chi-square=0.00 df=0					
Test for overall effect=0.74 p=0.5					
02 Intravenous Streptokinase vs control					
ASK 1996	31 /174	18 / 166		12.8	1.76 [0.96, 3.22]
MAST-E 1996	53 /156	28 / 154		18.2	2.20 [1.36, 3.75]
MAST-I 1995	30 /157	20 / 156		12.8	1.60 [0.87, 2.92]
Subtotal (95% CI)	114 /487	66 / 470		43.8	1.90 [1.37, 2.63]
Test for heterogeneity chi-square=0.84 df=2 p=0.6573					
Test for overall effect=3.84 p=0.0001					
03 Intravenous tPA vs control					
ECASS 1995	37 /313	26 / 307		17.2	1.44 [0.80, 2.43]
ECASS II 1998	25 /409	20 / 391		12.9	1.21 [0.66, 2.20]
Haley 1993	1 /14	3 / 13		1.1	0.30 [0.04, 2.39]
Mori 1992	2 /19	2 / 12		1.0	0.59 [0.07, 4.91]
Subtotal (95% CI)	65 /755	51 / 723		32.2	1.24 [0.85, 1.81]
Test for heterogeneity chi-square=2.61 df=3 p=0.4549					
Test for overall effect=1.10 p=0.3					
04 Intravenous Streptokinase + oral aspirin vs oral aspirin					
MAST-I 1995	53 /156	16 / 153		16.3	3.86 [2.26, 6.59]
Subtotal (95% CI)	53 /156	16 / 153		16.3	3.86 [2.26, 6.59]
Test for heterogeneity chi-square=0.00 df=0					
Test for overall effect=4.06 p<0.00001					
Total (95% CI)	255 /1715	141 / 1500		100.0	1.81 [1.46, 2.24]
Test for heterogeneity chi-square=15.64 df=8 p=0.0478					
Test for overall effect=5.38 p<0.00001					

.1   .2   1   5   10
Favours treatment   Favours control

Figure 5.1   Forest plot showing the effects of *any thrombolytic agent vs control* within 6 h of onset of ischaemic stroke on *early death (within 7–10 days of randomisation) from all causes*. Reproduced from Wardlaw *et al.* (2003), with permission from the authors and John Wiley & Sons Limited. Copyright Cochrane Library, reproduced with permission.

Early fatal intracranial haemorrhage

Thrombolysis within 6 h of onset of ischaemic stroke was associated with a significant 5-fold increase in fatal intracranial haemorrhage (5.2% thrombolysis, 0.9% control; OR: 4.34, 95% CI: 3.14–5.99; $2P < 0.000001$) (Fig. 5.2) (Wardlaw *et al.*, 2003). There was no significant heterogeneity among the trials ($P = 0.71$).

For every 1000 patients treated with *rt-PA*, there was an excess of 25 (95% CI: 13–44) fatal intracranial haemorrhages per 1000 patients (OR: 3.60, 95% CI: 2.28–5.68) compared with control, whereas for every 1000 patients treated with *SK*, there were 92 (95% CI: 65–120) extra fatal intracranial haemorrhages (OR: 6.03, 95% CI: 3.47–10.47) (Fig. 5.2). Furthermore, compared with SK (alone), the combination of SK and aspirin was associated with an excess of fatal intracranial haemorrhage (OR: 2.2, 95% CI: 1.0–5.5). And compared with aspirin alone, the combination of SK and aspirin was associated with an excess of fatal intracranial haemorrhage (OR: 4.56, 95% CI: 1.62–12.84) (Fig. 5.2) (Wardlaw *et al.*, 2003).

Early symptomatic (including fatal) intracranial haemorrhage

Thrombolytic therapy was also associated with a highly significant 3-fold increase in early symptomatic intracranial haemorrhage (8.7% thrombolysis, 2.5% control; OR: 3.37, 95% CI: 2.68–4.22; $2P < 0.00001$), equivalent to an excess of 58 (95% CI: 36–85) symptomatic intracranial haemorrhages per 1000 patients treated (Fig. 5.3). There was no heterogeneity between thrombolytic agents or trials ($P = 0.15$).

In trials using rt-PA, there were 62 (95% CI: 40–90) extra symptomatic intracranial haemorrhages per 1000 patients treated with rt-PA compared with control (OR: 3.13, 95% CI: 2.34–4.19; $P < 0.00001$) with no heterogeneity among the trials ($P = 0.11$) (Fig. 5.3).

Death at the end of patient follow-up at 3–6 months

At the end of patient follow-up (usually 3–6 months), patients allocated thrombolytic therapy had an increased odds of death (18.2% thrombolysis, 15.2% control; OR: 1.33, 95% CI: 1.15–1.53; $P = 0.002$), representing an extra 41 (95% CI: 19–63) deaths per 1000 patients treated with thrombolysis compared with control (Fig. 5.4). There was considerable heterogeneity among the trials ($P = 0.003$).

Death and dependency at the end of patient follow-up

Despite an excess early hazard, thrombolysis administered up to 6 h after ischaemic stroke was associated with a significant reduction in death or dependency (modified Rankin score (mRS) 3–6) at the end of follow-up 3–6 months after randomisation (53.3% thrombolysis, 58.0% control; OR: 0.84, 95% CI: 0.75–0.95; $2P = 0.004$) (Wardlaw *et al.*, 2003). This represents 43 (95% CI: 13–71) fewer dead or dependent patients per 1000 treated with thrombolysis compared with control (Fig. 5.5).

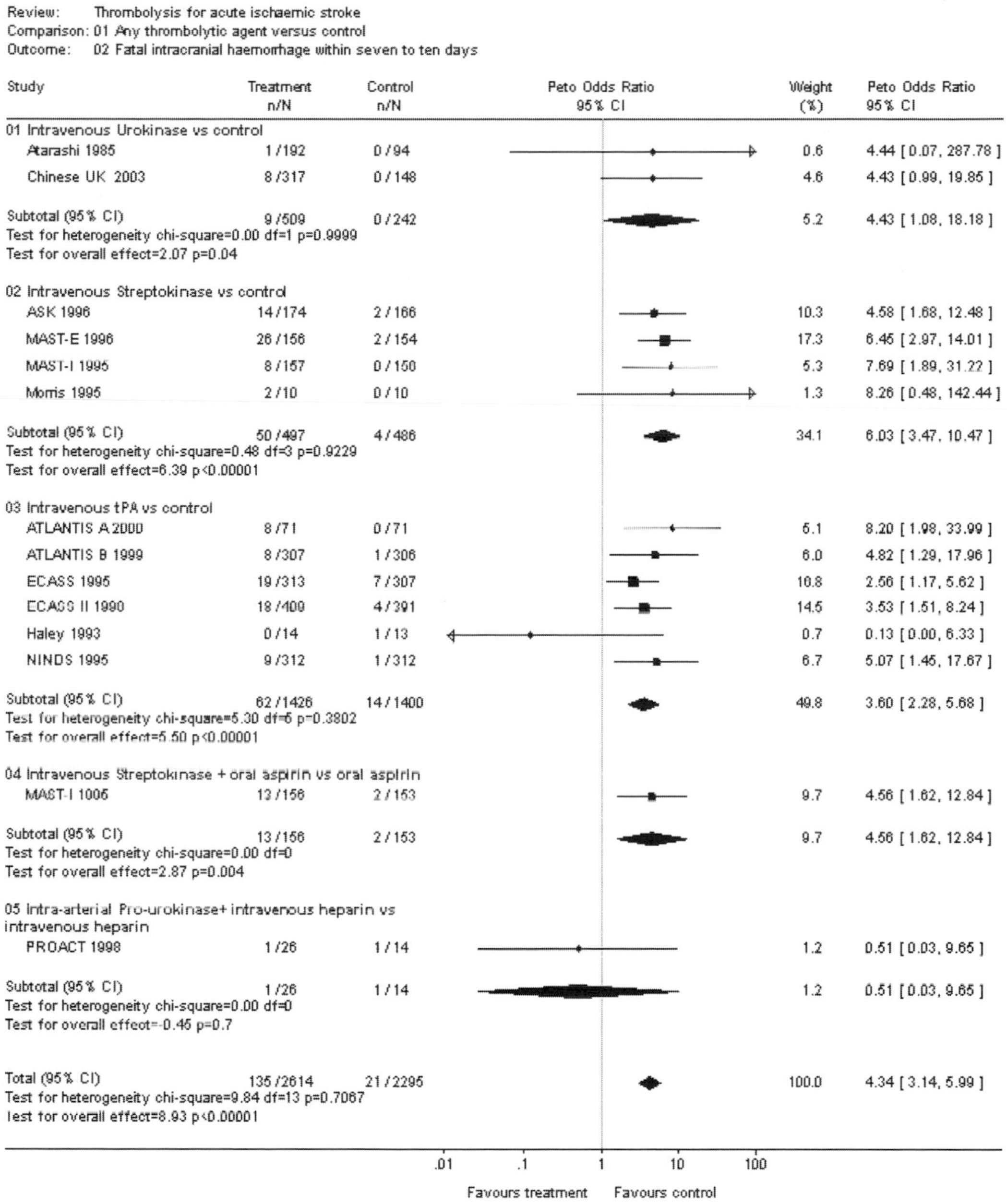

Review: Thrombolysis for acute ischaemic stroke
Comparison: 01 Any thrombolytic agent versus control
Outcome: 02 Fatal intracranial haemorrhage within seven to ten days

Study	Treatment n/N	Control n/N	Peto Odds Ratio 95% CI	Weight (%)	Peto Odds Ratio 95% CI
01 Intravenous Urokinase vs control					
Atarashi 1985	1/192	0/94		0.6	4.44 [0.07, 287.78]
Chinese UK 2003	8/317	0/148		4.6	4.43 [0.99, 19.85]
Subtotal (95% CI)	9/509	0/242		5.2	4.43 [1.08, 18.18]
Test for heterogeneity chi-square=0.00 df=1 p=0.9999					
Test for overall effect=2.07 p=0.04					
02 Intravenous Streptokinase vs control					
ASK 1996	14/174	2/166		10.3	4.58 [1.68, 12.48]
MAST-E 1996	26/156	2/154		17.3	6.45 [2.97, 14.01]
MAST-I 1995	8/157	0/150		5.3	7.69 [1.89, 31.22]
Morris 1995	2/10	0/10		1.3	8.26 [0.48, 142.44]
Subtotal (95% CI)	50/497	4/486		34.1	6.03 [3.47, 10.47]
Test for heterogeneity chi-square=0.48 df=3 p=0.9229					
Test for overall effect=6.39 p<0.00001					
03 Intravenous tPA vs control					
ATLANTIS A 2000	8/71	0/71		5.1	8.20 [1.98, 33.99]
ATLANTIS B 1999	8/307	1/306		6.0	4.82 [1.29, 17.96]
ECASS 1995	19/313	7/307		16.8	2.56 [1.17, 5.62]
ECASS II 1990	18/409	4/391		14.5	3.53 [1.51, 8.24]
Haley 1993	0/14	1/13		0.7	0.13 [0.00, 6.33]
NINDS 1995	9/312	1/312		6.7	5.07 [1.45, 17.67]
Subtotal (95% CI)	62/1426	14/1400		49.8	3.60 [2.28, 5.68]
Test for heterogeneity chi-square=5.30 df=6 p=0.3802					
Test for overall effect=5.50 p<0.00001					
04 Intravenous Streptokinase + oral aspirin vs oral aspirin					
MAST-I 1995	13/156	2/153		9.7	4.56 [1.62, 12.84]
Subtotal (95% CI)	13/156	2/153		9.7	4.56 [1.62, 12.84]
Test for heterogeneity chi-square=0.00 df=0					
Test for overall effect=2.87 p=0.004					
05 Intra-arterial Pro-urokinase+ intravenous heparin vs intravenous heparin					
PROACT 1998	1/26	1/14		1.2	0.51 [0.03, 9.65]
Subtotal (95% CI)	1/26	1/14		1.2	0.51 [0.03, 9.65]
Test for heterogeneity chi-square=0.00 df=0					
Test for overall effect=-0.45 p=0.7					
Total (95% CI)	135/2614	21/2295		100.0	4.34 [3.14, 5.99]
Test for heterogeneity chi-square=9.84 df=13 p=0.7067					
Test for overall effect=8.93 p<0.00001					

.01   .1   1   10   100

Favours treatment   Favours control

Figure 5.2   Forest plot showing the effects of *any thrombolytic agent vs control* within 6 h of onset of ischaemic stroke on *early fatal intracranial haemorrhage (within 7–10 days of randomisation)*. Reproduced from Wardlaw *et al.* (2003), with permission from the authors and John Wiley & Sons Limited. Copyright Cochrane Library, reproduced with permission.

Review: Thrombolysis for acute ischaemic stroke
Comparison: 01 Any thrombolytic agent versus control
Outcome: 03 Symptomatic (including fatal) intracranial haemorrhage within seven to ten days

Study	Treatment n/N	Control n/N	Peto Odds Ratio 95% CI	Weight (%)	Peto Odds Ratio 95% CI
01 Intravenous Urokinase vs control					
x Abe 1981	0 /54	0 /53		0.0	Not estimable
Atarashi 1985	1 /192	1 /94		0.6	0.46 [0.02, 8.81]
Chinese UK 2003	12 /317	3 /148		4.2	1.75 [0.58, 5.29]
Ohtomo 1985	0 /169	1 /181		0.3	0.14 [0.00, 7.31]
Subtotal (95% CI)	13 /732	5 /476		5.1	1.28 [0.47, 3.48]
Test for heterogeneity chi-square=1.96 df=2 p=0.3746					
Test for overall effect=0.48 p=0.6					
02 Intravenous Streptokinase vs control					
ASK 1996	22 /174	4 /166		8.0	4.24 [1.91, 9.43]
MAST-E 1996	33 /156	4 /154		10.9	5.81 [2.93, 11.53]
MAST-I 1995	10 /157	1 /156		3.6	5.39 [1.62, 17.91]
Morris 1995	2 /10	0 /10		0.6	8.26 [0.48, 142.44]
Subtotal (95% CI)	67 /497	9 /486		23.2	5.20 [3.25, 8.32]
Test for heterogeneity chi-square=0.46 df=3 p=0.9286					
Test for overall effect=6.86 p<0.00001					
03 Intravenous tPA vs control					
ATLANTIS A 2000	8 /71	0 /71		2.5	8.20 [1.98, 33.99]
ATLANTIS B 1999	21 /307	4 /306		8.0	4.10 [1.84, 9.13]
ECASS 1995	62 /313	20 /307		23.8	3.18 [2.00, 5.06]
ECASS II 1998	36 /409	13 /391		15.4	2.59 [1.45, 4.61]
Haley 1993	0 /14	1 /13		0.3	0.13 [0.00, 6.33]
JTSG 1993	4 /51	5 /47		2.8	0.72 [0.18, 2.81]
Mori 1992	2 /19	1 /12		0.9	1.27 [0.12, 14.12]
NINDS 1995	20 /312	2 /312		7.1	5.44 [2.32, 12.73]
Subtotal (95% CI)	153 /1496	46 /1459		60.9	3.13 [2.34, 4.19]
Test for heterogeneity chi-square=11.84 df=7 p=0.106					
Test for overall effect=7.71 p<0.00001					
04 Intravenous Streptokinase + oral aspirin vs oral aspirin					
MAST-I 1995	15 /156	3 /153		5.7	4.02 [1.55, 10.40]
Subtotal (95% CI)	15 /156	3 /153		5.7	4.02 [1.55, 10.40]
Test for heterogeneity chi-square=0.00 df=0					
Test for overall effect=2.87 p=0.004					
05 Intra-arterial Pro-urokinase+ intravenous heparin vs intravenous heparin					
PROACT 1998	4 /26	2 /14		1.6	1.09 [0.18, 6.56]
PROACT 2 1999	12 /121	1 /59		3.6	3.39 [1.02, 11.24]
Subtotal (95% CI)	16 /147	3 /73		5.2	2.39 [0.88, 6.47]
Test for heterogeneity chi-square=1.06 df=1 p=0.3025					
Test for overall effect=1.71 p=0.09					
Total (95% CI)	264 /3028	66 /2647		100.0	3.37 [2.68, 4.22]
Test for heterogeneity chi-square=23.01 df=17 p=0.1489					
Test for overall effect=10.50 p<0.00001					

.01   .1   1   10   100

Favours treatment   Favours control

Figure 5.3   Forest plot showing the effects of *any thrombolytic agent vs control* within 6 h of ischaemic stroke on *early symptomatic (including fatal) intracranial haemorrhage (within 7–10 days of randomisation)*. Reproduced from Wardlaw *et al.* (2003), with permission from the authors and John Wiley & Sons Limited. Copyright Cochrane Library, reproduced with permission.

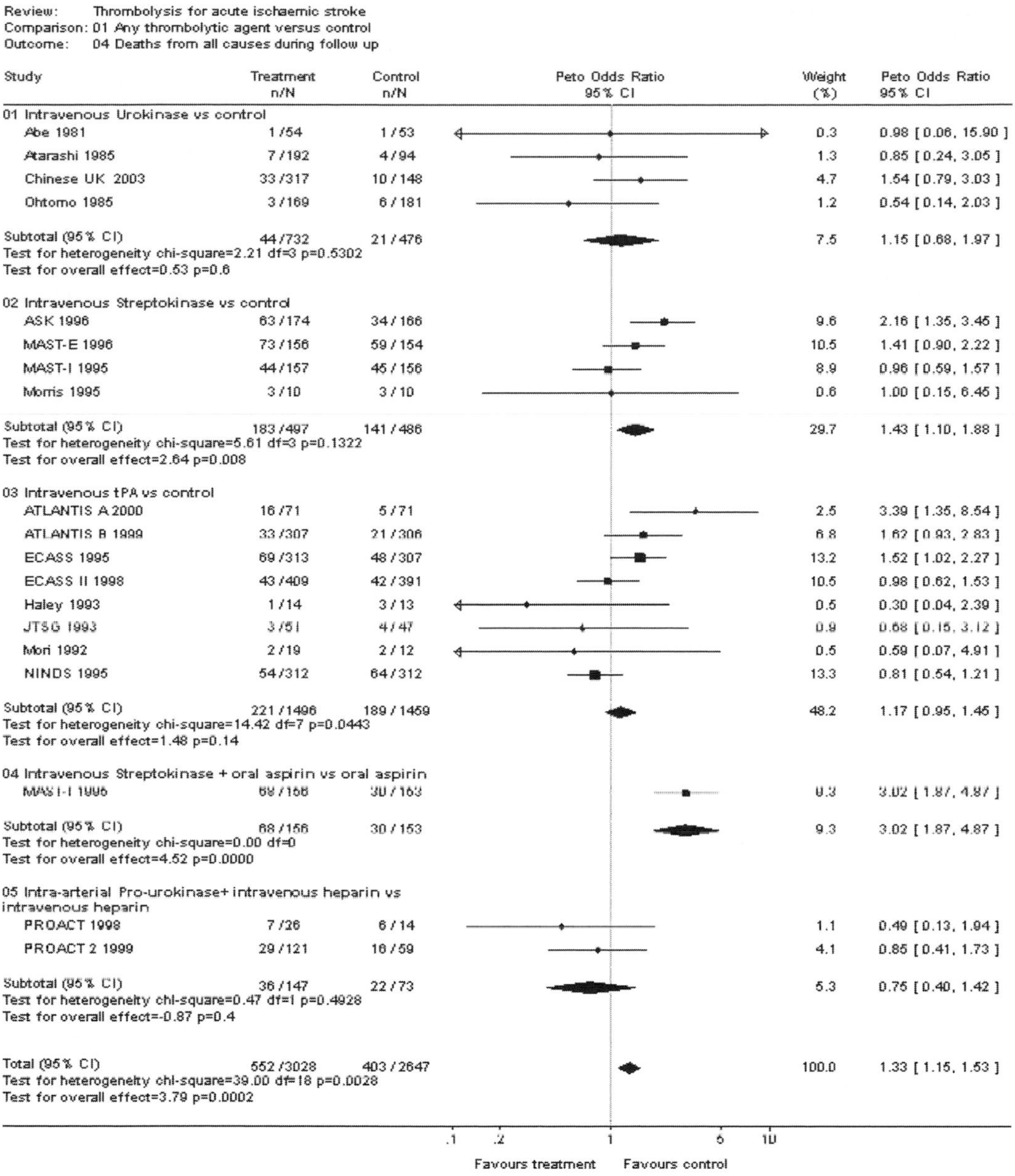

Review: Thrombolysis for acute ischaemic stroke
Comparison: 01 Any thrombolytic agent versus control
Outcome: 04 Deaths from all causes during follow up

Study	Treatment n/N	Control n/N	Peto Odds Ratio 95% CI	Weight (%)	Peto Odds Ratio 95% CI
01 Intravenous Urokinase vs control					
Abe 1981	1 /54	1 /53		0.3	0.98 [0.06, 15.90]
Atarashi 1985	7 /192	4 /94		1.3	0.85 [0.24, 3.05]
Chinese UK 2003	33 /317	10 /148		4.7	1.54 [0.79, 3.03]
Ohtomo 1985	3 /169	6 /181		1.2	0.54 [0.14, 2.03]
Subtotal (95% CI)	44 /732	21 /476		7.5	1.15 [0.68, 1.97]
Test for heterogeneity chi-square=2.21 df=3 p=0.5302					
Test for overall effect=0.53 p=0.6					
02 Intravenous Streptokinase vs control					
ASK 1996	63 /174	34 /166		9.6	2.16 [1.35, 3.45]
MAST-E 1996	73 /156	59 /154		10.5	1.41 [0.90, 2.22]
MAST-I 1995	44 /157	45 /156		8.9	0.96 [0.59, 1.57]
Morris 1995	3 /10	3 /10		0.6	1.00 [0.15, 6.45]
Subtotal (95% CI)	183 /497	141 /486		29.7	1.43 [1.10, 1.88]
Test for heterogeneity chi-square=5.61 df=3 p=0.1322					
Test for overall effect=2.64 p=0.008					
03 Intravenous tPA vs control					
ATLANTIS A 2000	16 /71	5 /71		2.5	3.39 [1.35, 8.54]
ATLANTIS B 1999	33 /307	21 /306		6.8	1.62 [0.93, 2.83]
ECASS 1995	69 /313	48 /307		13.2	1.52 [1.02, 2.27]
ECASS II 1998	43 /409	42 /391		10.5	0.98 [0.62, 1.53]
Haley 1993	1 /14	3 /13		0.5	0.30 [0.04, 2.39]
JTSG 1993	3 /51	4 /47		0.9	0.68 [0.15, 3.12]
Mori 1992	2 /19	2 /12		0.5	0.59 [0.07, 4.91]
NINDS 1995	54 /312	64 /312		13.3	0.81 [0.54, 1.21]
Subtotal (95% CI)	221 /1496	189 /1459		48.2	1.17 [0.95, 1.45]
Test for heterogeneity chi-square=14.42 df=7 p=0.0443					
Test for overall effect=1.48 p=0.14					
04 Intravenous Streptokinase + oral aspirin vs oral aspirin					
MAST-I 1995	68 /156	30 /153		9.3	3.02 [1.87, 4.87]
Subtotal (95% CI)	68 /156	30 /153		9.3	3.02 [1.87, 4.87]
Test for heterogeneity chi-square=0.00 df=0					
Test for overall effect=4.52 p=0.0000					
05 Intra-arterial Pro-urokinase+ intravenous heparin vs intravenous heparin					
PROACT 1998	7 /26	6 /14		1.1	0.49 [0.13, 1.94]
PROACT 2 1999	29 /121	16 /59		4.1	0.85 [0.41, 1.73]
Subtotal (95% CI)	36 /147	22 /73		5.3	0.75 [0.40, 1.42]
Test for heterogeneity chi-square=0.47 df=1 p=0.4928					
Test for overall effect=-0.87 p=0.4					
Total (95% CI)	552 /3028	403 /2647		100.0	1.33 [1.15, 1.53]
Test for heterogeneity chi-square=39.00 df=18 p=0.0028					
Test for overall effect=3.79 p=0.0002					

.1   .2   1   5   10

Favours treatment   Favours control

Figure 5.4   Forest plot showing the effects of *any thrombolytic agent vs control* within 6 h of onset of ischaemic stroke on *death from all causes during follow-up.* Reproduced from Wardlaw *et al.* (2003), with permission from the authors and John Wiley & Sons Limited. Copyright Cochrane Library, reproduced with permission.

There was no significant heterogeneity of treatment effect among the trials ($P = 0.09$), indicating that the favourable treatment effect was qualitatively the same (i.e. in the same direction) in all trials. This is reflected in the subgroup of six trials using i.v. rt-PA ($n = 2830$ patients) where there was a similar reduction in death or

Review: Thrombolysis for acute ischaemic stroke
Comparison: 01 Any thrombolytic agent versus control
Outcome: 05 Death or dependency at the end of follow-up

Study	Treatment n/N	Control n/N	Peto Odds Ratio 95% CI	Weight (%)	Peto Odds Ratio 95% CI
01 Intravenous Urokinase vs control					
Chinese UK 2003	127 /317	61 / 148		8.8	0.95 [0.64, 1.42]
Subtotal (95% CI)	127 /317	61 / 148		8.8	0.95 [0.64, 1.42]
Test for heterogeneity chi-square=0.00 df=0					
Test for overall effect=-0.24 p=0.8					
02 Intravenous Streptokinase vs control					
ASK 1996	84 /174	74 / 166		7.7	1.16 [0.76, 1.78]
MAST-E 1996	124 /156	126 / 154		4.4	0.86 [0.49, 1.51]
MAST-I 1995	97 /157	106 / 156		6.5	0.76 [0.48, 1.21]
Morris 1995	6 /10	5 / 10		0.5	1.47 [0.26, 8.18]
Subtotal (95% CI)	311 /497	311 / 486		19.0	0.94 [0.72, 1.24]
Test for heterogeneity chi-square=2.06 df=3 p=0.5607					
Test for overall effect=-0.41 p=0.7					
03 Intravenous tPA vs control					
ATLANTIS A 2000	64 /71	56 / 71		1.7	2.35 [0.95, 5.82]
ATLANTIS B 1999	141 /307	135 / 306		13.7	1.08 [0.78, 1.48]
ECASS 1995	171 /313	185 / 307		13.7	0.79 [0.58, 1.09]
ECASS II 1998	187 /409	211 / 391		18.1	0.72 [0.55, 0.95]
Mori 1992	11 /19	10 / 12		0.6	0.32 [0.07, 1.48]
NINDS 1995	155 /312	192 / 312		13.9	0.62 [0.45, 0.85]
Subtotal (95% CI)	729 /1431	789 / 1399		61.7	0.80 [0.69, 0.93]
Test for heterogeneity chi-square=13.23 df=5 p=0.0214					
Test for overall effect=-2.97 p=0.003					
04 Intravenous Streptokinase + oral aspirin vs oral aspirin					
MAST-I 1995	99 /156	94 / 153		6.6	1.09 [0.69, 1.73]
Subtotal (95% CI)	99 /156	94 / 153		6.6	1.09 [0.69, 1.73]
Test for heterogeneity chi-square=0.00 df=0					
Test for overall effect=0.37 p=0.7					
05 Intra-arterial Pro-urokinase + intravenous heparin vs intravenous heparin					
PROACT 1998	18 /26	11 / 14		0.7	0.63 [0.15, 2.66]
PROACT 2 1999	73 /121	44 / 59		3.3	0.54 [0.28, 1.03]
Subtotal (95% CI)	91 /147	55 / 73		3.9	0.55 [0.31, 1.00]
Test for heterogeneity chi-square=0.04 df=1 p=0.8367					
Test for overall effect=-1.97 p=0.05					
Total (95% CI)	1357 /2548	1310 / 2259		100.0	0.84 [0.75, 0.95]
Test for heterogeneity chi-square=20.07 df=13 p=0.0934					
Test for overall effect=-2.88 p=0.004					

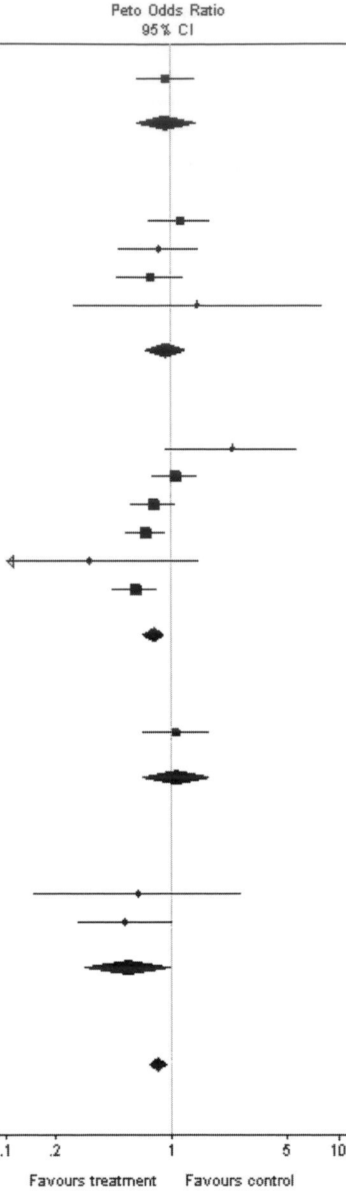

.1   .2   1   5   10

Favours treatment   Favours control

Figure 5.5   Forest plot showing the effects of *any thrombolytic agent vs control* within 6 h of onset of ischaemic stroke on *death or dependency at the end of follow-up.* Reproduced from Wardlaw *et al.* (2003), with permission from the authors and John Wiley & Sons Limited. Copyright Cochrane Library, reproduced with permission.

dependency (OR: 0.80, 95% CI: 0.69–0.93; $2P = 0.003$), equivalent to 55 (95% CI: 18–92) fewer dead or dependent patients per 1000 treated. However, there was significant heterogeneity of the treatment effect among trials using rt-PA ($P = 0.02$).

Results for subgroups of patients and thrombolytic therapies

Subgroup analyses were undertaken to explore whether the heterogeneity between the trials may have been due to variations in time to treatment, thrombolytic drug used, the concomitant use of aspirin and heparin, and the severity of the stroke (both between trials and between treatment groups within trials).

Patients treated with any thrombolytic drug *within 3 h* of ischaemic stroke

Death

Data from 10 trials involving 1338 patients (of which the National Institute of Neurological Disorders and Stroke (NINDS) 1995 trial contributes 624 patients (47%)) indicate that thrombolysis with any thrombolytic drug *within 3 h* of ischaemic stroke was also associated with a modest, non-statistically significant excess risk of *death* (20.9% thrombolysis with all agents, 19.4% control; OR: 1.13, 95% CI: 0.86–1.48), equivalent to 20 extra deaths per 1000 patients treated (95% CI: 23 less to 69 more) compared with control (Fig. 5.6) (Wardlaw *et al.*, 2003). There was statistically significant heterogeneity among the trials ($P = 0.0008$).

Among the trials which reported data for treatment within 3 h and after 3 h, the effects on death were similar when thrombolytic treatment was given within 3 h (OR: 1.58, 95% CI: 1.08–2.31) and between 3 and 6 h (OR: 1.59, 95% CI: 1.32–1.92) after stroke (Fig. 5.7) (Wardlaw *et al.*, 2003).

Death or dependency

For patients treated with any thrombolytic agent *within 3 h* of ischaemic stroke, data from six trials indicate that allocation to any thrombolytic therapy was more effective in reducing *death or dependency* (49.7% thrombolysis with all agents, 60.3% control; OR: 0.66, 95% CI: 0.53–0.83; $2P = 0.0003$), equivalent to 102 (95% CI: 45–157) fewer dead or dependent patients per 1000 patients treated within 3 h with thrombolysis compared with control (Fig. 5.8) (Wardlaw *et al.*, 2003).

Among the trials which reported data for treatment within 3 h and after 3 h, the effects of death and dependency were similar when thrombolytic treatment was given within 3 h (OR: 0.71, 95% CI: 0.52–0.96) or between 3 and 6 h (OR: 0.95, 95% CI: 0.82–1.10), although there was a trend towards better outcome with earlier treatment (Fig. 5.9) (Wardlaw *et al.*, 2003).

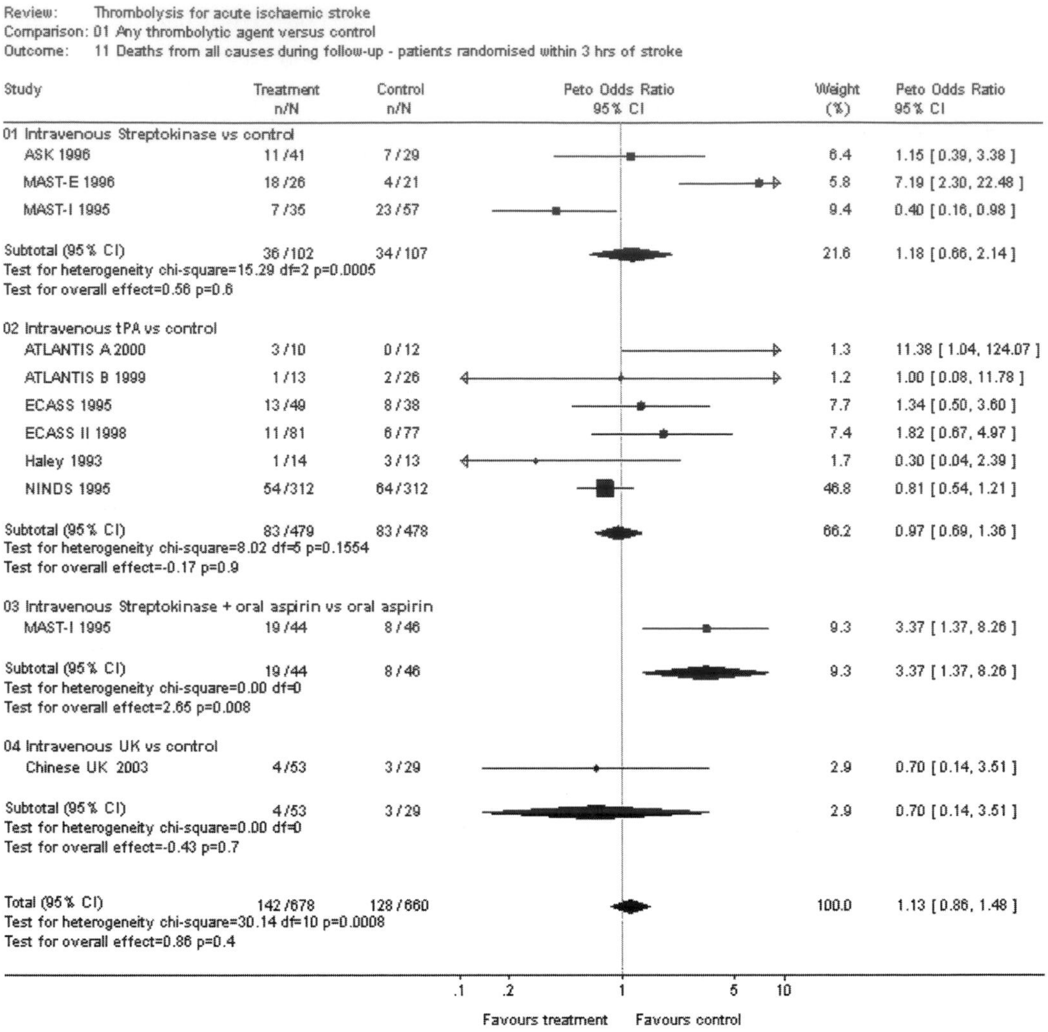

Figure 5.6   Forest plot showing the effects of *any thrombolytic agent vs control within 3 h* of onset of ischaemic stroke on *death from all causes during follow-up.* Reproduced from Wardlaw *et al.* (2003), with permission from the authors and John Wiley & Sons Limited. Copyright Cochrane Library, reproduced with permission.

Patients treated with rt-PA *within 3 h* of ischaemic stroke

Death

For patients treated with *rt-PA within 3 h*, there was no difference in *deaths* (OR: 0.97, 95% CI: 0.69–1.36; $P = 0.9$); for every 1000 patients treated, there were no fewer or more deaths (95% CI: 49 fewer to 47 more) (Fig. 5.6).

Among the trials which reported data for treatment within 3 h and after 3 h, the effects on death were similar for patients treated within 3 h with rt-PA (OR: 1.75,

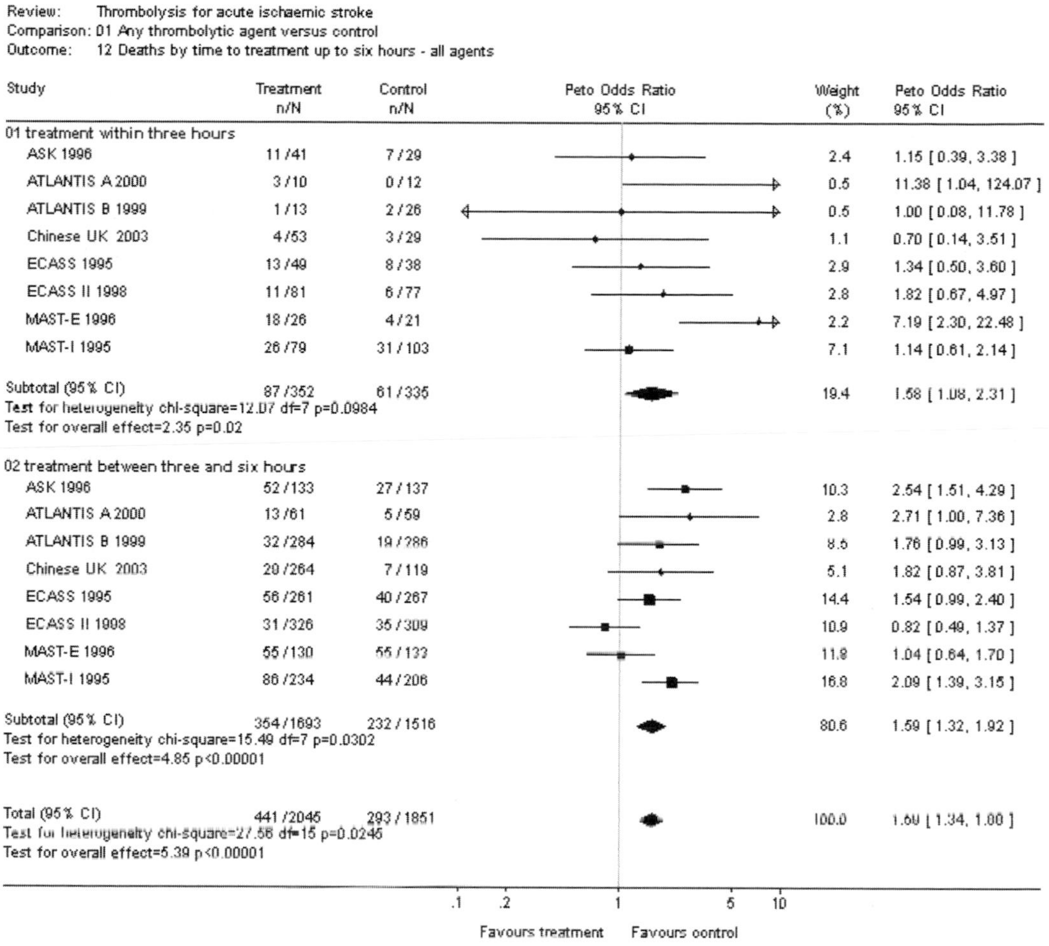

Review: Thrombolysis for acute ischaemic stroke
Comparison: 01 Any thrombolytic agent versus control
Outcome: 12 Deaths by time to treatment up to six hours - all agents

Study	Treatment n/N	Control n/N	Peto Odds Ratio 95% CI	Weight (%)	Peto Odds Ratio 95% CI
01 treatment within three hours					
ASK 1996	11/41	7/29		2.4	1.15 [0.39, 3.38]
ATLANTIS A 2000	3/10	0/12		0.5	11.38 [1.04, 124.07]
ATLANTIS B 1999	1/13	2/26		0.5	1.00 [0.08, 11.78]
Chinese UK 2003	4/53	3/29		1.1	0.70 [0.14, 3.51]
ECASS 1995	13/49	8/38		2.9	1.34 [0.50, 3.60]
ECASS II 1998	11/81	6/77		2.8	1.82 [0.67, 4.97]
MAST-E 1996	18/26	4/21		2.2	7.19 [2.30, 22.48]
MAST-I 1995	26/79	31/103		7.1	1.14 [0.61, 2.14]
Subtotal (95% CI)	87/352	61/335		19.4	1.58 [1.08, 2.31]
Test for heterogeneity chi-square=12.07 df=7 p=0.0984					
Test for overall effect=2.35 p=0.02					
02 treatment between three and six hours					
ASK 1996	52/133	27/137		10.3	2.54 [1.51, 4.29]
ATLANTIS A 2000	13/61	5/59		2.8	2.71 [1.00, 7.36]
ATLANTIS B 1999	32/284	19/286		8.5	1.76 [0.99, 3.13]
Chinese UK 2003	20/264	7/119		5.1	1.82 [0.87, 3.81]
ECASS 1995	56/261	40/267		14.4	1.54 [0.99, 2.40]
ECASS II 1998	31/326	35/309		10.9	0.82 [0.49, 1.37]
MAST-E 1996	55/130	55/133		11.9	1.04 [0.64, 1.70]
MAST-I 1995	86/234	44/206		16.8	2.09 [1.39, 3.15]
Subtotal (95% CI)	354/1693	232/1516		80.6	1.59 [1.32, 1.92]
Test for heterogeneity chi-square=15.49 df=7 p=0.0302					
Test for overall effect=4.85 p<0.00001					
Total (95% CI)	441/2045	293/1851		100.0	1.60 [1.34, 1.90]
Test for heterogeneity chi-square=27.56 df=15 p=0.0245					
Test for overall effect=5.39 p<0.00001					

.1   .2   1   5   10

Favours treatment   Favours control

Figure 5.7   Forest plot showing the effects of *any thrombolytic agent vs control* within 6 h of onset of ischaemic stroke on *death from all causes during follow-up, according to time to treatment up to 6 h*. Reproduced from Wardlaw *et al.* (2003), with permission from the authors and John Wiley & Sons Limited. Copyright Cochrane Library, reproduced with permission.

95% CI: 0.91–3.36) and between 3 and 6 h (OR: 1.38, 95% CI: 1.05–1.82) (Fig. 5.10) (Wardlaw *et al.*, 2003).

Symptomatic intracerebral haemorrhage

Data from four rt-PA trials indicate that there was an excess of symptomatic intracerebral haemorrhage (ICH) with rt-PA within 3 h (OR: 3.40, 95% CI: 1.48–7.84) (Fig. 5.11). This was not different to the increase in symptomatic haemorrhages in patients randomised to rt-PA between 3 and 6 h (OR: 3.14, 95% CI: 2.21–4.47).

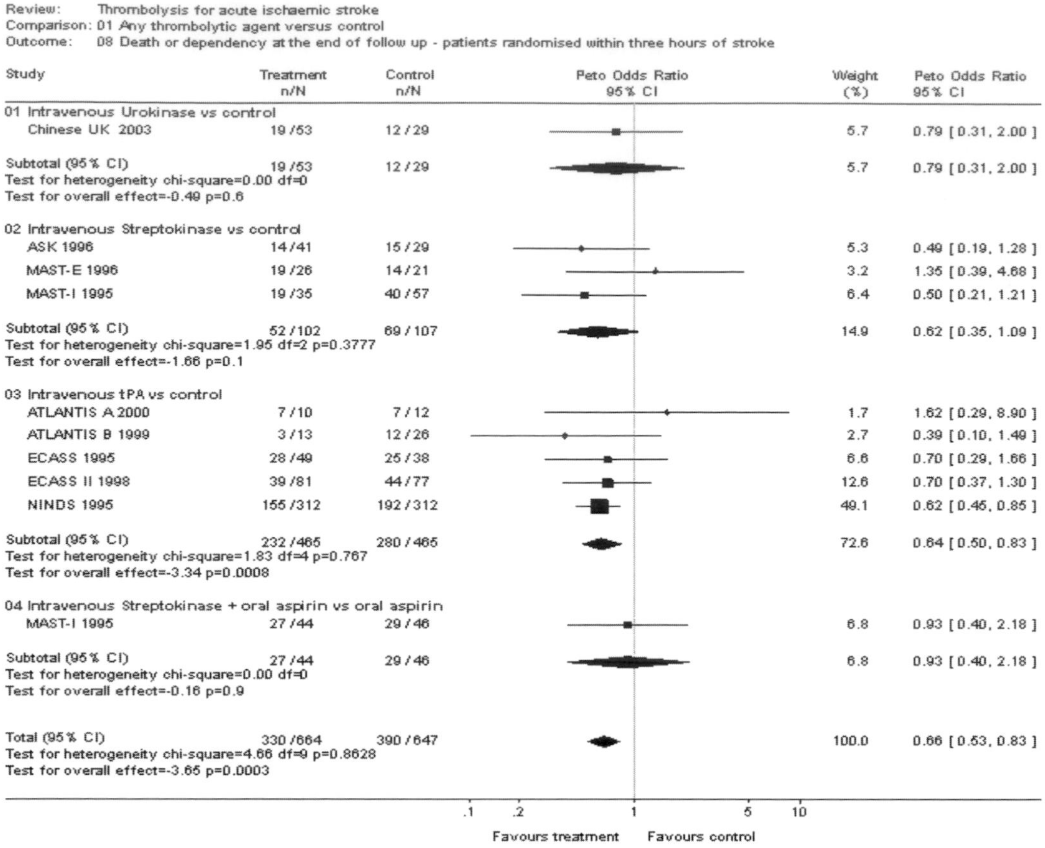

Review: Thrombolysis for acute ischaemic stroke
Comparison: 01 Any thrombolytic agent versus control
Outcome: 08 Death or dependency at the end of follow up - patients randomised within three hours of stroke

Study	Treatment n/N	Control n/N	Peto Odds Ratio 95% CI	Weight (%)	Peto Odds Ratio 95% CI
01 Intravenous Urokinase vs control					
Chinese UK 2003	19 /53	12 / 29		5.7	0.79 [0.31, 2.00]
Subtotal (95% CI)	19 /53	12 / 29		5.7	0.79 [0.31, 2.00]
Test for heterogeneity chi-square=0.00 df=0					
Test for overall effect=-0.49 p=0.6					
02 Intravenous Streptokinase vs control					
ASK 1996	14 /41	15 / 29		5.3	0.49 [0.19, 1.28]
MAST-E 1996	19 /26	14 / 21		3.2	1.35 [0.39, 4.68]
MAST-I 1995	19 /35	40 / 57		6.4	0.50 [0.21, 1.21]
Subtotal (95% CI)	52 /102	69 / 107		14.9	0.62 [0.35, 1.09]
Test for heterogeneity chi-square=1.95 df=2 p=0.3777					
Test for overall effect=-1.66 p=0.1					
03 Intravenous tPA vs control					
ATLANTIS A 2000	7 /10	7 / 12		1.7	1.62 [0.29, 8.90]
ATLANTIS B 1999	3 /13	12 / 26		2.7	0.39 [0.10, 1.49]
ECASS 1995	28 /49	25 / 38		6.6	0.70 [0.29, 1.66]
ECASS II 1998	39 /81	44 / 77		12.6	0.70 [0.37, 1.30]
NINDS 1995	155 /312	192 / 312		49.1	0.62 [0.45, 0.85]
Subtotal (95% CI)	232 /465	280 / 465		72.6	0.64 [0.50, 0.83]
Test for heterogeneity chi-square=1.83 df=4 p=0.767					
Test for overall effect=-3.34 p=0.0008					
04 Intravenous Streptokinase + oral aspirin vs oral aspirin					
MAST-I 1995	27 /44	29 / 46		6.8	0.93 [0.40, 2.18]
Subtotal (95% CI)	27 /44	29 / 46		6.8	0.93 [0.40, 2.18]
Test for heterogeneity chi-square=0.00 df=0					
Test for overall effect=-0.16 p=0.9					
Total (95% CI)	330 /664	390 / 647		100.0	0.66 [0.53, 0.83]
Test for heterogeneity chi-square=4.66 df=9 p=0.8628					
Test for overall effect=-3.65 p=0.0003					

.1   .2   1   5   10

Favours treatment   Favours control

Figure 5.8   Forest plot showing the effects of *any thrombolytic agent vs control within 3 h* of onset of ischaemic stroke on *death or dependency and the end of follow-up.* Reproduced from Wardlaw *et al.* (2003), with permission from the authors and John Wiley & Sons Limited. Copyright Cochrane Library, reproduced with permission.

Death or dependency

For patients treated with rt-PA *within 3 h* of ischaemic stroke, allocation to early rt-PA was more effective in reducing *death or dependency* (OR: 0.64, 95% CI: 0.5–0.83) (Fig. 5.8) (Wardlaw *et al.*, 2003).

Comparing early treatment within 3 h with later treatment within 3–6 h, the effect of treatment with rt-PA on death and dependency was similar when given within 3 h (OR: 0.69, 95% CI: 0.44–1.09) and more than 3 h after stroke (OR: 0.88, 95% CI: 0.73–1.06) (Fig. 5.12). This indirect comparison of the association between time to treatment and outcome may be confounded by some other factor(s), such as stroke severity.

However, a pooled analysis of the ATLANTIS (Alteplase Thrombolysis for Acute Noninterventional Therapy in Ischemic Stroke) trial, European Cooperative Acute

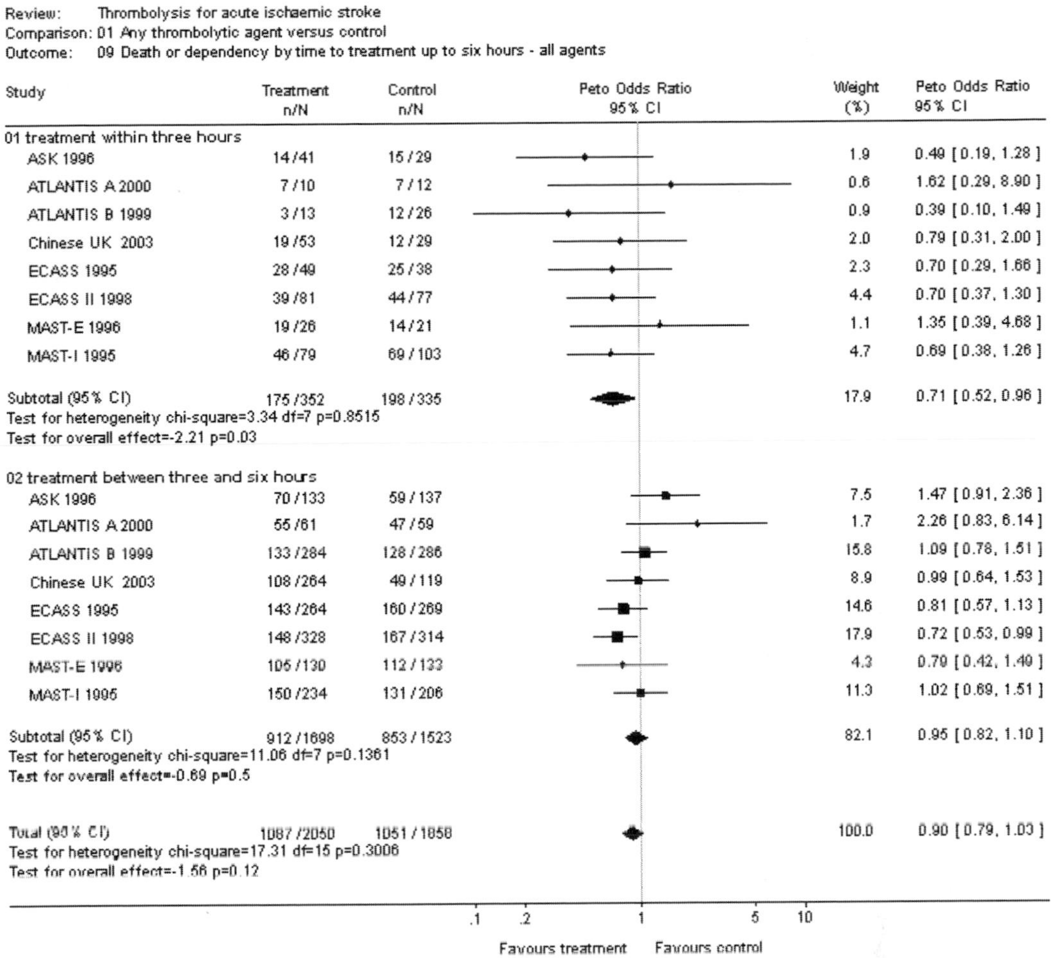

Review: Thrombolysis for acute ischaemic stroke
Comparison: 01 Any thrombolytic agent versus control
Outcome: 09 Death or dependency by time to treatment up to six hours - all agents

Study	Treatment n/N	Control n/N	Peto Odds Ratio 95% CI	Weight (%)	Peto Odds Ratio 95% CI
01 treatment within three hours					
ASK 1996	14/41	15/29		1.9	0.49 [0.19, 1.28]
ATLANTIS A 2000	7/10	7/12		0.6	1.62 [0.29, 8.90]
ATLANTIS B 1999	3/13	12/26		0.9	0.39 [0.10, 1.49]
Chinese UK 2003	19/53	12/29		2.0	0.79 [0.31, 2.00]
ECASS 1995	28/49	25/38		2.3	0.70 [0.29, 1.66]
ECASS II 1998	39/81	44/77		4.4	0.70 [0.37, 1.30]
MAST-E 1996	19/26	14/21		1.1	1.35 [0.39, 4.68]
MAST-I 1995	46/79	69/103		4.7	0.69 [0.38, 1.26]
Subtotal (95% CI)	175/352	198/335		17.9	0.71 [0.52, 0.96]

Test for heterogeneity chi-square=3.34 df=7 p=0.8515
Test for overall effect=-2.21 p=0.03

Study	Treatment n/N	Control n/N	Peto Odds Ratio 95% CI	Weight (%)	Peto Odds Ratio 95% CI
02 treatment between three and six hours					
ASK 1996	70/133	59/137		7.5	1.47 [0.91, 2.36]
ATLANTIS A 2000	55/61	47/59		1.7	2.26 [0.83, 6.14]
ATLANTIS B 1999	133/284	128/286		15.8	1.09 [0.78, 1.51]
Chinese UK 2003	108/264	49/119		8.9	0.99 [0.64, 1.53]
ECASS 1995	143/264	160/269		14.6	0.81 [0.57, 1.13]
ECASS II 1998	148/328	167/314		17.9	0.72 [0.53, 0.99]
MAST-E 1996	105/130	112/133		4.3	0.79 [0.42, 1.49]
MAST-I 1995	150/234	131/206		11.3	1.02 [0.69, 1.51]
Subtotal (95% CI)	912/1698	853/1523		82.1	0.95 [0.82, 1.10]

Test for heterogeneity chi-square=11.06 df=7 p=0.1361
Test for overall effect=-0.69 p=0.5

| Total (95% CI) | 1087/2050 | 1051/1858 | | 100.0 | 0.90 [0.79, 1.03] |

Test for heterogeneity chi-square=17.31 df=15 p=0.3006
Test for overall effect=-1.56 p=0.12

.1   .2   1   5   10

Favours treatment   Favours control

Figure 5.9   Forest plot showing the effects of *any thrombolytic agent vs control* within 6 h of onset of ischaemic stroke on *death or dependency from all causes during follow-up, according to time to treatment up to 6 h.* Reproduced from Wardlaw *et al.* (2003), with permission from the authors and John Wiley & Sons Limited. Copyright Cochrane Library, reproduced with permission.

Stroke Study (ECASS) and NINDS rt-PA stroke trials indicated that the sooner that rt-PA is given to stroke patients the greater the benefit, especially if started within 90 min (the ATLANTIS, ECASS and NINDS rt-PA Study Group Investigators, 2004). The odds of a favourable outcome at 3 months increased as the interval from stroke onset to start of treatment (onset to treatment time (OTT)) decreased ($P = 0.005$). The odds of a favourable outcome were 2.8 (95% CI: 1.8–4.50) for 0–90 min, 1.6 (1.1–2.2) for 91–180 min, 1.4 (1.1–1.9) for 181–270 min, and 1.2 (0.9–1.5) for 271–360 min in favour of the rt-PA group. Haemorrhage was not associated with OTT, but was associated with rt-PA treatment and increasing age.

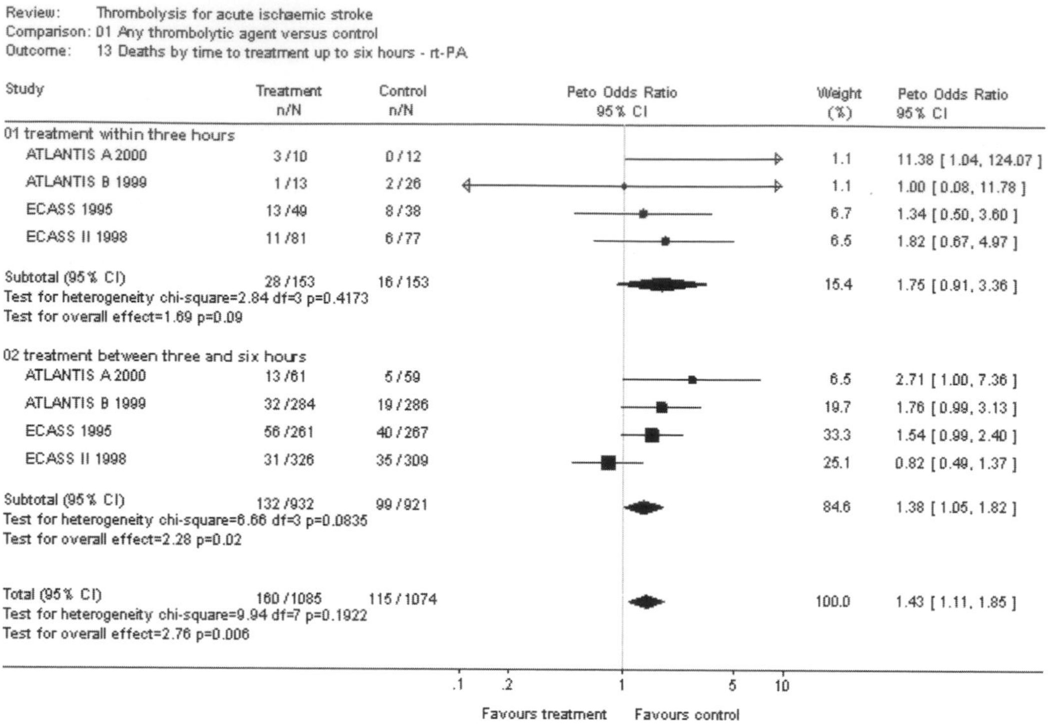

Review: Thrombolysis for acute ischaemic stroke
Comparison: 01 Any thrombolytic agent versus control
Outcome: 13 Deaths by time to treatment up to six hours - rt-PA

Study	Treatment n/N	Control n/N	Peto Odds Ratio 95% CI	Weight (%)	Peto Odds Ratio 95% CI
01 treatment within three hours					
ATLANTIS A 2000	3 / 10	0 / 12		1.1	11.38 [1.04, 124.07]
ATLANTIS B 1999	1 / 13	2 / 26		1.1	1.00 [0.08, 11.78]
ECASS 1995	13 / 49	8 / 38		6.7	1.34 [0.50, 3.60]
ECASS II 1998	11 / 81	6 / 77		6.5	1.82 [0.67, 4.97]
Subtotal (95% CI)	28 / 153	16 / 153		15.4	1.75 [0.91, 3.36]
Test for heterogeneity chi-square=2.84 df=3 p=0.4173					
Test for overall effect=1.69 p=0.09					
02 treatment between three and six hours					
ATLANTIS A 2000	13 / 61	5 / 59		6.5	2.71 [1.00, 7.36]
ATLANTIS B 1999	32 / 284	19 / 286		19.7	1.76 [0.99, 3.13]
ECASS 1995	56 / 261	40 / 267		33.3	1.54 [0.99, 2.40]
ECASS II 1998	31 / 326	35 / 309		25.1	0.82 [0.49, 1.37]
Subtotal (95% CI)	132 / 932	99 / 921		84.6	1.38 [1.05, 1.82]
Test for heterogeneity chi-square=6.66 df=3 p=0.0835					
Test for overall effect=2.28 p=0.02					
Total (95% CI)	160 / 1085	115 / 1074		100.0	1.43 [1.11, 1.85]
Test for heterogeneity chi-square=9.94 df=7 p=0.1922					
Test for overall effect=2.76 p=0.006					

.1   .2   1   5   10

Favours treatment   Favours control

Figure 5.10   Forest plot showing the effects of *t-PA vs control* within 6 h of onset of ischaemic stroke on *death at end of follow-up according to time to treatment up to 6 h.* Reproduced from Wardlaw *et al.* (2003), with permission from the authors and John Wiley & Sons Limited. Copyright Cochrane Library, reproduced with permission.

Different thrombolytic drugs

Different thrombolytic agents (rt-PA vs UK; tissue-cultured UK vs conventional UK) were compared directly in three trials ($n = 688$ patients) (Mielke *et al.*, 2004). No statistically significant difference was shown between different thrombolytic drugs tested.

Indirect, non-random comparisons suggest that trials testing i.v. rt-PA may be associated with slightly less hazard and more benefit than other drugs when given up to 6 h after stroke, but these are non-random comparisons – death within the first 10 days (OR: 1.24, 95% CI: 0.85–1.81), death at the end of follow-up (OR: 1.17, 95% CI: 0.95–1.45), dead or dependent at the end of follow-up (OR: 0.80, 95% CI: 0.69–0.93) (Wardlaw *et al.*, 2003).

Desmoteplase

Another thrombolytic agent, which is being evaluated currently, is recombinant desmodus salivary plasminogen activator α-1 (rDSPA α-1 or desmoteplase). It is theoretically attractive because of its high fibrin specificity, nonactivation by β-amyloid,

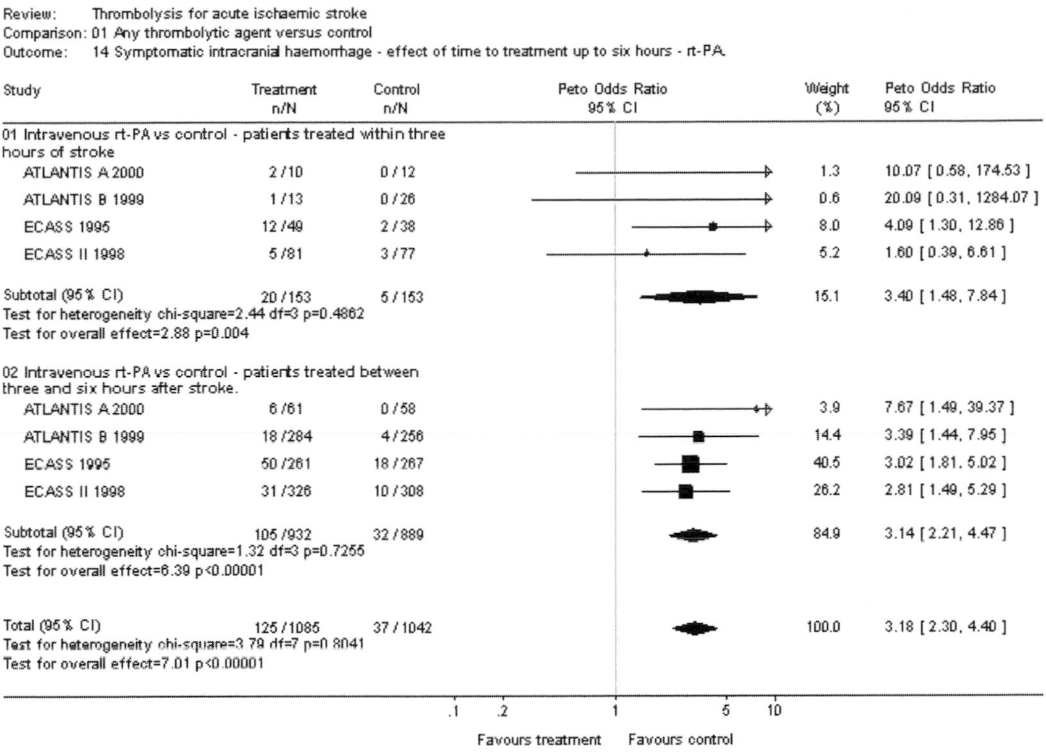

Review: Thrombolysis for acute ischaemic stroke
Comparison: 01 Any thrombolytic agent versus control
Outcome: 14 Symptomatic intracranial haemorrhage - effect of time to treatment up to six hours - rt-PA

Study	Treatment n/N	Control n/N	Peto Odds Ratio 95% CI	Weight (%)	Peto Odds Ratio 95% CI
01 Intravenous rt-PA vs control - patients treated within three hours of stroke					
ATLANTIS A 2000	2 / 10	0 / 12		1.3	10.07 [0.58, 174.53]
ATLANTIS B 1999	1 / 13	0 / 26		0.6	20.09 [0.31, 1284.07]
ECASS 1995	12 / 49	2 / 38		8.0	4.09 [1.30, 12.86]
ECASS II 1998	5 / 81	3 / 77		5.2	1.60 [0.39, 6.61]
Subtotal (95% CI)	20 / 153	5 / 153		15.1	3.40 [1.48, 7.84]

Test for heterogeneity chi-square=2.44 df=3 p=0.4862
Test for overall effect=2.88 p=0.004

02 Intravenous rt-PA vs control - patients treated between three and six hours after stroke.					
ATLANTIS A 2000	6 / 61	0 / 58		3.9	7.67 [1.49, 39.37]
ATLANTIS B 1999	18 / 284	4 / 256		14.4	3.39 [1.44, 7.95]
ECASS 1995	50 / 261	18 / 267		40.5	3.02 [1.81, 5.02]
ECASS II 1998	31 / 326	10 / 308		26.2	2.81 [1.49, 5.29]
Subtotal (95% CI)	105 / 932	32 / 889		84.9	3.14 [2.21, 4.47]

Test for heterogeneity chi-square=1.32 df=3 p=0.7255
Test for overall effect=6.39 p<0.00001

Total (95% CI)	125 / 1085	37 / 1042		100.0	3.18 [2.30, 4.40]

Test for heterogeneity chi-square=3.79 df=7 p=0.8041
Test for overall effect=7.01 p<0.00001

.1   .2   1   5   10

Favours treatment   Favours control

Figure 5.11   Forest plot showing the effects of *t-PA vs control* within 6 h of onset of ischaemic stroke on *symptomatic intracranial haemorrhage* during follow-up according to *time to treatment*. Reproduced from Wardlaw *et al.* (2003), with permission from the authors and John Wiley & Sons Limited. Copyright Cochrane Library, reproduced with permission.

long terminal half-life and absence of neurotoxicity compared with rt-PA (Liberatore *et al.*, 2003; Reddrop *et al.*, 2005).

The Desmoteplase in Acute Ischaemic Stroke Trial (DIAS) was a double-blind, placebo-controlled, randomised, dose-finding phase II trial which showed that i.v. desmoteplase in doses of 62.5 µg/kg ($n = 15$ patients), 90 µg/kg ($n = 15$ patients) and 125 µg/kg ($n = 15$ patients), administered 3–9 h after acute ischaemic stroke in 45 patients with focal cerebral perfusion/diffusion mismatch was associated with a higher rate of reperfusion (up to 71% with 125 µg/kg vs 19.2% with placebo, $P = 0.0012$), and better clinical outcome at 90 days (up to 60% with 125 µg/kg vs 22.2% with placebo, $P = 0.009$) compared with 11 patients assigned placebo. Symptomatic intracranial haemorrhage occurred in one of the 45 patients assigned desmoteplase and none of the 11 patients assigned placebo (Hacke *et al.*, 2005). These data support the concept of a wider therapeutic window for thrombolysis beyond 3 and even 6 h, but the findings need to be confirmed in larger phase III clinical trials, which are being planned.

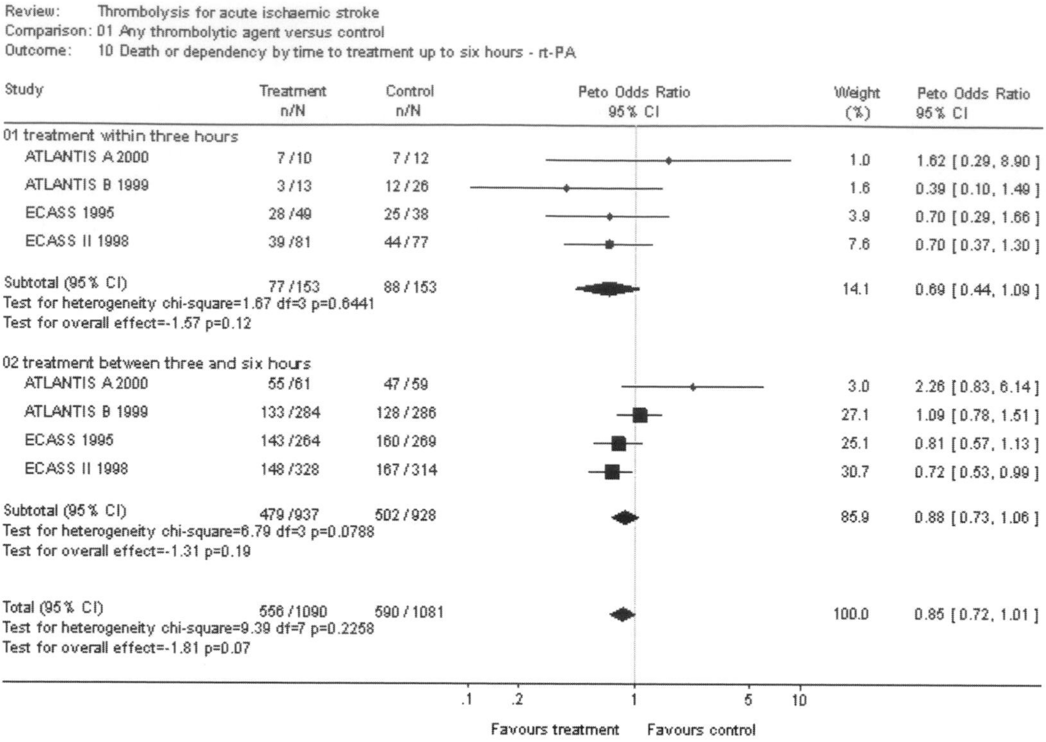

Review: Thrombolysis for acute ischaemic stroke
Comparison: 01 Any thrombolytic agent versus control
Outcome: 10 Death or dependency by time to treatment up to six hours - rt-PA

Study	Treatment n/N	Control n/N	Peto Odds Ratio 95% CI	Weight (%)	Peto Odds Ratio 95% CI
01 treatment within three hours					
ATLANTIS A 2000	7 / 10	7 / 12		1.0	1.62 [0.29, 8.90]
ATLANTIS B 1999	3 / 13	12 / 26		1.6	0.39 [0.10, 1.49]
ECASS 1995	28 / 49	25 / 38		3.9	0.70 [0.29, 1.66]
ECASS II 1998	39 / 81	44 / 77		7.6	0.70 [0.37, 1.30]
Subtotal (95% CI)	77 / 153	88 / 153		14.1	0.69 [0.44, 1.09]
Test for heterogeneity chi-square=1.67 df=3 p=0.6441					
Test for overall effect=-1.57 p=0.12					
02 treatment between three and six hours					
ATLANTIS A 2000	55 / 61	47 / 59		3.0	2.26 [0.83, 6.14]
ATLANTIS B 1999	133 / 284	128 / 286		27.1	1.09 [0.78, 1.51]
ECASS 1995	143 / 264	160 / 269		25.1	0.81 [0.57, 1.13]
ECASS II 1998	148 / 328	167 / 314		30.7	0.72 [0.53, 0.99]
Subtotal (95% CI)	479 / 937	502 / 928		85.9	0.88 [0.73, 1.06]
Test for heterogeneity chi-square=6.79 df=3 p=0.0788					
Test for overall effect=-1.31 p=0.19					
Total (95% CI)	556 / 1090	590 / 1081		100.0	0.85 [0.72, 1.01]
Test for heterogeneity chi-square=9.39 df=7 p=0.2258					
Test for overall effect=-1.81 p=0.07					

.1   .2   1   5   10

Favours treatment   Favours control

Figure 5.12 Forest plot showing the effects of *t-PA vs control* within 6 h of onset of ischaemic stroke on *death or dependency at the end of follow-up, according to time to treatment up to 6 h.* Reproduced from Wardlaw *et al.* (2003), with permission from the authors and John Wiley & Sons Limited. Copyright Cochrane Library, reproduced with permission.

Different thrombolytic doses

Different doses (of rt-PA or UK) were compared in seven trials ($n = 1072$ patients) (Mielke *et al.*, 2004). A higher dose of thrombolytic therapy was associated with a 3-fold increase in fatal intracranial haemorrhages (OR: 3.25; 95% CI: 1.32–7.97) compared with a lower dose of the same agent (based on 16 events among 539 higher-dose patients and four events among 533 lower-dose patients in seven trials). There was no statistically significant difference in early deaths (OR: 1.01, 95% CI: 0.58–1.74) or late deaths (OR: 0.94, 95% CI: 0.58–1.53) between higher and lower doses. Data were inadequate to assess the effect of dose on functional outcome.

The limited evidence suggests that higher doses of thrombolytic agents may lead to higher rates of bleeding, but it is uncertain whether lower doses are more effective than higher doses (or whether one agent is better than another, or which route of administration is best in acute ischaemic stroke (see below)).

Different routes of administration

Intra-arterial (i.a.) thrombolysis

Intra-arterial (i.a.) thrombolysis involves traversing the cervicocephalic arterial tree with an endovascular microcatheter delivery system. The catheter port is positioned immediately within and adjacent to the symptomatic thrombus and thrombolytic agents are infused directly into the clot. The potential advantage is that it allows high concentrations of lytic agent to be applied to the clot while minimising systemic exposure.

Early open studies suggested that i.a. thrombolysis achieves higher recanalisation rates than i.v. thrombolysis. The first randomised phase III trial of i.a. thrombolysis, the Prolyse in Acute Cerebral Thromboembolism II (PROACT II) trial, confirmed these earlier observations, and showed that i.a. recombinant pro-UK 9 mg for 120 min combined with i.v. heparin vs i.v. heparin alone, started within 6 h of onset (median 5.3 h) of symptoms of M1 or M2 middle cerebral artery occlusion, was associated with higher recanalisation rates (partial: 66% pro-UK vs 18% control, complete: 19% pro-UK vs 2% control) and a non-significant trend towards improved clinical outcomes, with acceptable haemorrhage rates (Furlan *et al.*, 1999). These results are consistent with those of the first PROACT trial (Figs 5.3–5.5) (Furlan *et al.*, 1996).

Overall the odds of symptomatic intracranial haemorrhage within 7–10 days of pro-UK treatment was increased by 2.39 (95% CI: 0.88–6.47) compared with control (Fig. 5.3). At final follow-up, allocation to i.a. pro-UK was associated with no significant reduction in death (OR: 0.75, 95% CI: 0.40–1.42) (Fig. 5.4) and a non-significant trend towards a reduction in death and dependency (OR: 0.55, 95% CI: 0.31–1.00) (Fig. 5.5).

One pilot trial (the Emergency Management of Stroke Bridging Trial) compared different routes of administration (i.v. plus i.a. rt-PA vs i.a. rt-PA alone, $n = 35$ patients) but the results were inconclusive (Lewandowski *et al.*, 1999).

Concomitant antithrombotic drugs

There is some evidence that antithrombotic drugs given with, or soon after, thrombolysis may increase the risk of death (Fig. 5.1). Non randomised comparisons suggest an adverse (haemorrhagic) interaction between thrombolytic and antithrombotic therapies (Fig. 5.13). There was a trend towards increased case fatality the earlier that concomitant antithrombotic drug therapy was introduced; OR: 1.95 when all patients received antithrombotic drugs within 24 h of thrombolysis; 1.27 when some patients received antithrombotic drugs within 24 h; 1.14 when no patients received antithrombotic drugs within 24 h but some thereafter; and 0.89 when no patients received antithrombotic drugs within the first 10–14 days (Fig. 5.13).

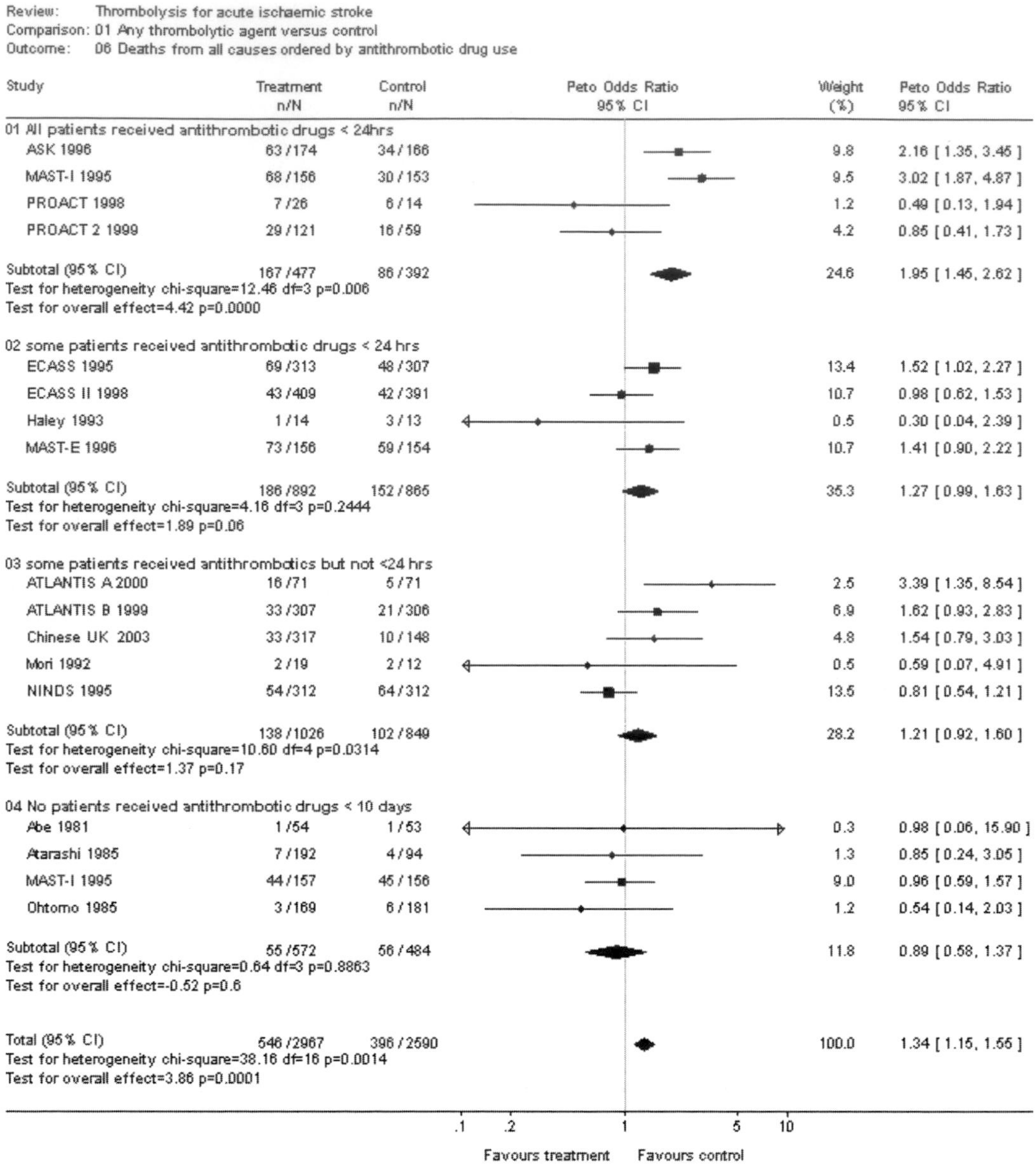

Review: Thrombolysis for acute ischaemic stroke
Comparison: 01 Any thrombolytic agent versus control
Outcome: 06 Deaths from all causes ordered by antithrombotic drug use

Study	Treatment n/N	Control n/N	Peto Odds Ratio 95% CI	Weight (%)	Peto Odds Ratio 95% CI
01 All patients received antithrombotic drugs < 24hrs					
ASK 1996	63 /174	34 /166		9.8	2.16 [1.35, 3.46]
MAST-I 1995	68 /156	30 /153		9.5	3.02 [1.87, 4.87]
PROACT 1998	7 /26	6 /14		1.2	0.49 [0.13, 1.94]
PROACT 2 1999	29 /121	16 /59		4.2	0.85 [0.41, 1.73]
Subtotal (95% CI)	167 /477	86 /392		24.6	1.95 [1.45, 2.62]
Test for heterogeneity chi-square=12.46 df=3 p=0.006					
Test for overall effect=4.42 p=0.0000					
02 some patients received antithrombotic drugs < 24 hrs					
ECASS 1995	69 /313	48 /307		13.4	1.52 [1.02, 2.27]
ECASS II 1998	43 /409	42 /391		10.7	0.98 [0.62, 1.53]
Haley 1993	1 /14	3 /13		0.5	0.30 [0.04, 2.39]
MAST-E 1996	73 /156	59 /154		10.7	1.41 [0.90, 2.22]
Subtotal (95% CI)	186 /892	152 /865		35.3	1.27 [0.99, 1.63]
Test for heterogeneity chi-square=4.16 df=3 p=0.2444					
Test for overall effect=1.89 p=0.06					
03 some patients received antithrombotics but not <24 hrs					
ATLANTIS A 2000	16 /71	5 /71		2.5	3.39 [1.35, 8.54]
ATLANTIS B 1999	33 /307	21 /306		6.9	1.62 [0.93, 2.83]
Chinese UK 2003	33 /317	10 /148		4.8	1.54 [0.79, 3.03]
Mori 1992	2 /19	2 /12		0.5	0.59 [0.07, 4.91]
NINDS 1995	54 /312	64 /312		13.5	0.81 [0.54, 1.21]
Subtotal (95% CI)	138 /1026	102 /849		28.2	1.21 [0.92, 1.60]
Test for heterogeneity chi-square=10.60 df=4 p=0.0314					
Test for overall effect=1.37 p=0.17					
04 No patients received antithrombotic drugs < 10 days					
Abe 1981	1 /54	1 /53		0.3	0.98 [0.06, 15.90]
Atarashi 1985	7 /192	4 /94		1.3	0.85 [0.24, 3.05]
MAST-I 1995	44 /157	45 /156		9.0	0.96 [0.59, 1.57]
Ohtomo 1985	3 /169	6 /181		1.2	0.54 [0.14, 2.03]
Subtotal (95% CI)	55 /572	56 /484		11.8	0.89 [0.58, 1.37]
Test for heterogeneity chi-square=0.64 df=3 p=0.8863					
Test for overall effect=-0.52 p=0.6					
Total (95% CI)	546 /2967	396 /2590		100.0	1.34 [1.15, 1.55]
Test for heterogeneity chi-square=38.16 df=16 p=0.0014					
Test for overall effect=3.86 p=0.0001					

.1   .2   1   5   10

Favours treatment   Favours control

Figure 5.13 Forest plot showing the effects of *any thrombolytic agent vs control* within 6 h of onset of ischaemic stroke on *death at the end of follow-up, according to time to antithrombotic drug use.* Reproduced from Wardlaw *et al.* (2003), with permission from the authors and John Wiley & Sons Limited. Copyright Cochrane Library, reproduced with permission.

Concomitant neuroprotection

The Clomethiazole Acute Stroke Study in tissue-type plasminogen activator-treated stroke (CLASS-T) was a pilot study which aimed to explore the safety and feasibility of administering the combination of a thrombolytic and neuroprotective drug in acute ischaemic stroke (Lyden *et al.*, 2001). A total of 190 patients were all treated with 0.9 mg/kg t-PA within 3 h of ischaemic stroke and then randomised to receive within 12 h of onset either clomethiazole 68 mg/kg i.v. over 24 h ($n = 97$) or placebo ($n = 93$). Patients were followed for 90 days and there were no significant differences in serious adverse events, but sedation was reported by 42% of clomethiazole patients and 13% of placebo patients. The authors concluded that the combination paradigm proved feasible and safe, but that future studies must endeavour to administer both therapies promptly, rather than the delayed administration of neuroprotection that occurred in CLASS-T.

Concomitant transcranial Doppler ultrasound

Ultrasound is believed to have a thrombolytic capacity that can be used for pure mechanical thrombolysis (with high intensities (>2 W/cm^2)) or improvement of enzyme-mediated thrombolysis (with lower intensities) (Daffertshofer and Hennerici, 2003).

A small phase II RCT suggests that continuous 2-MHz, single-element pulsed-wave transcranial Doppler (TCD) ultrasonography that is aimed at residual obstructive intracranial blood flow may help expose thrombi to t-PA and enhance the thrombolytic activity of t-PA. Among 126 patients randomly assigned to receive continuous ultrasonography (63 patients) or placebo (63 patients), complete recanalisation or dramatic clinical recovery within 2 h after the administration of a t PA bolus occurred in 31 patients in the treatment group (49%) compared with 19 patients in the control group (30%; $P = 0.03$) (Alexandrov *et al.*, 2004). At 3 months, a favourable outcome (modified Rankin scale score of 0 or 1) was achieved in 22 of the 53 patients in the treatment group who were eligible for follow-up (42%) and 14 of 49 in the control group (29%; $P = 0.20$).

Concomitant mechanical clot disruption

Uncontrolled case series suggest that arterial recanalisation following thrombolytic therapy may be improved by mechanical clot penetration (with a microwire or microcatheter) or more aggressive mechanical clot disruption (e.g. by balloon angioplasty, stent deployment, or use of a snare device). (Noser *et al.*, 2005). Further evaluation by RCTs is required.

Prognostic factors

Clinical

Tabular data were not available from the published trial results in sufficient detail to assess the effect of other potential prognostic factors (besides time to treatment and the type of thrombolytic agent), such as age and stroke severity.

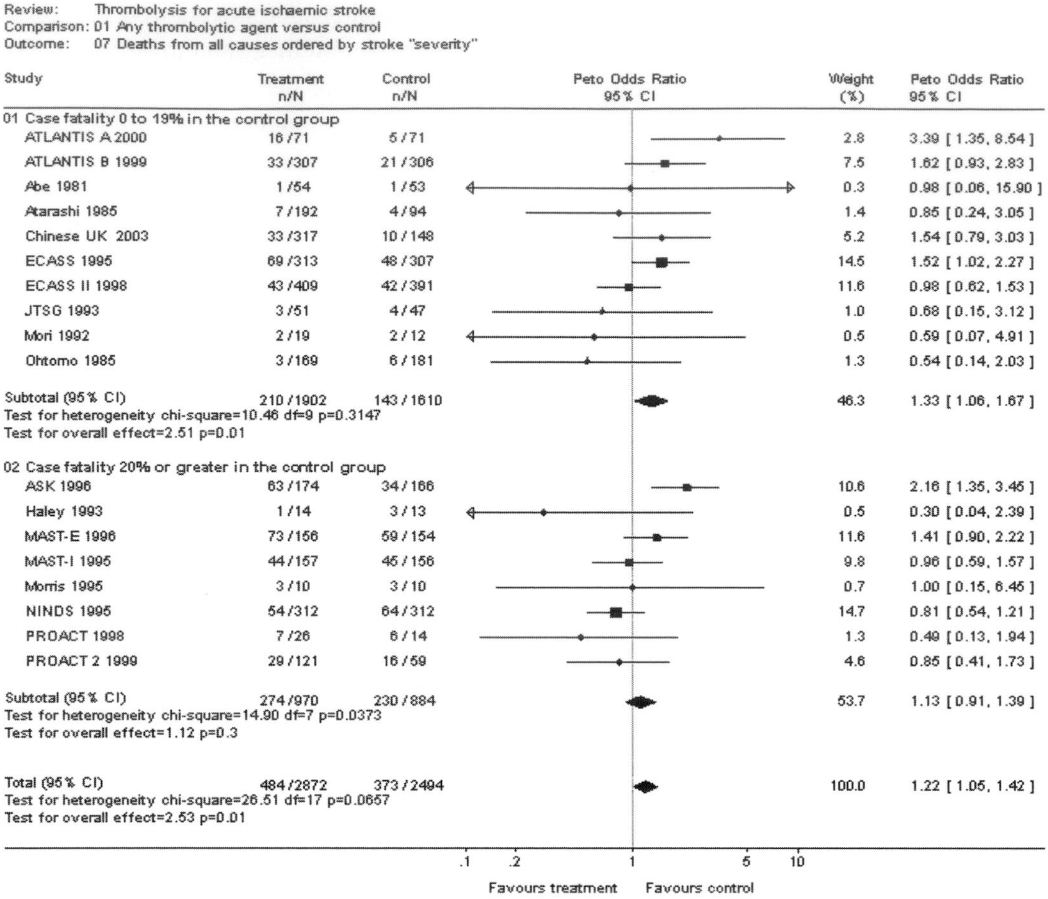

Review: Thrombolysis for acute ischaemic stroke
Comparison: 01 Any thrombolytic agent versus control
Outcome: 07 Deaths from all causes ordered by stroke "severity"

Study	Treatment n/N	Control n/N	Peto Odds Ratio 95% CI	Weight (%)	Peto Odds Ratio 95% CI
01 Case fatality 0 to 19% in the control group					
ATLANTIS A 2000	16 / 71	5 / 71		2.8	3.39 [1.35, 8.54]
ATLANTIS B 1999	33 / 307	21 / 306		7.5	1.62 [0.93, 2.83]
Abe 1981	1 / 54	1 / 53		0.3	0.98 [0.06, 15.90]
Atarashi 1985	7 / 192	4 / 94		1.4	0.85 [0.24, 3.05]
Chinese UK 2003	33 / 317	10 / 148		5.2	1.54 [0.79, 3.03]
ECASS 1995	69 / 313	48 / 307		14.5	1.52 [1.02, 2.27]
ECASS II 1998	43 / 409	42 / 391		11.6	0.98 [0.62, 1.53]
JTSG 1993	3 / 51	4 / 47		1.0	0.68 [0.15, 3.12]
Mori 1992	2 / 19	2 / 12		0.5	0.59 [0.07, 4.91]
Ohtomo 1985	3 / 169	6 / 181		1.3	0.54 [0.14, 2.03]
Subtotal (95% CI)	210 / 1902	143 / 1610		46.3	1.33 [1.06, 1.67]
Test for heterogeneity chi-square=10.46 df=9 p=0.3147					
Test for overall effect=2.51 p=0.01					
02 Case fatality 20% or greater in the control group					
ASK 1996	63 / 174	34 / 166		10.6	2.16 [1.35, 3.45]
Haley 1993	1 / 14	3 / 13		0.5	0.30 [0.04, 2.39]
MAST-E 1996	73 / 156	59 / 154		11.6	1.41 [0.90, 2.22]
MAST-I 1995	44 / 157	45 / 156		9.8	0.96 [0.59, 1.57]
Morris 1995	3 / 10	3 / 10		0.7	1.00 [0.15, 6.45]
NINDS 1995	54 / 312	64 / 312		14.7	0.81 [0.54, 1.21]
PROACT 1998	7 / 26	6 / 14		1.3	0.49 [0.13, 1.94]
PROACT 2 1999	29 / 121	16 / 59		4.6	0.85 [0.41, 1.73]
Subtotal (95% CI)	274 / 970	230 / 884		53.7	1.13 [0.91, 1.39]
Test for heterogeneity chi-square=14.90 df=7 p=0.0373					
Test for overall effect=1.12 p=0.3					
Total (95% CI)	484 / 2872	373 / 2494		100.0	1.22 [1.05, 1.42]
Test for heterogeneity chi-square=26.51 df=17 p=0.0657					
Test for overall effect=2.53 p=0.01					

.1   .2   1   5   10

Favours treatment   Favours control

Figure 5.14   Forest plot showing the effects of *any thrombolytic agent vs control* within 6 h of onset of ischaemic stroke on *death at the end of follow-up, according to the severity of the stroke, as defined by case fatality < or ≥ 20%*. Reproduced from Wardlaw *et al.* (2003), with permission from the authors and John Wiley & Sons Limited. Copyright Cochrane Library, reproduced with permission.

Figure 5.14 shows that the odds of death associated with thrombolytic therapy was consistently increased by about 20–30% in patients with less severe stroke (as defined by a low-case fatality <20% in the control group) and more severe stroke (as defined by a high-case fatality ≥20% in the control group), but more data are required to refine this analysis. A re-analysis of the NINDS trial showed that imbalances in stroke severity at baseline among the treatment and control group did not alter the conclusions of the study (Ingall *et al.*, 2004; Kwiatkowski *et al.*, 2005; Magid *et al.*, 2005).

Observational cohort studies have identified increasing age and disturbances of consciousness as risk factors for increased in-hospital mortality, and elevated blood glucose concentration, cortical involvement, increasing stroke severity, increasing time to thrombolytic therapy, and lack of improvement at 24 h as independent predictors of poor outcome and death at 3 months in patients with acute ischaemic stroke treated with thrombolytic therapy (Table 5.1) (Alvarez-Sabín et al., 2004; Heuschmann et al., 2004; Saposnik et al., 2004).

CT brain imaging

Data from some RCTs and observational studies suggest that plain CT brain scan signs of major infarction which involves more than one-third of the middle cerebral artery territory predicts an increased risk of symptomatic intracranial haemorrhage after thrombolysis. However, it is neither sensitive nor specific, and the interrater reliability among physicians involved in acute stroke care is less than ideal (Kalafut et al., 2000; Wardlaw and Farrell, 2004). Furthermore, other studies have not found that visible infarction involving more than a third of the territory of the middle cerebral artery is associated significantly and independently with an adverse outcome (Patel et al., 2001; Gilligan et al., 2002).

A CT scoring system (the Alberta Stroke Program Early CT Score (ASPECTS)) is a simple and reliable method of quantifying early ischaemic changes on pre-treatment CT scan, like an 'electrocardiogram (ECG) of the brain', in patients with acute ischaemic stroke (Barber et al., 2000; Coutts et al., 2004). It is a 10-point scale that grades the extent of ischaemic change within 10 regions of the territory of the middle cerebral artery. Each normal region is scored as 1, and each region showing signs of ischaemia is scored as 0. It helps observers to recognise visible infarction, and the score is reported to accurately predict risk of symptomatic intracranial haemorrhage and functional outcome in ischaemic stroke patients treated with i.v. and i.a. thrombolytic therapy (Barber et al., 2000; Hill et al., 2003). However, the signs are subtle and patients may be wrongly denied an effective treatment on the basis of a poorly identified sign that remains to be externally validated in multiple data sets.

MRI

MRI can provide a perfusion-weighted image (PWI) which reveals the region of brain which is underperfused and 'at risk', and if severe, may represent core, irreversibly infarcted tissue (Shih et al., 2003). Improved brain perfusion, as measured on MRI by a decrease in hypoperfusion volume on mean transit time map of more than 30% at 2 h after t-PA administration, has been reported to be an early marker of long-term clinical benefit thrombolytic therapy (Chalela et al., 2004; Hjort et al., 2005).

MRI can also provide a diffusion-weighted image (DWI) which has been thought to identify the core of early infarction. However, because diffusion abnormalities may be reversible, and normalise, it is likely that they often include both irreversibly infarcted tissue and penumbra (Kidwell et al., 2002, 2003). Nevertheless, it continues to be hypothesised that a mismatch between the acute PWI lesion and the (smaller) DWI lesion may represent the ischaemic penumbra of potentially salvageable brain (Hjort *et al.*, 2005). Clinical trials, such as Echoplanar Imaging Thrombolysis Evaluation Trial (EPITHET) (see below), are evaluating whether patients with a PWI/DWI mismatch are likely to benefit clinically from early reperfusion (Alberts *et al.*, 1999; Warach, 2002, 2003; Schellinger *et al.*, 2003; Wardlaw and Farrell, 2004). If confirmed, a further challenge will be to optimise the availability and feasibility of undertaking MRI brain scans within the first few hours of stroke onset in sick, dysphasic, disorientated and claustrophobic patients with acute stroke.

CT angiography, MR angiography, TCD

Patient selection for thrombolysis may also be improved by proof of arterial occlusion by means of non-invasive imaging, such as CT angiography, MR angiography, and TCD. TCD allows detection of intracranial thrombemboli, and monitoring permits the determination of reperfusion (Schellinger *et al.*, 2003; Warach, 2003). It may also facilitate clot lysis (see above).

Thrombolysis in clinical practice

The Canadian Activase for Stroke Effectiveness Study

The Canadian Activase for Stroke Effectiveness Study (CASES) is a prospective observational cohort study which was designed to fulfil the requirements of the Canadian Health Protection Branch for regulatory approval of rt-PA for acute stroke. It aims to monitor the safety of rt-PA in routine care, assess whether the results of the NINDS trial could be translated into routine practice in Canada, and identify predictors of benefit and harm associated with rt-PA. The 60 centres included both academic (45%) and community (55%) hospitals, and most treating physicians were neurologists (Hill *et al.*, 2005).

Within the first 2.5 years of rt-PA use in Canada, a total of 1135 patients were recruited, of whom 30 were lost to follow up at 90 days. Cranial CT scans, pre- and post-treatment were reviewed for 766 patients.

Patients were similar to those enrolled in the NINDS study in terms of mean age (72 years) and mean National Institute of Health Stroke Scale (NIHSS) score (14, range 2–40) but fewer had hypertension (50% vs 61%), diabetes (16% vs 20%), smoking (15% vs 31%) and congestive heart failure (7% vs 17%) (Teal, 2004).

The time from stroke onset to needle was 155 min (median), and from door to needle was 85 min (median) (Hill *et al.*, 2005). The breakdown was 56 min (median) from onset to presentation at the hospital emergency room (ER), 36 min from ER to CT scan and 44 min from CT to needle.

Anaphylactic reactions or angioedema (e.g. hemi-orolingual) occurred in 15 (1.3%, 95% CI: 0.7–2.2%) patients, of whom two required intubation to protect their airway. These were more common in patients taking angiotensin converting enzyme inhibitors (Hill *et al.*, 2003, 2005).

Table 5.1. Independent predictors of a good outcome (mRS 0–2) at 90 days after rt-PA in CASES.

Variable	Hazard ratio for good outcome
• Less severe stroke as measured by NIHSS score	0.58 per 5 point increment
• Younger age	0.78 per 10 year increment
• Less ischaemic change on CT scan as measured by the ASPECTS score	1.25 per 2 point increment
• Normal blood glucose	0.53 if Blood Glucose Level
• Shorter onset to needle time	(BGL) > 8.0 mmol/l

Early symptomatic ICH occurred in 52 patients, realising a rate of 4.6% (95% CI: 3.4%–6.0%) of patients in CASES (6.4% in NINDS). The 90 day mortality for these 52 patients was 81% compared with 22.3% (95% CI: 20.0–25.0%) for the whole cohort. The rate of ICH was significantly increased if there were protocol violations (mainly time violations), and there was a non-significant trend to increase ICH in patients with increased time to treatment, particularly beyond 3 h. Risk of bleeding was not related to stroke severity, although patients with less severe strokes had better outcomes (see below).

An excellent outcome (mRS 0–1) at 90 days was recorded in 32% of patients. After adjusting for baseline variables, to make them comparable with those of the NINDS study, almost 37% of patients had an excellent outcome, which was similar to the NINDS patients treated with rt-PA.

The independent predictors of a good outcome (mRS 0–2) are shown in Table 5.1.

The Safe Implementation of Thrombolysis in Stroke-MOnitoring STudy

The Safe Implementation of Thrombolysis in Stroke-MOnitoring STudy (SITS-MOST) is the post-marketing surveillance study required by the Committee for Proprietary Medicinal Products (CPMP) of the European Agency for the Evaluation of Medicinal products (EMEA) in Europe, as a condition for the approval of thrombolysis with rt-PA within 3 h of onset of acute ischaemic stroke. It began in January 2003, and by 8 September 2004, 1652 had been registered from 161 active clinical centres in 13 countries of Europe. Each month, an average of 83 patients have been registered, and the rate is increasing (106 in the last month). In 2003, 20% of all SITS-MOST centres were new centres without previous experience of thrombolysis. In 2004, this proportion had increased to 40%, and they had recruited 24% of all patients (Toni, 2004).

Every 6 months, the data are reported to the EMEA and a statement is published at the study web site (www.acutestroke.org). The most recent report stated that the main outcome variables for safety – symptomatic intracranial haemorrhage at 36 h (≥ 4 points reduction in NIHSS score and parenchymal haematoma type 2 (von Kummer))

Table 5.2. Summary of the relative and absolute benefits and hazards of thrombolytic therapy within 6 h (above) and 3 h (below), and also of rt-PA (italics).

Outcome events	Thrombolysis within 6 h (%)	Control (%)	OR	95% CI of OR	Absolute risk per 1000 patients treated (95% CI)	Heterogeneity (P)
Early (≤10 days)						
Death	14.9	9.4	1.81	1.46–2.24	+59 (21 to 108)	0.048
(rt-PA)			*1.24*	*0.8–1.81*	*+15 (−10 to +50)*	*NS*
Fatal intracranial haemorrhage	5.2	0.9	4.34	3.14–5.99	+44	0.71
(rt-PA)			*3.60*	*2.28–5.68*	*+25 (13 to 44)*	*0.38*
Symptomatic intracranial haemorrhage	8.7	2.5	3.37	2.68–4.22	+58 (36 to 85)	0.15
(rt-PA)			*3.13*	*2.34–4.19*	*+62 (40 to 90)*	*0.11*
At final follow-up (3–6 months)						
Death	18.2	15.2	1.33	1.15–1.53	+41 (19 to 63)	0.0028
(rt-PA)			*1.17*	*0.95–1.45*	*+19 (−6 to +48)*	*0.04*
Death or dependency	53.3	58.0	0.84	0.75–0.95	−43 (−13 to −71)	0.093
(rt-PA)			*0.80*	*0.69–0.93*	*−55 (−18 to −92)*	*0.02*

Outcome events	Thrombolysis within 3 h (%)	Control (%)	OR	95% CI of OR	Absolute risk per 1000 patients treated (95% CI)	Heterogeneity (P)
At final follow-up (3–6 months)						
Death	20.9	19.4	1.13	0.86–1.48	+20 (−23 to +69)	0.0008
(rt-PA)			*0.97*	*0.69–1.36*	*−1 (−49 to +47)*	
Death or dependency	49.7	60.3	0.66	0.53–0.83	−102 (−45 to −157)	0.86
(rt-PA)			*0.64*	*0.54–0.83*		

and mortality at 3 months; and efficacy: independence in activities of daily living at 3 months after treatment – were comparable with corresponding results from RCTs.

It is planned that this phase IV study will cease in December 2005.

Comment

Interpretation of the data

These data indicate that thrombolytic therapy for acute ischaemic stroke is very much like carotid endarterectomy for recently symptomatic severe carotid stenosis (see Chapter 12). Both are associated with a net early hazard and a net greater longer-term benefit, and the challenges are to identify which patients are likely to benefit, to not benefit, and to be harmed.

Overall, thrombolytic therapy given within 6 h of ischaemic stroke appears to result in a significant net reduction in the proportion of patients dead or dependent in activities of daily living at 3–6 months follow-up, irrespective of how dependency is defined (Wardlaw et al., 2000). This is despite a net increase in early deaths (within the first 7–10 days) and late deaths (at follow-up at 3–6 months), mostly from fatal intracranial haemorrhage (Table 5.2).

The greatest amount of data are available for i.v. rt-PA (alteplase; 0.9 mg/kg over 1 h), which was associated with fewer deaths and more patients avoiding death or dependent survival than was i.v. SK (there are fewer data for i.v. UK, and the pro-UK data were from i.a. trials). However, there was heterogeneity among the trials for some outcomes, and uncertainties remain regarding:

- the optimum clinical and radiological criteria to identify the patients most likely to benefit and least likely to be harmed;
- the duration of the therapeutic time window;
- the optimum thrombolytic agent, dose and route of administration;
- the role (if any) and timing of concomitant antithrombotic therapy.

Implications for clinical practice

The trial evidence is promising but limited (Wardlaw et al., 2003, Warlow and Wardlaw, 2003). As a result, guidelines vary. The Royal College of Physicians of London recommends that alteplase should be used only in the context of randomised trials, and both the US and Canadian emergency guidelines for physicians are similarly cautious. In contrast, alteplase has been approved in North America and several other countries in Europe and Australia, albeit with tight criteria. In these countries, rates of use in routine clinical practice have remained low.

Although the data do not support the widespread use of thrombolytic therapy in routine clinical practice at present, they do justify the use of thrombolytic therapy with i.v. rt-PA in countries where a therapeutic licence exists for this indication, in highly

Table 5.3. Suggested guidelines for the use of i.v. rt-PA in ischaemic stroke.

- Thrombolysis with i.v. rt-PA should be considered in all patients with a definite ischaemic stroke who present within 3 h of onset and have a measurable neurological deficit.
- Thrombolytic therapy should only be administered by clinicians with expertise in stroke medicine, who have access to a suitable stroke service, with facilities for immediately identifying and managing haemorrhagic complications
- Thrombolysis should be avoided in cases where the CT brain scan suggests substantial (e.g. multilobar) early changes of major infarction (e.g. oedema, sulcal effacement, mass effect)
- Other exclusion criteria:

Past history
  - Intracranial haemorrhage at any time in the past
  - Heparin exposure in preceding 48 h and partial thromboplastin time not normal
  - Arterial puncture or non-compressible site within previous 7 days
  - Gastrointestinal, urinary or any bleeding; deep biopsy, surgery, internal injury, or wound within previous 21 days that could increase the risk of unmanageable (e.g. by local pressure) bleeding
  - Stroke, serious head injury or myocardial infarction in previous 3 months

Current (i.e. pretreatment)
  - First seizure at stroke onset (i.e. the diagnosis could be a 'Todd's Paresis', not a stroke)
  - Neurological deficits are mild
  - Neurological condition is improving rapidly
  - Systolic BP >180 mmHg or diastolic BP >110 mmHg
  - Oral anticoagulant use, advanced liver disease, or advanced right heart failure and International Normalised Ratio (INR) >1.4
  - Platelet count <80 × 10^9/l
  - Prolonged partial thromboplastin time
  - Blood glucose <2.8 mmol/l (50 mg/dl) or >22 mmol/l (400 mg/dl)
- Caution in patients with severe stroke (NIHSS score >22)
- Discuss potential treatment benefits and adverse effects with patient and family before treatment
- Recommended dose of rt-PA is 0.9 mg/kg up to a maximum of 90 mg, the first 10% of the dose as a bolus over 1 min, the rest as an infusion over 60 min
- Perform neurologic assessments every 15 min during infusion of rt-PA, every 30 min for the next 6 h, and every 60 min for the next 16 h. If severe headache, acute hypertension, or nausea and vomiting occur, discontinue the infusion and obtain an emergency CT brain scan
- Measure BP every 15 min for 2 h, every 30 min for 6 h, and every 60 min for 16 h; repeat measurements more frequently if systolic BP is >180 mmHg or diastolic BP is >105 mmHg, and administer antihypertensive drugs as needed to maintain BP at or below those levels

NB. There is no reliable evidence that current use of antiplatelet therapy is a contraindication.

Appendix 1

Schedule for potential rt-PA candidate
1. Establish i.v. access
2. Bloods: full blood count (FBC), glucose, urea and electrolytes (U&E), activated partial thromboplastin time (APTT), INR, blood group and screen

Table 5.3. (*Cont.*)

3. Check BP
4. Arrange urgent CT brain
5. Ask family to stay
6. Quick, but adequate history and general physical and neurological examination
7. Estimate (or ask) weight
8. If BP >180/110: Treat, see below

If eligible:

1. Discuss potential risks and benefits of treatment with patient (if not dysphasic) and family
2. Insert indwelling urine catheter before rt-PA, if required (do not catheterise in first 90 min after starting rt-PA)
3. Start treatment in emergency department (ED) and inform Stroke Unit
4. rt-PA is compatible with sodium chloride 0.9%, not with glucose containing fluids or with fluids containing preservatives
5. Continue to check BP every 15 min in first 2 h (see Appendix 1)
6. Hourly observations of GCS, pupils, BP and pulse for first 24 h
7. No punctures of arteries or large veins in first 24 h
8. Preferably no nasogastric tube in first 24 h
9. No antiplatetet therapy or anti-coagulants in first 24 h
10. Admit stroke unit

Appendix 2

rt-PA dose checking table (Note: Exact dose must be calculated for each patient)

Body weight (kg)	Total volume (ml)	Vials	Bolus volume (ml) over 1–2 min	Infusion volume (ml) over 60 min
40	36	1	3.6	32.4
50	45	1	4.5	40.5
60	54	2	5.4	48.6
70	63	2	6.3	56.7
80	72	2	7.2	64.8
90	81	2	8.1	72.9
100 or more	90	2	9.0	81.0

rt-PA reconstitution and administration

Reconstitution

Patients 55 kg or less: Use one 50 mg vial.   Note: costs per vial: Euros 600

Patients >55 kg use two 50 mg vials

1. Reconstitute each vial with 50 ml of water for injection from the accompanying vial by use of the transfer cannula in the packet, resulting in a concentration of 1 mg/ml rt-PA
2. Introduce the transfer cannula vertically into the stopper and through the mark at its centre

Table 5.3. (*Cont.*)

3. If slight foaming occurs, allow the vial to stand for several minutes to allow dissipation of large bubbles

4. Do not shake vigorously

Administration

Bolus: 0.09 ml/kg i.v. push over 1–2 min

Infusion: 0.81 ml/kg i.v. over 60 min

                The infusion volume should be placed in a burette

Appendix 3

Management of high BP after thrombolysis

BP monitoring first 24 h:

0–2 h: every 15 min after initiation of infusion

2–8 h: every 30 min after initiation of infusion

8–24 h: every 60 min after initiation of infusion

During treatment with glyceryl trinitrate (GTN) infusion: every 15 min

Maintain BP <180/110

If at two readings 10 min apart:

1. Systolic BP >180–230 mmHg, or diastolic BP >110–120 mmHg
   - GTN infusion 50 mg/100 ml 5% dextrose, start at 6–10 ml/h, titrate until BP <180/110
     (6 ml/h = 50 µg/min)
   - May need to diminish dose quickly; after switching off, effect gone in minutes
   - Note: GTN dissolved in glucose containing fluid, whereas rt-PA is *not* compatible with glucose
     containing fluids. Needs to be administered via separate i.v. line

   If still high: Consider admission high dependency unit (HDU) or intensive care unit (ICU) for treatment
   with nitroprusside i.v. 0.5–10 µg/kg/min
2. Systolic BP >230 mmHg or, diastolic BP >140 mmHg
   - Admission to HDU or ICU

If sudden rise in BP: suspect intracranial haemorrhage, discontinue rt-PA, organise urgent CT brain

Appendix 4

Management of intracranial haemorrhage after thrombolysis

Suspect intracranial haemorrhage if:

1. Acute neurological deterioration
2. New headache
3. Nausea or vomiting
4. Acute increase in BP

If intracranial haemorrhage is suspected:

1. Discontinue rt-PA administration
2. Organise urgent CT brain
3. Bloods: FBC, APTT, INR, fibrinogen, cross match
4. Call haematologist to provisionally request cryoprecipitate and platelets

Table 5.3. (Cont.)

If haemorrhage:

5. Administer cryoprecipitate 1 unit/10 kg body weight and platelets 6–12 units
6. If rt-PA is still circulating at the time of the bleeding onset *and* immediate control of bleeding is required: consider antifibrinolytic therapy (e.g. i.v. aminocaproic acid 0.1 g/kg over 30 min or aprotinin 2 million kallikrein inhibitory units over 30 min), while awaiting cryoprecipitate
7. Consult neurosurgeon if decompressive surgery indicated
8. Recheck FBC, APTT, INR, fibrinogen after administration of cryoprecipitate and platelets, and target further administration of cryoprecipitate if fibrinogen levels remain <1.0 g/l, in consultation with haematologist

In case of bleeding elsewhere, cease rt-PA and investigate and treat as clinically indicated. The principles regarding use of cryoprecipitate, platelets and antifibrinolytic therapy are the same. In additon: call blood bank to arrange cross-match in case transfusion of fresh frozen plasma is required.

Consult gastroenterologist or urologist as clinically indicated.

---

selected patients, and in organised and experienced stroke care centres with staff and facilities for rapid and accurate assessment, intervention, monitoring and management of any complications in accordance with current guidelines (an example is given in Table 5.3) (Sandercock *et al.*, 2004; Adams *et al.*, 2005). One lesson learnt from the early North American experience is that treating patients who violate the guidelines outlined in Table 5.3 is associated with excess risk and poor patient outcome (Buchan *et al.*, 2000). Active centres should be prepared to undertake prospective, systematic and rigorous audit as part of a national register, as in CASES and SITS-MOST. This will ensure that stroke patients have access to this effective (yet risky) treatment, that stroke physicians gain experience and expertise in its use and that quality control and patient selection continues to be optimised by correlation of baseline demographic, clinical, imaging and treatment data with early and long-term patient outcome.

The efficient and equitable delivery of thrombolysis also must overcome several pre-hospital and in-hospital barriers, including education of the public to recognise symptoms of stroke and seek urgent help by calling the ambulance first rather than the family doctor; paramedical training; very well-organised systems to bring patients with suspected acute stroke to hospital quickly; efficient well-trained 'brain attack' teams to look after patients once they arrive and to direct management in remote community hospitals (by telephone or telemedicine) (Frey *et al.*, 2005; Audebert *et al.*, 2005); and sufficient spare capacity in imaging and high-dependency care to deal with cases at once, within minutes (Sandercock *et al.*, 2002; Kwan *et al.*, 2004).

Due to the many uncertainties about thrombolysis, some clinicians may only wish to use thrombolytic therapy in highly selected patients under licence conditions, others who are concerned about the definite risks may choose not to use the treatment at all, and others only in the context of a randomised trial (e.g. the International Stroke Trial-3, see below).

Implications for researchers

As stated above, the burning question is no longer whether thrombolysis (and carotid endarterectomy) is effective, but *in whom* it is effective, in whom it is ineffective and in whom it is dangerous. At present it is not known exactly which combination of clinical and imaging features reliably identify patients who will benefit and be harmed by thrombolysis. It is also not known what is the optimal thrombolytic agent, dose, half-life, and route of administration, nor the most effective concomitant neuroprotective, antithrombotic and antihypertensive regime, if any (Warlow and Wardlaw, 2003). Furthermore, the therapeutic time window remains to be established; patients do not magically change from Cinderellas to witches as the clock strikes 3 h (Caplan, 2002).

Further large-scale randomised trials are needed, and are underway (Internet Stroke Centre: http://www.strokecenter.org/trials/) to compare thrombolytic therapy with control in patients with acute ischaemic stroke to perform the following:

(a) Identify which categories of patient are most likely to benefit (and which are harmed), especially the elderly (age >75 years) in whom the data on the effects of thrombolysis are very sparse.

(b) Identify the therapeutic time window; optimal thrombolytic agent, dose, half-life and route of administration; and the most effective concomitant therapies, if any.

(c) Determine whether a combination of an 'ECG of the brain' (e.g. the 'ASPECTS' score on CT brain scan, or findings on DWI and perfusion MR brain imaging) and a 'troponin of the brain' (e.g. S100B or neurone specific enolase), can reliably identify the ischaemic penumbra and the amount of brain infarcted, and improve risk stratification and targeting of thrombolytic treatment to patients with still viable ischaemic brain who are most likely to benefit (Donnan and Davis, 2002; Foerch *et al.*, 2003; Oh *et al.*, 2003; Davis *et al.*, 2005). And, to identify factors, possibly such as increasing stroke severity and blood pressure (BP), and old microbleeds on gradient-echo T2*-weighted MRI, that may help identify patients who are most likely to be harmed by haemorrhagic complications (Nighoghossian *et al.*, 2002).

(d) Confirm whether the advantage to thrombolytic therapy in terms of the reduction in death and dependency at 3 months does indeed persist to 6 months and beyond, as suggested by one trial.

(e) Determine reliably the effects on long-term survival (i.e. one year and beyond).

(f) Identify means of minimising the hazard without reducing the benefit.

(g) Provide clearer evidence that when used in a wider range of hospitals, thrombolytic therapy is associated with a definite net benefit.

Ongoing clinical trials of reperfusion therapies

Third International Stroke Trial

The Third International Stroke Trial (IST-3) is an international, multicentre, RCT of i.v. rt-PA within 6 h of onset of acute ischaemic stroke with blinded outcome assessment (www.ist3.com) (Kane *et al.*, 2004).

It is projected that 6000 patients with acute ischaemic stroke of less than 6 h duration will be randomly allocated to 'immediate rt-PA' or to avoid treatment with rt-PA. Patients allocated to 'immediate rt-PA' are to receive rt-PA in a total dose of 0.9 mg/kg of body weight up to a maximum of 90 mg (an immediate i.v. bolus of 10% of the calculated dose over 1–2 min, followed without delay by the rest of the infusion given over the next 60 min). Patients allocated 'control' must avoid treatment with rt-PA and should receive stroke care in exactly the same clinical environment as those allocated 'immediate rt-PA.' Both treatment groups must have their BP monitored according to the IST-3 protocol and both groups should receive the same general supportive care.

Initial clinical follow-up will be at 7 days, hospital discharge, transfer to another hospital or death, whichever occurs first. A repeat CT scan is repeated between 24 and 48 h to identify any intracranial haemorrhage, cerebral infarction, oedema or midline shift. The primary outcome is the proportion of patients alive and independent at 6 months (Modified Rankin Scale score of 0, 1 or 2). Secondary outcomes will include:

(a) Events within 7 days: deaths from any cause; symptomatic intracranial haemorrhage (fatal or non-fatal); any intracranial haemorrhage (including asymptomatic bleeds on repeat CT); severe extracranial haemorrhage (i.e. fatal, severe enough to require transfusion or operation, or an absolute decrease in haemoglobin $\geqslant$5 g/dl or a decrease in haematocrit of $\geqslant$15% or bleeding associated with persistent or serious disability).

(b) Status at 6 months: number of patients dead from any cause, alive but dependent, and making a complete recovery; and Health Related Quality of Life (HRQoL), measured with the postal questionnaire version of the EuroQol.

(c) The same outcomes as (b) at 18 months and annually thereafter.

All baseline and follow-up, brain images will be sent to the international co-ordinating centre and anonymised, digitised and archived. Images will be presented to an international panel of expert readers by means of a web-based system developed and successfully piloted in the Acute Candesartan Cilexetil thErapy in Stroke Survivors (ACCESS) study (http://www.neuroimage.co.uk/).

With a total international sample size of 6000 patients, the trial will have >99.9% power to detect an absolute difference of 10% in the proportion of patients dead or dependent at 6 months after treatment ($\alpha = 0.001$), and this power would permit reliable subgroup analyses. A trial of this size could detect a smaller, but still clinically worthwhile benefit of as little as a 3% absolute difference in the primary outcome (80% power, at $\alpha = 0.05$).

ECASS (European Cooperative Acute Stroke Study)

This is a placebo-controlled trial of alteplase (rt-PA) in acute ischaemic hemispheric stroke where thrombolysis is initiated between 3 and 4 h after stroke onset. The trial is scheduled to randomise 800 patients between April 2003 and October 2005 (www.strokecenter.org/trials/).

EPITHET (EchoPlanar Imaging Thrombolytic Evaluation Trial)

This is a double blind, placebo-controlled, randomised trial of t-PA vs placebo in 100 patients within 6 h from ischaemic stroke symptom onset. The primary aim is to determine whether the presence and extent of the ischaemic penumbra in acute stroke, as measured by DWI-PWI mismatch on echoplanar MR brain imaging, will predict patients most likely to respond to t-PA (within 3–6 h) and as measured by DWI ('infarct core') expansion in follow-up imaging. The primary outcome is the degree of expansion of the ischaemic lesion core between acute and outcome studies. Secondary outcomes include haemorrhagic transformation detected by MRI at day 3, the proportion of patients achieving an NIHSS improvement of more than 11 points (acute to outcome), and brain infarct volume at 3 months (www.astn.org.au/epithet/index.html) (Davis *et al.*, 2005).

The DEFUSE (DWI Evolution for Understanding Stroke Etiology) study

This is an open label trial of 80 patients in the USA aimed at identifying PWI and DWI measures that predict response to tPA in the 3–6 hour time window. It is not randomised.

The SYNTHESIS trial (Local vs systemic thrombolysis for acute stroke)

The SYNTHESIS trial aims to determine whether i.a. rt-PA (0.9 mg/kg, max 90 mg) infused over 60 min within 6 h of ischaemic stroke is more effective than i.v. rt-PA (0.9 mg/kg, max 90 mg) administered within 3 h of onset in increasing the proportion of independent survivors at 3 months among 350 patients with acute ischaemic stroke (Ciccone *et al.*, 2004).

The MR RESCUE (MR and Recanalisation of Stroke Clots Undergoing Embolectomy) trial

This is evaluating mechanical thrombolysis up to 8 hours in patients with PWI/DWI mismatch.

DIAS II (Desmotoplase In Acute Stroke) trial

Promising results have been reported with the use of desmoteplase up to 9 h after ischaemic stroke (see above) (Hacke *et al.*, 2005), and a subsequent RCT is in progress.

The CLEAR (Combined approach to Lysis utilising Eptifibatide And rt-PA in acute ischaemic stroke) trial

Some preliminary evidence suggests that low-dose rt-PA combined with an antiplatelet agent, such as body weight adjusted platelet glycoprotein IIb/IIIa receptor antagonists like tirofiban may be safe and effective but further trials are necessary (Seitz *et al.*, 2004). The safety of a glycoprotein IIb/IIIa antagonist, eptifibatide in combination with low-dose rt-PA (0.3 mg/kg and 0.45 mg/kg) is being examined in the Combined approach to Lysis utilising Eptifibatide And rt-PA in acute ischaemic stroke (CLEAR) trial. The CLEAR trial is a randomised, double-blind, sequential, doseescalation safety study of the combination of i.v. eptifibatide and i.v. low-dose rt-PA in 100 acute ischaemic stroke patients within 3 h of symptom onset (Pancioli *et al.*, 2004).

The ROSIE (Reopro Retavase Reperfusion Of Stroke Safety Study Imaging Evaluation)
This is evaluating the efficacy and safety of abciximab and reteplase in acute ischaemic stroke with *MRI* evidence of a perfusion deficit, 3–24 h after onset, by measurement of reperfusion (Warach and Davis, 2003; Dunn and Warach, 2005).

The combined cytoprotection t-PA trial
The combination of rt-PA and neuroprotection (caffeinol 8 mg/kg, ethanol 0.4 g/kg and hypothermia (femoral-based catheter cooling system)) is being evaluated in 25 patients within 5 h of onset of cortical ischaemic stroke the combined cytoprotection t-PA trial (Labiche *et al.*, 2004).

The MR and Recanalisation of Stroke Clots Using Embolectomy (MR RESCUE) trial
The MR RESCUE trial aims to determine whether diffusion–perfusion MRI can identify patients who will benefit from mechanical embolectomy with the Concentric Clot Retriever within 8 h of onset of symptoms of acute ischaemic stroke. A total of 120 patients will be randomised to embolectomy vs standard medical care and followed for 90 days for handicap as measured by the modified Rankis scale (Kidwell *et al.*, 2005).

SUMMARY

Thrombolysis with i.v. recombinant tissue-plasminogen activator (alteplase; 0.9 mg/kg over 1 h) increases survival free of disability for a few, highly selected patients who can be assessed and treated within 3 h of onset of symptoms. However, treatment is also risky, and associated with a one in 20 chance of fatal intracranial haemorrhage.

The trial evidence is limited, so guidelines vary. Caution is expressed by the North American guidelines for emergency physicians and the Royal College of Physicians of London, which recommends that alteplase should be used only in the context of randomised trials. In contrast, alteplase has been approved by the regulatory authorities in many countries, but with strict criteria. However, even in countries where it is accepted, rates of use in routine clinical practice are still low.

Large-scale trials are needed to answer several important questions reliably, such as the precise duration of the therapeutic time window in which the benefits outweigh the risks; the optimum selection criteria; the best agent, dose and route of administration; and how cost-effective is the treatment. Trials are underway to clarify these issues.

Intra-arterial thrombolysis and mechanical clot removal from large arteries are technically feasible options for the few centres with appropriate skills and resources, but further trials are needed to establish their place in wider practice.

Augmentation of cerebral blood flow: fibrinogen-depleting agents, haemodilution and pentoxifylline

Fibrinogen-depleting agents

Fibrinogen-depleting agents (defibrinogenating enzymes) reduce fibrinogen in blood plasma and therefore reduce blood viscosity and increase blood flow.

Evidence

Death

A systematic review of five randomised-controlled trials (RCTs) of fibrinogen-depleting agents (ancrod: four trials, defibrase: one trial) involving 2926 patients with acute ischaemic stroke revealed that random assignment to fibrinogen-depleting agents was associated with no statistically significant difference in death from all causes during the scheduled treatment period compared with control (relative risk (RR): 0.71, 95% confidence interval (CI): 0.44–1.13), or at the end of follow-up (RR: 0.98, 95% CI: 0.78–1.24) (Fig. 6.1) (Liu *et al.*, 2003, 2004).

Symptomatic intracranial haemorrhage

Fibrinogen-depleting agents were associated with a non-significant excess of symptomatic intracranial haemorrhages at the end of the treatment period (RR: 2.64, 95% CI: 0.96–7.30, $2P = 0.06$) (Fig. 6.2) (Liu *et al.*, 2003).

Death or dependency

Random allocation to a fibrinogen-depleting agents was associated with a moderate reduction in the proportion of patients who were dead or dependent at the end of follow-up (RR: 0.90, 95% CI: 0.82–0.98, $2P = 0.02$) (Fig. 6.3) (Liu *et al.*, 2003).

Comments

Interpretation of the evidence

The Cochrane systematic review included the Stroke Treatment with Ancrod Trial (STAT) in which ancrod was given within 3 h of onset of ischaemic stroke and continued for 5 days (Sherman, *et al.*, 2000, see p 432, 433), but it did not have access

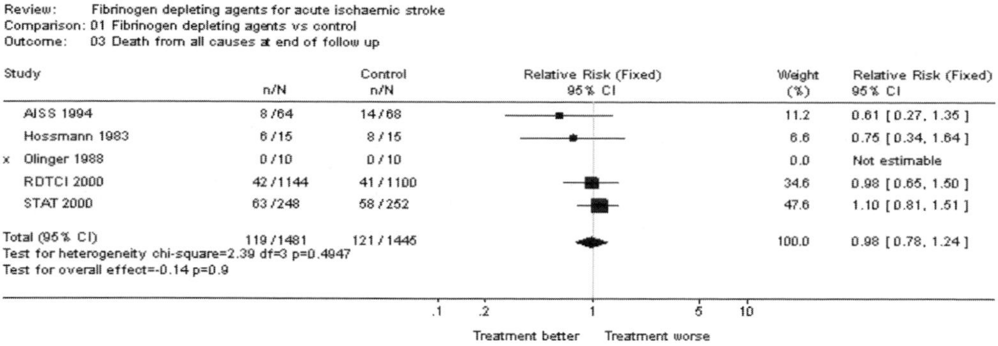
Review: Fibrinogen depleting agents for acute ischaemic stroke
Comparison: 01 Fibrinogen depleting agents vs control
Outcome: 03 Death from all causes at end of follow up
Study
n/N
Control n/N
Relative Risk (Fixed) 95% CI
Weight (%)
Relative Risk (Fixed) 95% CI
AISS 1994 8/64 14/68 11.2 0.61 [0.27, 1.35]
Hossmann 1983 6/15 8/15 6.6 0.75 [0.34, 1.64]
x Olinger 1988 0/10 0/10 0.0 Not estimable
RDTCI 2000 42/1144 41/1100 34.6 0.98 [0.65, 1.50]
STAT 2000 63/248 58/252 47.6 1.10 [0.81, 1.51]
Total (95% CI) 119/1481 121/1445 100.0 0.98 [0.78, 1.24]
Test for heterogeneity chi-square=2.39 df=3 p=0.4947
Test for overall effect=-0.14 p=0.9
.1 .2 1 5 10
Treatment better Treatment worse

Figure 6.1 Forest plot showing the effects of *any fibrinogen-depleting agent vs control* for acute ischaemic stroke on *death at the end of follow-up*. Reproduced from Liu *et al.* (2003), with permission from the authors and John Wiley & Sons Limited. Copyright Cochrane Library, reproduced with permission.

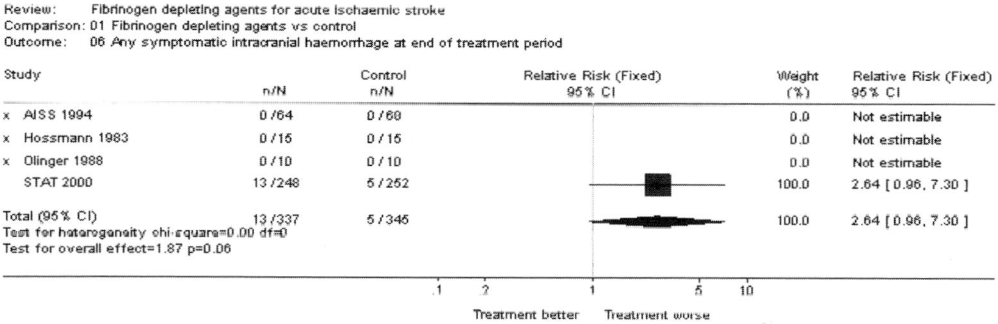
Review: Fibrinogen depleting agents for acute ischaemic stroke
Comparison: 01 Fibrinogen depleting agents vs control
Outcome: 06 Any symptomatic intracranial haemorrhage at end of treatment period
Study
n/N
Control n/N
Relative Risk (Fixed) 95% CI
Weight (%)
Relative Risk (Fixed) 95% CI
x AISS 1994 0/64 0/68 0.0 Not estimable
x Hossmann 1983 0/15 0/15 0.0 Not estimable
x Olinger 1988 0/10 0/10 0.0 Not estimable
STAT 2000 13/248 5/252 100.0 2.64 [0.96, 7.30]
Total (95% CI) 13/337 5/345 100.0 2.64 [0.96, 7.30]
Test for heterogeneity chi-square=0.00 df=0
Test for overall effect=1.87 p=0.06
.1 .2 1 5 10
Treatment better Treatment worse

Figure 6.2 Forest plot showing the effects of *any fibrinogen-depleting agent vs control* for acute ischaemic stroke on *any symptomatic intracranial haemorrhage at the end of the treatment period*. Reproduced from Liu *et al.* (2003), with permission from the authors and John Wiley & Sons Limited. Copyright Cochrane Library, reproduced with permission.

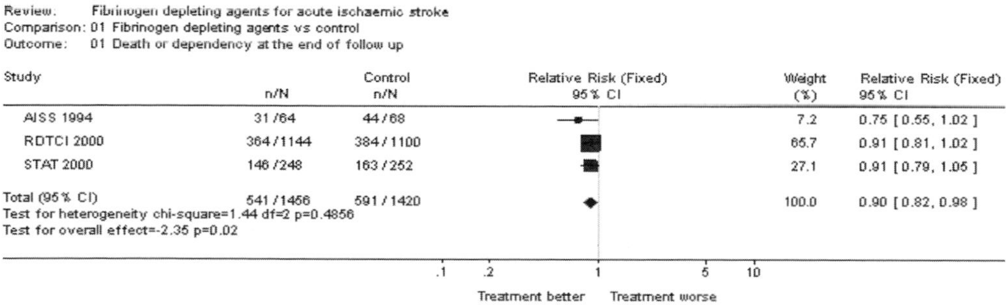
Review: Fibrinogen depleting agents for acute ischaemic stroke
Comparison: 01 Fibrinogen depleting agents vs control
Outcome: 01 Death or dependency at the end of follow up
Study
n/N
Control n/N
Relative Risk (Fixed) 95% CI
Weight (%)
Relative Risk (Fixed) 95% CI
AISS 1994 31/64 44/68 7.2 0.75 [0.55, 1.02]
RDTCI 2000 364/1144 384/1100 65.7 0.91 [0.81, 1.02]
STAT 2000 146/248 163/252 27.1 0.91 [0.79, 1.05]
Total (95% CI) 541/1456 591/1420 100.0 0.90 [0.82, 0.98]
Test for heterogeneity chi-square=1.44 df=2 p=0.4856
Test for overall effect=-2.35 p=0.02
.1 .2 1 5 10
Treatment better Treatment worse

Figure 6.3 Forest plot showing the effects of *any fibrinogen-depleting agent vs control* for acute ischaemic stroke on *death or dependency at the end of follow-up*. Reproduced from Liv *et al.* (2003), with permission from the authors and John Wiley & Sons Limited. Copyright Cochrane Library, reproduced with permission.

to unpublished data from ESTAT, a European trial testing ancrod treatment (European STAT) in a 6-h time window, which was terminated prematurely because it did not confirm the findings of the STAT trial in the USA.

Implications for practice

Fibrinogen-depleting agents are promising but cannot presently be recommended for use in acute ischaemic stroke outside the setting of clinical trials.

Implications for research

More data, particularly the results of the unpublished ESTAT trial, are needed before more reliable conclusions can be drawn. Further trials should test simpler fixed-dose regimens if this therapy is to be used widely.

Haemodilution

Evidence

A systematic review identified 18 RCTs trials of haemodilution therapy for acute ischaemic stroke (Asplund, 2002). Ten trials used plasma volume expander alone, and eight trials a combination of venesection and plasma volume expander. The plasma volume expander was dextran 40 in 12 trials, hydroxyethyl starch (HES) in five trials and albumin in one trial. Two trials tested haemodilution in combination with another therapy. Evaluation was blinded in 11 trials.

Death

Random assignment to haemodilution did not significantly reduce deaths within the first 4 weeks compared with control (odds ratio (OR): 1.09, 95% CI: 0.86–1.38) or within 3–6 months (OR: 1.01, 95% CI: 0.84–1.22) (Fig. 6.4).

Death or dependency

Random assignment to haemodilution did not significantly reduce death or dependency or institutionalisation at the end of follow-up (OR: 0.98, 95% CI: 0.84–1.15) (Fig. 6.5). The results were similar in confounded and unconfounded trials, and in trials of isovolaemic and hypervolaemic haemodilution. Although no statistically significant benefits were documented for any particular type of haemodiluting agents, the statistical power to detect effects of HES and albumin was weak.

Venous thromboembolism

Six trials reported venous thromboembolic events. There was a tendency towards reduction in deep venous thrombosis and/or pulmonary embolism at 3–6 months follow-up (OR: 0.59, 95% CI: 0.33–1.06) (Fig. 6.6) (Asplund, 2002). There was no increased risk of serious cardiac events among haemodiluted patients.

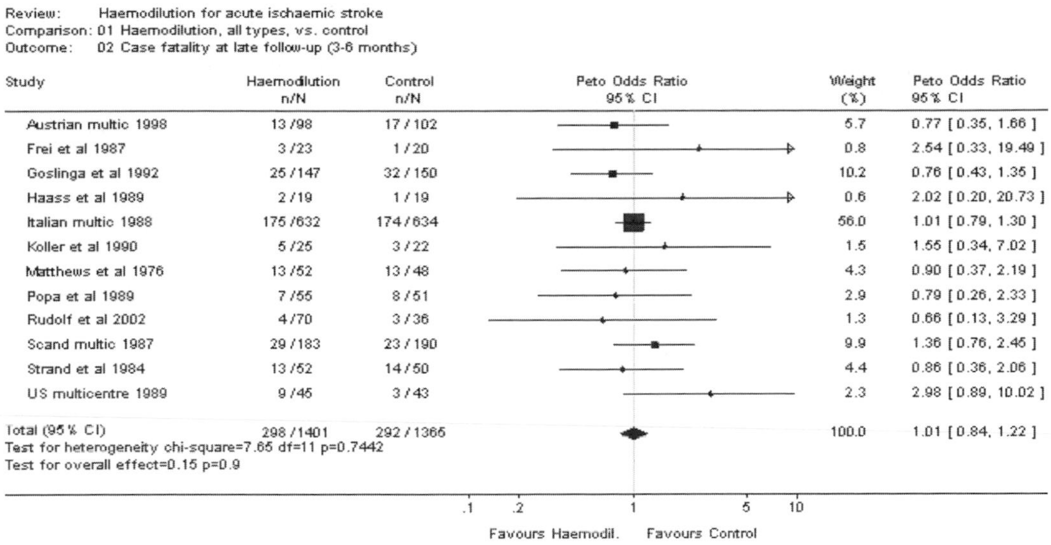

Review: Haemodilution for acute ischaemic stroke
Comparison: 01 Haemodilution, all types, vs. control
Outcome: 02 Case fatality at late follow-up (3-6 months)

Study	Haemodilution n/N	Control n/N	Peto Odds Ratio 95% CI	Weight (%)	Peto Odds Ratio 95% CI
Austrian multic 1998	13 /98	17 / 102		5.7	0.77 [0.35, 1.66]
Frei et al 1987	3 /23	1 / 20		0.8	2.54 [0.33, 19.49]
Goslinga et al 1992	25 /147	32 / 150		10.2	0.76 [0.43, 1.35]
Haass et al 1989	2 /19	1 / 19		0.6	2.02 [0.20, 20.73]
Italian multic 1988	175 /632	174 /634		56.0	1.01 [0.79, 1.30]
Koller et al 1990	5 /25	3 / 22		1.5	1.55 [0.34, 7.02]
Matthews et al 1976	13 /52	13 / 48		4.3	0.90 [0.37, 2.19]
Popa et al 1989	7 /55	8 / 51		2.9	0.79 [0.26, 2.33]
Rudolf et al 2002	4 /70	3 / 36		1.3	0.66 [0.13, 3.29]
Scand multic 1987	29 /183	23 / 190		9.9	1.36 [0.76, 2.45]
Strand et al 1984	13 /52	14 /50		4.4	0.86 [0.36, 2.06]
US multicentre 1989	9 /45	3 / 43		2.3	2.98 [0.89, 10.02]
Total (95% CI)	298 /1401	292 / 1366		100.0	1.01 [0.84, 1.22]

Test for heterogeneity chi-square=7.65 df=11 p=0.7442
Test for overall effect=0.15 p=0.9

.1   .2   1   5   10

Favours Haemodil.   Favours Control

Figure 6.4   Forest plot showing the effects of *any haemodilution agent vs control* for acute ischaemic stroke on *case fatality at the end of follow-up*. Reproduced from Asplund (2002), with permission from the authors and John Wiley & Sons Limited. Copyright Cochrane Library, reproduced with permission.

Review.   Haemodilution for acute ischaemic stroke
Comparison: 01 Haemodilution, all types, vs. control
Outcome: 03 Dead or dependent/institutionalised at 3-6 months

Study	Haemodilution n/N	Control n/N	Peto Odds Ratio 95% CI	Weight (%)	Peto Odds Ratio 95% CI
Austrian multic 1998	68 /98	77 / 102		6.6	0.74 [0.40, 1.37]
Goslinga et al 1992	78 /147	87 / 150		12.1	0.82 [0.52, 1.29]
Italian multic 1988	343 /632	331 /634		52.0	1.09 [0.87, 1.35]
Koller et al 1990	10 /25	11 / 22		1.9	0.67 [0.22, 2.10]
Matthews et al 1976	24 /52	18 / 48		4.1	1.42 [0.64, 3.13]
Rudolf et al 2002	28 /70	20 / 36		3.9	0.54 [0.24, 1.20]
Scand multic 1987	85 /183	76 / 190		15.1	1.30 [0.86, 1.96]
Strand et al 1984	18 /52	28 /50		4.2	0.43 [0.20, 0.92]
Total (95% CI)	654 /1259	648 / 1232		100.0	0.98 [0.84, 1.15]

Test for heterogeneity chi-square=11.93 df=7 p=0.103
Test for overall effect=-0.19 p=0.8

.1   .2   1   5   10

Favours Haemodil.   Favours Control

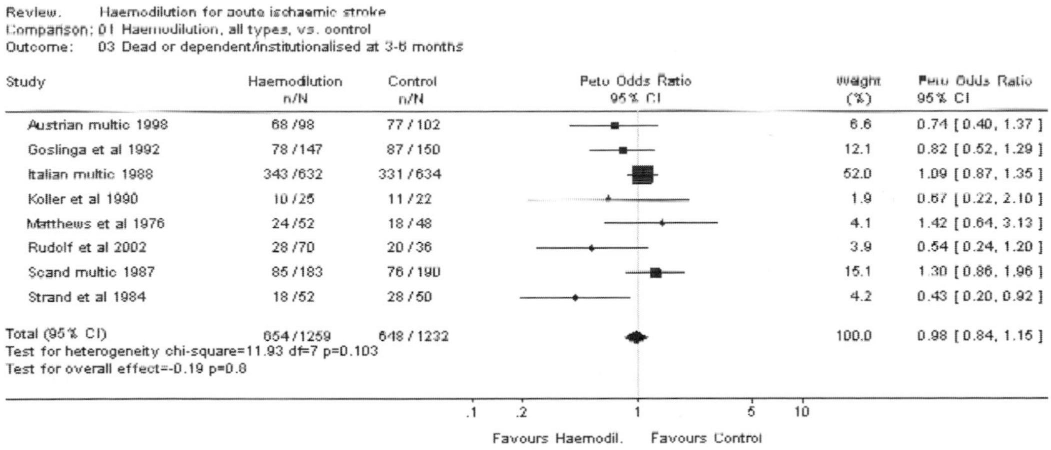

Figure 6.5   Forest plot showing the effects of *any haemodilution agent vs control* for acute ischaemic stroke on *death or dependency or institutionalisation at the end of follow-up*. Reproduced from Asplund (2002), with permission from the authors and John Wiley & Sons Limited. Copyright Cochrane Library, reproduced with permission.

Allergic reactions

Haemodilution was associated with a significant increase in anaphylactic reactions (OR: 7.36, 95% CI: 1.48–36) (Fig. 6.7). The absolute increase was 0.5% (i.e. on in 200) (Asplund, 2002).

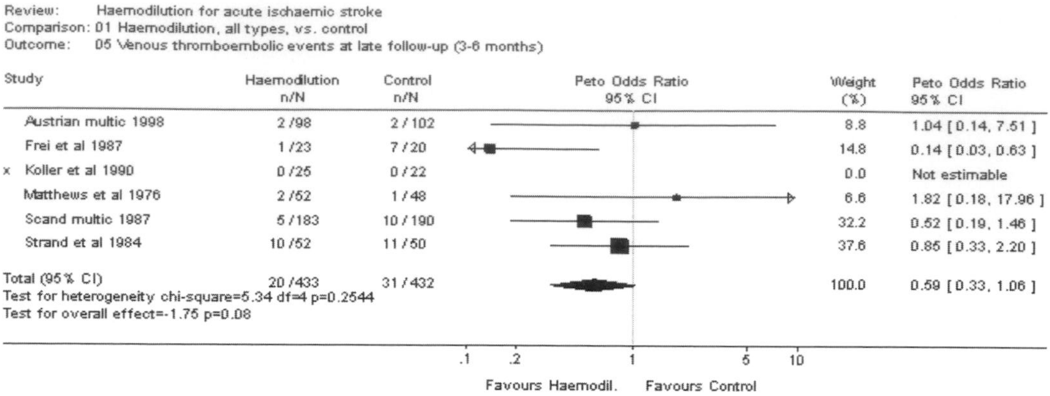

Review: Haemodilution for acute ischaemic stroke
Comparison: 01 Haemodilution, all types, vs. control
Outcome: 05 Venous thromboembolic events at late follow-up (3-6 months)

Study	Haemodilution n/N	Control n/N	Peto Odds Ratio 95% CI	Weight (%)	Peto Odds Ratio 95% CI
Austrian multic 1998	2 /98	2 / 102		8.8	1.04 [0.14, 7.51]
Frei et al 1987	1 /23	7 / 20		14.8	0.14 [0.03, 0.63]
x Koller et al 1990	0 /25	0 / 22		0.0	Not estimable
Matthews et al 1976	2 /52	1 / 48		6.6	1.82 [0.18, 17.96]
Scand multic 1987	5 /183	10 / 190		32.2	0.52 [0.19, 1.46]
Strand et al 1984	10 /52	11 / 50		37.6	0.85 [0.33, 2.20]
Total (95% CI)	20 /433	31 /432		100.0	0.59 [0.33, 1.06]

Test for heterogeneity chi-square=5.34 df=4 p=0.2544
Test for overall effect=-1.75 p=0.08

.1   .2   1   5   10

Favours Haemodil.   Favours Control

Figure 6.6   Forest plot showing the effects of *any haemodilution agent vs control* for acute ischaemic stroke on *venous thromboembolic events* at the end of follow-up. Reproduced from Asplund (2002), with permission from the authors and John Wiley & Sons Limited. Copyright Cochrane Library, reproduced with permission.

Review: Haemodilution for acute ischaemic stroke
Comparison: 01 Haemodilution, all types, vs. control
Outcome: 06 Anaphylactic (or anaphylactic-like) reactions

Study	Haemodilution n/N	Control n/N	Peto Odds Ratio 95% CI	Weight (%)	Peto Odds Ratio 95% CI
x Austrian multic 1998	0 /98	0 / 102		0.0	Not estimable
x Gilroy et al 1969	0 /46	0 / 54		0.0	Not estimable
Italian multic 1988	2 /632	0 / 634		33.4	7.42 [0.46, 118.83]
x Koller et al 1990	0 /25	0 / 22		0.0	Not estimable
x Rudolf et al 2002	0 /70	0 / 36		0.0	Not estimable
Scand multic 1987	1 /183	0 / 190		16.7	7.68 [0.15, 387.20]
Spudis et al 1973	1 /30	0 / 29		16.7	7.15 [0.14, 360.41]
Strand et al 1984	2 /52	0 / 50		33.1	7.25 [0.46, 117.61]
Total (95% CI)	6 /1136	0 /1117		100.0	7.36 [1.48, 36.58]

Test for heterogeneity chi-square=0.00 df=3 p=1.0
Test for overall effect=2.44 p=0.01

.1   .2   1   5   10

Favours Haemodil.   Favours Control

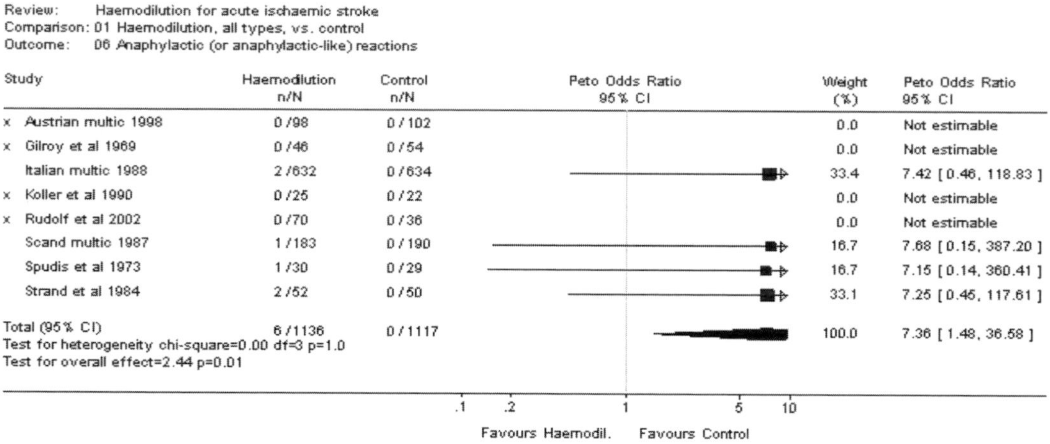

Figure 6.7   Forest plot showing the effects of *any haemodilution agent vs control* for acute ischaemic stroke on *anaphylactic reactions* at the end of the treatment period. Reproduced from Asplund (2002), with permission from the authors and John Wiley & Sons Limited. Copyright Cochrane Library, reproduced with permission.

Comments

Interpretation of the evidence

The overall results of the Cochrane Review are compatible both with modest benefit and moderate harm of haemodilution therapy for acute ischaemic stroke.

Implications for practice

Haemodilution has not been proven to improve survival or functional outcome and has no current place in acute stroke management.

Pentoxifylline

Pentoxifylline, propentofylline and pentifylline are methylxanthine derivatives. They increase blood flow by promoting vasodilatation. They also inhibit thromboxane A2 synthesis (and thus platelet aggregation) and decrease the release of free radicals.

Evidence

Death

A systematic review of five RCTs (four trials testing pentoxifylline in 763 patients, and one trial testing propentofylline in 30 patients) found that there was a non-significant trend towards a reduction in the odds of early death (within 4 weeks) among patients allocated a methylxanthine compared with control (OR: 0.64, 95% CI: 0.41–1.02) (Bath and Bath-Hextall, 2004). This effect was mainly due to a single trial of pentoxifylline reporting a highly significant reduction in early deaths. There was no significant difference in late deaths (beyond 4 weeks) (OR: 0.70, 95% CI: 0.13–3.68).

Death or disability

Two trials reported early death or disability and overall there was a non-significant trend toward a reduction in death or disability among patients allocated a methylxanthine compared with control (OR: 0.49, 95% CI: 0.20–1.20) (Bath and Bath-Hextall, 2004).

Comments

There is not enough reliable evidence to adequately assess the effectiveness and safety of methylxanthines for acute ischaemic stroke.

> **SUMMARY**
>
> Fibrinogen-depleting agents are promising but cannot presently be recommended for use in acute ischaemic stroke outside the setting of clinical trials.
>
> Haemodilution has not been proven to improve survival or functional outcome and has no current place in acute stroke management.
>
> There is not enough reliable evidence to adequately assess the effectiveness and safety of methylxanthines, such as pentoxifylline for acute ischaemic stroke.

Neuroprotection

Rationale

Normally, cerebral blood flow (CBF) is maintained by cerebral autoregulation at about 50 ml blood/100 g brain/min.

In acute ischaemic stroke, a cerebral artery is occluded or there is a reduction in perfusion distal to a severe stenosis, resulting in focal brain ischaemia and infarction. As the regional CBF falls, the regional lack of oxygen and glucose results in a time- and flow-dependent cascade characterised by a fall in energy (adenosine triphosphate, ATP) production. Neuronal function is affected in two stages. The first threshold is at a blood flow of about 20 ml blood/100 g brain/min, below which neuronal electrical function is compromised, but is recoverable. If blood flow falls below the second critical threshold of 10 ml blood/100 g brain/min, there is excessive release from pre-synaptic vesicles, and impaired reuptake, of excitatory amino acid (EAA) neurotransmitters such as glutamate. Neuronal glutamate receptors are overstimulated (excitotoxicity), free radicals are generated, spreading damage occurs, aerobic mitochondrial metabolism fails, inefficient anaerobic metabolism of glucose takes over, and lactic acidosis evolves. Energy-dependent homoeostatic mechanisms of maintaining cellular ions fail, potassium leaks out of cells, and sodium, water and calcium enters cells leading to cytotoxic oedema and calcium-induced mitochondrial failure, respectively (Lee *et al.*, 1999). If severe ischaemia (blood flow below 10 ml blood/100 g brain/min) is sustained, irreversible neuronal damage occurs and neuronal cell apoptosis and necrosis ensue.

The recognition of two thresholds of CBF and stages of neuronal failure led to the concept of the ischaemic penumbra as an area of brain surrounding the infarcted core which has reached the reversible stage of neuronal electrical failure (i.e. it is electrically quiescent) but has not passed into the second irreversible stage of failure of cellular homoeostasis.

Pre-clinical and neuroimaging studies indicate that the untreated penumbra deteriorates over time (Baird *et al.*, 1997; Ginsberg, 1997). This concept is supported

Table 7.1. Drugs to protect brain tissue (neuroprotective agents).

EAA (glutamate) antagonists	Free radical scavengers: antioxidants
AMPA receptor antagonists	Ebselen
Kainate receptor antagonist	Tirilazad
SYM 2081	NXY-059 (Cerovive)
NMDA receptor antagonists	**Growth factors**
	Fibroblast growth factor
• Competitive NMDA antagonists	**Leucocyte adhesion and infiltration**
CGS 19755 (Selfotel)	**inhibitors**
	R6.5 (Enlimomab) anti-ICAM antibody
• NMDA channel blockers	Hu23F2G (LeukArrest)
Aptiganel (Cerestat)	UK-279,276
CP-101,606	**Nitric oxide inhibitors**
Dextrorphan	Lubeluzole
Dextromethorphan	**Opioid antagonists**
Magnesium	Naloxone
Memantine	Nalmefene
MK-801	**Phosphatidylcholine precursors**
NPS 1506	Citicoline (CDP-choline)
Remacemide	**Serotonin agonists**
• Glycine site antagonists	Bay x 3072
ACEA 1021	**Sodium channel blockers**
GV 150526	Fosphenytoin
• Polyamine site antagonists	Lubeluzole
Eliprodil	619C89
Ifenprodil	**Potassium channel openers**
GABA antagonists	BMS-204352
Clomethiazole	**Mechanism(s) unknown or uncertain**
Calcium channel antagonists	Gangliosides
Nimodipine	Piracetam
Flunarazine	Lubeluzole

by *post hoc* analysis of the National Institute of Neurological Disorders and Stroke (NINDS) recombinant tissue plasminogen activator (rt-PA) trial which showed greater benefits of thrombolysis with earlier treatment (Marler, 2000). It remains unknown however just how long ischaemic human brain may survive, and therefore the time window for therapeutic intervention. This will probably vary among individual patients and be influenced by several factors, and not just the severity of the ischaemia. Nevertheless, since a large proportion of stroke-induced neuronal death develops over many hours, it is possible that the time window may be longer than currently appreciated.

The potential role of neuroprotective therapy is to support the ischaemic penumbra whilst endogenous, with or without exogenous, thrombolysis endeavours to restore CBF.

There are several drugs which aim to protect brain tissue (neuroprotective agents), some of which are listed in Table 7.1.

EAA (glutamate) antagonists

Focal cerebral ischaemia causes excess release of EAA neurotransmitters, particularly glutamate, from pre-synaptic vesicles and prevents normal reuptake of glutamate, resulting in very high synaptic concentrations of glutamate. Glutamate is toxic in neuronal cell culture and *in vivo*. It acts at post-synaptic receptors, notably the N-methyl-D-aspartate (NMDA) receptor complex (to promote entry of calcium and sodium into neurones) and the α-amino-3-hydroxy-5-methylisoxazole-4-propionic acid (AMPA) receptor (to promote principally sodium entry). Resultant cellular depolarisation and calcium overload activates intracellular second messenger systems with consequent cell death.

In pre-clinical models of stroke, antagonists of glutamate release or of post-synaptic glutamate receptors significantly reduce the volume of histological neuronal infarction, and improve functional recovery, even when administered up to several hours after the onset of ischaemia (Muir and Lees, 2003). Drugs that modulate EAA toxicity (EAA antagonists) encompass a diversity of pharmacological agents and a number of potential mechanisms of action, including principally inhibition of glutamate release, NMDA receptor antagonism and AMPA receptor antagonism. The NMDA receptor itself has multiple modulatory sites that are amenable to pharmacological modification. Furthermore, many of these drugs also have ancillary properties which may influence both their efficacy and safety (Muir and Lees, 2003).

Evidence

A systematic review of randomised-controlled trials (RCTs) of EAA antagonists vs control in acute ischaemic stroke revealed that there were 29 RCTs involving a total of 10,802 patients which could contribute to an efficacy analysis (Fig. 7.1). Time to treatment averaged under 5 h in many trials, although only a minority of patients were treated in 3 h or less after stroke onset. There was no substantial heterogeneity of outcome amongst individual drugs, or of drug classes either for the primary efficacy analysis (death or dependence) or for mortality at final follow-up (Muir and Lees, 2003).

Death or dependency

Random allocation to an EAA antagonist was associated with no significant effect on death or dependence at final follow-up compared with control (odds ratio (OR): 1.04, 95% confidence interval (CI): 0.96–1.12) (Fig. 7.1). There was a trend towards heterogeneity of outcome amongst individual drugs ($P = 0.05$) (Muir and Lees, 2003).

Death

Random allocation to an EAA antagonist was associated with no significant effect on death at final follow-up compared with control (OR: 1.01, 95% CI: 0.92–1.11) (Fig. 7.2). There was no heterogeneity among the trials ($P = 0.92$) (Muir and Lees, 2003).

Subgroup analyses

Drug classes   The effect of ion channel modulators on death or dependence (OR: 1.02, 95% CI: 0.90–1.16) and NMDA antagonists on death or dependence (OR: 1.05, 95% CI: 0.95–1.16) did not differ from the principal analysis including all compounds (Fig. 7.3). However, trends towards heterogeneity for death or dependence (but not mortality) among both ion channel modulators (Chi-squared = 11.3, d.f. = 6, $P = 0.08$) and NMDA antagonists (Chi-squared = 15.1, d.f. = 9, $P = 0.09$) suggested that broad classification into these modes of action may be inappropriate. Individual drug analysis may be more informative.

Individual drugs   Allocation to one of three NMDA antagonists was associated with non-statistically significant trends for increased mortality – selfotel (OR: 1.18 [0.81–1.73]), aptiganel (OR: 1.32 [0.92–1.91]) and gavestinel (OR: 1.12 [0.95–1.32]) (Fig. 7.2). Aptiganel was also associated with a trend towards worse functional outcome (OR: 1.20 [0.88–1.65]) (Fig. 7.1).

Exploratory analysis of NMDA antagonists with psychotomimetic side effects at the doses studied vs those without psychotomimetic effects disclosed no effect on death or dependency (OR: 1.01, 95% CI: 0.81–1.26) (Fig. 7.4), but a trend towards higher mortality with psychotomimetic drugs (aptiganel and selfotel) (OR: 1.25, 95% CI: 0.96–1.64) (Fig. 7.5).

Lubeluzole

Lubeluzole is a benzothiazole derivative that has shown neuroprotective properties in different experimental models inhibiting glutamate release, nitric oxide (NO) synthesis and blocking voltage-gated sodium and calcium ion channels.

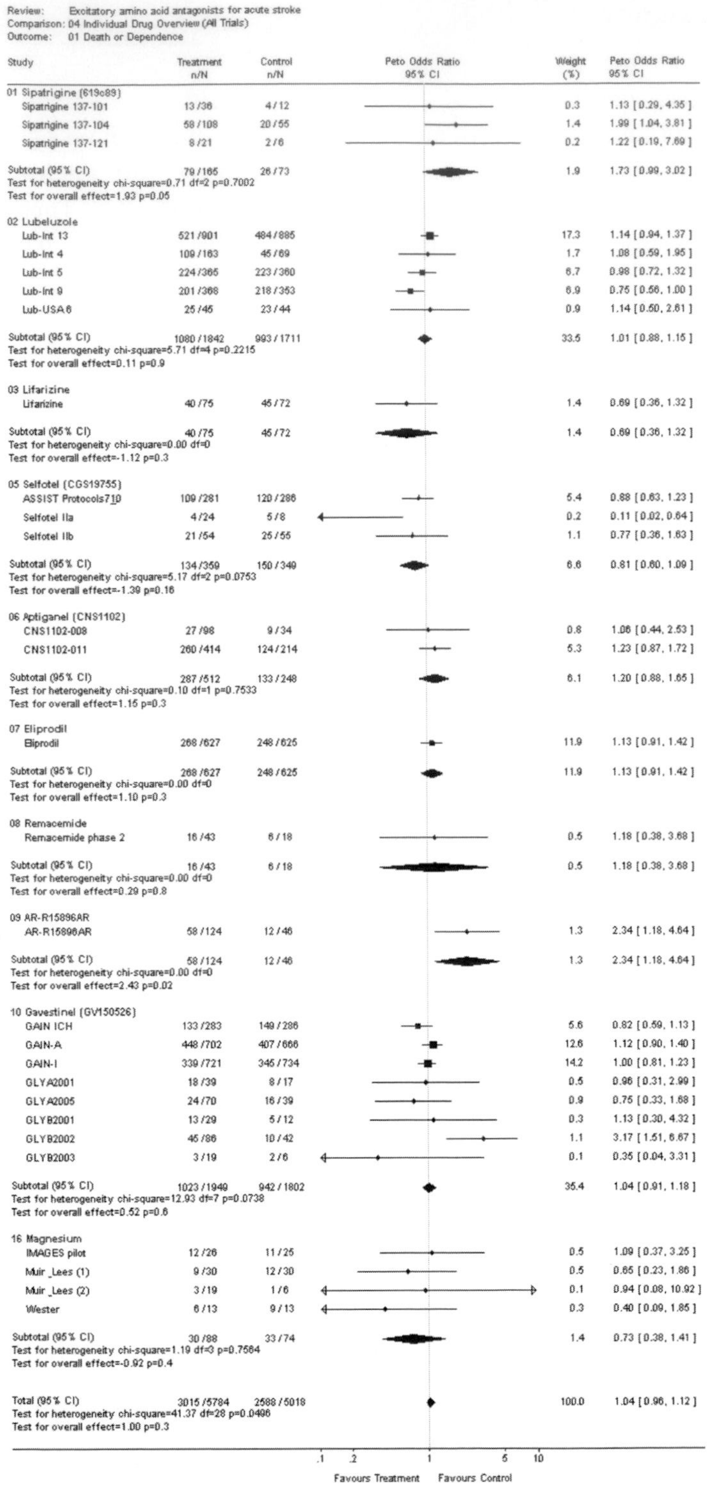

Review: Excitatory amino acid antagonists for acute stroke
Comparison: 04 Individual Drug Overview (All Trials)
Outcome: 01 Death or Dependence

Study	Treatment n/N	Control n/N	Peto Odds Ratio 95% CI	Weight (%)	Peto Odds Ratio 95% CI
01 Sipatrigine (619c89)					
Sipatrigine 137-101	13 /36	4 / 12		0.3	1.13 [0.29, 4.35]
Sipatrigine 137-104	58 /108	20 / 55		1.4	1.99 [1.04, 3.81]
Sipatrigine 137-121	8 /21	2 / 6		0.2	1.22 [0.19, 7.69]
Subtotal (95% CI)	79 /165	26 / 73		1.9	1.73 [0.99, 3.02]
Test for heterogeneity chi-square=0.71 df=2 p=0.7002					
Test for overall effect=1.93 p=0.05					
02 Lubeluzole					
Lub-Int 13	521 /901	484 / 885		17.3	1.14 [0.94, 1.37]
Lub-Int 4	109 /163	45 / 69		1.7	1.08 [0.59, 1.95]
Lub-Int 5	224 /365	223 / 360		8.7	0.98 [0.72, 1.32]
Lub-Int 9	201 /366	218 / 353		6.9	0.75 [0.56, 1.00]
Lub-USA 6	25 /45	23 / 44		0.9	1.14 [0.50, 2.61]
Subtotal (95% CI)	1080 /1842	993 / 1711		33.5	1.01 [0.88, 1.15]
Test for heterogeneity chi-square=5.71 df=4 p=0.2215					
Test for overall effect=0.11 p=0.9					
03 Lifarizine					
Lifarizine	40 /75	45 / 72		1.4	0.69 [0.36, 1.32]
Subtotal (95% CI)	40 /75	45 / 72		1.4	0.69 [0.36, 1.32]
Test for heterogeneity chi-square=0.00 df=0					
Test for overall effect=-1.12 p=0.3					
05 Selfotel (CGS19755)					
ASSIST Protocols710	109 /281	120 / 286		5.4	0.88 [0.63, 1.23]
Selfotel IIa	4 /24	5 / 8		0.2	0.11 [0.02, 0.64]
Selfotel IIb	21 /54	25 / 55		1.1	0.77 [0.36, 1.63]
Subtotal (95% CI)	134 /359	150 / 349		6.6	0.81 [0.60, 1.09]
Test for heterogeneity chi-square=5.17 df=2 p=0.0753					
Test for overall effect=-1.39 p=0.16					
06 Aptiganel (CNS1102)					
CNS1102-008	27 /98	9 / 34		0.8	1.06 [0.44, 2.53]
CNS1102-011	260 /414	124 / 214		5.3	1.23 [0.87, 1.72]
Subtotal (95% CI)	287 /512	133 / 248		6.1	1.20 [0.88, 1.65]
Test for heterogeneity chi-square=0.10 df=1 p=0.7533					
Test for overall effect=1.15 p=0.3					
07 Eliprodil					
Eliprodil	268 /627	248 / 625		11.9	1.13 [0.91, 1.42]
Subtotal (95% CI)	268 /627	248 / 625		11.9	1.13 [0.91, 1.42]
Test for heterogeneity chi-square=0.00 df=0					
Test for overall effect=1.10 p=0.3					
08 Remacemide					
Remacemide phase 2	16 /43	6 / 18		0.5	1.18 [0.38, 3.68]
Subtotal (95% CI)	16 /43	6 / 18		0.5	1.18 [0.38, 3.68]
Test for heterogeneity chi-square=0.00 df=0					
Test for overall effect=0.29 p=0.8					
09 AR-R15896AR					
AR-R15896AR	58 /124	12 / 46		1.3	2.34 [1.18, 4.64]
Subtotal (95% CI)	58 /124	12 / 46		1.3	2.34 [1.18, 4.64]
Test for heterogeneity chi-square=0.00 df=0					
Test for overall effect=2.43 p=0.02					
10 Gavestinel (GV150526)					
GAIN ICH	133 /283	149 / 286		5.6	0.82 [0.59, 1.13]
GAIN-A	448 /702	407 / 666		12.6	1.12 [0.90, 1.40]
GAIN-I	339 /721	345 / 734		14.2	1.00 [0.81, 1.23]
GLYA2001	18 /39	8 / 17		0.5	0.96 [0.31, 2.99]
GLYA2005	24 /70	16 / 39		0.9	0.75 [0.33, 1.68]
GLYB2001	13 /29	5 / 12		0.3	1.13 [0.30, 4.32]
GLYB2002	45 /86	10 / 42		1.1	3.17 [1.51, 6.67]
GLYB2003	3 /19	2 / 6		0.1	0.35 [0.04, 3.31]
Subtotal (95% CI)	1023 /1949	942 / 1802		35.4	1.04 [0.91, 1.18]
Test for heterogeneity chi-square=12.93 df=7 p=0.0738					
Test for overall effect=0.52 p=0.6					
16 Magnesium					
IMAGES pilot	12 /26	11 / 25		0.5	1.09 [0.37, 3.25]
Muir_Lees (1)	9 /30	12 / 30		0.5	0.65 [0.23, 1.86]
Muir_Lees (2)	3 /19	1 / 6		0.1	0.94 [0.08, 10.92]
Wester	6 /13	9 / 13		0.3	0.40 [0.09, 1.85]
Subtotal (95% CI)	30 /88	33 / 74		1.4	0.73 [0.38, 1.41]
Test for heterogeneity chi-square=1.19 df=3 p=0.7564					
Test for overall effect=-0.92 p=0.4					
Total (95% CI)	3015 /5784	2588 / 5018		100.0	1.04 [0.96, 1.12]
Test for heterogeneity chi-square=41.37 df=28 p=0.0496					
Test for overall effect=1.00 p=0.3					

.1   .2   1   5   10

Favours Treatment   Favours Control

Figure 7.1   Forest plot showing the effects of *all EAAs vs control* for acute ischaemic stroke on *death or dependency at the end of follow-up*. Reproduced from Muir and Lees (2003), with permission from the authors and John Wiley & Sons Limited. Copyright Cochrane Library, reproduced with permission.

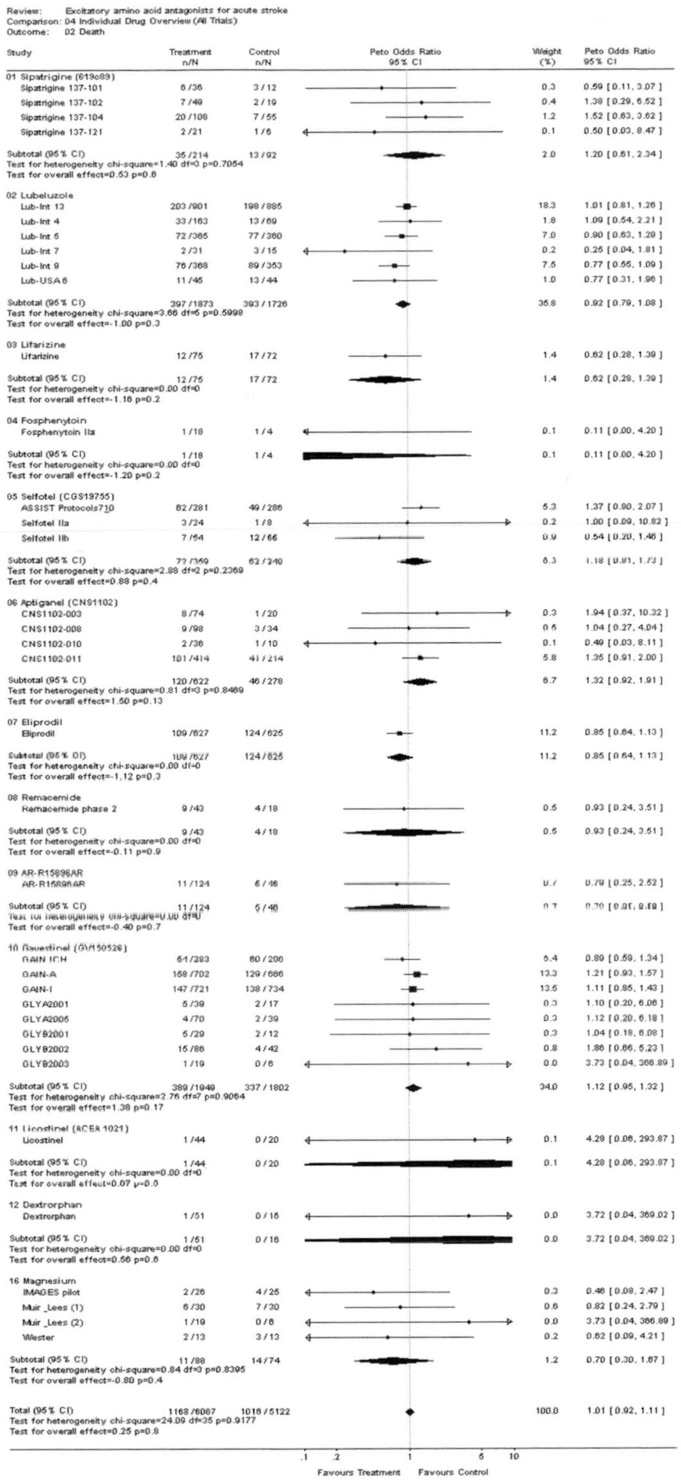

Review: Excitatory amino acid antagonists for acute stroke
Comparison: 04 Individual Drug Overview (All Trials)
Outcome: 02 Death

Study	Treatment n/N	Control n/N	Peto Odds Ratio 95% CI	Weight (%)	Peto Odds Ratio 95% CI
01 Sipatrigine (619c89)					
Sipatrigine 137-101	6 /36	3 /12		0.3	0.59 [0.11, 3.07]
Sipatrigine 137-102	7 /49	2 /19		0.4	1.38 [0.29, 6.52]
Sipatrigine 137-104	20 /108	7 /55		1.2	1.52 [0.63, 3.62]
Sipatrigine 137-121	2 /21	1 /6		0.1	0.50 [0.03, 8.47]
Subtotal (95% CI)	35 /214	13 /92		2.0	1.20 [0.61, 2.34]
Test for heterogeneity chi-square=1.40 df=3 p=0.7054					
Test for overall effect=0.53 p=0.6					
02 Lubeluzole					
Lub-Int 13	203 /901	198 /885		18.3	1.01 [0.81, 1.26]
Lub-Int 4	33 /163	13 /69		1.8	1.09 [0.54, 2.21]
Lub-Int 5	72 /385	77 /380		7.0	0.90 [0.63, 1.29]
Lub-Int 7	2 /31	3 /15		0.2	0.25 [0.04, 1.81]
Lub-Int 9	76 /368	89 /353		7.5	0.77 [0.55, 1.09]
Lub-USA 6	11 /44	13 /44		1.0	0.77 [0.31, 1.96]
Subtotal (95% CI)	397 /1873	393 /1726		35.8	0.92 [0.79, 1.08]
Test for heterogeneity chi-square=3.66 df=5 p=0.5998					
Test for overall effect=-1.00 p=0.3					
03 Lifarizine					
Lifarizine	12 /75	17 /72		1.4	0.62 [0.28, 1.39]
Subtotal (95% CI)	12 /75	17 /72		1.4	0.62 [0.28, 1.39]
Test for heterogeneity chi-square=0.00 df=0					
Test for overall effect=-1.16 p=0.2					
04 Fosphenytoin					
Fosphenytoin IIa	1 /18	1 /4		0.1	0.11 [0.00, 4.20]
Subtotal (95% CI)	1 /18	1 /4		0.1	0.11 [0.00, 4.20]
Test for heterogeneity chi-square=0.00 df=0					
Test for overall effect=-1.20 p=0.2					
05 Selfotel (CGS19755)					
ASSIST Protocols710	62 /281	49 /286		5.3	1.37 [0.90, 2.07]
Selfotel IIa	3 /24	1 /8		0.2	1.00 [0.09, 10.82]
Selfotel IIb	7 /54	12 /66		0.9	0.54 [0.20, 1.46]
Subtotal (95% CI)	72 /359	62 /340		6.3	1.18 [0.81, 1.73]
Test for heterogeneity chi-square=2.88 df=2 p=0.2369					
Test for overall effect=0.88 p=0.4					
06 Aptiganel (CNS1102)					
CNS1102-003	8 /74	1 /20		0.3	1.94 [0.37, 10.32]
CNS1102-008	9 /98	3 /34		0.5	1.04 [0.27, 4.04]
CNS1102-010	2 /36	1 /10		0.1	0.49 [0.03, 8.11]
CNS1102-011	101 /414	41 /214		5.8	1.35 [0.91, 2.00]
Subtotal (95% CI)	120 /622	46 /278		6.7	1.32 [0.92, 1.91]
Test for heterogeneity chi-square=0.81 df=3 p=0.8469					
Test for overall effect=1.50 p=0.13					
07 Eliprodil					
Eliprodil	109 /827	124 /625		11.2	0.85 [0.64, 1.13]
Subtotal (95% CI)	109 /827	124 /625		11.2	0.85 [0.64, 1.13]
Test for heterogeneity chi-square=0.00 df=0					
Test for overall effect=-1.12 p=0.3					
08 Remacemide					
Remacemide phase 2	9 /43	4 /18		0.5	0.93 [0.24, 3.51]
Subtotal (95% CI)	9 /43	4 /18		0.5	0.93 [0.24, 3.51]
Test for heterogeneity chi-square=0.00 df=0					
Test for overall effect=-0.11 p=0.9					
09 AR-R15896AR					
AR-R15896AR	11 /124	6 /46		0.7	0.70 [0.25, 2.52]
Subtotal (95% CI)	11 /124	6 /46		0.7	0.70 [0.25, 2.52]
Test for heterogeneity chi-square=0.00 df=0					
Test for overall effect=-0.40 p=0.7					
10 Gavestinel (GV150526)					
GAIN ICH	61 /293	60 /200		5.4	0.89 [0.59, 1.34]
GAIN-A	168 /702	129 /686		13.3	1.21 [0.93, 1.57]
GAIN-I	147 /721	138 /734		13.5	1.11 [0.85, 1.43]
GLYA2001	5 /39	2 /17		0.3	1.10 [0.20, 6.08]
GLYA2005	4 /70	2 /39		0.3	1.12 [0.20, 6.18]
GLYB2001	5 /29	2 /12		0.3	1.04 [0.18, 6.08]
GLYB2002	15 /86	4 /42		0.8	1.86 [0.66, 5.23]
GLYB2003	1 /19	0 /6		0.0	3.73 [0.04, 366.89]
Subtotal (95% CI)	389 /1949	337 /1802		34.0	1.12 [0.95, 1.32]
Test for heterogeneity chi-square=2.76 df=7 p=0.9064					
Test for overall effect=1.38 p=0.17					
11 Licostinel (ACEA 1021)					
Licostinel	1 /44	0 /20		0.1	4.28 [0.06, 293.87]
Subtotal (95% CI)	1 /44	0 /20		0.1	4.28 [0.06, 293.87]
Test for heterogeneity chi-square=0.00 df=0					
Test for overall effect=0.07 p=0.5					
12 Dextrorphan					
Dextrorphan	1 /51	0 /16		0.0	3.72 [0.04, 369.02]
Subtotal (95% CI)	1 /51	0 /16		0.0	3.72 [0.04, 369.02]
Test for heterogeneity chi-square=0.00 df=0					
Test for overall effect=0.56 p=0.6					
16 Magnesium					
IMAGES pilot	2 /26	4 /25		0.3	0.46 [0.08, 2.47]
Muir_Lees (1)	6 /30	7 /30		0.6	0.82 [0.24, 2.79]
Muir_Lees (2)	1 /19	0 /8		0.0	3.73 [0.04, 366.89]
Wester	2 /13	3 /13		0.2	0.62 [0.09, 4.21]
Subtotal (95% CI)	11 /88	14 /74		1.2	0.70 [0.30, 1.67]
Test for heterogeneity chi-square=0.84 df=3 p=0.8395					
Test for overall effect=-0.80 p=0.4					
Total (95% CI)	1168 /6087	1016 /5122		100.0	1.01 [0.92, 1.11]
Test for heterogeneity chi-square=24.09 df=35 p=0.9177					
Test for overall effect=0.25 p=0.8					

.1   .2   1   5   10
Favours Treatment   Favours Control

Figure 7.2 Forest plot showing the effects of *all EAAs vs control* for acute ischaemic stroke on *death at the end of follow-up*. Reproduced from Muir and Lees (2003), with permission from the authors and John Wiley & Sons Limited. Copyright Cochrane Library, reproduced with permission.

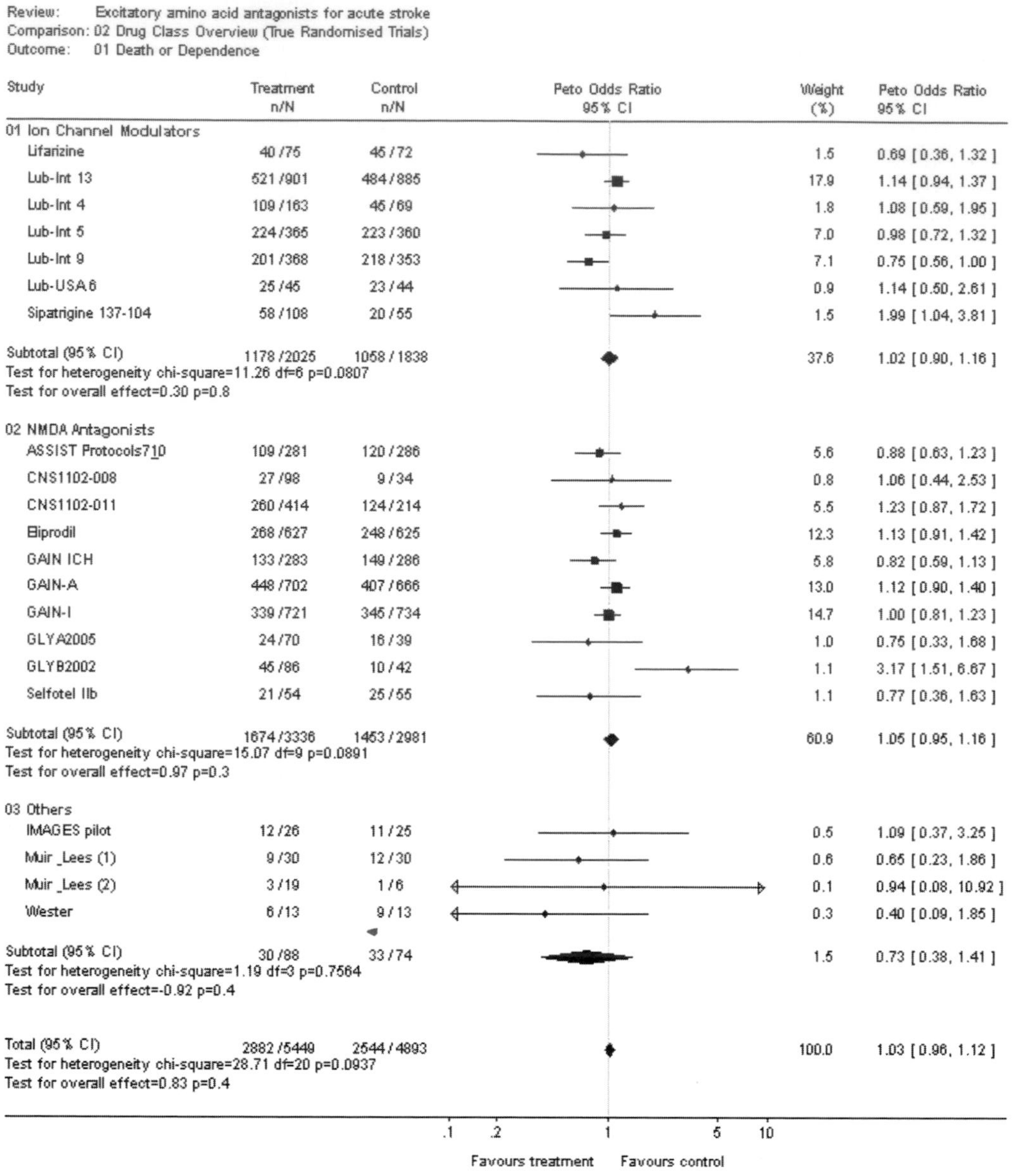

Review: Excitatory amino acid antagonists for acute stroke
Comparison: 02 Drug Class Overview (True Randomised Trials)
Outcome: 01 Death or Dependence

Study	Treatment n/N	Control n/N	Peto Odds Ratio 95% CI	Weight (%)	Peto Odds Ratio 95% CI
01 Ion Channel Modulators					
Lifarizine	40 /75	45 /72		1.5	0.69 [0.36, 1.32]
Lub-Int 13	521 /901	484 /885		17.9	1.14 [0.94, 1.37]
Lub-Int 4	109 /163	45 /69		1.8	1.08 [0.59, 1.95]
Lub-Int 5	224 /365	223 /360		7.0	0.98 [0.72, 1.32]
Lub-Int 9	201 /368	218 /353		7.1	0.75 [0.56, 1.00]
Lub-USA 6	25 /45	23 /44		0.9	1.14 [0.50, 2.61]
Sipatrigine 137-104	58 /108	20 /55		1.5	1.99 [1.04, 3.81]
Subtotal (95% CI)	1178 /2025	1058 / 1838		37.6	1.02 [0.90, 1.16]

Test for heterogeneity chi-square=11.26 df=6 p=0.0807
Test for overall effect=0.30 p=0.8

02 NMDA Antagonists					
ASSIST Protocols7 10	109 /281	120 /286		5.6	0.88 [0.63, 1.23]
CNS1102-008	27 /98	9 /34		0.8	1.06 [0.44, 2.53]
CNS1102-011	260 /414	124 /214		5.5	1.23 [0.87, 1.72]
Eliprodil	268 /627	248 /625		12.3	1.13 [0.91, 1.42]
GAIN ICH	133 /283	149 /286		5.8	0.82 [0.59, 1.13]
GAIN-A	448 /702	407 /666		13.0	1.12 [0.90, 1.40]
GAIN-I	339 /721	345 /734		14.7	1.00 [0.81, 1.23]
GLYA2005	24 /70	16 /39		1.0	0.75 [0.33, 1.68]
GLYB2002	46 /86	10 /42		1.1	3.17 [1.51, 6.67]
Selfotel IIb	21 /54	25 /55		1.1	0.77 [0.36, 1.63]
Subtotal (95% CI)	1674 /3336	1453 /2981		60.9	1.05 [0.95, 1.16]

Test for heterogeneity chi-square=15.07 df=9 p=0.0891
Test for overall effect=0.97 p=0.3

03 Others					
IMAGES pilot	12 /26	11 /25		0.5	1.09 [0.37, 3.25]
Muir _Lees (1)	9 /30	12 /30		0.6	0.65 [0.23, 1.86]
Muir _Lees (2)	3 /19	1 /6		0.1	0.94 [0.08, 10.92]
Wester	6 /13	9 /13		0.3	0.40 [0.09, 1.85]
Subtotal (95% CI)	30 /88	33 /74		1.5	0.73 [0.38, 1.41]

Test for heterogeneity chi-square=1.19 df=3 p=0.7564
Test for overall effect=-0.92 p=0.4

| Total (95% CI) | 2882 /5449 | 2544 / 4893 | | 100.0 | 1.03 [0.96, 1.12] |

Test for heterogeneity chi-square=28.71 df=20 p=0.0937
Test for overall effect=0.83 p=0.4

.1   .2   1   5   10

Favours treatment   Favours control

Figure 7.3   Forest plot showing the effects of *all EAAs vs control* for acute ischaemic stroke on *death or dependency at the end of follow-up, according to drug class*. Reproduced from Muir and Lees (2003), with permission from the authors and John Wiley & Sons Limited. Copyright Cochrane Library, reproduced with permission.

Evidence

There have been five randomised unconfounded trials comparing intravenous (i.v.) lubeluzole with placebo or open control in patients with a clinical syndrome definitely considered as an acute stroke in whom computed tomographical (CT)

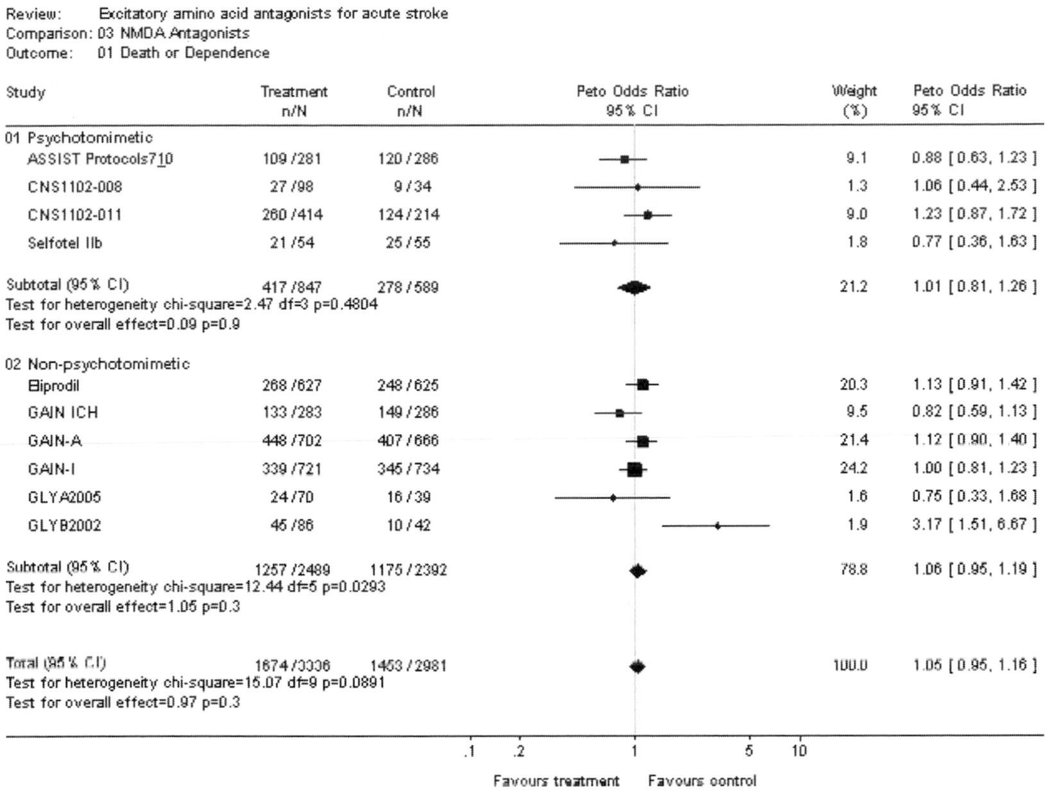

Review: Excitatory amino acid antagonists for acute stroke
Comparison: 03 NMDA Antagonists
Outcome: 01 Death or Dependence

Study	Treatment n/N	Control n/N	Peto Odds Ratio 95% CI	Weight (%)	Peto Odds Ratio 95% CI
01 Psychotomimetic					
ASSIST Protocols710	109 /281	120 /286		9.1	0.88 [0.63, 1.23]
CNS1102-008	27 /98	9 /34		1.3	1.06 [0.44, 2.53]
CNS1102-011	260 /414	124 /214		9.0	1.23 [0.87, 1.72]
Selfotel IIb	21 /54	25 /55		1.8	0.77 [0.36, 1.63]
Subtotal (95% CI)	417 /847	278 /589		21.2	1.01 [0.81, 1.26]
Test for heterogeneity chi-square=2.47 df=3 p=0.4804					
Test for overall effect=0.09 p=0.9					
02 Non-psychotomimetic					
Eliprodil	268 /627	248 /625		20.3	1.13 [0.91, 1.42]
GAIN ICH	133 /283	149 /286		9.5	0.82 [0.59, 1.13]
GAIN-A	448 /702	407 /666		21.4	1.12 [0.90, 1.40]
GAIN-I	339 /721	345 /734		24.2	1.00 [0.81, 1.23]
GLYA2005	24 /70	16 /39		1.6	0.75 [0.33, 1.68]
GLYB2002	45 /86	10 /42		1.9	3.17 [1.51, 6.67]
Subtotal (95% CI)	1257 /2489	1175 /2392		78.8	1.06 [0.95, 1.19]
Test for heterogeneity chi-square=12.44 df=5 p=0.0293					
Test for overall effect=1.05 p=0.3					
Total (95% CI)	1674 /3336	1453 /2981		100.0	1.05 [0.95, 1.16]
Test for heterogeneity chi-square=15.07 df=9 p=0.0891					
Test for overall effect=0.97 p=0.3					

.1   .2   1   5   10

Favours treatment   Favours control

Figure 7.4   Forest plot showing the effects of *NMDA receptor antagonists vs control* for acute ischaemic stroke on *death or dependency at the end of follow-up*. Reproduced from Muir and Lees (2003), with permission from the authors and John Wiley & Sons Limited. Copyright Cochrane Library, reproduced with permission.

scanning showed an infarct or was normal (Gandolfo *et al.*, 2002). Lubeluzole given at the doses of 5, 10 and 20 mg/day for 5 days was tested against a placebo-control group in a total of 3510 patients.

There was no evidence that lubeluzole given at any dose either reduced the odds of death from all causes (OR: 0.92, 95% CI: 0.79–1.08) (Fig. 7.2) or reduced the odds of being dead or dependent at the end of follow-up (OR: 1.01, 95% CI: 0.88–1.15) (Fig. 7.1).

However, when given at any dose, lubeluzole was associated with a significant excess of heart-conduction disorders (QT prolonged >450 ms) at the end of follow-up (OR: 1.43, 95% CI: 1.09–1.88) (Fig. 7.6).

Comment

Lubeluzole, given in the acute phase of ischaemic stroke, is not associated with a significant reduction of death or dependency at the end of scheduled follow-up

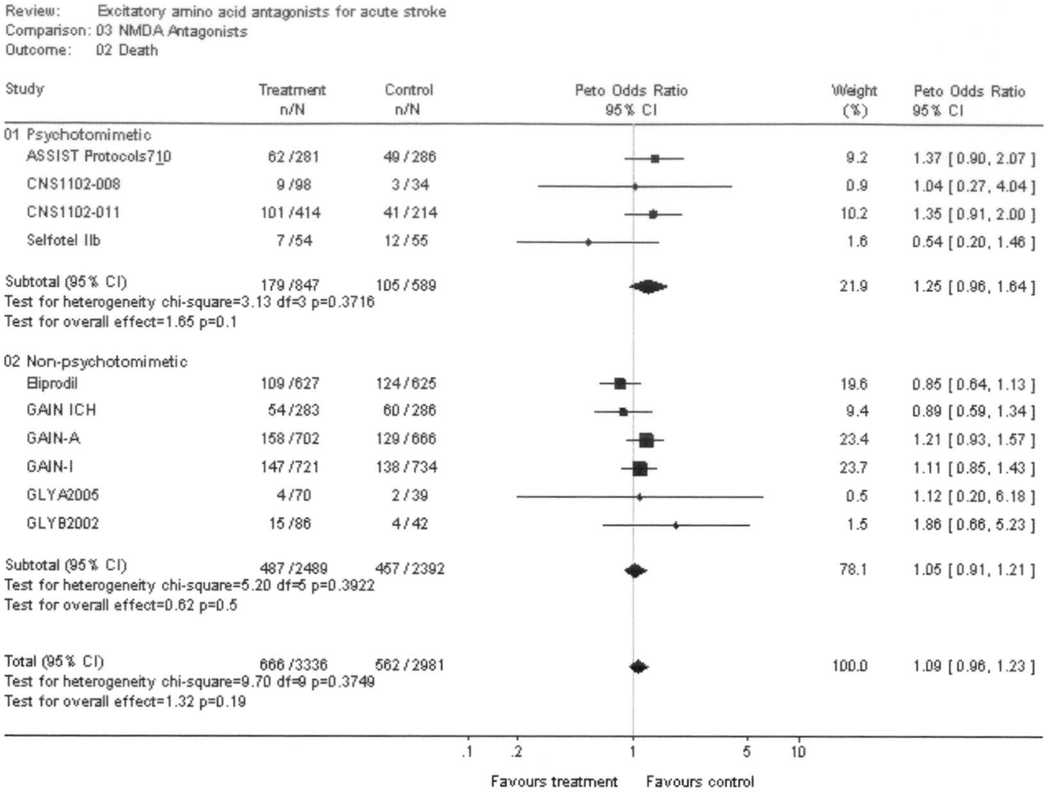

Figure 7.5   Forest plot showing the effects of *NMDA receptor antagonists vs control* for acute
ischaemic stroke on *death at the end of follow-up*. Reproduced from Muir and Lees
(2003), with permission from the authors and John Wiley & Sons Limited. Copyright
Cochrane Library, reproduced with permission.

period but seems to be associated with a significant increase of heart-conduction
disorders (QT prolonged >450 ms).

Magnesium

Magnesium is neuroprotective in animal models of stroke. Potential neuroprotective effects have been identified in preterm perinatal hypoxic injury (Crowther
et al., 2003). The mechanism of neuroprotection by magnesium is uncertain but
increasing magnesium concentration reduces pre-synaptic release of the neuro-
transmitter glutamate, blocks glutamatergic NMDA receptors, potentiates adenosine
action, improves mitochondrial calcium buffering and blocks calcium entry via
voltage-gated channels. Furthermore, it has cardiovascular effects, notably enhanced
cerebral perfusion after middle cerebral artery occlusion and raised cardiac output.
Magnesium is an attractive neuroprotective agent because of low cost and apparent
safety.

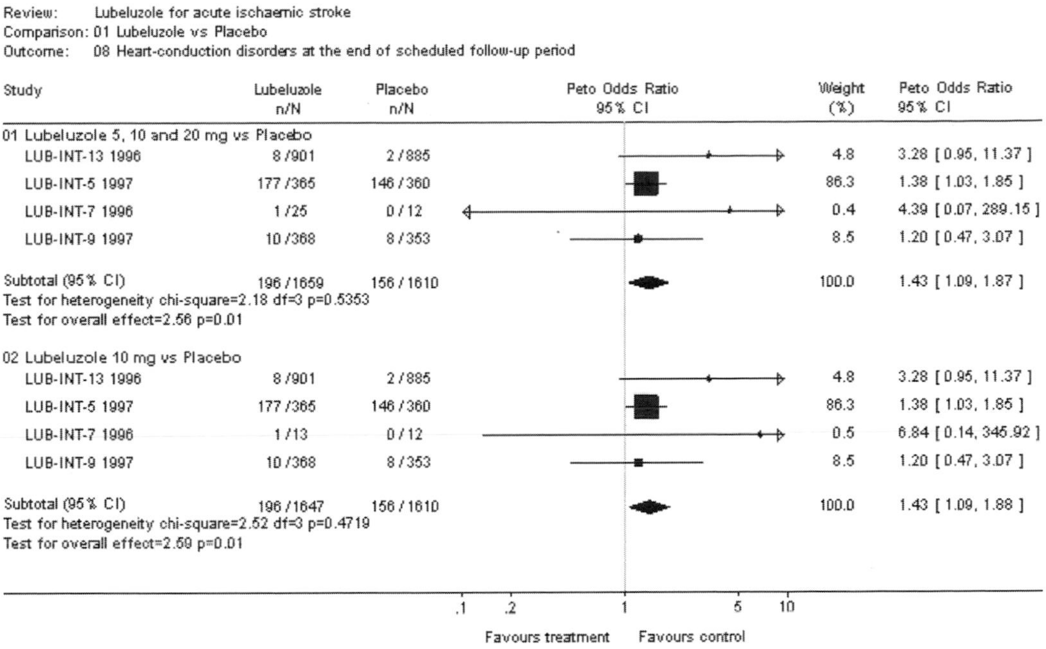

Review: Lubeluzole for acute ischaemic stroke
Comparison: 01 Lubeluzole vs Placebo
Outcome: 08 Heart-conduction disorders at the end of scheduled follow-up period

Study	Lubeluzole n/N	Placebo n/N	Peto Odds Ratio 95% CI	Weight (%)	Peto Odds Ratio 95% CI
01 Lubeluzole 5, 10 and 20 mg vs Placebo					
LUB-INT-13 1996	8 /901	2 /885		4.8	3.28 [0.95, 11.37]
LUB-INT-5 1997	177 /365	146 /360		86.3	1.38 [1.03, 1.85]
LUB-INT-7 1996	1 /25	0 /12		0.4	4.39 [0.07, 289.15]
LUB-INT-9 1997	10 /368	8 /353		8.5	1.20 [0.47, 3.07]
Subtotal (95% CI)	196 /1659	156 /1610		100.0	1.43 [1.09, 1.87]
Test for heterogeneity chi-square=2.18 df=3 p=0.5353					
Test for overall effect=2.56 p=0.01					
02 Lubeluzole 10 mg vs Placebo					
LUB-INT-13 1996	8 /901	2 /885		4.8	3.28 [0.95, 11.37]
LUB-INT-5 1997	177 /365	146 /360		86.3	1.38 [1.03, 1.85]
LUB-INT-7 1996	1 /13	0 /12		0.5	6.84 [0.14, 345.92]
LUB-INT-9 1997	10 /368	8 /353		8.5	1.20 [0.47, 3.07]
Subtotal (95% CI)	196 /1647	156 /1610		100.0	1.43 [1.09, 1.88]
Test for heterogeneity chi-square=2.52 df=3 p=0.4719					
Test for overall effect=2.59 p=0.01					

.1   .2   1   5   10

Favours treatment   Favours control

Figure 7.6   Forest plot showing the effects of *lubeluzole vs control* for acute ischaemic stroke on *heart-conduction disorders at the end of follow-up*. Reproduced from Gandolfo *et al.* (2002), with permission from the authors and John Wiley & Sons Limited. Copyright Cochrane Library, reproduced with permission.

Evidence

A systematic review of several small clinical pilot trials of magnesium in stroke suggested potential benefit; the OR for death or disability was 0.73, but with wide 95% CI: 0.38–1.41 (Fig. 7.1) (Muir and Lees, 2003).

The Intravenous Magnesium Efficacy in Stroke (IMAGES) trial randomised 2589 patients within 12 h of acute stroke to receive 16 mmol $MgSO_4$ i.v. over 15 min and then 65 mmol over 24 h, or matching placebo. For the primary outcome measure (a global endpoint statistic incorporating dichotomous outcomes on both Barthel and Rankin scores, and expressed as the common OR for death or disability at day 90), random assignment to magnesium was not associated with any improvement (OR: 0.95, 95% CI: 0.80–1.13, $P = 0.59$) (Intravenous Magnesium Efficacy in Stroke (IMAGES) Investigators, 2004). Mortality was slightly higher in the magnesium-treated group than in the placebo group (hazard ratio 1.18, 95% CI: 0.97–1.42, $P = 0.098$). Pre-specified subgroup analyses showed the results were consistent among patients randomised within 6 h and beyond 6 h (i.e. between 6 and 12 h) after stroke, and in patients with ischaemic and non-ischaemic stroke. However, benefit of magnesium was seen in patients with non-cortical stroke

(OR: 0.75, 95% CI: 0.58–0.97, $P = 0.011$), which was an unanticipated finding, because greater benefit had been expected among patients with cortical stroke. An exploratory *post hoc* analysis also revealed that patients with higher initial blood pressures (BP) had improved outcomes, and that treatment with magnesium was associated with mild reduction in systolic and diastolic BP throughout the study infusion ($P < 0.0001$ compared with placebo 0.25, 12 and 24 h after infusion started). Mean BP reduction between baseline and 24 h was 4/3 mmHg lower than placebo.

Comment

There is no evidence from reliable RCTs that magnesium, given within 12 h of acute stroke, in the dose of 16 mmol $MgSO_4$ i.v. over 15 min and then 65 mmol over 24 h, reduces the chances of death or disability significantly.

However, there are several caveats to this statement. Firstly, that magnesium may have exerted some neuroprotective effects and these may have been negated by a concurrent harmful acute BP-lowering effect of magnesium. Although modest, the lower BP in the acute stage may have compromised perfusion in the ischaemic penumbra, where cerebral autoregulation is impaired. Secondly, there is no evidence that the magnesium actually reached its target, the ischaemic penumbra. Consequently, the efficacy of magnesium, when combined with reperfusion therapies, remains to be explored. Thirdly, magnesium may be of benefit if given early in acute stroke, within 3 h of onset; only 3% of patients randomised in IMAGES were treated within 3 h of onset. A trial of i.v. magnesium as a pre-hospital treatment, in the field (Field Administration of Stroke Therapy – Magnesium, FAST-MAG), is under way (Saver *et al.*, 2004). Fourthly, magnesium may only be neuroprotective if administered in association with a period of post-ischaemic hypothermia. Furthermore, magnesium sulphate may, in turn, facilitate the rate of hypothermia via surface cooling because of its antishivering and vasodilatory properties (Schmid-Elsaesser *et al.*, 1999; Zweifler *et al.*, 2004). Finally, magnesium may also be of benefit in patients with particular types of stroke such as subcortical lacunar stroke (Goldstein, 2004; Zivin, 2004).

Comment

There is no evidence of significant benefit or harm from drugs modulating EAA action. Reduction of death or dependence by 12% or more has been excluded for gavestinel and lubeluzole, which contribute most of the data for this review. Although numbers of patients are too small to confirm or refute a trend towards increased mortality with some NMDA antagonists, further development of these agents is unlikely (unless coupled with reperfusion ± other adjunct therapies perhaps).

Gamma-aminobutyric acid antagonists

Clomethiazole

Clomethiazole is a neuroprotectant that enhances gamma-aminobutyric acid (GABA$_A$) receptor activity, and thereby causes hyperpolarisation of neuronal membranes to prevent the excitotoxic effects of glutamate, including ligand and voltage-gated calcium influx. Clomethiazole has been shown to reduce ischaemia-induced cerebral damage and clinically relevant behavioural abnormalities in rodents and primates at plasma concentrations of 3.5–19 μmol/l (Lyden *et al.*, 2002).

Evidence

The efficacy and safety of 75 mg/kg clomethiazole administered within 12 h of stroke onset was evaluated in a large placebo-controlled study in Europe and Canada, the CLomethiazole Acute Stroke Study (CLASS) (Wahlgren *et al.*, 1999). The study failed to show a significant benefit overall when comparing the proportion of disabled patients as measured by the Barthel Index (BI). However, an apparent benefit of clomethiazole was seen in a *post hoc* analysis of a subgroup of patients having a clinical syndrome of major stroke: total anterior circulation syndrome (TACS). The subgroup analysis from CLASS generated a second trial (CLASS in Ischemic stroke, CLASS-I) designed to test the hypothesis that clomethiazole administered within 12 h of stroke onset is effective in patients with major acute ischaemic stroke (Lyden *et al.*, 2002). A total of 1198 patients with major ischaemic stroke and a combination of limb weakness, higher cortical dysfunction and visual field deficits were randomly assigned to clomethiazole (68 mg/kg i.v over 24 h) or placebo. The study drug was initiated within 12 h of symptom onset. Functional outcome and neurological recovery were assessed at days 7, 30 and 90, with the proportion of patients with a BI score ⩾60/100 at last follow-up as the primary outcome measure.

The patients were randomly assigned equally, and the two treatment groups were well matched for baseline characteristics, including stroke severity (mean National Institutes of Health Stroke Scale score 16.9 ± 5.2). Ninety-six per cent were classified as TACS. The proportion of patients reaching a BI score ⩾60/100 was 42% in the clomethiazole-treated group and 46% in the placebo-treated group (OR: 0.81, 95% CI: 0.62–1.05, $P = 0.11$). There was no evidence of efficacy on any secondary outcome variables (modified Rankin Score, National Institutes of Health Stroke Scale, Scandinavian Stroke Scale and 30-day CT infarct volumes) compared with placebo. Subgroup analysis showed a similar lack of treatment effect in patients treated early (<6 h) and in those treated later (6–12 h).

Clomethiazole was well tolerated. Sedation was the most common adverse event, found in about half of all the clomethiazole-treated patients compared with 10% of placebo-treated patients.

Comment

Clomethiazole does not improve outcome in patients with major ischaemic stroke when given in isolation (Hankey, 2002).

Calcium channel antagonists

Massive calcium influx into ischaemic brain cells is a final common pathway leading to cell death (Lee *et al.*, 1999). Animal experiments have indicated that calcium antagonists administered after cerebral ischaemia may be effective in reducing infarct volume and lead to improvements in neurological outcome (Horn and Limburg, 2000, 2001). Furthermore, nimodipine was shown to be effective in decreasing the occurrence of death and disability (poor outcome) after aneurysmal and traumatic subarachnoid haemorrhage (SAH) in humans (see Chapter 18; Horn and Limburg, 2000, 2001). Nimodipine and other calcium antagonists may act as neuroprotective drugs by diminishing the influx of calcium ions through the voltage-sensitive calcium channels.

Evidence

Death or dependency

A systematic review of 22 RCTs which recorded functional outcome at the end of follow-up in a total of 6877 patients revealed that random allocation to treatment with a calcium channel antagonists was associated with no significant difference in death and dependency at end of follow-up compared with control (OR: 1.07, 95% CI: 0.97–1.18) (Fig. 7.7) (Horn and Limburg, 2000, 2001). There was significant heterogeneity among the trials ($P = 0.044$).

Death

Among 7522 patients randomised in 28 RCTs, random assignment to treatment with a calcium antagonist was associated with a non-statistically significant trend towards more deaths in the calcium antagonist-treated group compared with control (OR: 1.10, 95% CI: 0.98–1.23) (Fig. 7.8). For the drug flunarazine, there was a statistically significant increase in mortality (OR: 1.45, 95% CI: 1.01–2.09) (Fig. 7.8).

Recurrent stroke

Among the nine RCTs which reported stroke recurrences, there was no difference in the proportion of recurrent strokes between calcium antagonists and placebo (OR: 0.92, 95% CI: 0.56–1.52), but the CI are wide (Fig. 7.9).

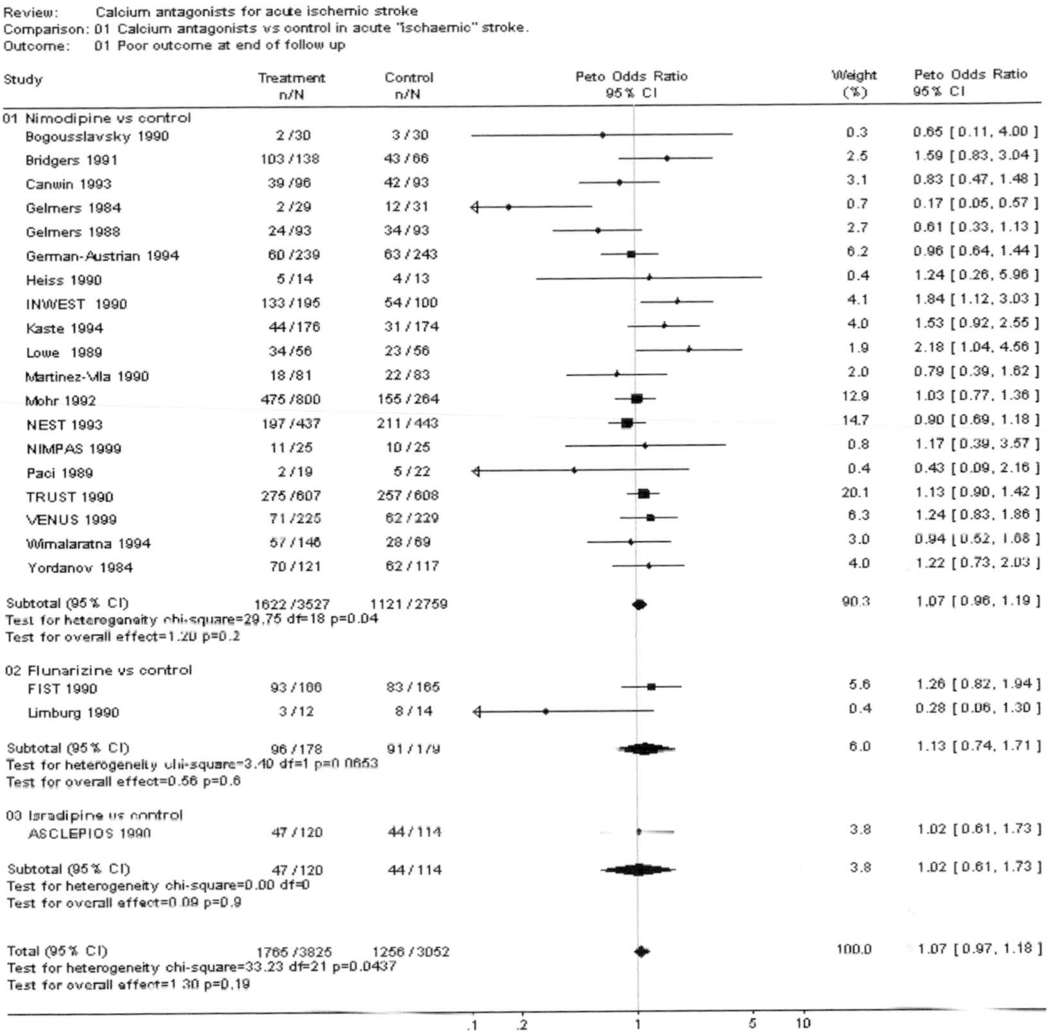

Review: Calcium antagonists for acute ischemic stroke
Comparison: 01 Calcium antagonists vs control in acute "ischaemic" stroke.
Outcome: 01 Poor outcome at end of follow up

Study	Treatment n/N	Control n/N	Peto Odds Ratio 95% CI	Weight (%)	Peto Odds Ratio 95% CI
01 Nimodipine vs control					
Bogousslavsky 1990	2 / 30	3 / 30		0.3	0.65 [0.11, 4.00]
Bridgers 1991	103 / 138	43 / 66		2.5	1.59 [0.83, 3.04]
Canwin 1993	39 / 96	42 / 93		3.1	0.83 [0.47, 1.48]
Gelmers 1984	2 / 29	12 / 31		0.7	0.17 [0.05, 0.57]
Gelmers 1988	24 / 93	34 / 93		2.7	0.61 [0.33, 1.13]
German-Austrian 1994	60 / 239	63 / 243		6.2	0.96 [0.64, 1.44]
Heiss 1990	5 / 14	4 / 13		0.4	1.24 [0.26, 5.96]
INWEST 1990	133 / 195	54 / 100		4.1	1.84 [1.12, 3.03]
Kaste 1994	44 / 176	31 / 174		4.0	1.53 [0.92, 2.55]
Lowe 1989	34 / 56	23 / 56		1.9	2.18 [1.04, 4.56]
Martinez-Vila 1990	18 / 81	22 / 83		2.0	0.79 [0.39, 1.62]
Mohr 1992	475 / 800	155 / 264		12.9	1.03 [0.77, 1.36]
NEST 1993	197 / 437	211 / 443		14.7	0.90 [0.69, 1.18]
NIMPAS 1999	11 / 25	10 / 25		0.8	1.17 [0.39, 3.57]
Paci 1989	2 / 19	5 / 22		0.4	0.43 [0.09, 2.16]
TRUST 1990	275 / 607	257 / 608		20.1	1.13 [0.90, 1.42]
VENUS 1999	71 / 225	62 / 229		6.3	1.24 [0.83, 1.86]
Wimalaratna 1994	57 / 146	28 / 69		3.0	0.94 [0.52, 1.68]
Yordanov 1984	70 / 121	62 / 117		4.0	1.22 [0.73, 2.03]
Subtotal (95% CI)	1622 / 3527	1121 / 2759		90.3	1.07 [0.96, 1.19]
Test for heterogeneity chi-square=29.75 df=18 p=0.04					
Test for overall effect=1.20 p=0.2					
02 Flunarizine vs control					
FIST 1990	93 / 166	83 / 165		5.6	1.26 [0.82, 1.94]
Limburg 1990	3 / 12	8 / 14		0.4	0.28 [0.06, 1.30]
Subtotal (95% CI)	96 / 178	91 / 179		6.0	1.13 [0.74, 1.71]
Test for heterogeneity chi-square=3.40 df=1 p=0.0653					
Test for overall effect=0.56 p=0.6					
03 Isradipine vs control					
ASCLEPIOS 1990	47 / 120	44 / 114		3.8	1.02 [0.61, 1.73]
Subtotal (95% CI)	47 / 120	44 / 114		3.8	1.02 [0.61, 1.73]
Test for heterogeneity chi-square=0.00 df=0					
Test for overall effect=0.09 p=0.9					
Total (95% CI)	1765 / 3825	1256 / 3052		100.0	1.07 [0.97, 1.18]
Test for heterogeneity chi-square=33.23 df=21 p=0.0437					
Test for overall effect=1.30 p=0.19					

.1   .2   1   5   10

Figure 7.7   Forest plot showing the effects of *all calcium channel antagonists vs control* for acute ischaemic stroke on *death or dependency at the end of follow-up*. Reproduced from Horn and Limburg (2000), with permission from the authors and John Wiley & Sons Limited. Copyright Cochrane Library, reproduced with permission.

Adverse events

Overall, there was no significant excess of adverse events among patients allocated calcium antagonists compared with controls (OR: 1.19, 95% CI: 0.97–1.47) (Fig. 7.10). However, there was highly significant heterogeneity among the trials ($P = 0.0004$), mainly due to the clear increase in adverse events among patients treated with flunarazine (33% flunarazine vs 10% control, OR: 3.73, 95% CI: 2.21–6.29). This was mainly due to an excess of superficial thrombophlebitis in the flunarazine group (Fig. 7.10).

Review: Calcium antagonists for acute ischemic stroke
Comparison: 01 Calcium antagonists vs control in acute "ischaemic" stroke.
Outcome: 02 Death at end of follow up

Study	Treatment n/N	Control n/N	Peto Odds Ratio 95% CI	Weight (%)	Peto Odds Ratio 95% CI
01 Nimodipine vs control					
Bogousslavsky 1990	0 /30	1 /30		0.1	0.14 [0.00, 6.82]
Bridgers 1991	37 /138	12 /66		2.8	1.60 [0.81, 3.18]
Canwin 1993	29 /96	33 /93		3.6	0.79 [0.43, 1.44]
Capon 1983	1 /30	2 /30		0.2	0.50 [0.05, 5.02]
Gelmers 1984	2 /29	5 /31		0.5	0.41 [0.09, 1.98]
Gelmers 1988	16 /93	27 /93		2.8	0.52 [0.26, 1.02]
German-Austrian 1994	49 /239	45 /243		6.5	1.13 [0.72, 1.78]
Heiss 1990	5 /14	4 /13		0.5	1.24 [0.26, 5.96]
INWEST 1990	83 /195	33 /100		5.4	1.49 [0.91, 2.44]
Kaste 1994	29 /176	22 /174		3.7	1.36 [0.75, 2.46]
Lowe 1989	15 /56	12 /56		1.8	1.34 [0.56, 3.17]
Martinez-Vila 1990	15 /81	20 /83		2.4	0.72 [0.34, 1.51]
Mohr 1992	120 /800	42 /264		8.8	0.93 [0.63, 1.37]
NEST 1993	105 /437	103 /443		13.6	1.04 [0.77, 1.42]
NIMPAS 1999	3 /25	3 /25		0.5	1.00 [0.18, 5.41]
x Paci 1989	0 /19	0 /22		0.0	Not estimable
x Sherman 1986	0 /11	0 /11		0.0	Not estimable
TRUST 1990	173 /607	150 /608		20.3	1.22 [0.94, 1.57]
Uzunur 1995	6 /50	7 /50		1.0	0.84 [0.26, 2.68]
VENUS 1999	30 /225	32 /229		4.6	0.95 [0.55, 1.62]
Wimalaratna 1994	40 /146	24 /69		3.4	0.70 [0.38, 1.31]
Yordanov 1984	44 /121	36 /117		4.6	1.28 [0.75, 2.20]
Subtotal (95% CI)	**802 /3618**	**613 /2850**		**87.1**	**1.06 [0.94, 1.20]**

Test for heterogeneity chi-square=17.47 df=19 p=0.5582
Test for overall effect=0.96 p=0.3

02 Flunarizine vs control					
FIST 1990	59 /166	41 /165		6.0	1.66 [1.04, 2.65]
Komhuber 1993	25 /215	20 /218		3.5	1.30 [0.70, 2.41]
Limburg 1990	3 /12	5 /14		0.5	0.62 [0.12, 3.17]
Subtotal (95% CI)	**87 /393**	**66 /397**		**9.9**	**1.45 [1.01, 2.09]**

Test for heterogeneity chi-square=1.48 df=2 p=0.4769
Test for overall effect=2.01 p=0.04

03 Isradipine vs control					
ASCLEPIOS 1990	21 /120	19 /114		2.8	1.06 [0.54, 2.09]
Subtotal (95% CI)	**21 /120**	**19 /114**		**2.8**	**1.06 [0.54, 2.09]**

Test for heterogeneity chi-square=0.00 df=0
Test for overall effect=0.17 p=0.9

04 Any other agent vs control					
x Lisk 1993	0 /5	0 /6		0.0	Not estimable
Oczkowski 1989	1 /9	1 /10		0.2	1.12 [0.06, 19.46]
Subtotal (95% CI)	**1 /14**	**1 /16**		**0.2**	**1.12 [0.06, 19.46]**

Test for heterogeneity chi-square=0.00 df=0
Test for overall effect=0.08 p=0.9

Total (95% CI)	**911 /4145**	**699 /3377**		**100.0**	**1.10 [0.98, 1.23]**

Test for heterogeneity chi-square=21.50 df=24 p=0.609
Test for overall effect=1.56 p=0.12

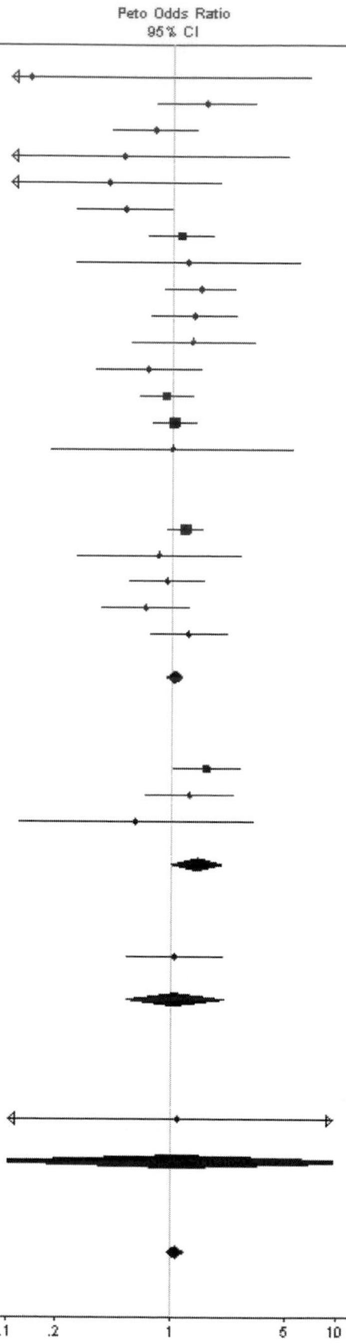

                    .1   .2   1   5   10

Figure 7.8   Forest plot showing the effects of *all calcium channel antagonists vs control* for acute
ischaemic stroke on *death at the end of follow-up*. Reproduced from Horn and Limburg
(2000), with permission from the authors and John Wiley & Sons Limited. Copyright
Cochrane Library, reproduced with permission.

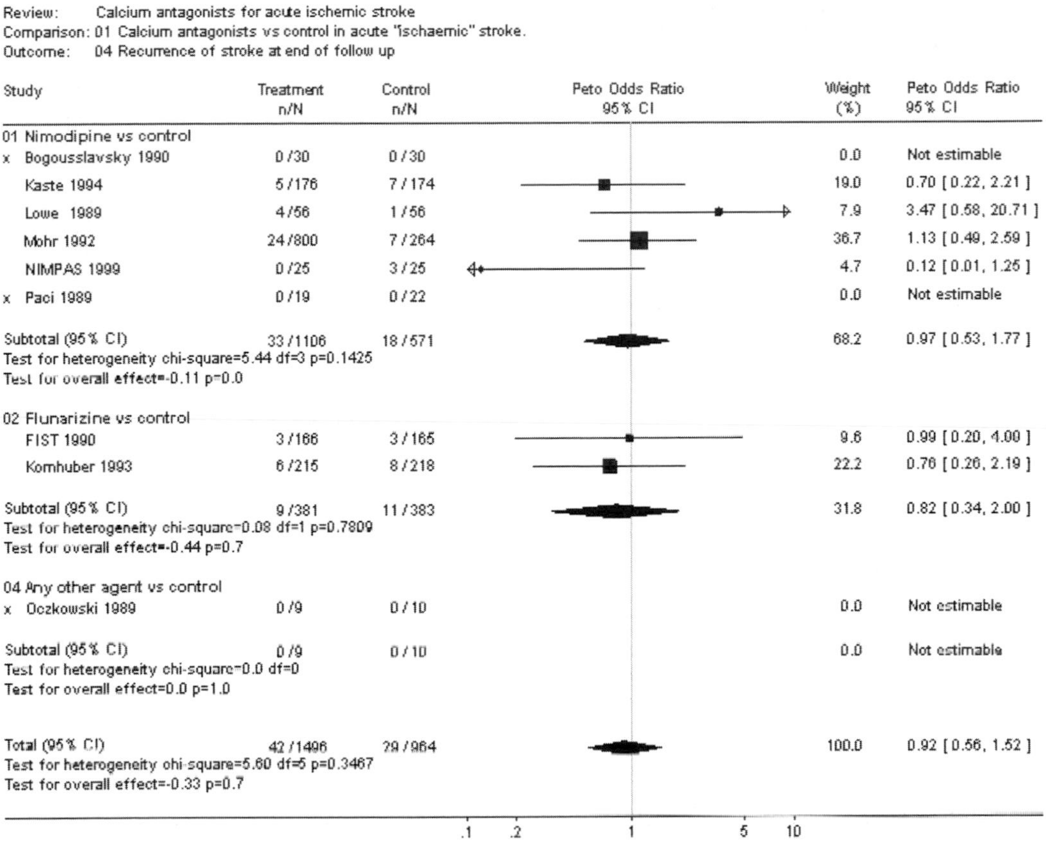

Review: Calcium antagonists for acute ischemic stroke
Comparison: 01 Calcium antagonists vs control in acute "ischaemic" stroke.
Outcome: 04 Recurrence of stroke at end of follow up

Study	Treatment n/N	Control n/N	Peto Odds Ratio 95% CI	Weight (%)	Peto Odds Ratio 95% CI
01 Nimodipine vs control					
x Bogousslavsky 1990	0 /30	0 /30		0.0	Not estimable
Kaste 1994	5 /176	7 /174		19.0	0.70 [0.22, 2.21]
Lowe 1989	4 /56	1 /56		7.9	3.47 [0.58, 20.71]
Mohr 1992	24 /800	7 /264		36.7	1.13 [0.49, 2.59]
NIMPAS 1999	0 /25	3 /25		4.7	0.12 [0.01, 1.25]
x Paci 1989	0 /19	0 /22		0.0	Not estimable
Subtotal (95% CI)	33 /1106	18 /571		68.2	0.97 [0.53, 1.77]
Test for heterogeneity chi-square=5.44 df=3 p=0.1425					
Test for overall effect=-0.11 p=0.0					
02 Flunarizine vs control					
FIST 1990	3 /166	3 /165		9.6	0.99 [0.20, 4.00]
Kornhuber 1993	6 /215	8 /218		22.2	0.76 [0.26, 2.19]
Subtotal (95% CI)	9 /381	11 /383		31.8	0.82 [0.34, 2.00]
Test for heterogeneity chi-square=0.08 df=1 p=0.7809					
Test for overall effect=-0.44 p=0.7					
04 Any other agent vs control					
x Oczkowski 1989	0 /9	0 /10		0.0	Not estimable
Subtotal (95% CI)	0 /9	0 /10		0.0	Not estimable
Test for heterogeneity chi-square=0.0 df=0					
Test for overall effect=0.0 p=1.0					
Total (95% CI)	42 /1496	29 /964		100.0	0.92 [0.56, 1.52]
Test for heterogeneity chi-square=5.60 df=5 p=0.3467					
Test for overall effect=-0.33 p=0.7					

.1   .2   1   5   10

Figure 7.9   Forest plot showing the effects of *all calcium channel antagonists vs control* for acute ischaemic stroke on *recurrent stroke at the end of follow-up*. Reproduced from Horn and Limburg (2000), with permission from the authors and John Wiley & Sons Limited. Copyright Cochrane Library, reproduced with permission.

Hypotension during treatment period   In six trials in which episodes of hypotension (sufficient to stop treatment) were mentioned, there was a non-significant trend for an increase in hypotensive episodes among patients allocated calcium antagonists compared with control (2.0% vs 1.4%, OR: 1.37, 95% CI: 0.70–2.67).

Mean systolic BP during or at end of treatment   In three trials, data were presented in a way that allowed analysis. The mean BP in the treated groups was on average 2 mmHg lower than control (Fig. 7.11) (Horn and Limburg, 2000).

Publication status

A very conspicuous difference in outcomes was present between the 15 trials that were officially published in a peer-reviewed journal and the 4 trials that were not or had only been published as abstracts. The published trials did not show an

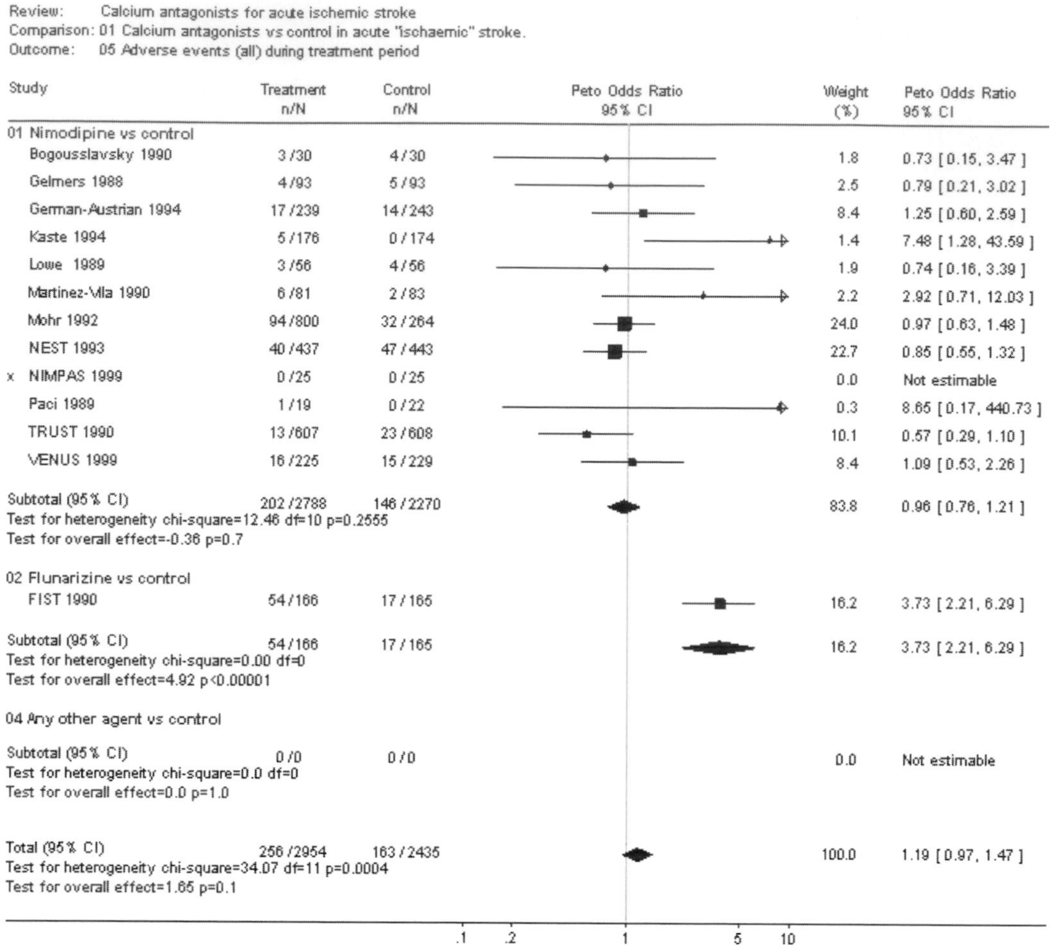

Review: Calcium antagonists for acute ischemic stroke
Comparison: 01 Calcium antagonists vs control in acute "ischaemic" stroke.
Outcome: 05 Adverse events (all) during treatment period

Study	Treatment n/N	Control n/N	Peto Odds Ratio 95% CI	Weight (%)	Peto Odds Ratio 95% CI
01 Nimodipine vs control					
Bogousslavsky 1990	3 /30	4 /30		1.8	0.73 [0.15, 3.47]
Gelmers 1988	4 /93	5 /93		2.5	0.79 [0.21, 3.02]
German-Austrian 1994	17 /239	14 /243		8.4	1.25 [0.60, 2.59]
Kaste 1994	5 /176	0 /174		1.4	7.48 [1.28, 43.59]
Lowe 1989	3 /56	4 /56		1.9	0.74 [0.16, 3.39]
Martinez-Vila 1990	6 /81	2 /83		2.2	2.92 [0.71, 12.03]
Mohr 1992	94 /800	32 /264		24.0	0.97 [0.63, 1.48]
NEST 1993	40 /437	47 /443		22.7	0.85 [0.55, 1.32]
x NIMPAS 1999	0 /25	0 /25		0.0	Not estimable
Paci 1989	1 /19	0 /22		0.3	8.65 [0.17, 440.73]
TRUST 1990	13 /607	23 /608		10.1	0.57 [0.29, 1.10]
VENUS 1999	16 /225	15 /229		8.4	1.09 [0.53, 2.26]
Subtotal (95% CI)	202 /2788	146 /2270		83.8	0.96 [0.76, 1.21]

Test for heterogeneity chi-square=12.46 df=10 p=0.2555
Test for overall effect=-0.36 p=0.7

02 Flunarizine vs control					
FIST 1990	54 /166	17 /165		16.2	3.73 [2.21, 6.29]
Subtotal (95% CI)	54 /166	17 /165		16.2	3.73 [2.21, 6.29]

Test for heterogeneity chi-square=0.00 df=0
Test for overall effect=4.92 p<0.00001

04 Any other agent vs control

| **Subtotal (95% CI)** | 0 /0 | 0 /0 | | 0.0 | Not estimable |

Test for heterogeneity chi-square=0.0 df=0
Test for overall effect=0.0 p=1.0

| **Total (95% CI)** | 256 /2954 | 163 /2435 | | 100.0 | 1.19 [0.97, 1.47] |

Test for heterogeneity chi-square=34.07 df=11 p=0.0004
Test for overall effect=1.65 p=0.1

```
        .1    .2          1          5    10
```

Figure 7.10   Forest plot showing the effects of *all calcium channel antagonists vs control* for acute ischaemic stroke on *adverse events during the treatment period*. Reproduced from Horn and Limburg (2000), with permission from the authors and John Wiley & Sons Limited. Copyright Cochrane Library, reproduced with permission.

overall effect of active treatment (OR: 1.03, 95% CI: 0.92–1.15) on poor outcome (Fig. 7.12). Unpublished trials, on the contrary, were associated with a significantly deleterious effect of active treatment; the overall OR was 1.33 (95% CI: 1.00–1.79).

Comment

This systematic review of all available data failed to demonstrate a reduction in death and dependency after treatment with calcium antagonists in acute stroke (OR: 1.07, 95% CI: 0.97–1.18). There is therefore no evidence to justify the routine use of calcium antagonists in patients with an acute stroke. Further studies in acute

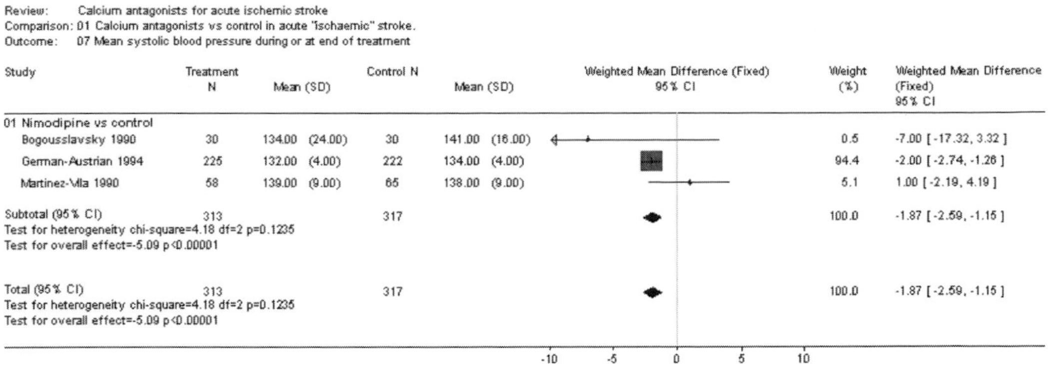

Review: Calcium antagonists for acute ischemic stroke
Comparison: 01 Calcium antagonists vs control in acute "ischaemic" stroke.
Outcome: 07 Mean systolic blood pressure during or at end of treatment

Study	Treatment N	Mean (SD)	Control N	Mean (SD)	Weighted Mean Difference (Fixed) 95% CI	Weight (%)	Weighted Mean Difference (Fixed) 95% CI
01 Nimodipine vs control							
Bogousslavsky 1990	30	134.00 (24.00)	30	141.00 (16.00)		0.5	-7.00 [-17.32, 3.32]
German-Austrian 1994	225	132.00 (4.00)	222	134.00 (4.00)		94.4	-2.00 [-2.74, -1.26]
Martinez-Vila 1990	58	139.00 (9.00)	65	138.00 (9.00)		5.1	1.00 [-2.19, 4.19]
Subtotal (95% CI)	313		317			100.0	-1.87 [-2.59, -1.15]
Test for heterogeneity chi-square=4.18 df=2 p=0.1235							
Test for overall effect=-5.09 p<0.00001							
Total (95% CI)	313		317			100.0	-1.87 [-2.59, -1.15]
Test for heterogeneity chi-square=4.18 df=2 p=0.1235							
Test for overall effect=-5.09 p<0.00001							

-10   -5   0   5   10

Figure 7.11   Forest plot showing the effects of *all calcium channel antagonists vs control* for acute ischaemic stroke on *mean systolic BP during or at the end of the treatment period*. Reproduced from Horn and Limburg (2000), with permission from the authors and John Wiley & Sons Limited. Copyright Cochrane Library, reproduced with permission.

ischaemic stroke with calcium antagonists acting on voltage-sensitive calcium channels do not seem to be justified (unless coupled with other therapies perhaps).

Free radical scavengers: antioxidants

Tirilazad

Tirilazad mesylate (U-74006F, 'Freedox'®, Pharmacia & Upjohn) is a lipid soluble synthetic, non-glucocorticoid, 21-aminosteroid (or lazaroid). Its proposed mechanism of action is to inhibit iron-dependent lipid peroxidation within membranes. These effects are mediated through:

(i)   free radical scavenging of lipid peroxyl and hydroxyl groups,
(ii) reducing the formation of hydroxyl radicals,
(iii) decreasing membrane phospholipid fluidity,
(iv) maintaining endogenous antioxidant levels (especially vitamins E and C).

Tirilazad is neuroprotective in animal models of ischaemic stroke and improved outcome in two of four phase III studies in SAH. It is licensed for this indication in some countries (The Tirilazad International Steering Committee, 2000, 2001).

Evidence

A systematic review identified six RCTs (four published, two unpublished) assessing tirilazad in 1757 patients with presumed acute ischaemic stroke; all were double-blind and placebo-controlled in design (The Tirilazad International Steering Committee, 2000, 2001).

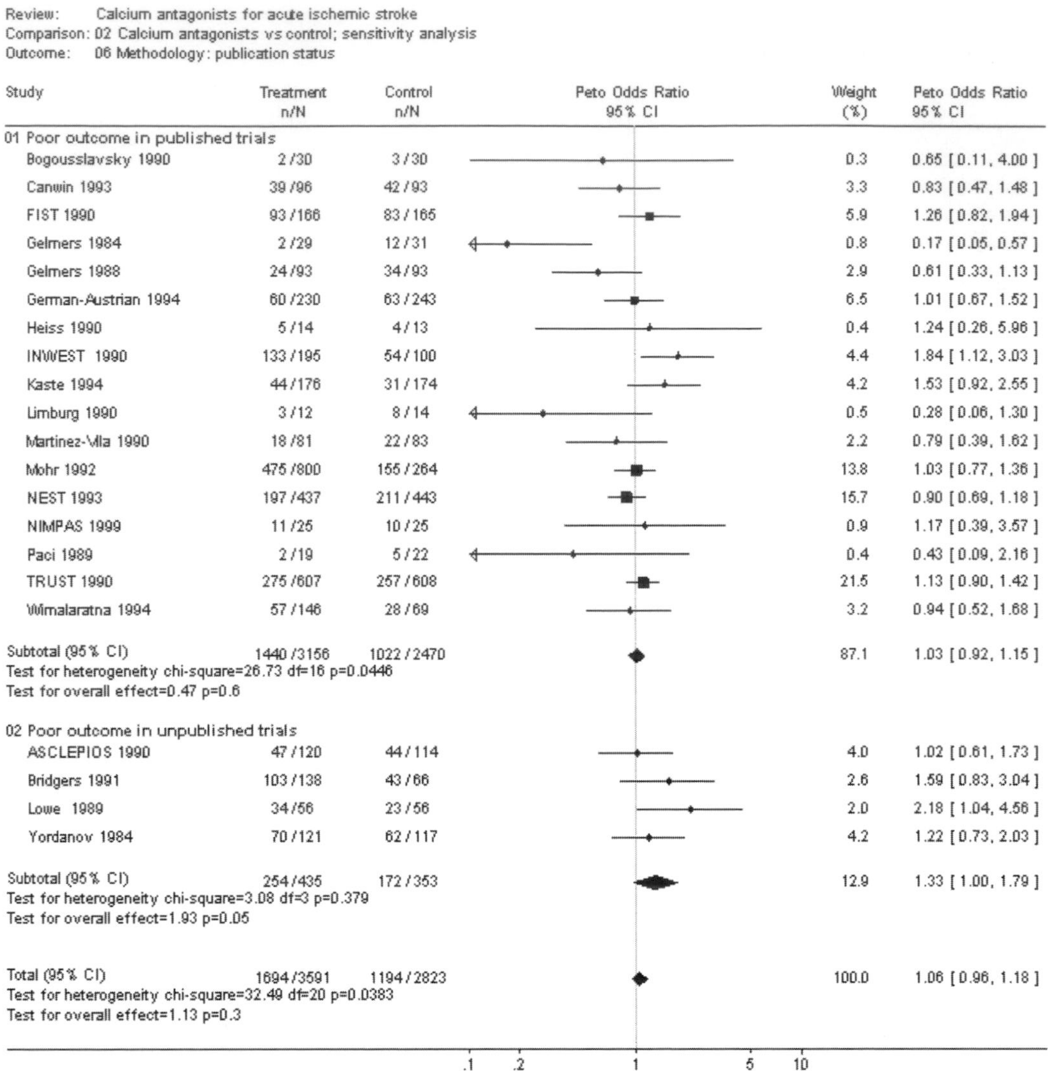

Review: Calcium antagonists for acute ischemic stroke
Comparison: 02 Calcium antagonists vs control; sensitivity analysis
Outcome: 06 Methodology: publication status

Study	Treatment n/N	Control n/N	Peto Odds Ratio 95% CI	Weight (%)	Peto Odds Ratio 95% CI
01 Poor outcome in published trials					
Bogousslavsky 1990	2/30	3/30		0.3	0.65 [0.11, 4.00]
Canwin 1993	39/96	42/93		3.3	0.83 [0.47, 1.48]
FIST 1990	93/166	83/165		5.9	1.26 [0.82, 1.94]
Gelmers 1984	2/29	12/31		0.8	0.17 [0.05, 0.57]
Gelmers 1988	24/93	34/93		2.9	0.61 [0.33, 1.13]
German-Austrian 1994	60/230	63/243		6.5	1.01 [0.67, 1.52]
Heiss 1990	5/14	4/13		0.4	1.24 [0.26, 5.96]
INWEST 1990	133/195	54/100		4.4	1.84 [1.12, 3.03]
Kaste 1994	44/176	31/174		4.2	1.53 [0.92, 2.55]
Limburg 1990	3/12	8/14		0.5	0.28 [0.06, 1.30]
Martinez-Vila 1990	18/81	22/83		2.2	0.79 [0.39, 1.62]
Mohr 1992	475/800	155/264		13.8	1.03 [0.77, 1.36]
NEST 1993	197/437	211/443		15.7	0.90 [0.69, 1.18]
NIMPAS 1999	11/25	10/25		0.9	1.17 [0.39, 3.57]
Paci 1989	2/19	5/22		0.4	0.43 [0.09, 2.16]
TRUST 1990	275/607	257/608		21.5	1.13 [0.90, 1.42]
Wimalaratna 1994	57/146	28/69		3.2	0.94 [0.52, 1.68]
Subtotal (95% CI)	1440/3156	1022/2470		87.1	1.03 [0.92, 1.15]
Test for heterogeneity chi-square=26.73 df=16 p=0.0446					
Test for overall effect=0.47 p=0.6					
02 Poor outcome in unpublished trials					
ASCLEPIOS 1990	47/120	44/114		4.0	1.02 [0.61, 1.73]
Bridgers 1991	103/138	43/66		2.6	1.59 [0.83, 3.04]
Lowe 1989	34/56	23/56		2.0	2.18 [1.04, 4.56]
Yordanov 1984	70/121	62/117		4.2	1.22 [0.73, 2.03]
Subtotal (95% CI)	254/435	172/353		12.9	1.33 [1.00, 1.79]
Test for heterogeneity chi-square=3.08 df=3 p=0.379					
Test for overall effect=1.93 p=0.05					
Total (95% CI)	1694/3591	1194/2823		100.0	1.06 [0.96, 1.18]
Test for heterogeneity chi-square=32.49 df=20 p=0.0383					
Test for overall effect=1.13 p=0.3					

.1   .2   1   5   10

Figure 7.12   Forest plot showing the effects of *all calcium channel antagonists vs control* for acute
ischaemic stroke on *death or dependency according to publication status*. Reproduced
from Horn and Limburg (2000), with permission from the authors and John Wiley & Sons
Limited. Copyright Cochrane Library, reproduced with permission.

Death
Tirilazad did not alter early case fatality (OR: 1.11, 95% CI: 0.79–1.56) or end-
of-trial case fatality (OR: 1.12, 95% CI: 0.88–1.44) (Fig. 7.13).

Death or dependency
Tirilazad increased the odds of being dead or disabled by about one-fifth, though
the result was only just statistically significant at the $P = 0.05$ level. The OR was

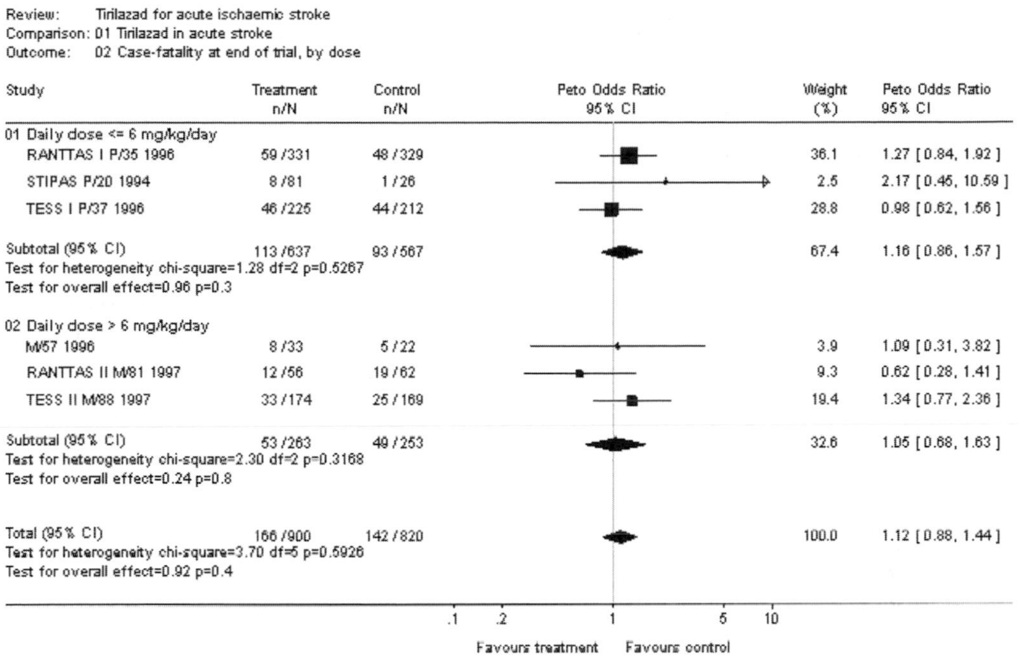

Review: Tirilazad for acute ischaemic stroke
Comparison: 01 Tirilazad in acute stroke
Outcome: 02 Case-fatality at end of trial, by dose

Study	Treatment n/N	Control n/N	Peto Odds Ratio 95% CI	Weight (%)	Peto Odds Ratio 95% CI
01 Daily dose <= 6 mg/kg/day					
RANTTAS I P/35 1996	59 /331	48 /329		36.1	1.27 [0.84, 1.92]
STIPAS P/20 1994	8 /81	1 /26		2.5	2.17 [0.45, 10.59]
TESS I P/37 1996	46 /225	44 /212		28.8	0.98 [0.62, 1.56]
Subtotal (95% CI)	113 /637	93 /567		67.4	1.16 [0.86, 1.57]
Test for heterogeneity chi-square=1.28 df=2 p=0.5267					
Test for overall effect=0.96 p=0.3					
02 Daily dose > 6 mg/kg/day					
M/57 1996	8 /33	5 /22		3.9	1.09 [0.31, 3.82]
RANTTAS II M/81 1997	12 /56	19 /62		9.3	0.62 [0.28, 1.41]
TESS II M/88 1997	33 /174	25 /169		19.4	1.34 [0.77, 2.36]
Subtotal (95% CI)	53 /263	49 /253		32.6	1.05 [0.68, 1.63]
Test for heterogeneity chi-square=2.30 df=2 p=0.3168					
Test for overall effect=0.24 p=0.8					
Total (95% CI)	166 /900	142 /820		100.0	1.12 [0.88, 1.44]
Test for heterogeneity chi-square=3.70 df=5 p=0.5926					
Test for overall effect=0.92 p=0.4					

```
        .1    .2         1         5    10
           Favours treatment   Favours control
```

Figure 7.13   Forest plot showing the effects of *tirilazad vs control* for acute ischaemic stroke on *case fatality at the end of the trial*. Reproduced from The Tirilazad International Steering Committee (2001), with permission from the authors and John Wiley & Sons Limited. Copyright Cochrane Library, reproduced with permission.

similar whether the expanded BI (EBI) or Glasgow Outcome Scale were used to assess outcome (OR: 1.23, 95% CI: 1.01–1.51; OR: 1.23, 95% CI: 1.01–1.50, respectively) (Fig. 7.14). Functional outcome (EBI) was significantly worse in pre-specified subgroups of patients: females (OR: 1.46, 95% CI: 1.08–1.98) and subjects receiving low-dose tirilazad (OR: 1.31, 95% CI: 1.03–1.67); a non-significant worse outcome was also seen in patients with mild-moderate stroke (OR: 1.40, 95% CI: 0.99–1.98).

Phlebitis
Tirilazad significantly increased the odds of infusion site phlebitis (OR: 2.81, 95% CI: 2.14–3.69) (Fig. 7.15).

Comment

Tirilazad mesylate increased the combined endpoint of 'death or disability' by about one-fifth, but did not alter case fatality, when given to patients with acute ischaemic stroke. Further trials of tirilazad are not warranted (unless combined with other adjunct therapies, such as reperfusion, perhaps).

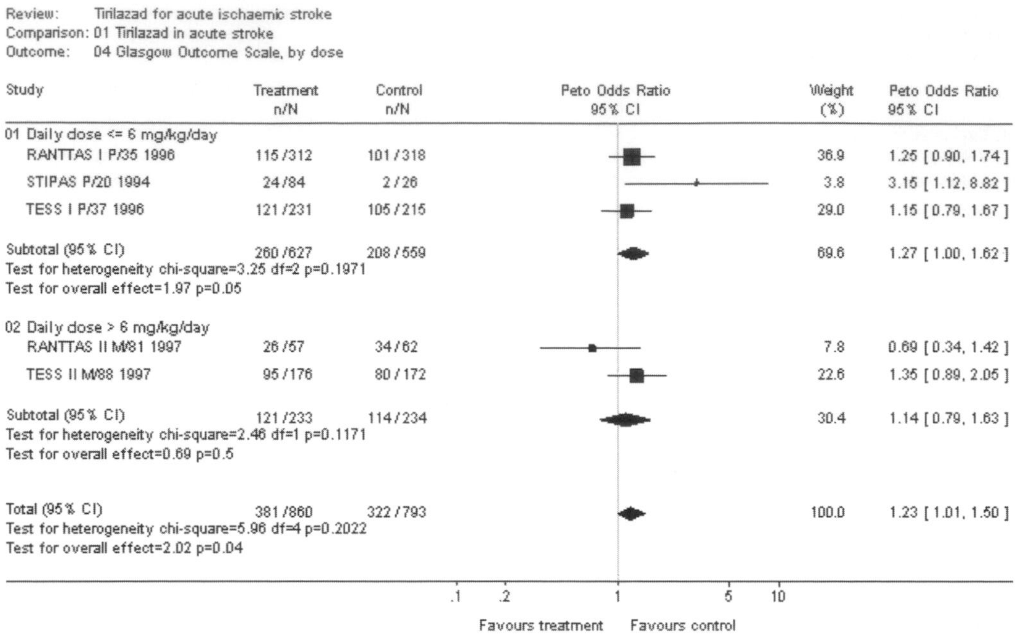

Review: Tirilazad for acute ischaemic stroke
Comparison: 01 Tirilazad in acute stroke
Outcome: 04 Glasgow Outcome Scale, by dose

Study	Treatment n/N	Control n/N	Peto Odds Ratio 95% CI	Weight (%)	Peto Odds Ratio 95% CI
01 Daily dose <= 6 mg/kg/day					
RANTTAS I P/35 1996	115/312	101/318		36.9	1.25 [0.90, 1.74]
STIPAS P/20 1994	24/84	2/26		3.8	3.15 [1.12, 8.82]
TESS I P/37 1996	121/231	105/215		29.0	1.15 [0.79, 1.67]
Subtotal (95% CI)	260/627	208/559		69.6	1.27 [1.00, 1.62]
Test for heterogeneity chi-square=3.25 df=2 p=0.1971					
Test for overall effect=1.97 p=0.05					
02 Daily dose > 6 mg/kg/day					
RANTTAS II M/81 1997	26/57	34/62		7.8	0.69 [0.34, 1.42]
TESS II M/88 1997	95/176	80/172		22.6	1.35 [0.89, 2.05]
Subtotal (95% CI)	121/233	114/234		30.4	1.14 [0.79, 1.63]
Test for heterogeneity chi-square=2.46 df=1 p=0.1171					
Test for overall effect=0.69 p=0.5					
Total (95% CI)	381/860	322/793		100.0	1.23 [1.01, 1.50]
Test for heterogeneity chi-square=5.96 df=4 p=0.2022					
Test for overall effect=2.02 p=0.04					

.1   .2   1   5   10

Favours treatment   Favours control

Figure 7.14   Forest plot showing the effects of *tirilazad vs control* for acute ischaemic stroke on *functional outcome as measured by the Glasgow Outcome Scale.* Reproduced from The Tirilazad International Steering Committee (2001), with permission from the authors and John Wiley & Sons Limited. Copyright Cochrane Library, reproduced with permission.

NXY-059 (Cerovive)

NXY-059 (cerovive) is a free-radical trapping agent.

Evidence

The SAINT I trial (Stroke-Acute Ischemic-NXY-059 (cerovive) Treatment) randomised 1722 patients within 6 h of onset of acute ischaemic stroke to placebo or a 1 h loading dose, followed by 71 h infusion of NXY-059 (cerovive) and followed patients for 90 days (www.strokecenter.org/trials/trialdetail.aspx?tid=537). The analysis of 847 patients assigned placebo and 858 patients assigned NXY-059, who actually received the treatment, showed active treatment with NXY-059 was associated with a significant reduction in disability as measured by the modified Rankin scale, at day 90 ($P = 0.038$).

Comment

The reproducibility and clinical significance of the promising results of SAINT-I are being assessed in the ongoing SAINT II trial (involving more than 3000 patients) and the CHANT (Cerebral Hemorrhage And NXY-059 Treatment) trial.

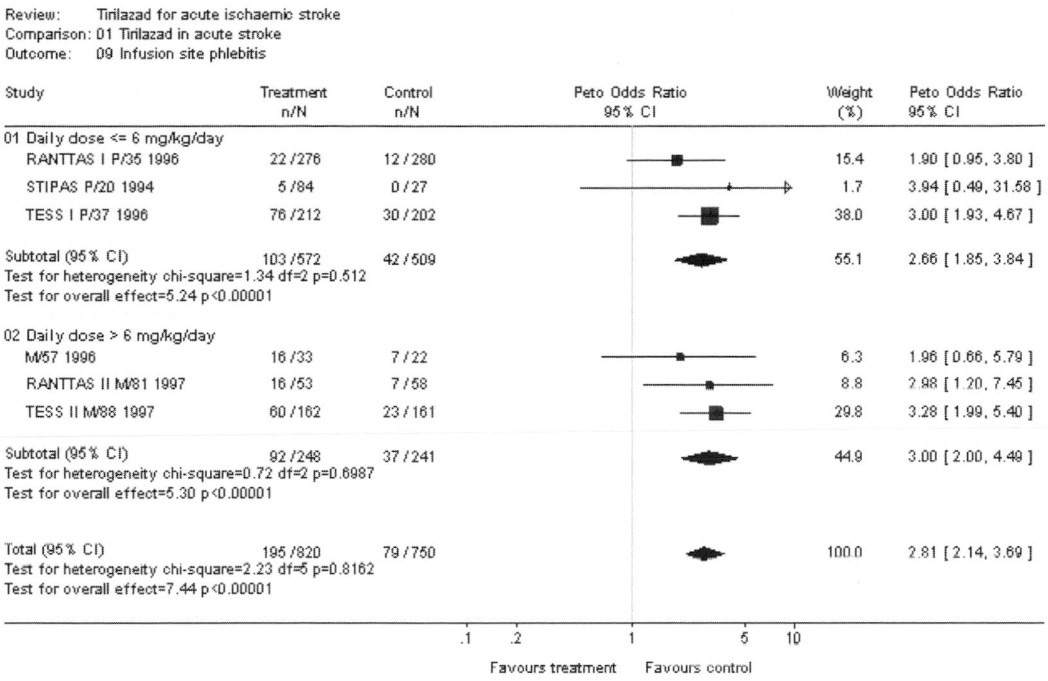

Review: Tirilazad for acute ischaemic stroke
Comparison: 01 Tirilazad in acute stroke
Outcome: 09 Infusion site phlebitis

Study	Treatment n/N	Control n/N	Peto Odds Ratio 95% CI	Weight (%)	Peto Odds Ratio 95% CI
01 Daily dose <= 6 mg/kg/day					
RANTTAS I P/35 1996	22 /276	12 / 280		15.4	1.90 [0.95, 3.80]
STIPAS P/20 1994	5 /84	0 / 27		1.7	3.94 [0.49, 31.58]
TESS I P/37 1996	76 /212	30 / 202		38.0	3.00 [1.93, 4.67]
Subtotal (95% CI)	103 /572	42 / 509		55.1	2.66 [1.85, 3.84]
Test for heterogeneity chi-square=1.34 df=2 p=0.512					
Test for overall effect=5.24 p<0.00001					
02 Daily dose > 6 mg/kg/day					
M/57 1996	16 /33	7 / 22		6.3	1.96 [0.66, 5.79]
RANTTAS II M/81 1997	16 /53	7 / 58		8.8	2.98 [1.20, 7.45]
TESS II M/88 1997	60 /162	23 / 161		29.8	3.28 [1.99, 5.40]
Subtotal (95% CI)	92 /248	37 / 241		44.9	3.00 [2.00, 4.49]
Test for heterogeneity chi-square=0.72 df=2 p=0.6987					
Test for overall effect=5.30 p<0.00001					
Total (95% CI)	195 /820	79 / 750		100.0	2.81 [2.14, 3.69]
Test for heterogeneity chi-square=2.23 df=5 p=0.8162					
Test for overall effect=7.44 p<0.00001					

.1   .2   1   5   10

Favours treatment   Favours control

Figure 7.15   Forest plot showing the effects of *tirilazad vs control* for acute ischaemic stroke on *infusion site phlebitis*. Reproduced from The Tirilazad International Steering Committee (2001), with permission from the authors and John Wiley & Sons Limited. Copyright Cochrane Library, reproduced with permission.

Growth factors

Fibroblast growth factor

Trafermin (basic fibroblast growth factor) has been shown to reduce infarct volume in acute ischaemic stroke models, and to promote functional recovery and new synapse formation when given to animals with completed cerebral infarction.

Evidence

Trafermin (basic fibroblast growth factor) has been compared with placebo in the European–Australian Fiblast (Trafermin) trial (Bogousslavsky *et al.*, 2002). This was a double-blind, placebo-controlled trial in 286 stroke patients who were randomised within 6 h of stroke onset. Patients were randomised to receive 5 or 10 mg of trafermin or placebo i.v. infused over 24 h. The primary efficacy outcome was a categorised combination of the Barthel and Rankin scales assessed at 90 days.

The 286 patients had been enrolled at 55 sites in 11 countries when the sponsor directed that enrolment be stopped because an interim (futility) analysis of efficacy data predicted too small a chance of demonstrating a statistically significant benefit after recruitment of the planned 900 patients.

Patients randomly assigned to 5 mg of trafermin had a slight but non-significant advantage over placebo (OR: 1.2, 95% CI: 0.72–2.00, $P = 0.48$); and patients randomly assigned to 10 mg of trafermin had a non-significant disadvantage (OR: 0.74, 95% CI: 0.44–1.22, $P = 0.24$). Mortality rates at 90 days were 17% in the 5-mg group, 24% in the 10-mg group and 18% in the placebo group.

Treatment with trafermin was associated with an increase in leucocytosis and a decrease in BP: mean decrease in systolic BP from baseline was 19 mmHg in the 5-mg group, 22 mmHg in the 10-mg group and 8 mmHg in the placebo group.

In a *post hoc* subgroup analysis, patients in the 5-mg group treated more than 5 h after the onset of symptoms showed an apparent advantage over placebo (OR: 2.1, 95% CI: 1.00–4.41, $P = 0.044$; after age adjustment: OR: 1.9, 95% CI: 0.91–4.13, $P = 0.08$).

Comment

There are not enough data from RCTs to reliably determine the safety and effectiveness of trafermin in patients with acute stroke.

Leucocyte adhesion and infiltration inhibitors

In experimental models, inflammation contributes to ischaemic brain injury. This begs the question of whether modulating the inflammatory response may improve functional recovery in stroke patients.

Anti-intercellular adhesion molecule antibody

Enlimomab (R6.5) is a murine intercellular adhesion molecule-1 (ICAM-1) antibody which reduces leucocyte adhesion to the endothelial wall, and infarct size in experimental stroke studies. The mechanism is thought to be reducing reperfusion-induced inflammation and neuronal injury after stroke.

Evidence

The Enlimomab Acute Stroke Trial randomised 625 patients with ischaemic stroke to either enlimomab ($n = 317$) or placebo ($n = 308$) within 6 h of stroke onset. Treatment was given over 5 days (Enlimomab Acute Stroke Trial Investigators, 2001).

At day 90, the modified Rankin Scale score (the primary outcome for efficacy) was worse in patients treated with enlimomab than with placebo ($P = 0.004$). Fewer patients had symptom-free recovery on enlimomab than placebo ($P = 0.004$), and more died (22.2 vs 16.2%). The negative effect of enlimomab was apparent on days 5, 30 and 90 of treatment ($P = 0.005$). There were significantly more adverse events with enlimomab treatment than placebo, primarily infections and fever. Patients experiencing fever were more likely to have a poor outcome or die.

Comment

This trial suggests that anti-ICAM therapy with enlimomab is not an effective treatment for ischaemic stroke and may significantly worsen stroke outcome.

UK-279,276 (neutrophil inhibitory factor)

This is a recombinant glycoprotein with selective binding to the CD11b integrin of MAX-1 (CD11b/CD18). It has been shown to reduce neutrophil infiltration and brain infarct volume in transient (2-h) rat middle cerebral artery occlusion models when administered within 4 h after onset of ischaemia.

Evidence

The Acute Stroke Therapy by Inhibition of Neutrophils (ASTIN) study was an adaptive phase II dose–response-finding proof-of-concept study to establish whether UK-279,276 (neutrophil inhibitory factor) improves recovery after acute ischaemic stroke (Krams *et al.*, 2003). It was stopped for futility after a total of 966 acute stroke patients had been treated within 6 h of symptom onset because of no favourable effect of the treatment in the primary outcome measure – a change from baseline to day 90 on the Scandinavian Stroke Scale. There were also no serious adverse effects.

Phosphatidylcholine precursor

Citicoline

Citicoline (or cytidine-5′-diphosphocholine, CDP-choline), a compound normally present in all cells in the body, is both a neuroprotective drug, when administered exogenously, and an intermediate in membrane phosphatide biosynthesis.

Evidence

There have been four clinical trials of oral citicoline administered within 24 h of onset of moderate to severe ischaemic stroke, in various doses (500, 1000 and 2000 mg), and continued for six weeks, in a total of 1372 patients (583 allocated placebo, 789 allocated citicoline).

Results of an exploratory, post-hoc meta-analysis indicate that recovery (combining the National Institutes of Health Stroke Study (NIHSS) $\leqslant 1$, modified Rankin Scale score $\leqslant 1$ and BI score $\geqslant 95$) at 3 months was 25.2% among patients allocated citicoline and 20.2% among patients allocated placebo (OR: 1.33, 95% CI: 1.10–1.62, $P = 0.0034$) (Figs 7.16 and 7.17) (Dávalos *et al.*, 2002).

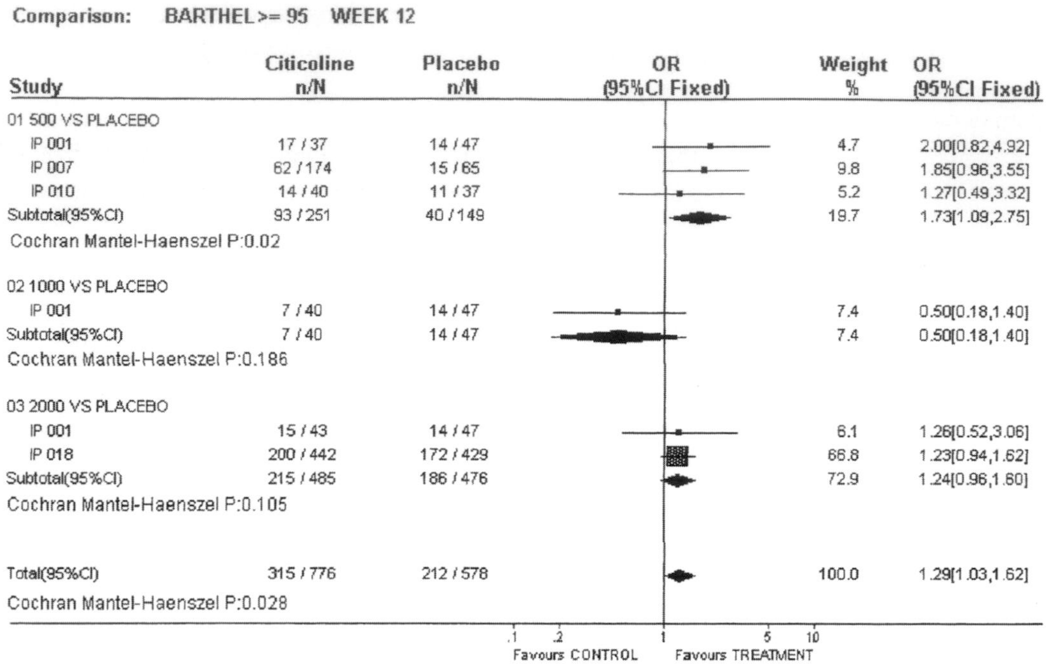

Comparison: BARTHEL >= 95 WEEK 12

Study	Citicoline n/N	Placebo n/N	OR (95%CI Fixed)	Weight %	OR (95%CI Fixed)
01 500 VS PLACEBO					
IP 001	17 / 37	14 / 47		4.7	2.00[0.82,4.92]
IP 007	62 / 174	15 / 65		9.8	1.85[0.96,3.55]
IP 010	14 / 40	11 / 37		5.2	1.27[0.49,3.32]
Subtotal(95%CI)	93 / 251	40 / 149		19.7	1.73[1.09,2.75]
Cochran Mantel-Haenszel P:0.02					
02 1000 VS PLACEBO					
IP 001	7 / 40	14 / 47		7.4	0.50[0.18,1.40]
Subtotal(95%CI)	7 / 40	14 / 47		7.4	0.50[0.18,1.40]
Cochran Mantel-Haenszel P:0.186					
03 2000 VS PLACEBO					
IP 001	15 / 43	14 / 47		6.1	1.26[0.52,3.06]
IP 018	200 / 442	172 / 429		66.8	1.23[0.94,1.62]
Subtotal(95%CI)	215 / 485	186 / 476		72.9	1.24[0.96,1.60]
Cochran Mantel-Haenszel P:0.105					
Total(95%CI)	315 / 776	212 / 578		100.0	1.29[1.03,1.62]
Cochran Mantel-Haenszel P:0.028					

.1   .2   1   5   10

Favours CONTROL   Favours TREATMENT

Figure 7.16 Forest plot showing the effects of *citicoline vs placebo* for acute ischaemic stroke on *survival free of dependency* as defined by a BI score of >95/100 at 3 months after stroke. Reproduced from Dávalos *et al.* (2002), with permission from the authors and Lippincott, Williams and Wilkins.

A subgroup analysis suggested that the dose showing the largest difference with placebo was 2000 mg, with 27.9% of patients achieving recovery (OR: 1.38, 95% CI: 1.10–1.72, $P = 0.0043$).

The overall safety of citicoline was similar to placebo. However, significant excess differences were found in anxiety (citicoline, 13.7%; placebo, 9.9%; $P = 0.036$) and leg oedema (citicoline, 9.7%; placebo, 6.5%; $P = 0.032$). There were however significantly fewer cases of depression (citicoline, 22.5%; placebo, 27.4%; $P = 0.038$), falling down (citicoline, 12.6%; placebo, 18.7%; $P = 0.002$) and urinary incontinence (citicoline, 10.5%; placebo, 14.0%; $P = 0.047$).

Comment

These preliminary data suggest that treatment with oral citicoline within the first 24 h after symptom onset in patients with moderate to severe stroke increases the probability of complete recovery at 3 months. A new trial to confirm these results should be conducted.

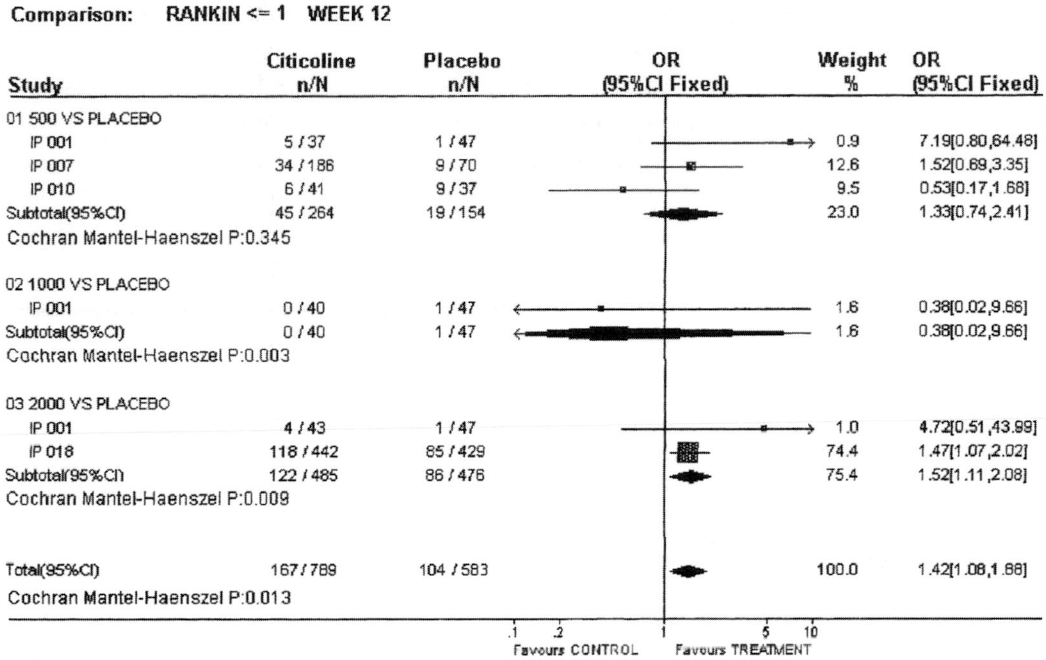

Comparison: RANKIN <= 1   WEEK 12

Study	Citicoline n/N	Placebo n/N	OR (95%CI Fixed)	Weight %	OR (95%CI Fixed)
01 500 VS PLACEBO					
IP 001	5 / 37	1 / 47		0.9	7.19[0.80,64.48]
IP 007	34 / 186	9 / 70		12.6	1.52[0.69,3.35]
IP 010	6 / 41	9 / 37		9.5	0.53[0.17,1.68]
Subtotal(95%CI)	45 / 264	19 / 154		23.0	1.33[0.74,2.41]
Cochran Mantel-Haenszel P:0.345					
02 1000 VS PLACEBO					
IP 001	0 / 40	1 / 47		1.6	0.38[0.02,9.66]
Subtotal(95%CI)	0 / 40	1 / 47		1.6	0.38[0.02,9.66]
Cochran Mantel-Haenszel P:0.003					
03 2000 VS PLACEBO					
IP 001	4 / 43	1 / 47		1.0	4.72[0.51,43.99]
IP 018	118 / 442	85 / 429		74.4	1.47[1.07,2.02]
Subtotal(95%CI)	122 / 485	86 / 476		75.4	1.52[1.11,2.08]
Cochran Mantel-Haenszel P:0.009					
Total(95%CI)	167 / 789	104 / 583		100.0	1.42[1.08,1.88]
Cochran Mantel-Haenszel P:0.013					

```
        .1    .2         1        5   10
          Favours CONTROL   Favours TREATMENT
```

Figure 7.17   Forest plot showing the effects of *citicoline vs placebo* for acute ischaemic stroke on *survival free of dependency* as defined by a modified Rankin Scale Score of ≤1 at 3 months after stroke. Reproduced from Dávalos *et al.* (2002), with permission from the authors and Lippincott, Williams and Wilkins

Mechanism(s) unknown or uncertain

Gangliosides

Gangliosides may have a protective effect on the central and peripheral nervous systems.

Evidence

A systematic review of 13 placebo-controlled, randomised trials of purified mono-sialoganglioside GM1 in 2265 patients with acute (within 15 days) ischaemic stroke revealed that allocation to a ganglioside was associated with a non-significant reduction in the odds of death at the end of follow-up (15–180 days) of 9% (95% CI: −13% to 27%) (Fig. 7.18) (Candelise and Ciccone, 2000, 2002).

There was no significant difference in mortality among patients treated early (within 48 h) and those receiving delayed treatment despite a trend to greater benefit with delayed treatment (Fig. 7.19).

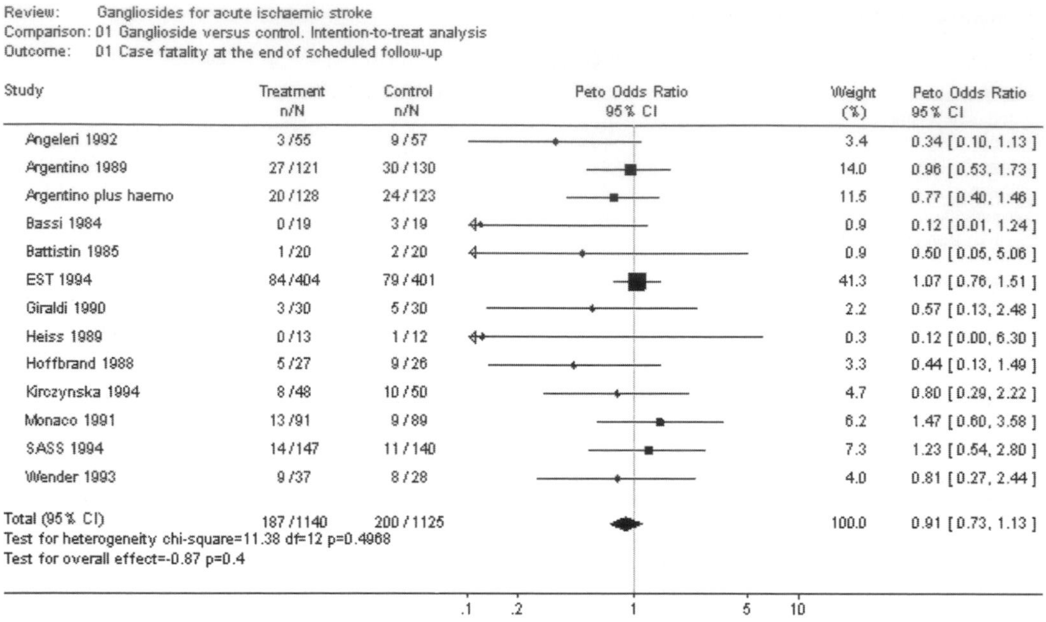

Review: Gangliosides for acute ischaemic stroke
Comparison: 01 Ganglioside versus control. Intention-to-treat analysis
Outcome: 01 Case fatality at the end of scheduled follow-up

Study	Treatment n/N	Control n/N	Peto Odds Ratio 95% CI	Weight (%)	Peto Odds Ratio 95% CI
Angeleri 1992	3 /55	9 /57		3.4	0.34 [0.10, 1.13]
Argentino 1989	27 /121	30 /130		14.0	0.96 [0.53, 1.73]
Argentino plus haemo	20 /128	24 /123		11.5	0.77 [0.40, 1.46]
Bassi 1984	0 /19	3 /19		0.9	0.12 [0.01, 1.24]
Battistin 1985	1 /20	2 /20		0.9	0.50 [0.05, 5.06]
EST 1994	84 /404	79 /401		41.3	1.07 [0.76, 1.51]
Giraldi 1990	3 /30	5 /30		2.2	0.57 [0.13, 2.48]
Heiss 1989	0 /13	1 /12		0.3	0.12 [0.00, 6.30]
Hoffbrand 1988	5 /27	9 /26		3.3	0.44 [0.13, 1.49]
Kirczynska 1994	8 /48	10 /50		4.7	0.80 [0.29, 2.22]
Monaco 1991	13 /91	9 /89		6.2	1.47 [0.60, 3.58]
SASS 1994	14 /147	11 /140		7.3	1.23 [0.54, 2.80]
Wender 1993	9 /37	8 /28		4.0	0.81 [0.27, 2.44]
Total (95% CI)	187 /1140	200 /1125		100.0	0.91 [0.73, 1.13]

Test for heterogeneity chi-square=11.38 df=12 p=0.4968
Test for overall effect=-0.87 p=0.4

.1   .2   1   5   10

Figure 7.18   Forest plot showing the effects of *gangliosides vs control* for acute ischaemic stroke on *case fatality at the end of the scheduled follow-up*. Reproduced from Candelise and Ciccone (2000), with permission from the authors and John Wiley & Sons Limited. Copyright Cochrane Library, reproduced with permission.

Among the three trials which also recorded disability as an outcome measure, random allocation to treatment with gangliosides was not associated with any improvement in BI score (weighted mean difference 2.1; 95% CI: −4.8 to 8.9).

In two trials, eight patients exposed to gangliosides experienced adverse effects that led to discontinuation of ganglioside treatment; seven had skin reactions and one developed Guillain–Barré syndrome.

Comment

There is not enough evidence to conclude that gangliosides are beneficial in acute stroke. Caution is warranted because of reports of sporadic cases of Guillain–Barré syndrome after ganglioside therapy.

Piracetam

Piracetam has neuroprotective and antithrombotic effects which may help to reduce death and disability in people with acute stroke.

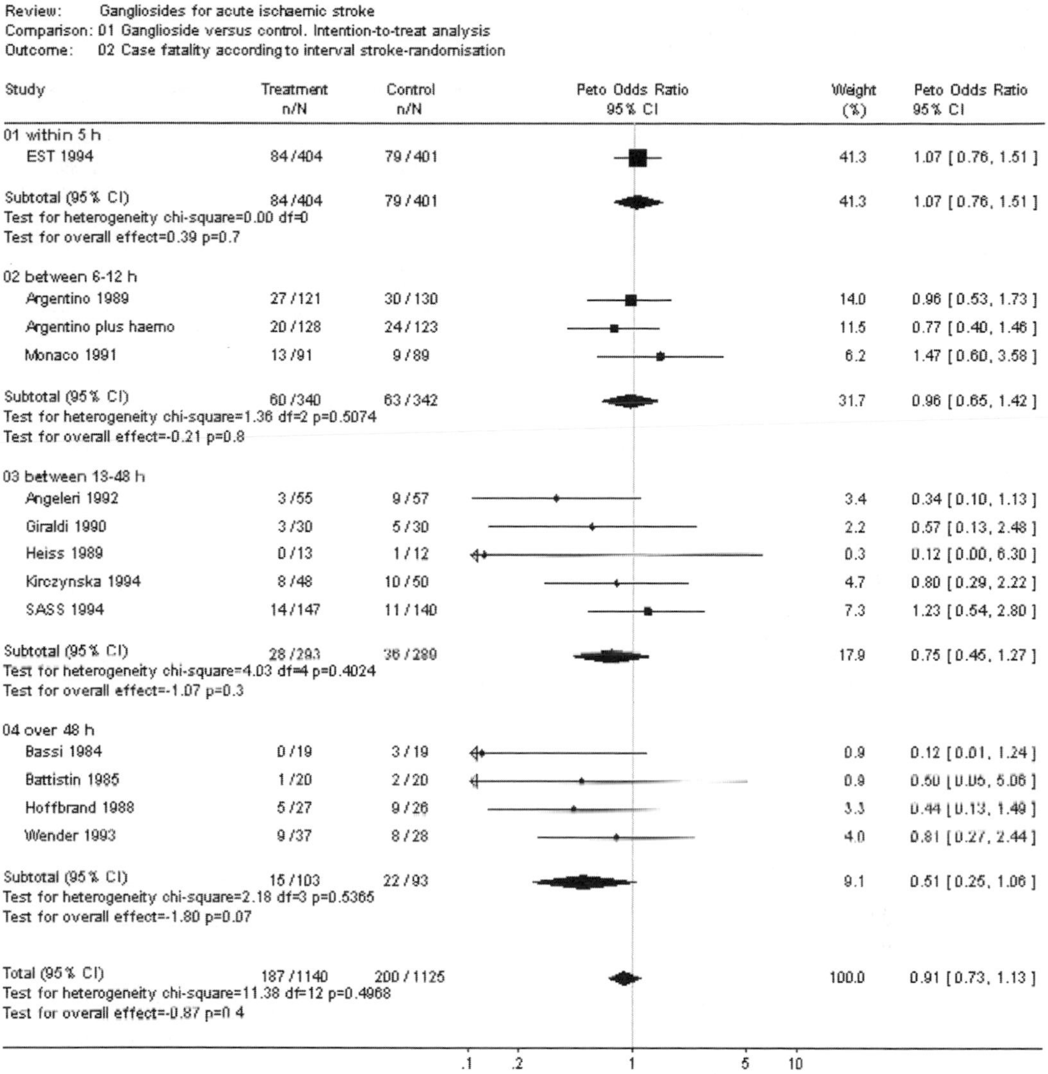

Review: Gangliosides for acute ischaemic stroke
Comparison: 01 Ganglioside versus control. Intention-to-treat analysis
Outcome: 02 Case fatality according to interval stroke-randomisation

Study	Treatment n/N	Control n/N	Peto Odds Ratio 95% CI	Weight (%)	Peto Odds Ratio 95% CI
01 within 5 h					
EST 1994	84/404	79/401		41.3	1.07 [0.76, 1.51]
Subtotal (95% CI)	84/404	79/401		41.3	1.07 [0.76, 1.51]
Test for heterogeneity chi-square=0.00 df=0					
Test for overall effect=0.39 p=0.7					
02 between 6-12 h					
Argentino 1989	27/121	30/130		14.0	0.96 [0.53, 1.73]
Argentino plus haemo	20/128	24/123		11.5	0.77 [0.40, 1.46]
Monaco 1991	13/91	9/89		6.2	1.47 [0.60, 3.58]
Subtotal (95% CI)	60/340	63/342		31.7	0.96 [0.65, 1.42]
Test for heterogeneity chi-square=1.36 df=2 p=0.5074					
Test for overall effect=-0.21 p=0.8					
03 between 13-48 h					
Angeleri 1992	3/55	9/57		3.4	0.34 [0.10, 1.13]
Giraldi 1990	3/30	5/30		2.2	0.57 [0.13, 2.48]
Heiss 1989	0/13	1/12		0.3	0.12 [0.00, 6.30]
Kirczynska 1994	8/48	10/50		4.7	0.80 [0.29, 2.22]
SASS 1994	14/147	11/140		7.3	1.23 [0.54, 2.80]
Subtotal (95% CI)	28/293	36/289		17.9	0.75 [0.45, 1.27]
Test for heterogeneity chi-square=4.03 df=4 p=0.4024					
Test for overall effect=-1.07 p=0.3					
04 over 48 h					
Bassi 1984	0/19	3/19		0.9	0.12 [0.01, 1.24]
Battistin 1985	1/20	2/20		0.9	0.50 [0.06, 5.06]
Hoffbrand 1988	5/27	9/26		3.3	0.44 [0.13, 1.49]
Wender 1993	9/37	8/28		4.0	0.81 [0.27, 2.44]
Subtotal (95% CI)	15/103	22/93		9.1	0.51 [0.25, 1.06]
Test for heterogeneity chi-square=2.18 df=3 p=0.5365					
Test for overall effect=-1.80 p=0.07					
Total (95% CI)	187/1140	200/1125		100.0	0.91 [0.73, 1.13]
Test for heterogeneity chi-square=11.38 df=12 p=0.4968					
Test for overall effect=-0.87 p=0.4					

```
        .1      .2              1           5      10
```

Figure 7.19   Forest plot showing the effects of *gangliosides vs control* for acute ischaemic stroke on *case fatality according to the time interval from stroke to randomisation*. Reproduced from Candelise and Ciccone (2000), with permission from the authors and John Wiley & Sons Limited. Copyright Cochrane Library, reproduced with permission.

Evidence

There have been three randomised trials comparing piracetam with control in patients within 48 h of onset of presumed acute ischaemic stroke and in which at least mortality was reported (Ricci *et al.*, 2002).

A total of 1002 people were randomised, with one trial contributing 93% of the data.

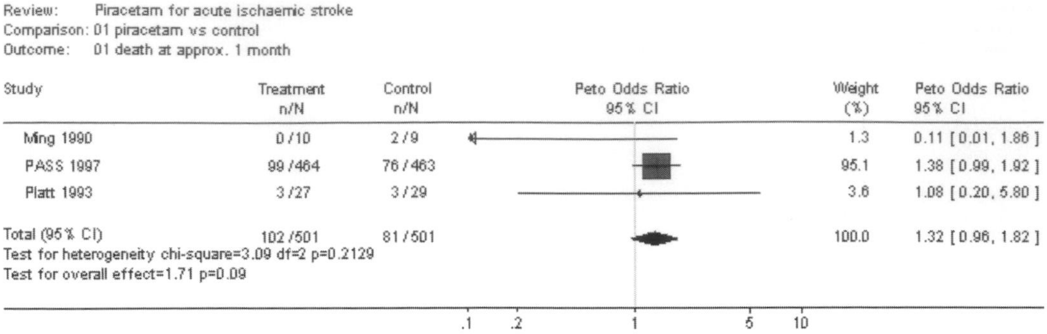

Review: Piracetam for acute ischaemic stroke
Comparison: 01 piracetam vs control
Outcome: 01 death at approx. 1 month

Study	Treatment n/N	Control n/N	Peto Odds Ratio 95% CI	Weight (%)	Peto Odds Ratio 95% CI
Ming 1990	0 /10	2 /9		1.3	0.11 [0.01, 1.86]
PASS 1997	99 /464	76 /463		95.1	1.38 [0.99, 1.92]
Platt 1993	3 /27	3 /29		3.6	1.08 [0.20, 5.80]
Total (95% CI)	102 /501	81 /501		100.0	1.32 [0.96, 1.82]

Test for heterogeneity chi-square=3.09 df=2 p=0.2129
Test for overall effect=1.71 p=0.09

.1   .2   1   5   10

Figure 7.20   Forest plot showing the effects of *piracetam vs control* for acute ischaemic stroke on *death at approximately 1 month after randomisation*. Reproduced from Ricci *et al.* (2002), with permission from the authors and John Wiley & Sons Limited. Copyright Cochrane Library, reproduced with permission.

Review: Piracetam for acute ischaemic stroke
Comparison: 03 death or dependency at 12 weeks
Outcome: 01 death or dependency at 12 weeks

Study	Treatment n/N	Control n/N	Peto Odds Ratio 95% CI	Weight (%)	Peto Odds Ratio 95% CI
PASS 1997	293 /460	294 /463		100.0	1.01 [0.77, 1.32]
Total (95% CI)	293 /460	294 /463		100.0	1.01 [0.77, 1.32]

Test for heterogeneity chi-square=0.00 df=0
Test for overall effect=0.06 p=1.0

.1   .2   1   5   10

Favours Treatment   Favours Control

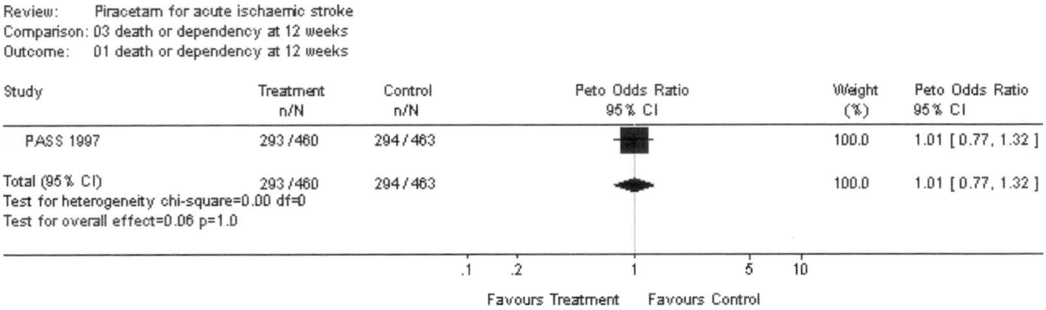

Figure 7.21   Forest plot showing the effects of *piracetam vs control* for acute ischaemic stroke on *death or dependency at 12 weeks after randomisation*. Reproduced from Ricci *et al.* (2002), with permission from the authors and John Wiley & Sons Limited. Copyright Cochrane Library, reproduced with permission.

Random assignment to treatment with piracetam was associated with a statistically non-significant increase in odds of death at 1 month (approximately 32% increase, 95% CI: 82% increase to 4% reduction). This trend was no longer apparent in the large trial after correction for imbalance in stroke severity.

Limited data showed no difference between the treatment and control groups for the proportion of patients dead (Fig. 7.20) or dead or dependent (Fig. 7.21).

Adverse effects were not reported.

Comment

There is some suggestion (but no statistically significant result) of an unfavourable effect of piracetam on early death, but this may have been caused by baseline differences in stroke severity in the trials. There is not enough evidence to assess the effect of piracetam on dependency.

Cooling therapy

Hypothermia decreases the cerebral metabolic rate and metabolic demand. While hypothermia (33°C) does not preserve high-energy phosphate (e.g. ATP, phosphocreatinine) or prevent accumulation of metabolic waste (e.g. lactate) it does confer histopathological protection from ischaemia. Moderate hypothermia is associated with a decrease in the extracellular levels of glutamate during ischaemia in rats and glycine in rabbits, and beneficial effects of hypothermia may be mediated, at least in part, by attenuation of release of EAAs (Correia *et al.*, 1999).

Profound hypothermia is already applied in neurosurgery and open-heart surgery to counter the effects of cerebral hypoxia. In severe closed head injury and cardiac arrest, moderate (33–32°C) hypothermia appears to improve outcome (Correia *et al.*, 1999; Bernard *et al.*, 2002; Hypothermia after cardiac arrest study group, 2002).

In acute stroke, a high body temperature has been associated with a worse prognosis (Reith *et al.*, 1996) (see Chapter 4) but it is not known if lowering temperature improves prognosis. Some temperature-lowering agents, like non-steroidal anti-inflammatory drugs, have antiplatelet activity and could increase the risk of bleeding in acute ischaemic and haemorrhagic stroke. Other risks associated with induced hypothermia are mainly sepsis, pneumonia and coagulopathy.

Evidence

There is currently no evidence from randomised trials to support the routine use of physical or chemical cooling therapy in acute stroke (Correia *et al.*, 1999).

Comment

Since experimental studies showed a neuroprotective effect of hypothermia in cerebral ischaemia, and hypothermia appears to improve the outcome in patients with severe closed head injury and cardiac arrest, trials with cooling therapy in acute stroke are warranted.

SUMMARY

Interpretation of the evidence

More than 11,000 patients have participated in more than 65 clinical trials of neuroprotective therapies and despite this enormous effort, none of the trials in the large number of compounds tested have provided convincing evidence of a clinic-ally and statistically significant benefit (with the possible exception of oral citicoline (Dávalos *et al.*, 2002)) and no compound has gained a product licence (Sandercock *et al.*, 2002; Muir and Lees, 2003). Furthermore, some have revealed dose-limiting intolerance and systemic adverse effects, such as excessive sedation and hypertension.

Implications for practice

There is no current role for neuroprotective drugs in acute stroke management because no agent has yet been found to have significant clinical benefits. Further use of any of these agents should occur only in the context of a clinical trial.

Implications for research

A series of conferences have analysed the possible reasons for this poor record and have led to consensus recommendations for the design of further studies (Finkelstein *et al.*, 1999; Albers *et al.*, 2001; Gladstone *et al.*, 2002; Fisher *et al.*, 2003). Many problems have been cited, ranging from the design and interpreta-tion of pre-clinical studies, their translation into rational designs for clinical trials, and the conduct and analysis of phase II dose-finding and toxicity studies and phase III efficacy trials.

Further clinical trials of new neuroprotective agents are justified if they can embrace many of the above concepts in their planning and design, and are of adequate sample size. Encouragingly, there are several such ongoing trials of neuro-protective therapies (Internet Stroke Centre: http://www.strokecenter.org/trials/).

In addition to further evaluating the promising benefits of oral citicoline, and perhaps other drugs in combination with reperfusion therapy, new therapies should also perhaps be developed and evaluated which target the white (as well as the grey) matter (Falcao *et al.*, 2004) and genes expressed by ischaemic brain cells. It is now recognised that the fate of neurones in ischaemic stroke is not only determined by the severity and duration of focal brain ischaemia, and the direct biochemical effects, but also by changes in the expression of genes by ischaemic cells. Genes are expressed by all cells and code for proteins that control many cel-lular functions including cell division and maturation, biochemical pathways and cell death. Ischaemic stroke results in an upregulation of several genes including heat shock proteins, trk B and sodium–calcium exchanger (NCX). NCX genes, for example, code for membrane proteins responsible for moving calcium in and out of cells, including neurones. Three different NCX genes are expressed in the brain: NCX1, NCX2 and NCX3. In the rat, ischaemia of the hippocampus reduces NCX2 gene expression. Identifying genes expressed in the brain following stroke and responsible for neuronal death or survival may provide therapeutic targets to reduce brain damage.

Treatment of brain oedema

Brain oedema sufficient to cause mass effect and compress adjacent brain structures (e.g. cerebrospinal fluid (CSF) pathways, long tracts, cranial nerves), or increase intracranial pressure (ICP) and lead to herniation, occurs in up to 10% of patients with ischaemic stroke, mainly those with large infarcts. Much of the brain swelling is due to cytotoxic oedema, which is related to ischaemic dysfunction of the cell membrane (e.g. sodium–potassium adenosine triphosphatase (ATPase) pump).

Cytotoxic brain oedema develops in the first few hours after the onset of ischaemic stroke and can be detected on magnetic resonance imaging (MRI) brain scan as a decrease in the apparent diffusion coefficient (ADC) of water. However, brain oedema is usually not sufficiently large in the first 24 h of the stroke to be clinically significant except among patients with large cerebellar infarcts. The MRI brain appearances of cytotoxic brain oedema (a reduction in ADC) lasts for 3–4 days, and then vasogenic oedema develops (Schlaug *et al.*, 1997). The complications of brain oedema usually peak at 3–5 days after ischaemic stroke.

The management of clinically significant brain oedema aims to:
- reduce mass effect and ICP,
- maintain adequate cerebral perfusion to avoid worsening of the brain ischaemia,
- prevent secondary brain injury from herniation.

Strategies to reduce mass effect and ICP include:
- elevate the head of the bed to 20–30 degrees to assist cerebral venous drainage;
- mild fluid restriction;
- avoid hypo-osmolar fluids, such as 5% dextrose in water, which may worsen oedema (Ropper and Shafran, 1984);
- avoid anti-hypertensive drugs that induce cerebral vasodilatation;
- Treat factors that exacerbate raised ICP:
  - hypoxia,
  - hypercarbia,
  - hyperthermia;
- hyperventilation (Gujjar *et al.*, 1998);

- osmotic diuretics;
- barbiturates (Schwab *et al.*, 1997);
- hypothermia (Schwab *et al.*, 1997);
- drainage of cerebrospinal fluid;
- surgical decompression.

Despite reports of success with these measures in anecdotal case reports and case series, there are few data from randomised-controlled trials (RCTs) to evaluate the safety and efficacy of the above measures. Furthermore, it has not been established if continuous ICP monitoring in these patients is of any value, apart from helping predict the patient's outcome and guiding the choice of therapies (Schwab *et al.*, 1996).

Hyperventilation

Hyperventilation sufficient to reduce PCO_2 by 5–10 mmHg can lower ICP by 25–30% (Gujjar *et al.*, 1998). As hyperventilation can lead to vasoconstriction that might compromise brain perfusion and aggravate ischaemia it should probably only be used as a temporary measure whilst preparing to intervene definitively to control brain oedema and ICP.

Corticosteroids

Evidence

Death

A systematic review of seven RCTs involving 453 people with acute ischaemic stroke revealed that compared with control, random assignment to corticosteroid treatment within 48 h of stroke onset made no difference to the odds of death within 1 month (odds ratio (OR): 0.94, 95% confidence interval (CI): 0.59–1.52) (Fig. 8.1) or 1 year (OR: 1.08, 95% CI: 0.68–1.72) (Fig. 8.2) (Qizilbash *et al.*, 2001).

Corticosteroids also do not improve survival after haemorrhagic stroke (Poungvarin *et al.*, 1987).

Adverse effects

The only adverse effects of corticosteroids reported were small numbers of gastro-intestinal bleeds, infections and deterioration of hyperglycaemia across both groups.

Comment

Interpretation of the evidence

The few RCTs do not provide evidence of a beneficial effect of corticosteroids in patients with acute ischaemic stroke on death, neurological impairment or functional outcome.

Review: Corticosteroids for acute ischaemic stroke
Comparison: 01 corticosteroids vs. placebo
Outcome: 02 Deaths within 1 month

Study	Treatment n/N	Control n/N	Peto Odds Ratio 95% CI	Weight (%)	Peto Odds Ratio 95% CI
Bauer 1973	2 /28	2 /26		5.6	0.92 [0.12, 6.96]
Gupta 1978	2 /13	2 /17		5.2	1.35 [0.17, 10.93]
Mulley 1978	25 /61	27 /57		43.6	0.77 [0.37, 1.60]
Norris 1976	7 /26	5 /27		14.1	1.60 [0.45, 5.73]
Norris 1986	13 /54	15 /59		31.5	0.93 [0.40, 2.18]
x Patten 1972	0 /17	0 /20		0.0	Not estimable
Total (95% CI)	49 /199	51 /206		100.0	0.94 [0.59, 1.52]

Test for heterogeneity chi-square=1.07 df=4 p=0.8995
Test for overall effect=-0.23 p=0.8

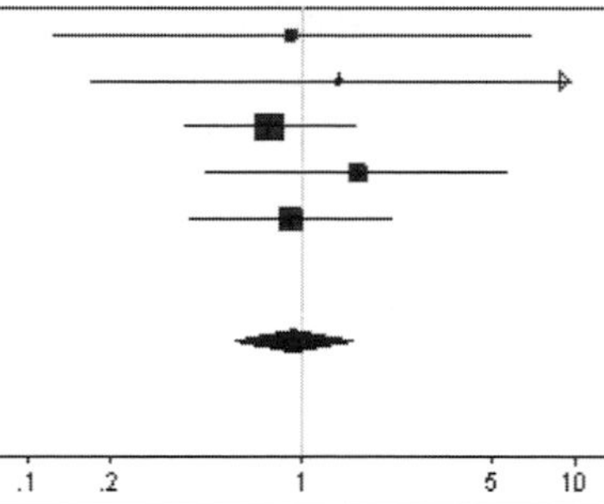

.1   .2   1   5   10

Figure 8.1   Forest plot showing the effects of *corticosteroids vs control* for acute ischaemic stroke on *death within 1 month of randomisation*. Reproduced from Qizilbash *et al.* (2001), with permission from the authors and John Wiley & Sons Limited. Copyright Cochrane Library, reproduced with permission.

Review: Corticosteroids for acute ischaemic stroke
Comparison: 01 corticosteroids vs. placebo
Outcome: 01 All deaths

Study	Treatment n/N	Control n/N	Peto Odds Ratio 95% CI	Weight (%)	Peto Odds Ratio 95% CI
Bauer 1973	2 /28	2 /26		5.2	0.92 [0.12, 6.96]
Gupta 1978	2 /13	2 /17		4.9	1.35 [0.17, 10.93]
McQueen 1978	12 /24	5 /24		15.5	3.49 [1.08, 11.24]
Mulley 1978	42 /61	45 /57		31.9	0.60 [0.26, 1.35]
Norris 1976	7 /26	6 /27		13.1	1.00 [0.45, 5.73]
Norris 1986	13 /54	15 /59		29.4	0.93 [0.40, 2.18]
x Patten 1972	0 /17	0 /20		0.0	Not estimable
Total (95% CI)	78 /223	74 /230		100.0	1.08 [0.68, 1.72]

Test for heterogeneity chi-square=6.43 df=5 p=0.2667
Test for overall effect=0.34 p=0.7

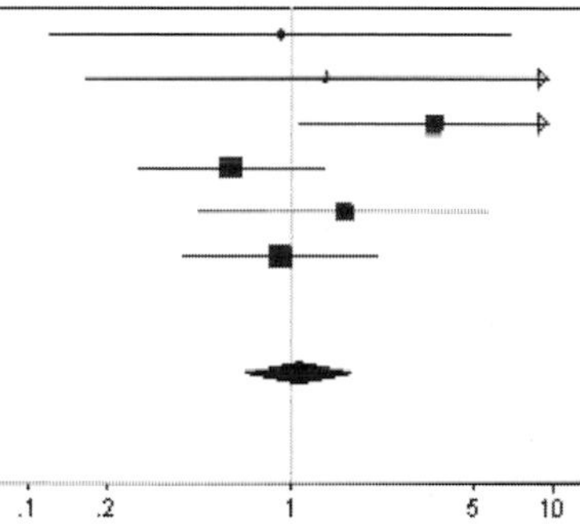

.1   .2   1   5   10

Figure 8.2   Forest plot showing the effects of *corticosteroids vs placebo* for acute ischaemic stroke on *death at the end of follow-up*. Reproduced from Qizilbash *et al.* (2001), with permission from the authors and John Wiley & Sons Limited. Copyright Cochrane Library, reproduced with permission.

Implications for practice

Corticosteroids should not be used in the routine management of brain oedema after acute ischaemic stroke.

Implications for research

As the amount of evidence is minimal, and there have been no recent large trials, it is possible that steroid therapy may be an effective therapy that has been discarded prematurely (Davis and Donnan, 2004; Norris, 2004; Poungvarin, 2004). Future research is required and should be of adequate sample size, and perhaps focus on patients with large infarcts and substantial cerebral oedema, the use of mega-doses of corticosteroids (e.g. methylprednisolone 500–1000 mg/day) which may be more effective on the vasogenic component of the oedema in large brain infarcts, and for a shorter duration to avoid potential adverse effects.

Osmotic diuretics

Osmotic diuretics are widely used in the treatment of cerebral oedema.

Frusemide

An acute intravenous (i.v.) bolus of 40 mg of frusemide is sometimes used as an adjunct therapy in patients whose neurological condition is rapidly deteriorating but it has not been evaluated in RCTs.

Mannitol

Mannitol is an osmotic agent and a free radical scavenger. Mannitol (0.25–0.5 g/kg, e.g. 20–30 g) i.v. over 20 min lowers ICP. It can be given every 6 h to a maximum daily dose of 2 g/kg (e.g. about 140 g in a 70 kg person).

Mannitol is thought to decrease ICP by decreasing overall brain water content and CSF volume, and by reducing blood volume by vasoconstriction (Winkler and Munoz-Ruiz, 1995). Mannitol may also improve cerebral perfusion by decreasing viscosity or by altering red blood cell rheology.

Evidence

Experimental

In several experimental models of ischaemic stroke, mannitol is reported to decrease cerebral oedema, infarct size and neurological deficit when administered within 6 h after stroke onset (Bereczki et al., 2000, 2001).

Subsequent imaging studies of changes in brain tissue volume indicate that mannitol preferentially reduces the water content and volume of non-infarcted brain in patients with ischaemic stroke (Videen et al., 2001), and it may accumulate in the injured brain tissue (Kaufmann and Carduso, 1992).

Clinical condition

A systematic review revealed only one unconfounded RCT in which 300 patients were randomised to one control and three treatment groups: a mixture of ergot alkaloids, dexamethasone or mannitol (Santambrogio et al., 1978; Bereczki et al., 2000, 2001). Of the 300 patients included, only 166 were included in the analysis, of whom 41 were allocated control and 36 mannitol, which was administered i.v.

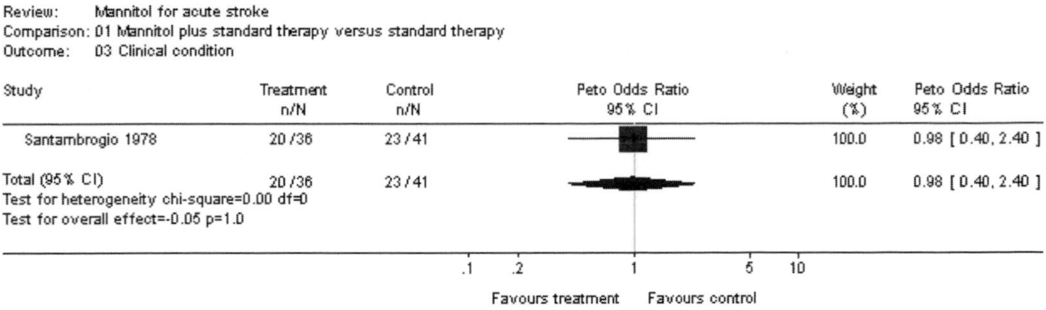

Review: Mannitol for acute stroke
Comparison: 01 Mannitol plus standard therapy versus standard therapy
Outcome: 03 Clinical condition

Study	Treatment n/N	Control n/N	Peto Odds Ratio 95% CI	Weight (%)	Peto Odds Ratio 95% CI
Santambrogio 1978	20 /36	23 /41		100.0	0.98 [0.40, 2.40]
Total (95% CI)	20 /36	23 /41		100.0	0.98 [0.40, 2.40]

Test for heterogeneity chi-square=0.00 df=0
Test for overall effect=-0.05 p=1.0

.1   .2   1   5   10

Favours treatment   Favours control

Figure 8.3   Forest plot showing the effects of *mannitol plus standard therapy vs standard therapy* for acute ischaemic stroke on *clinical condition* at the end of follow-up. Reproduced from Bereczki *et al.* (2001), with permission from the authors and John Wiley & Sons Limited. Copyright Cochrane Library, reproduced with permission.

once a day in a dose of 0.8–0.9 g/kg for 10 days. Among the 41 patients allocated control, 14 (34%) improved compared with 12 of the 36 patients allocated mannitol (33%) (OR: 0.98, 95% CI: 0.40–2.40). The clinical condition worsened among 18 of the 41 (44%) patients assigned control and 16 of the 36 (44%) patients assigned mannitol (Bereczki *et al.*, 2000, 2001) (Fig. 8.3). Case fatality, the proportion of dependent patients at the end of the follow-up and side effects were not reported and were not available from the investigators.

Adverse effects

The most common complications of mannitol therapy were fluid and electrolyte imbalances, cardiopulmonary oedema and rebound cerebral oedema (Bereczki *et al.*, 2000, 2001). Mannitol might cause kidney failure in therapeutic doses, and hypersensitivity reactions may also occur.

Comment

Interpretation of the evidence

There is not enough reliable evidence to determine whether mannitol is effective or ineffective in patients with cerebral oedema due to ischaemic or haemorrhagic stroke.

Implications for practice

Although a beneficial effect of mannitol in acute stroke cannot be excluded, and the use of mannitol in certain clinical conditions in selected cases of acute stroke might be appropriate (e.g. in those with a decreased level of consciousness), the routine use of mannitol in patients with acute stroke cannot be recommended.

Implications for research

The clinical efficacy of mannitol in acute stroke has not yet been properly evaluated. Based on some animal experiments and clinical observations, mannitol has effects

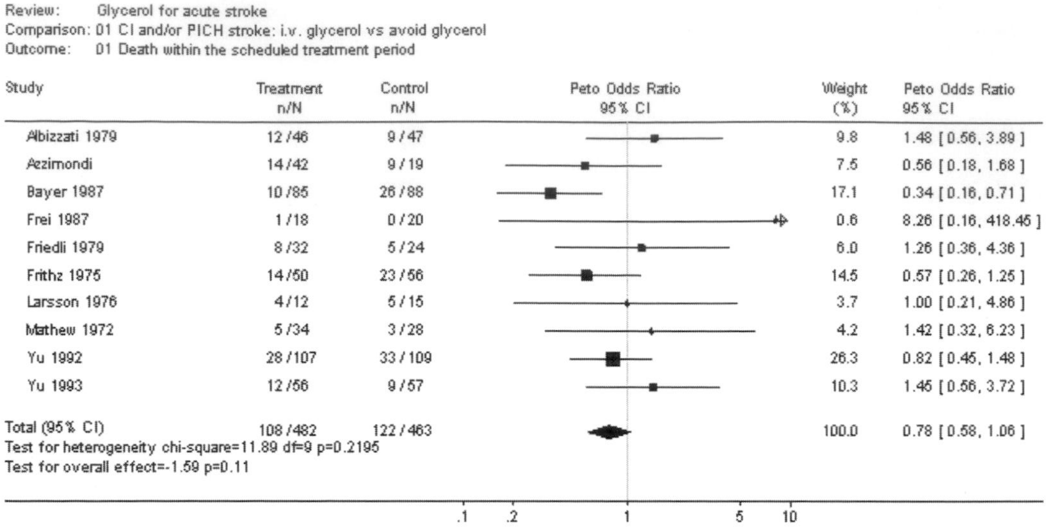

Review: Glycerol for acute stroke
Comparison: 01 CI and/or PICH stroke: i.v. glycerol vs avoid glycerol
Outcome: 01 Death within the scheduled treatment period

Study	Treatment n/N	Control n/N	Peto Odds Ratio 95% CI	Weight (%)	Peto Odds Ratio 95% CI
Albizzati 1979	12 /46	9 / 47		9.8	1.48 [0.56, 3.89]
Aczimondi	14 /42	9 / 19		7.5	0.56 [0.18, 1.68]
Bayer 1987	10 /85	26 / 88		17.1	0.34 [0.16, 0.71]
Frei 1987	1 /18	0 / 20		0.6	8.26 [0.16, 418.45]
Friedli 1979	8 /32	5 / 24		6.0	1.26 [0.36, 4.36]
Frithz 1975	14 /50	23 / 56		14.5	0.57 [0.26, 1.25]
Larsson 1976	4 /12	5 / 15		3.7	1.00 [0.21, 4.86]
Mathew 1972	5 /34	3 / 28		4.2	1.42 [0.32, 6.23]
Yu 1992	28 /107	33 / 109		26.3	0.82 [0.45, 1.48]
Yu 1993	12 /56	9 / 57		10.3	1.45 [0.56, 3.72]
Total (95% CI)	108 /482	122 / 463		100.0	0.78 [0.58, 1.06]

Test for heterogeneity chi-square=11.89 df=9 p=0.2195
Test for overall effect=-1.59 p=0.11

.1   .2   1   5   10

Figure 8.4   Forest plot showing the effects of *i.v. glycerol vs avoid glycerol* for acute stroke on *death within the scheduled treatment period.* Reproduced from Righetti *et al.* (2003), with permission from the authors and John Wiley & Sons Limited. Copyright Cochrane Library, reproduced with permission.

that might be beneficial in acute stroke. To prove this hypothesis, placebo-controlled unconfounded, properly randomised, clinical studies have to be designed and performed. In these studies the registration of early and late case fatality and of valid and reliable measures of dependency and disability are recommended.

Glycerol

A 10% solution of glycerol is a hyperosmolar agent that is claimed to reduce brain oedema, and is used commonly for this purpose in some countries such as Italy, Poland and China.

Evidence

A systematic review of 11 randomised trials comparing i.v. glycerol initiated within the first days after stroke onset with control revealed 10 trials involving a total 482 glycerol treated patients and 463 control patients in which an analysis of death during the scheduled treatment period was possible (Righetti *et al.*, 2003, 2004).

Death

Random allocation to glycerol was associated with a non-significant reduction in the odds of death within the scheduled treatment period (OR: 0.78, 95% CI: 0.58–1.06) (Fig. 8.4).

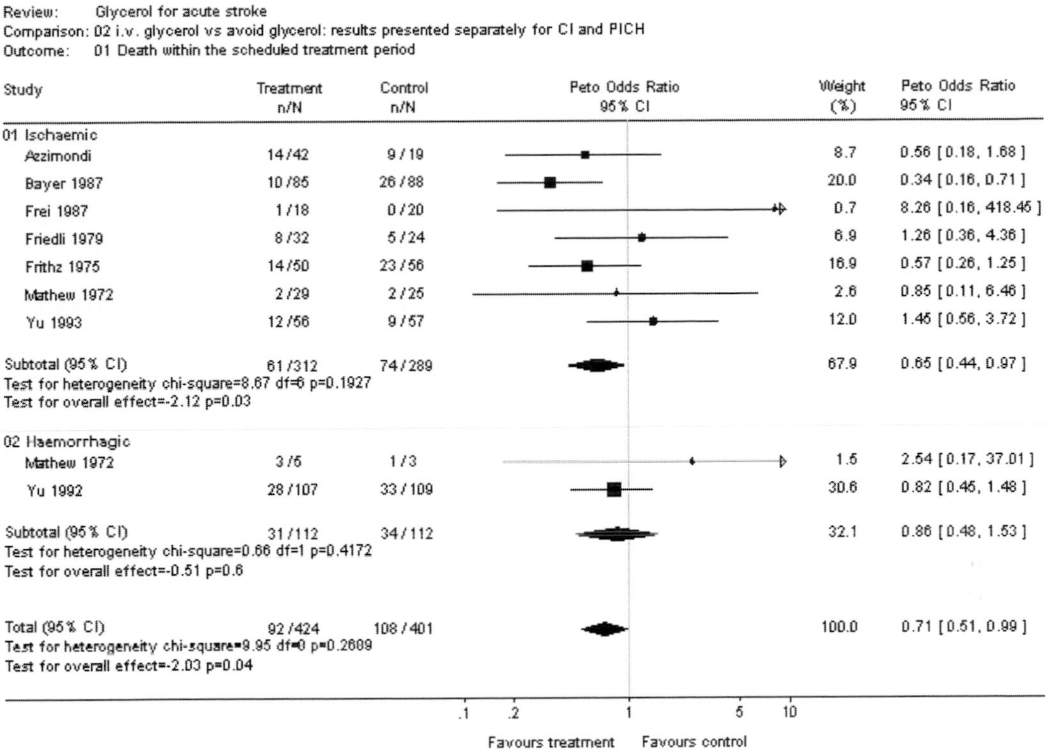

Review: Glycerol for acute stroke
Comparison: 02 i.v. glycerol vs avoid glycerol: results presented separately for CI and PICH
Outcome: 01 Death within the scheduled treatment period

Study	Treatment n/N	Control n/N	Peto Odds Ratio 95% CI	Weight (%)	Peto Odds Ratio 95% CI
01 Ischaemic					
Aezimondi	14/42	9/19		8.7	0.56 [0.18, 1.68]
Bayer 1987	10/85	26/88		20.0	0.34 [0.16, 0.71]
Frei 1987	1/18	0/20		0.7	8.26 [0.16, 418.46]
Friedli 1979	8/32	5/24		6.9	1.26 [0.36, 4.36]
Frithz 1975	14/50	23/56		16.9	0.57 [0.26, 1.25]
Mathew 1972	2/29	2/25		2.6	0.85 [0.11, 6.46]
Yu 1993	12/56	9/57		12.0	1.46 [0.56, 3.72]
Subtotal (95% CI)	61/312	74/289		67.9	0.65 [0.44, 0.97]
Test for heterogeneity chi-square=8.67 df=6 p=0.1927					
Test for overall effect=-2.12 p=0.03					
02 Haemorrhagic					
Mathew 1972	3/6	1/3		1.5	2.54 [0.17, 37.01]
Yu 1992	28/107	33/109		30.6	0.82 [0.45, 1.48]
Subtotal (95% CI)	31/112	34/112		32.1	0.86 [0.48, 1.53]
Test for heterogeneity chi-square=0.66 df=1 p=0.4172					
Test for overall effect=-0.51 p=0.6					
Total (95% CI)	92/424	108/401		100.0	0.71 [0.51, 0.99]
Test for heterogeneity chi-square=9.95 df=9 p=0.2689					
Test for overall effect=-2.03 p=0.04					

.1   .2   1   5   10

Favours treatment   Favours control

Figure 8.5   Forest plot showing the effects of *i.v. glycerol vs avoid glycerol* for acute stroke on *death within the scheduled treatment period, according to the pathological subtype of stroke.* Reproduced from Righetti *et al.* (2003), with permission from the authors and John Wiley & Sons Limited. Copyright Cochrane Library, reproduced with permission.

Among patients with ischaemic stroke, glycerol was associated with a significant reduction in the odds of death during the scheduled treatment period (OR: 0.65, 95% CI: 0.44–0.97) (Fig. 8.5).

At the end of the scheduled follow-up period, there was no significant difference in the odds of death (OR: 0.98, 95% CI: 0.73–1.31) (Fig. 8.6).

Death or dependency
Functional outcome was reported in only two studies, in which there was a non-significant trend toward more patients assigned glycerol who had a good outcome at the end of scheduled follow-up (OR: 0.73, 95% CI: 0.37–1.42) (Fig. 8.7).

Adverse effects
Haemolysis was the only relevant adverse effect of glycerol treatment.

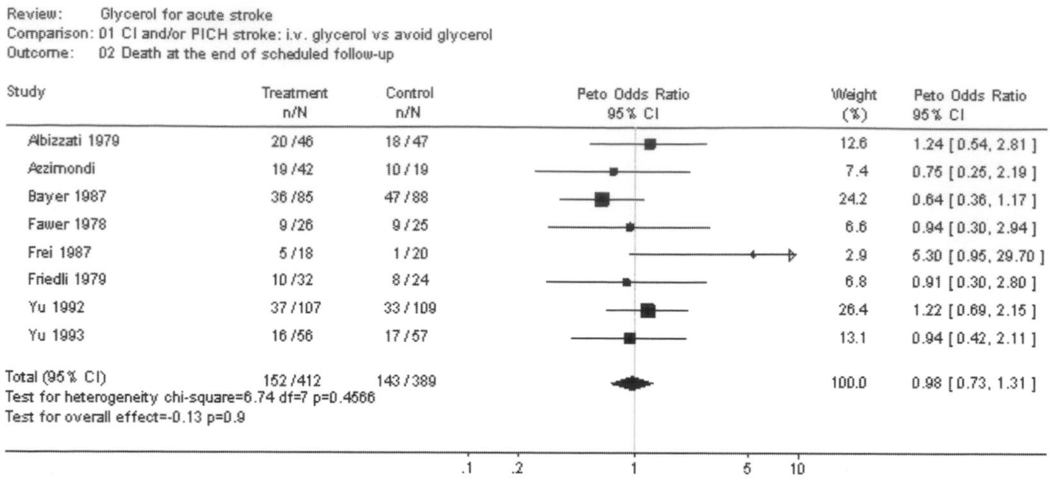

Review: Glycerol for acute stroke
Comparison: 01 CI and/or PICH stroke: i.v. glycerol vs avoid glycerol
Outcome: 02 Death at the end of scheduled follow-up

Study	Treatment n/N	Control n/N	Peto Odds Ratio 95% CI	Weight (%)	Peto Odds Ratio 95% CI
Albizzati 1979	20 /46	18 / 47		12.6	1.24 [0.54, 2.81]
Azzimondi	19 /42	10 / 19		7.4	0.75 [0.25, 2.19]
Bayer 1987	36 /85	47 /88		24.2	0.64 [0.36, 1.17]
Fawer 1978	9 /26	9 /25		6.6	0.94 [0.30, 2.94]
Frei 1987	5 /18	1 / 20		2.9	5.30 [0.95, 29.70]
Friedli 1979	10 /32	8 / 24		6.8	0.91 [0.30, 2.80]
Yu 1992	37 /107	33 / 109		26.4	1.22 [0.69, 2.15]
Yu 1993	16 /56	17 /57		13.1	0.94 [0.42, 2.11]
Total (95% CI)	152 /412	143 /389		100.0	0.98 [0.73, 1.31]

Test for heterogeneity chi-square=6.74 df=7 p=0.4566
Test for overall effect=-0.13 p=0.9

.1   .2   1   5   10

Figure 8.6   Forest plot showing the effects of *i.v. glycerol vs avoid glycerol* for acute stroke on *death at the end of the follow-up period*. Reproduced from Righetti *et al.* (2003), with permission from the authors and John Wiley & Sons Limited. Copyright Cochrane Library, reproduced with permission.

Review: Glycerol for acute stroke
Comparison: 01 CI and/or PICH stroke: i.v. glycerol vs avoid glycerol
Outcome: 03 Dead or disabled at end of scheduled follow-up

Study	Treatment n/N	Control n/N	Peto Odds Ratio 95% CI	Weight (%)	Peto Odds Ratio 95% CI
Azzimondi	35 /42	15 / 19		23.1	1.34 [0.33, 5.42]
Bayer 1987	66 /85	75 / 88		76.9	0.61 [0.28, 1.30]
Total (95% CI)	101 /127	90 / 107		100.0	0.73 [0.37, 1.42]

Test for heterogeneity chi-square=0.95 df=1 p=0.3302
Test for overall effect=-0.93 p=0.4

.1   .2   1   5   10

Favours treatment   Favours control

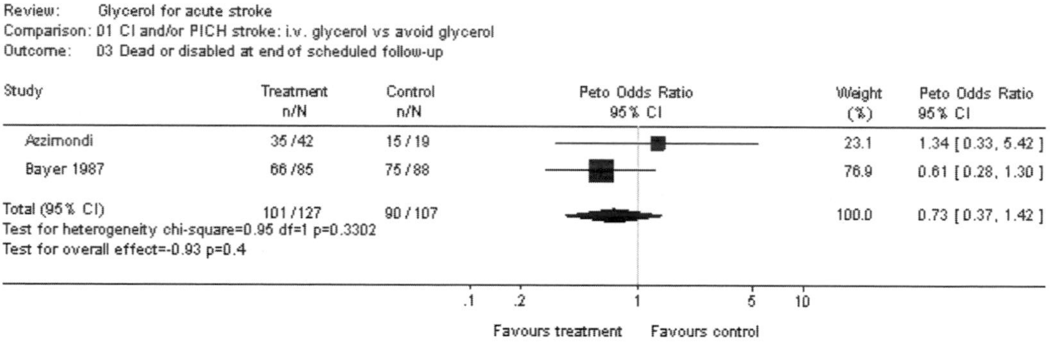

Figure 8.7   Forest plot showing the effects of *i.v. glycerol vs avoid glycerol* for acute stroke on *death or dependency at the end of the follow-up period.* Reproduced from Righetti *et al.* (2003), with permission from the authors and John Wiley & Sons Limited. Copyright Cochrane Library, reproduced with permission.

Comment

Interpretation of the evidence

These data suggest a favourable effect of glycerol treatment on short-term survival in patients with probable or definite ischaemic stroke, but the CI were wide and the magnitude of the treatment effect may be only minimal. Due to the relatively small number of patients, and that the trials were performed in the pre-CT era, the results must be interpreted cautiously. Furthermore, most patients included in the studies did not have impairment of consciousness.

Implications for practice

The lack of reliable evidence of benefit in long-term survival does not support the routine or selective use of glycerol treatment in patients with acute stroke.

Implications for research

As glycerol treatment is inexpensive, may be effective, and appears to be safe it should continue to be tested, but in much larger RCTs, perhaps restricted to patients who have clinical evidence of cerebral oedema, in which the long-term effects of treatment on disability, handicap and quality of life are reliably assessed.

Cerebrospinal fluid drainage

Drainage of CSF via an intra-ventricular catheter can rapidly lower ICP if hydrocephalus is present, but has not been evaluated in RCTs.

Surgical decompression

Surgical approaches to the treatment of symptomatic cerebral oedema seek to create space to accommodate the swollen brain. This can be accomplished by releasing the restriction of the cranial vault and dura or creating space within it by removing non-viable or non-essential brain tissue (Morley *et al.*, 2002). These strategies are described as 'external' or 'internal' decompression respectively. External decompression involves hemicraniectomy with or without duroplasty. Internal decompression involves the removal of brain tissue, either the infarcted region or non-eloquent regions of the brain. These techniques are sometimes combined. Despite the possible benefit, surgical therapy involves risks which may include secondary cerebral haemorrhage and brain herniation through the craniectomy defect (Morley *et al.*, 2002).

In the past few years, enthusiasm has developed for hemicraniectomy in patients with malignant cerebral infarcts; that is, those that involve the entire territory of the middle cerebral artery (MCA) or internal carotid artery (ICA) in one cerebral hemisphere. The mortality rate in these patients is very high without surgery, and most of those that do survive are disabled and dependent. Widespread decompression with removal of a large part of the hemicranium and opening of the dura mata can be lifesaving, particularly early in the course of the disease, before herniation. It is hypothesised that many such patients, particularly young ones, recover function more frequently than if they are not operated on.

Evidence

Two systematic reviews of studies comparing medical therapy plus decompressive surgery with medical therapy alone in patients with acute ischaemic stroke complicated by clinical and radiologically confirmed cerebral oedema identified no RCTs (Morley *et al.*, 2002, 2003; Gupta *et al.*, 2004).

Several observational studies reporting comparative data have been reported, along with a number of small series and single case reports. A recent analysis of the databases of eight neurosurgical departments in Germany identified 188 patients who underwent decompressive craniectomy for space occupying MCA infarction between 1996 and 2001 (Uhl *et al.*, 2004). The unadjusted 3, 6 and 12 month mortality rates were 7.9%, 37.6% and 43.8% respectively (median follow-up 26 weeks). In the 'best' multivariate model, age >50 years ($P < 0.02$) and the involvement of two or more vascular territories ($P < 0.01$) had an unfavourable impact on length of survival. The adjusted 6 month mortality was a low as 20.0% (no risk factor) and as high as 60% (two risk factors). The adverse prognostic significance of infarction in more than one vascular territory (i.e. beyond the MCA territory, such as additional anterior choroidal or anterior or posterior cerebral artery infarction) has also been reported in other studies (Maramattom *et al.*, 2004).

Comment

There is no evidence from RCTs to support the use of decompressive surgery for the treatment of cerebral oedema in acute ischaemic stroke.

Uncontrolled studies suggest that those most likely to benefit are younger patients with infarction confined to the MCA territory, who are developing brain oedema and deteriorating clinically (e.g. drowsy with bilateral ptosis (due to presumed pressure on the central oculomotor nucleus), but who do not have established signs of transtentorial herniation (e.g. are not unconscious), and who are operated on early rather than late (Brown, 2003; Donnan and Davis, 2003; Schwab and Hacke, 2003).

Evidence from ongoing RCTs is urgently needed to accurately assess the effect of decompressive surgery (Cockroft, 2004).

The Hemicraniectomy After Middle cerebral artery infarction with Life-threatening Edema Trial (HAMLET) trial started in September 2002 and aims to randomise 112 patients, up to 60 years of age with a space-occupying infarct in the territory of the MCA leading to a decrease in consciousness, to decompressive surgery (hemicraniectomy and duraplasty) followed by intensive care treatment, or conservative treatment, consisting of either intensive care treatment or 'standard' therapy on a stroke unit (Hofmeijer *et al.*, 2001; van der Worp *et al.*, 2004). The primary outcome measure is the modified Rankin scale score at 1 year. Recruitment is expected to be completed in 2007.

The Decompressive Craniectomy In Malignant middle cerebral artery infarcts (DECIMAL) trial had randomised 18 patients by November 2003 and aims to randomise 60 patients, aged 18–55 years, within 24 h of malignant MCA infarction to decompressive surgery (hemicraniectomy and duraplasty) plus best medical treatment or to best medical treatment alone (Vahedi *et al.*, 2004).

The Hemicraniectomy for Malignant Middle cerebral artery Infarcts (HeMMI) trial is an open randomised trial which had randomised 15 patients by November 2003 and aims to randomise 28 patients, aged 18–55 years, within 72 h of malignant MCA infarction to decompressive surgery (hemicraniectomy and duraplasty) plus best medical treatment or to best medical treatment alone (Jamora *et al.*, 2004).

HEADFIRST is another ongoing trial (Frank, 1999, 2000).

Ventriculostomy and suboccipital craniectomy

Ventriculostomy and suboccipital craniectomy, in conjunction with aggressive medical therapies, are reported to be effective in relieving hydrocephalus and brain-stem compression caused by large cerebellar infarction (and haemorrhage) in anec-dotal case studies and series, but data from RCTs are lacking (Chen *et al.*, 1992).

SUMMARY

Corticosteroids have no place in the management of cerebral oedema and increased ICP following ischaemic stroke (level 1 evidence).

Osmotherapy (mannitol, glycerol) and hyperventilation are recommended for patients whose condition is deteriorating secondary to increased ICP, including those with herniation syndromes (level IV).

External ventricular drainage or ventriculostomy can be used to treat increased ICP due to hydrocephalus (level III).

Surgical decompression and evacuation of large cerebellar infarction or haemorrhage that compresses the brainstem and causes hydrocephalus is justified (level III).

Surgical decompression of brain oedema associated with large hemispheric infarc-tion can be a lifesaving measure but the relative risks and benefits remain to be evaluated in ongoing RCTs.

Anticoagulation

The purpose of anticoagulation in patients with ischaemic stroke is to prevent recurrent ischaemic stroke and other serious vascular events (by preventing arterial thromboembolism and cardiogenic embolism) and to prevent venous thromboembolism.

Recurrent stroke

The risk of a recurrent stroke after ischaemic stroke or transient ischaemic attack (TIA) is about 10% within 1 week and 18% within the first 3 months in the community (Lovett *et al.*, 2003; Coull *et al.*, 2004; Hankey, 2005). This substantial early risk is 3-fold higher if the TIA or ischaemic stroke is caused by large artery disease, and 5-fold lower if the cause is small artery disease (Lovett *et al.*, 2004). The prevalence and level of other causal vascular risk factors also influence risk of recurrence (Hankey *et al.*, 1992; Kernan *et al.*, 2000; Dippel *et al.*, 2004).

About 50% of all recurrent ischaemic strokes and TIAs are probably due to atherothrombotic disease of the extracranial, or less commonly large intracranial arteries; about 20% arise from emboli from the heart; and about 25% are so-called lacunar infarcts, probably due to occlusion of one of the small, deep, perforating cerebral arteries (Warlow *et al.*, 2000).

The formation of thrombus on the subendothelial tissue of arteries (aorta and large extra- and intracranial arteries) and irregular endothelial surfaces of the cardiac and valvular endocardium depends on the initial formation of a platelet plug (by means of platelet adhesion, activation and aggregation) and the generation of a meshwork of fibrin (by means of the coagulation cascade).

Theoretically, anticoagulants and antiplatelet drugs should be effective in preventing recurrent ischaemic stroke, provided they can both be administered safely over a long period of time. Anticoagulants should theoretically work by inhibiting the formation of predominantly 'red' fibrin clots in areas of very reduced and stagnant blood flow, such as in cardiac chambers with impaired contractility (e.g. atrial fibrillation (AF), akinetic left ventricle) and in veins (e.g. paralysed leg). Antiplatelet drugs should theoretically work by inhibiting the formation of predominantly 'white' platelet clots in areas of high shear stress such as in arteries (e.g. carotid artery atherothrombosis). However, because the vascular lesions that cause ischaemic stroke are very heterogeneous, it is unlikely that any one drug or strategy will be dramatically effective in all aetiological subtypes of ischaemic stroke.

Venous thromboembolism

Deep venous thrombosis (DVT), diagnosed by means of radiolabelled fibrinogen leg scanning, develops in more than half of stroke patients with hemiparesis, but is clinically evident in less than 5% (see Chapter 4) (Warlow *et al.*, 1972; Warlow, 1978; Langhorne *et al.*, 2000).

Pulmonary embolism (PE), diagnosed at autopsy, is present in a substantial proportion of patients with fatal stroke, and accounts for about 10% of deaths after stroke, but is clinically evident in less than 2% of patients (see Chapter 4) (Warlow, 1978; Wijdicks and Scott, 1997).

Acute ischaemic stroke

Anticoagulation (heparins) vs control

Evidence

A systematic review identified 21 randomised-controlled trials (RCTs) comparing anticoagulant therapy with control in the early treatment of a total of 23,547 patients with acute ischaemic stroke (Gubitz *et al.*, 2004; Sandercock *et al.*, 2004). Twelve trials enrolled patients within 48 h of stroke onset, three within 72 h, four within 7 days and two within 14 days. The quality of the trials varied considerably.

The anticoagulants used were:

* standard unfractionated subcutaneous heparin (six trials);
* standard unfractionated intravenous heparin (two trials);
* low-molecular-weight heparins (LMWHs) (six trials: two dalteparin, two nadroparin, one tinzaparin and one CY 222);
* subcutaneous heparinoid (two trials: one danaparoid and one mesoglycan);
* intravenous heparinoid (one danaparoid trial);
* oral anticoagulants (two trials);
* thrombin inhibitors (two MD805 trials).

Thirteen trials routinely performed a computerised tomography (CT) head scan in all patients to rule out haemorrhage before randomisation (CESG, 1983; Duke, 1986; Tazaki, 1986; Turpie, 1987; Cazzato, 1989; Prins, 1989; Elias, 1990; Sandset, 1990; Tazaki, 1992; FISS, 1995; Pambianco, 1995; FISS-bis, 1998; TOAST, 1998).

Three trials performed CT in most patients (Duke, 1983; Vissinger, 1995; IST, 1997). In the International Stroke Trial (IST), 67% of patients were scanned before randomisation and 29% after randomisation, so that overall, 96% of patients were scanned. It is therefore likely that some patients with intracerebral haemorrhage were inadvertently included in the main analyses of this review. This may have biased the results against anticoagulation if the risks of anticoagulation are greater in those with intracerebral haemorrhage, although such a bias is unlikely given the relatively small numbers of patients with intracerebral haemorrhage involved in these trials. Therefore a sensitivity analysis was performed based on only those trials where all patients had CT scanning prior to randomisation (see below).

Death or dependency

Six RCTs involving a total of 21,966 patients found no evidence that anticoagulants reduced the odds of being dead or dependent at the end of follow-up compared with control (odds ratio (OR): 0.99, 95% confidence interval (CI): 0.93–1.04) (Fig. 9.1).

There was significant heterogeneity of treatment effect in the LMWH group ($P = 0.043$), which was chiefly attributable to one trial of 312 oriental patients (FISS, 1995). There was no obvious explanation other than the play of chance, or possibly ethnic differences in the study population, although the latter would seem to be unlikely. A subsequent trial (FISS-bis, 1998), designed to replicate the results of the FISS trial, did not show any clear benefit overall, suggesting that the FISS result was due to the play of chance. Another meta-analysis, confined to LMWHs and heparinoids in acute ischaemic stroke showed similar results (Bath *et al.*, 2000).

Pre-specified sensitivity analyses showed that the overall result for death and dependency (OR: 0.99, 95% CI: 0.93–1.04; Fig. 9.1) was consistent if:
- different types of anticoagulant were used: LMWH (OR: 0.85, 95% CI: 0.66–1.08) and heparinoid (TOAST, 1998) (OR: 0.92, 95% CI: 0.72–1.19);
- a CT head scan was performed before randomisation (OR: 1.01, 95% CI: 0.95–1.08), or after randomisation or not at all (OR: 1.01, 95% CI: 0.91–1.12);
- anticoagulants were added to aspirin during the treatment period (OR: 1.00, 95% CI: 0.92–1.09), or if anticoagulants alone were given during the treatment period (OR: 0.98, 95% CI: 0.91–1.06);
- low-fixed-dose anticoagulants were compared to control (OR: 1.00, 95% CI: 0.93–1.09), or if medium fixed-dose anticoagulants or adjusted-dose anticoagulants were compared to control (OR: 0.98, 95% CI: 0.91–1.05) during the treatment period;

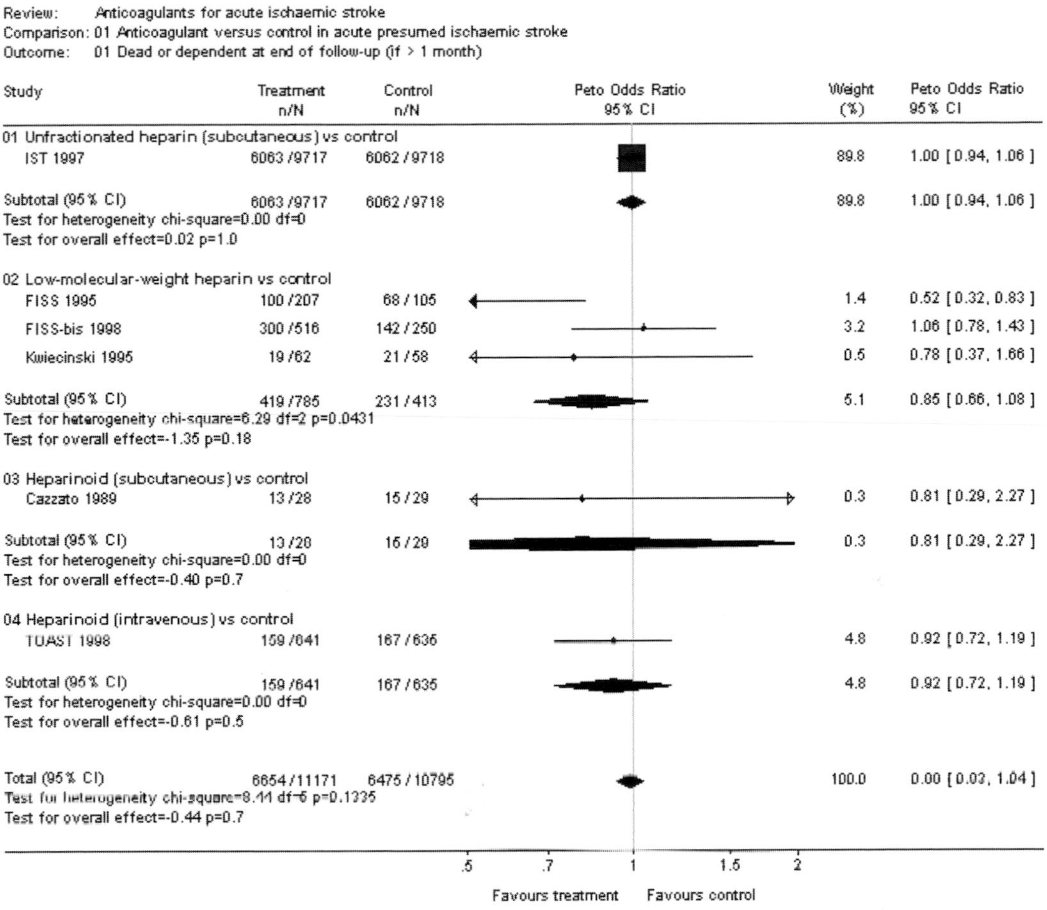

Review: Anticoagulants for acute ischaemic stroke
Comparison: 01 Anticoagulant versus control in acute presumed ischaemic stroke
Outcome: 01 Dead or dependent at end of follow-up (if > 1 month)

Study	Treatment n/N	Control n/N	Peto Odds Ratio 95% CI	Weight (%)	Peto Odds Ratio 95% CI
01 Unfractionated heparin (subcutaneous) vs control					
IST 1997	6063 /9717	6062 /9718		89.8	1.00 [0.94, 1.06]
Subtotal (95% CI)	6063 /9717	6062 /9718		89.8	1.00 [0.94, 1.06]
Test for heterogeneity chi-square=0.00 df=0					
Test for overall effect=0.02 p=1.0					
02 Low-molecular-weight heparin vs control					
FISS 1995	100 /207	68 / 105		1.4	0.52 [0.32, 0.83]
FISS-bis 1998	300 /516	142 / 250		3.2	1.06 [0.78, 1.43]
Kwiecinski 1995	19 /62	21 /58		0.5	0.78 [0.37, 1.66]
Subtotal (95% CI)	419 /785	231 /413		5.1	0.85 [0.66, 1.08]
Test for heterogeneity chi-square=6.29 df=2 p=0.0431					
Test for overall effect=-1.35 p=0.18					
03 Heparinoid (subcutaneous) vs control					
Cazzato 1989	13 /28	15 /29		0.3	0.81 [0.29, 2.27]
Subtotal (95% CI)	13 /28	15 /29		0.3	0.81 [0.29, 2.27]
Test for heterogeneity chi-square=0.00 df=0					
Test for overall effect=-0.40 p=0.7					
04 Heparinoid (intravenous) vs control					
TOAST 1998	159 /641	167 /635		4.8	0.92 [0.72, 1.19]
Subtotal (95% CI)	159 /641	167 /635		4.8	0.92 [0.72, 1.19]
Test for heterogeneity chi-square=0.00 df=0					
Test for overall effect=-0.61 p=0.5					
Total (95% CI)	6654 /11171	6475 /10795		100.0	0.00 [0.03, 1.04]
Test for heterogeneity chi-square=8.44 df=6 p=0.1335					
Test for overall effect=-0.44 p=0.7					

.5   .7   1   1.5   2

Favours treatment   Favours control

Figure 9.1   Forest plot showing the effects of *any anticoagulant vs control* in acute ischaemic stroke on *death or dependency at the end of follow-up*. Reproduced from Gubitz *et al.* (2004), with permission from the authors and John Wiley & Sons Limited. Copyright Cochrane Library, reproduced with permission.

- data from the IST were included (OR: 0.99, 95% CI: 0.94–1.05) or excluded (OR: 0.89, 95% CI: 0.74–1.06);
- if a cardiac source of embolism was suspected (OR: 1.00, 95% CI: 0.85–1.18) or not suspected (OR: 1.00, 95% CI: 0.94–1.06) to be the cause of the stroke (see below: page 186 (AF) and Chapter 15).

Death

Based on nine trials involving a total of 22,570 patients, there was no evidence that anticoagulant therapy reduced the odds of death from all causes (OR: 1.05, 95% CI: 0.98–1.12) at the end of follow-up (Fig. 9.2).

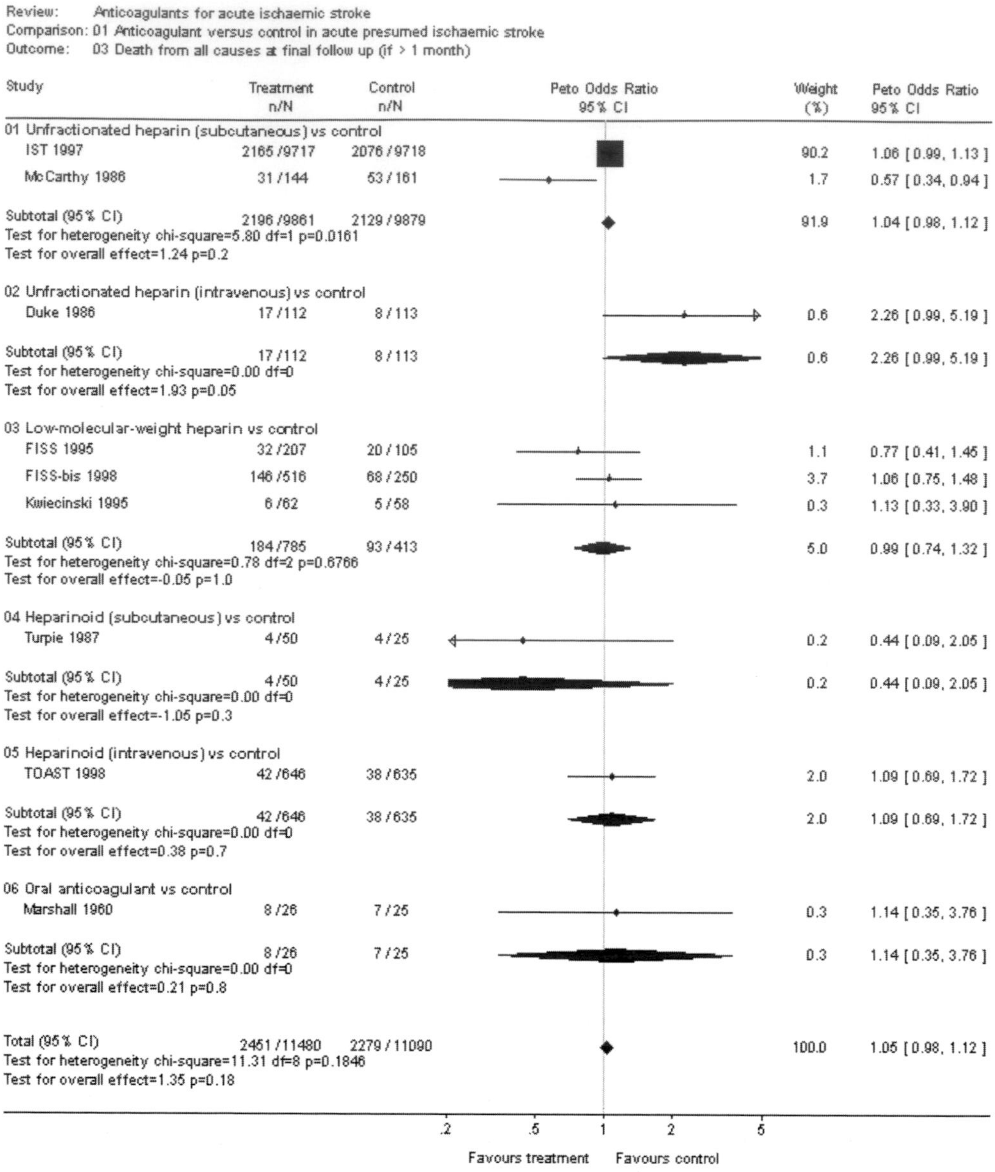

Review: Anticoagulants for acute ischaemic stroke
Comparison: 01 Anticoagulant versus control in acute presumed ischaemic stroke
Outcome: 03 Death from all causes at final follow up (if > 1 month)

Study	Treatment n/N	Control n/N	Peto Odds Ratio 95% CI	Weight (%)	Peto Odds Ratio 95% CI
01 Unfractionated heparin (subcutaneous) vs control					
IST 1997	2165 / 9717	2076 / 9718		90.2	1.06 [0.99, 1.13]
McCarthy 1986	31 / 144	53 / 161		1.7	0.57 [0.34, 0.94]
Subtotal (95% CI)	2196 / 9861	2129 / 9879		91.9	1.04 [0.98, 1.12]

Test for heterogeneity chi-square=5.80 df=1 p=0.0161
Test for overall effect=1.24 p=0.2

02 Unfractionated heparin (intravenous) vs control					
Duke 1986	17 / 112	8 / 113		0.6	2.26 [0.99, 5.19]
Subtotal (95% CI)	17 / 112	8 / 113		0.6	2.26 [0.99, 5.19]

Test for heterogeneity chi-square=0.00 df=0
Test for overall effect=1.93 p=0.05

03 Low-molecular-weight heparin vs control					
FISS 1995	32 / 207	20 / 105		1.1	0.77 [0.41, 1.45]
FISS-bis 1998	146 / 516	68 / 250		3.7	1.06 [0.75, 1.48]
Kwiecinski 1995	6 / 62	5 / 58		0.3	1.13 [0.33, 3.90]
Subtotal (95% CI)	184 / 785	93 / 413		5.0	0.99 [0.74, 1.32]

Test for heterogeneity chi-square=0.78 df=2 p=0.6766
Test for overall effect=-0.05 p=1.0

04 Heparinoid (subcutaneous) vs control					
Turpie 1987	4 / 50	4 / 25		0.2	0.44 [0.09, 2.05]
Subtotal (95% CI)	4 / 50	4 / 25		0.2	0.44 [0.09, 2.05]

Test for heterogeneity chi-square=0.00 df=0
Test for overall effect=-1.05 p=0.3

05 Heparinoid (intravenous) vs control					
TOAST 1998	42 / 646	38 / 635		2.0	1.09 [0.69, 1.72]
Subtotal (95% CI)	42 / 646	38 / 635		2.0	1.09 [0.69, 1.72]

Test for heterogeneity chi-square=0.00 df=0
Test for overall effect=0.38 p=0.7

06 Oral anticoagulant vs control					
Marshall 1960	8 / 26	7 / 25		0.3	1.14 [0.35, 3.76]
Subtotal (95% CI)	8 / 26	7 / 25		0.3	1.14 [0.35, 3.76]

Test for heterogeneity chi-square=0.00 df=0
Test for overall effect=0.21 p=0.8

Total (95% CI)	2451 / 11480	2279 / 11090		100.0	1.05 [0.98, 1.12]

Test for heterogeneity chi-square=11.31 df=8 p=0.1846
Test for overall effect=1.35 p=0.18

.2   .5   1   2   5

Favours treatment   Favours control

Figure 9.2   Forest plot showing the effects of *any anticoagulant vs control* in acute ischaemic stroke on *death at the end of follow-up.* Reproduced from Gubitz *et al.* (2004), with permission from the authors and John Wiley & Sons Limited. Copyright Cochrane Library, reproduced with permission.

Pre-specified sensitivity analyses showed that the overall result for death (OR: 1.05, 95% CI: 0.98–1.12) was consistent if:

- the different types of anticoagulant were used (Fig. 9.2);
- patients had a CT head scan before randomisation (OR: 1.06, 95% CI: 0.84–1.34), or after randomisation or not at all (OR: 1.04, 95% CI: 0.98–1.12);

- patients were randomised within 48 h (OR: 1.05, 95% CI: 0.98–1.12), and after 48 h (OR: 0.80, 95% CI: 0.31–2.05);
- data from the IST (1997) were included (OR: 1.05, 95% CI: 0.98–1.12) or excluded (OR: 0.95, 95% CI: 0.77–1.18).

Recurrent stroke

Ischaemic stroke   Eleven trials in 21,605 patients indicated that anticoagulant therapy for acute ischaemic stroke was associated with a statistically significant reduction in recurrent ischaemic stroke (OR: 0.76, 95% CI: 0.65–0.88), from 3.6% (388/10739) with control to 2.7% (300/10866) with anticoagulants, which translated into about nine fewer recurrent ischaemic strokes per 1000 patients treated (95% CI: 4–13 strokes avoided) (Fig. 9.3). The majority of the data (95%) were obtained from one trial (IST, 1997).

Haemorrhagic stroke   Fifteen trials in 22,794 patients indicated that immediate anticoagulant therapy was associated with a statistically significant increase in symptomatic intracranial haemorrhage (ICH) by more than 2-fold (OR: 2.52, 95% CI: 1.92–3.30), from 0.5% (54/11,198) with control to 1.4% (163/11,596) with heparin, which represented an absolute excess of nine ICHs per 1000 patients treated (95% CI: 6–11 per 1000) (Fig. 9.4).

Indirect comparisons of different types of anticoagulant indicated that there was no significant heterogeneity in the number of excess haemorrhages with different types of heparin (Fig. 9.4).

There was a dose-related increase in major ICH in patients treated with anticoagulants in the IST, with an increase in the absolute risk of bleeding from 0.3% to 0.7% to 1.8% for control, low dose (5000 U bid) and medium dose (12,500 U bid) of subcutaneous unfractionated heparin (UFH), respectively (IST, 1997).

There is the possibility of some bias within these data, as there may have been a lower threshold for re-scanning patients who had deteriorated clinically if they were known to be receiving anticoagulants (e.g. in the IST where treatment allocation was not blinded). In addition, even in blinded trials, a clinician is likely to be unblinded if bruising is observed at heparin injection sites. An unbiased assessment of the effect of anticoagulants on the occurrence of ICH would come from systematic studies, in which all patients undergo a CT scan before the beginning of treatment to exclude haemorrhage, and all survivors have a repeat CT scan at the end of the scheduled treatment period, regardless of their clinical status. In such an unbiased assessment, all patients who died during the study would also have to undergo an autopsy. Unfortunately, it has rarely been possible in RCTs to achieve repeat CT scans in all survivors, or autopsies in all deaths. Four trials in the Cochrane Review made a systematic attempt to detect both symptomatic and asymptomatic ICH in this way

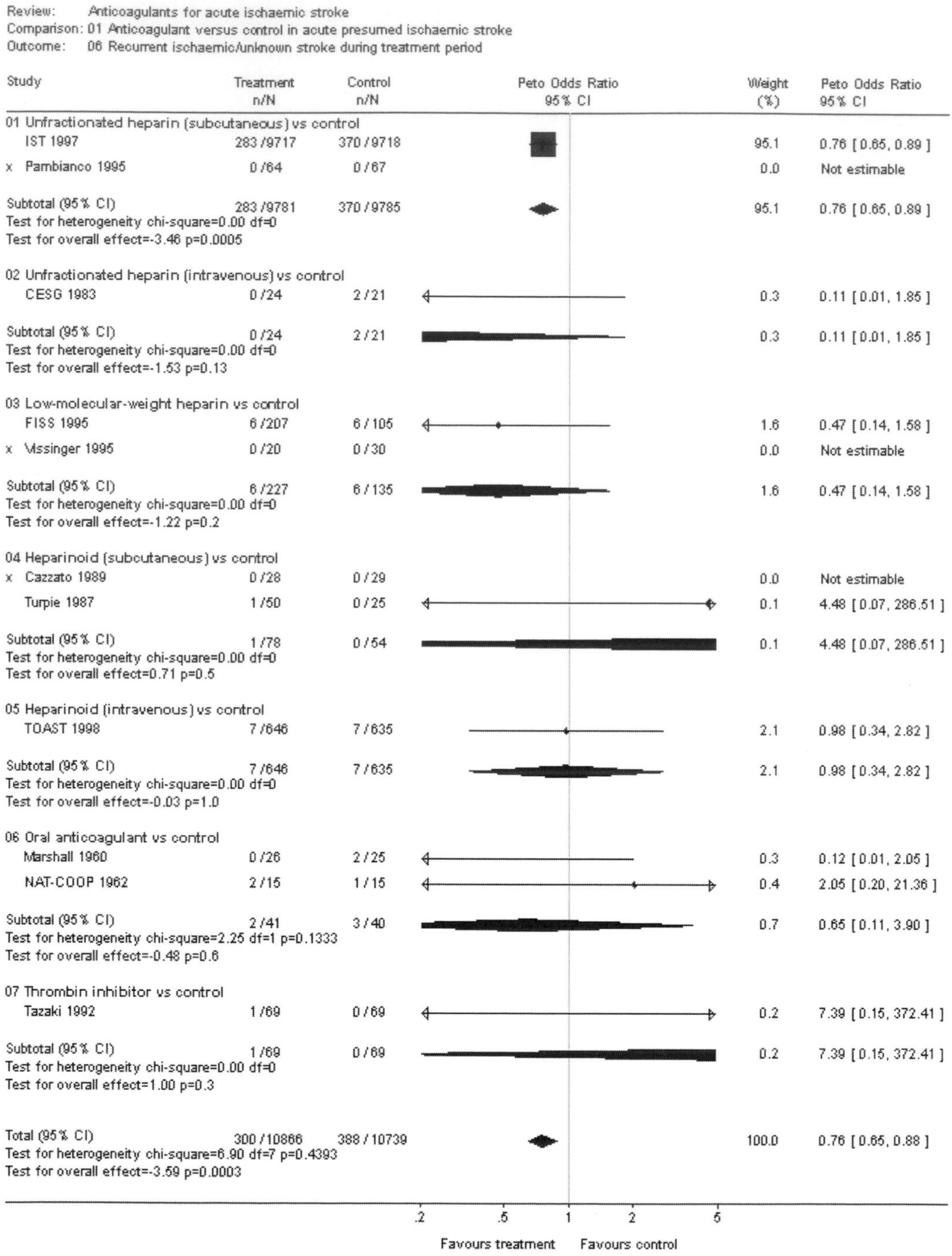

Review: Anticoagulants for acute ischaemic stroke
Comparison: 01 Anticoagulant versus control in acute presumed ischaemic stroke
Outcome: 06 Recurrent ischaemic/unknown stroke during treatment period

Figure 9.3   Forest plot showing the effects of *any anticoagulant vs control* in acute ischaemic stroke on *recurrent ischaemic/unknown stroke at the end of follow-up*. Reproduced from Gubitz *et al.* (2004), with permission from the authors and John Wiley & Sons Limited. Copyright Cochrane Library, reproduced with permission.

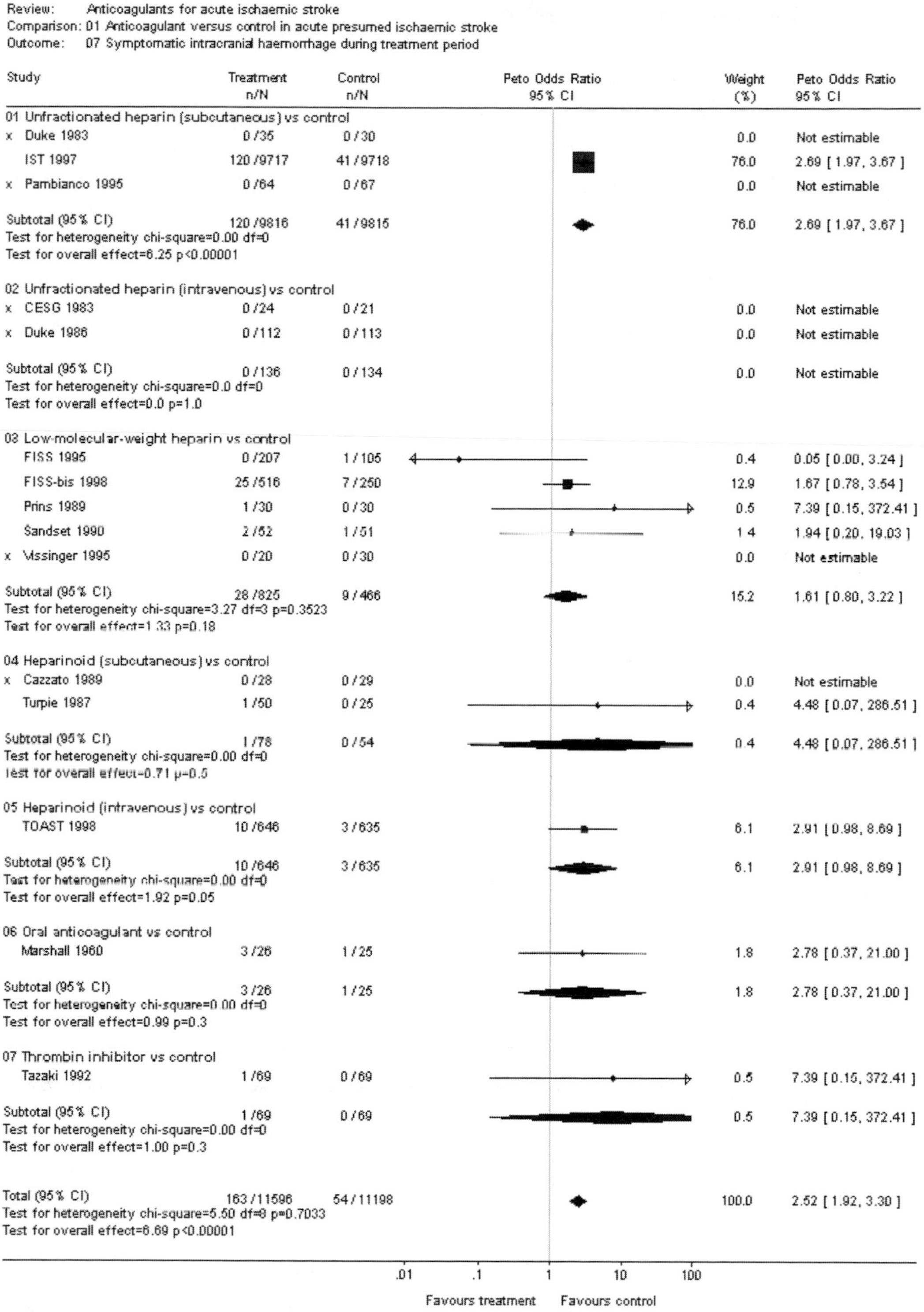

Review: Anticoagulants for acute ischaemic stroke
Comparison: 01 Anticoagulant versus control in acute presumed ischaemic stroke
Outcome: 07 Symptomatic intracranial haemorrhage during treatment period

Study	Treatment n/N	Control n/N	Peto Odds Ratio 95% CI	Weight (%)	Peto Odds Ratio 95% CI
01 Unfractionated heparin (subcutaneous) vs control					
x Duke 1983	0 /35	0 /30		0.0	Not estimable
IST 1997	120 /9717	41 /9718		76.0	2.69 [1.97, 3.67]
x Pambianco 1995	0 /64	0 /67		0.0	Not estimable
Subtotal (95% CI)	120 /9816	41 /9815		76.0	2.69 [1.97, 3.67]
Test for heterogeneity chi-square=0.00 df=0					
Test for overall effect=6.25 p<0.00001					
02 Unfractionated heparin (intravenous) vs control					
x CESG 1983	0 /24	0 /21		0.0	Not estimable
x Duke 1986	0 /112	0 /113		0.0	Not estimable
Subtotal (95% CI)	0 /136	0 /134		0.0	Not estimable
Test for heterogeneity chi-square=0.0 df=0					
Test for overall effect=0.0 p=1.0					
03 Low-molecular-weight heparin vs control					
FISS 1995	0 /207	1 /105		0.4	0.05 [0.00, 3.24]
FISS-bis 1998	25 /516	7 /250		12.9	1.67 [0.78, 3.54]
Prins 1989	1 /30	0 /30		0.5	7.39 [0.15, 372.41]
Sandset 1990	2 /52	1 /51		1.4	1.94 [0.20, 19.03]
x Vissinger 1995	0 /20	0 /30		0.0	Not estimable
Subtotal (95% CI)	28 /825	9 /466		15.2	1.61 [0.80, 3.22]
Test for heterogeneity chi-square=3.27 df=3 p=0.3523					
Test for overall effect=1.33 p=0.18					
04 Heparinoid (subcutaneous) vs control					
x Cazzato 1989	0 /28	0 /29		0.0	Not estimable
Turpie 1987	1 /50	0 /25		0.4	4.48 [0.07, 286.51]
Subtotal (95% CI)	1 /78	0 /54		0.4	4.48 [0.07, 286.51]
Test for heterogeneity chi-square=0.00 df=0					
Test for overall effect=0.71 p=0.5					
05 Heparinoid (intravenous) vs control					
TOAST 1998	10 /646	3 /635		6.1	2.91 [0.98, 8.69]
Subtotal (95% CI)	10 /646	3 /635		6.1	2.91 [0.98, 8.69]
Test for heterogeneity chi-square=0.00 df=0					
Test for overall effect=1.92 p=0.05					
06 Oral anticoagulant vs control					
Marshall 1960	3 /26	1 /25		1.8	2.78 [0.37, 21.00]
Subtotal (95% CI)	3 /26	1 /25		1.8	2.78 [0.37, 21.00]
Test for heterogeneity chi-square=0.00 df=0					
Test for overall effect=0.99 p=0.3					
07 Thrombin inhibitor vs control					
Tazaki 1992	1 /69	0 /69		0.5	7.39 [0.15, 372.41]
Subtotal (95% CI)	1 /69	0 /69		0.5	7.39 [0.15, 372.41]
Test for heterogeneity chi-square=0.00 df=0					
Test for overall effect=1.00 p=0.3					
Total (95% CI)	163 /11596	54 /11198		100.0	2.52 [1.92, 3.30]
Test for heterogeneity chi-square=5.50 df=8 p=0.7033					
Test for overall effect=6.69 p<0.00001					

.01 .1 1 10 100

Favours treatment   Favours control

Figure 9.4   Forest plot showing the effects of *any anticoagulant vs control* in acute ischaemic stroke on *symptomatic ICH at the end of follow-up*. Reproduced from Gubitz *et al.* (2004), with permission from the authors and John Wiley & Sons Limited. Copyright Cochrane Library, reproduced with permission.

(CESG, 1983; Prins, 1989; Sandset, 1990; FISS, 1995). The numbers of patients and events in these trials was small (symptomatic plus asymptomatic haemorrhages occuring in 20/266 (7.5%) patients allocated anticoagulant vs 27/264 (10.2%) patients allocated control. The estimate of risk of 'symptomatic plus asymptomatic' haemorrhage in these few small trials of anticoagulation with control is imprecise and inconclusive (OR: 0.76, 95% CI: 0.38–1.52).

Recurrent stroke of any type   Eleven RCTs involving 22,605 patients indicated that anticoagulation was not associated with a net reduction in the odds of recurrent stroke of any pathological type (OR: 0.97, 95% CI: 0.85–1.11) (Fig. 9.5). The majority of the data (93.6%) were obtained from one trial (IST, 1997).

An analysis of only fatal recurrent strokes or ICHs during the treatment period similarly demonstrated no net benefit from anticoagulants (OR: 0.98, 95% CI: 0.75–1.27).

Major extracranial haemorrhage (ECH)

Sixteen trials included data from 22,049 randomised patients (94.1% of patients included in the overall review) in whom data on major extracranial haemorrhage (defined as bleeding serious enough to cause death or require hospitalisation or transfusion) were recorded. Anticoagulation was associated with a significant 3-fold increase in major extracranial haemorrhage (OR: 2.99, 95% CI: 2.24–3.99), from 0.4% (42/10927) with control to 1.3% (143/11122) with anticoagulation, or about nine additional major extracranial haemorrhages per 1000 patients treated (95% CI: 7–12 additional haemorrhages) (Fig. 9.6).

There was a dose-related increase in major extracranial haemorrhage in patients treated with anticoagulant, with an increase in the absolute risk of bleeding from 0.3% to 0.4% to 1.4% for control, low dose (5000 U bid), and medium dose (12,500 U bid) of subcutaneous UFH, respectively (IST, 1997).

Deep vein thrombosis (DVT)

Ten RCTs contained data from 916 randomised patients (only 3.9% of patients included in the overall review) in whom the effect of anticoagulants on the occurrence of 'symptomatic or asymptomatic DVT' at the end of the treatment period was sought by:
  (i) I-125 fibrinogen scanning (Pince, 1981; Duke, 1983; McCarthy, 1986; Turpie, 1987; Prins, 1989; Elias, 1990; McCarthy, 1977);
 (ii) B mode and Doppler ultrasound (Pambianco, 1995);
(iii) X-ray contrast venography (Sandset, 1990; Vissinger, 1995).

Despite the small numbers of patients studied, it is possible to conclude reliably that anticoagulation was associated with a highly significant reduction in the odds of DVT (OR: 0.21, 95% CI: 0.15–0.29), from 44.3% (204/460) with control to 15.1% (69/456)

Review: Anticoagulants for acute ischaemic stroke
Comparison: 01 Anticoagulant versus control in acute presumed ischaemic stroke
Outcome: 08 Any recurrent stroke or symptomatic intracranial haemorrhage during treatment period or follow-up (> 1 month)

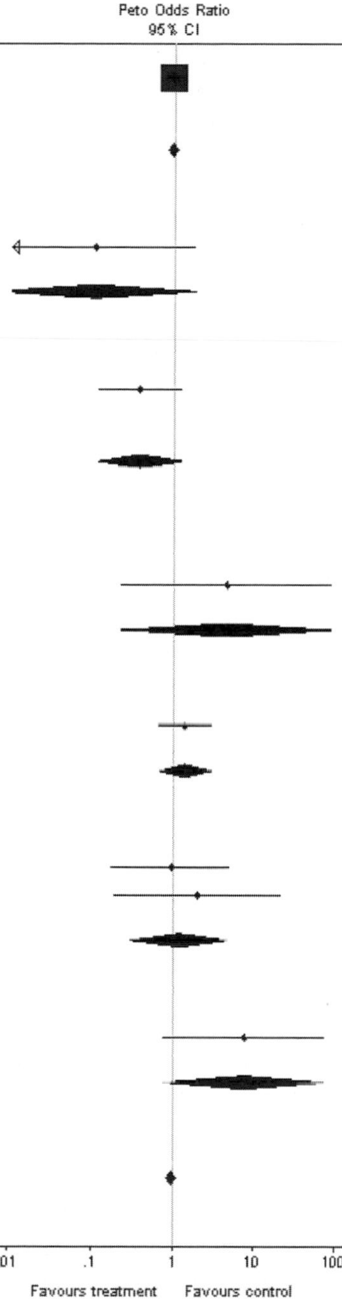

Figure 9.5 Forest plot showing the effects of *any anticoagulant vs control* in acute ischaemic stroke on *recurrent stroke of any type at the end of follow-up.* Reproduced from Gubitz *et al.* (2004), with permission from the authors and John Wiley & Sons Limited. Copyright Cochrane Library, reproduced with permission.

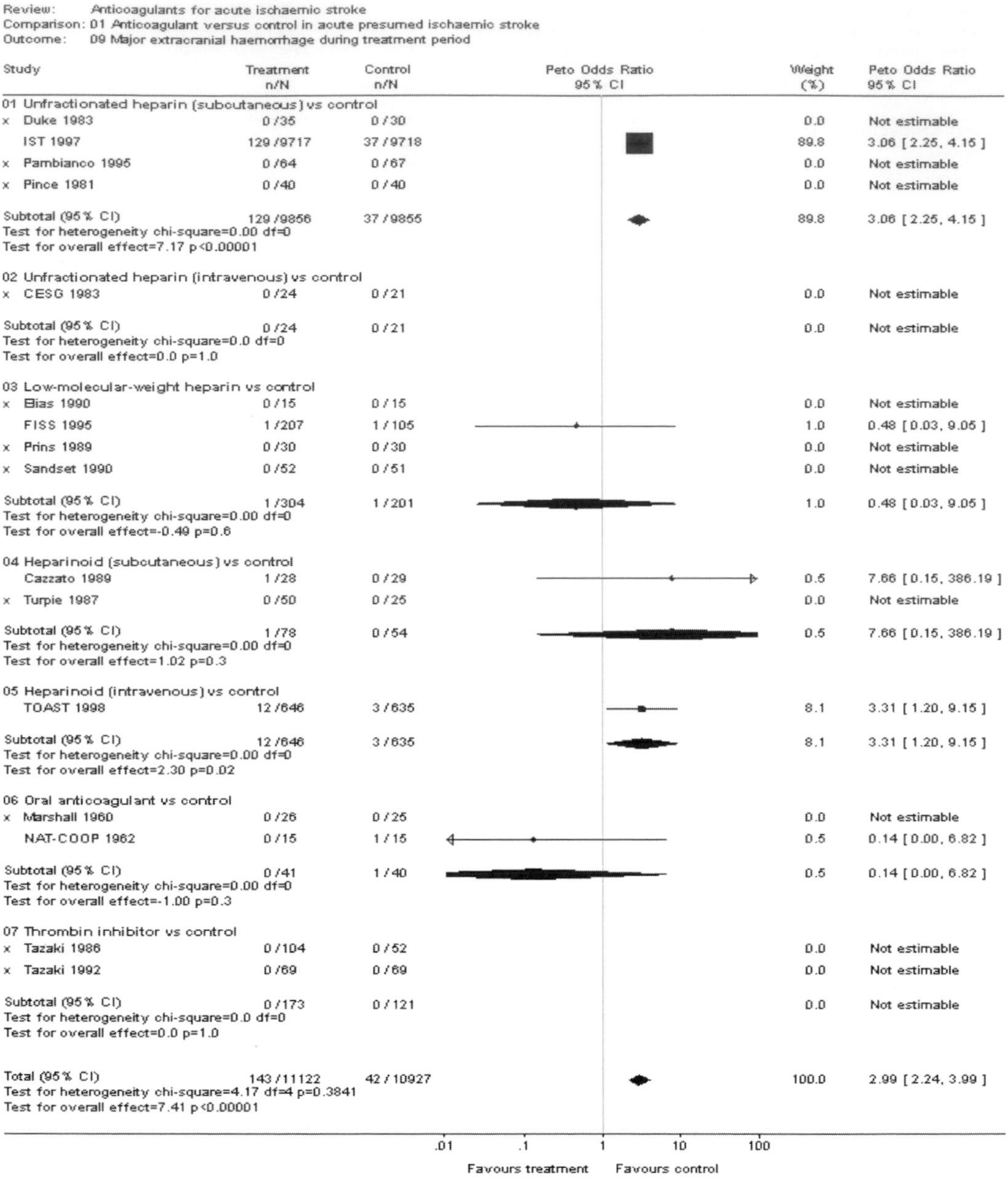

Review: Anticoagulants for acute ischaemic stroke
Comparison: 01 Anticoagulant versus control in acute presumed ischaemic stroke
Outcome: 09 Major extracranial haemorrhage during treatment period

Study	Treatment n/N	Control n/N	Peto Odds Ratio 95% CI	Weight (%)	Peto Odds Ratio 95% CI
01 Unfractionated heparin (subcutaneous) vs control					
x Duke 1983	0/35	0/30		0.0	Not estimable
IST 1997	129/9717	37/9718		89.8	3.06 [2.25, 4.15]
x Pambianco 1995	0/64	0/67		0.0	Not estimable
x Pince 1981	0/40	0/40		0.0	Not estimable
Subtotal (95% CI)	129/9856	37/9855		89.8	3.06 [2.25, 4.15]
Test for heterogeneity chi-square=0.00 df=0					
Test for overall effect=7.17 p<0.00001					
02 Unfractionated heparin (intravenous) vs control					
x CESG 1983	0/24	0/21		0.0	Not estimable
Subtotal (95% CI)	0/24	0/21		0.0	Not estimable
Test for heterogeneity chi-square=0.0 df=0					
Test for overall effect=0.0 p=1.0					
03 Low-molecular-weight heparin vs control					
x Bias 1990	0/15	0/15		0.0	Not estimable
FISS 1995	1/207	1/105		1.0	0.48 [0.03, 9.05]
x Prins 1989	0/30	0/30		0.0	Not estimable
x Sandset 1990	0/52	0/51		0.0	Not estimable
Subtotal (95% CI)	1/304	1/201		1.0	0.48 [0.03, 9.05]
Test for heterogeneity chi-square=0.00 df=0					
Test for overall effect=-0.49 p=0.6					
04 Heparinoid (subcutaneous) vs control					
Cazzato 1989	1/28	0/29		0.5	7.66 [0.15, 386.19]
x Turpie 1987	0/50	0/25		0.0	Not estimable
Subtotal (95% CI)	1/78	0/54		0.5	7.66 [0.15, 386.19]
Test for heterogeneity chi-square=0.00 df=0					
Test for overall effect=1.02 p=0.3					
05 Heparinoid (intravenous) vs control					
TOAST 1998	12/646	3/635		8.1	3.31 [1.20, 9.15]
Subtotal (95% CI)	12/646	3/635		8.1	3.31 [1.20, 9.15]
Test for heterogeneity chi-square=0.00 df=0					
Test for overall effect=2.30 p=0.02					
06 Oral anticoagulant vs control					
x Marshall 1960	0/26	0/25		0.0	Not estimable
NAT-COOP 1962	0/15	1/15		0.5	0.14 [0.00, 6.82]
Subtotal (95% CI)	0/41	1/40		0.5	0.14 [0.00, 6.82]
Test for heterogeneity chi-square=0.00 df=0					
Test for overall effect=-1.00 p=0.3					
07 Thrombin inhibitor vs control					
x Tazaki 1986	0/104	0/52		0.0	Not estimable
x Tazaki 1992	0/69	0/69		0.0	Not estimable
Subtotal (95% CI)	0/173	0/121		0.0	Not estimable
Test for heterogeneity chi-square=0.0 df=0					
Test for overall effect=0.0 p=1.0					
Total (95% CI)	143/11122	42/10927		100.0	2.99 [2.24, 3.99]
Test for heterogeneity chi-square=4.17 df=4 p=0.3841					
Test for overall effect=7.41 p<0.00001					

.01   .1   1   10   100

Favours treatment   Favours control

Figure 9.6   Forest plot showing the effects of *any anticoagulant vs control* in acute ischaemic stroke on *major extracranial haemorrhage during the treatment period.* Reproduced from Gubitz *et al.* (2004), with permission from the authors and John Wiley & Sons Limited. Copyright Cochrane Library, reproduced with permission.

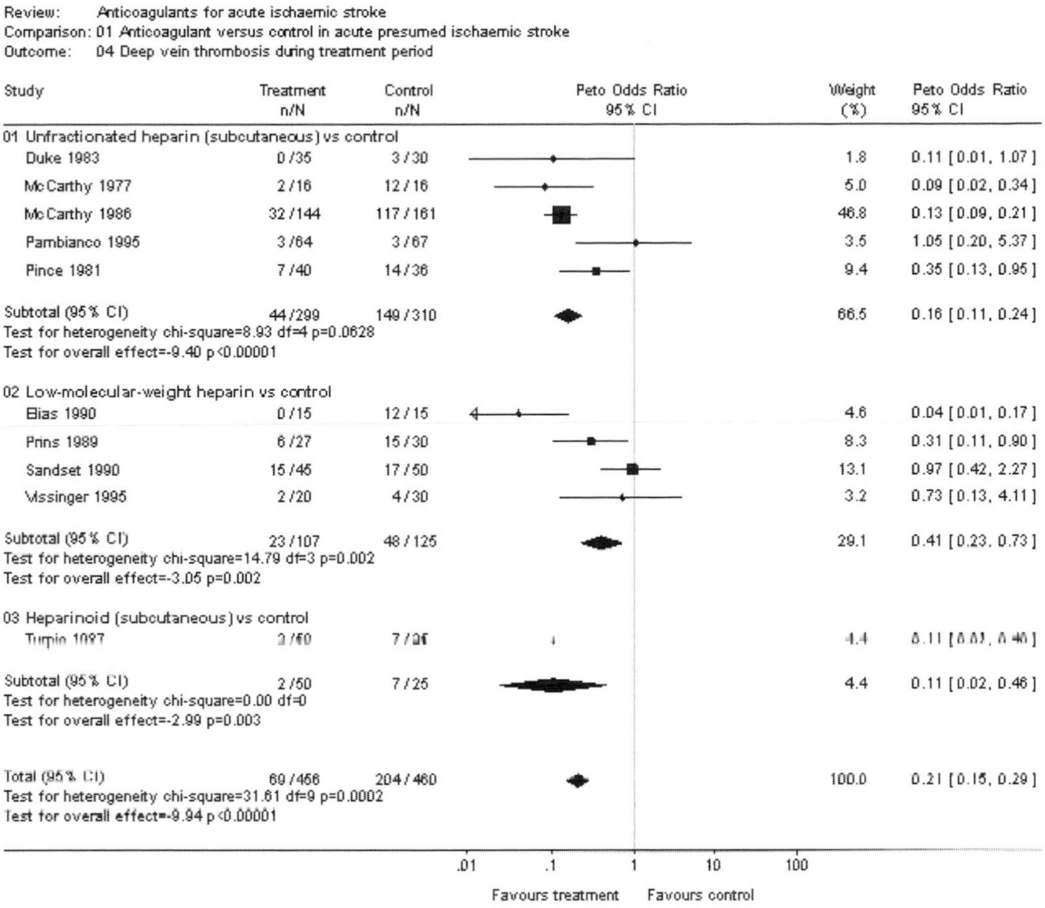

Review: Anticoagulants for acute ischaemic stroke
Comparison: 01 Anticoagulant versus control in acute presumed ischaemic stroke
Outcome: 04 Deep vein thrombosis during treatment period

Study	Treatment n/N	Control n/N	Peto Odds Ratio 95% CI	Weight (%)	Peto Odds Ratio 95% CI
01 Unfractionated heparin (subcutaneous) vs control					
Duke 1983	0 /35	3 /30		1.8	0.11 [0.01, 1.07]
McCarthy 1977	2 /16	12 /16		5.0	0.09 [0.02, 0.34]
McCarthy 1986	32 /144	117 /161		46.8	0.13 [0.09, 0.21]
Pambianco 1995	3 /64	3 /67		3.5	1.05 [0.20, 5.37]
Pince 1981	7 /40	14 /36		9.4	0.35 [0.13, 0.95]
Subtotal (95% CI)	44 /299	149 /310		66.5	0.16 [0.11, 0.24]
Test for heterogeneity chi-square=8.93 df=4 p=0.0628					
Test for overall effect=-9.40 p<0.00001					
02 Low-molecular-weight heparin vs control					
Elias 1990	0 /15	12 /15		4.6	0.04 [0.01, 0.17]
Prins 1989	6 /27	15 /30		8.3	0.31 [0.11, 0.90]
Sandset 1990	15 /46	17 /50		13.1	0.97 [0.42, 2.27]
Vissinger 1995	2 /20	4 /30		3.2	0.73 [0.13, 4.11]
Subtotal (95% CI)	23 /107	48 /125		29.1	0.41 [0.23, 0.73]
Test for heterogeneity chi-square=14.79 df=3 p=0.002					
Test for overall effect=-3.05 p=0.002					
03 Heparinoid (subcutaneous) vs control					
Turpie 1987	2 /50	7 /25		4.4	0.11 [0.02, 0.46]
Subtotal (95% CI)	2 /50	7 /25		4.4	0.11 [0.02, 0.46]
Test for heterogeneity chi-square=0.00 df=0					
Test for overall effect=-2.99 p=0.003					
Total (95% CI)	69 /456	204 /460		100.0	0.21 [0.16, 0.29]
Test for heterogeneity chi-square=31.61 df=9 p=0.0002					
Test for overall effect=-9.94 p<0.00001					

.01   .1   1   10   100

Favours treatment   Favours control

Figure 9.7   Forest plot showing the effects of *any anticoagulant vs control* in acute ischaemic stroke on *DVT during the treatment period.* Reproduced from Gubitz *et al.* (2004), with permission from the authors and John Wiley & Sons Limited. Copyright Cochrane Library, reproduced with permission.

with anticoagulation (Fig. 9.7). This result was equivalent to the prevention of DVT in about 281 patients for every 1000 patients treated (95% CI: 230–332 DVTs prevented). However, the majority of DVTs detected were subclinical and asymptomatic (Fig. 9.7).

There was significant heterogeneity in the results of the trials (Chi-square 31.61 (d.f. = 9), $P = 0.0002$). This appeared to be related to three trials which did not show any clear effect of anticoagulation on the odds of DVT (Sandset, 1990; Pambianco, 1995; Vissinger, 1995), and two trials which did (McCarthy, 1986; Elias, 1990). The three negative trials were the only trials which did not use I-125 fibrinogen scanning. One used ultrasound assessment (Pambianco, 1995); the other two used venography (Sandset, 1990; Vissinger, 1995).

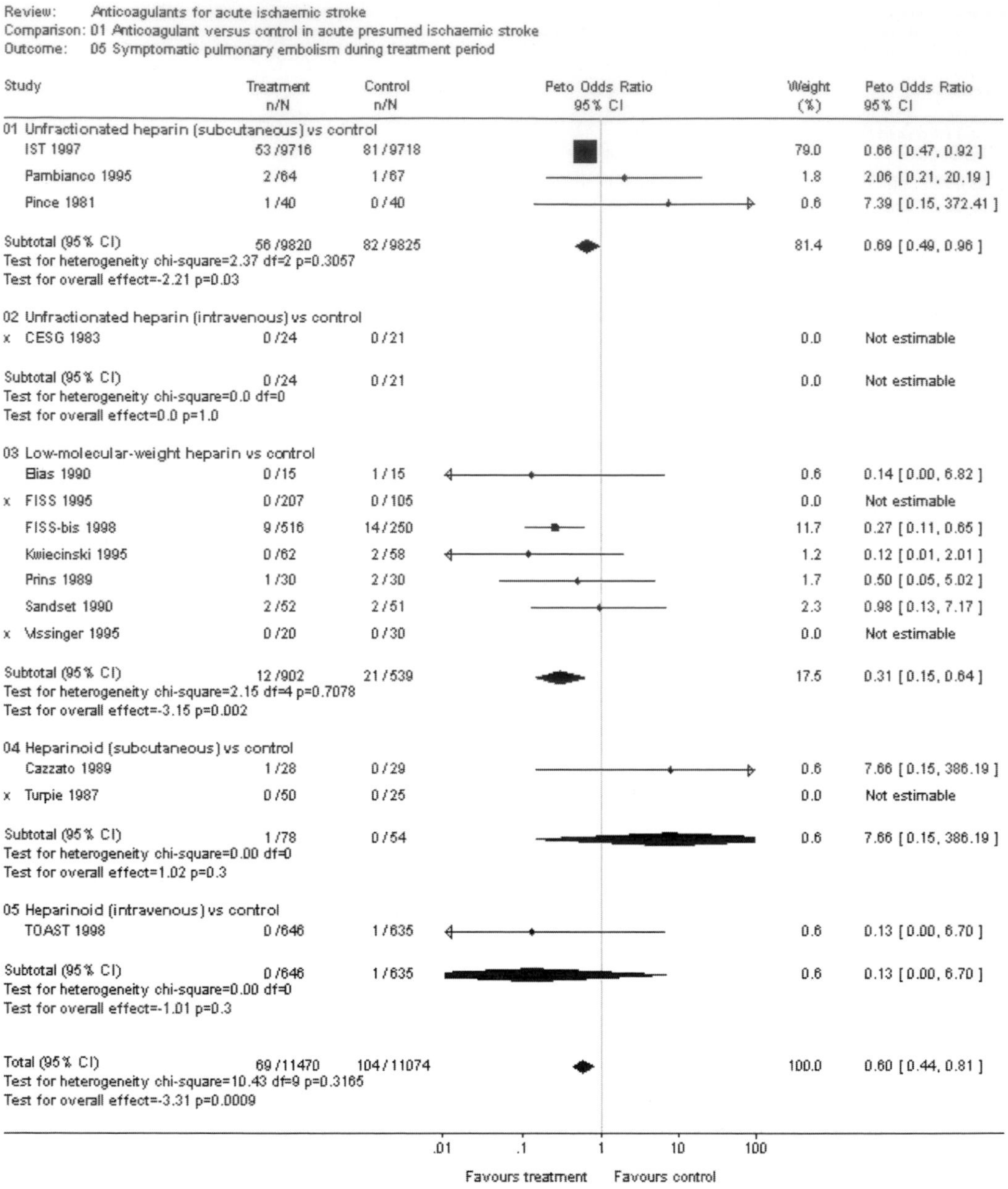

Review: Anticoagulants for acute ischaemic stroke
Comparison: 01 Anticoagulant versus control in acute presumed ischaemic stroke
Outcome: 05 Symptomatic pulmonary embolism during treatment period

Study	Treatment n/N	Control n/N	Peto Odds Ratio 95% CI	Weight (%)	Peto Odds Ratio 95% CI
01 Unfractionated heparin (subcutaneous) vs control					
IST 1997	53 /9716	81 /9718		79.0	0.66 [0.47, 0.92]
Pambianco 1995	2 /64	1 /67		1.8	2.06 [0.21, 20.19]
Pince 1981	1 /40	0 /40		0.6	7.39 [0.15, 372.41]
Subtotal (95% CI)	56 /9820	82 /9825		81.4	0.69 [0.49, 0.96]
Test for heterogeneity chi-square=2.37 df=2 p=0.3057					
Test for overall effect=-2.21 p=0.03					
02 Unfractionated heparin (intravenous) vs control					
x CESG 1983	0 /24	0 /21		0.0	Not estimable
Subtotal (95% CI)	0 /24	0 /21		0.0	Not estimable
Test for heterogeneity chi-square=0.0 df=0					
Test for overall effect=0.0 p=1.0					
03 Low-molecular-weight heparin vs control					
Elias 1990	0 /15	1 /15		0.6	0.14 [0.00, 6.82]
x FISS 1995	0 /207	0 /105		0.0	Not estimable
FISS-bis 1998	9 /516	14 /250		11.7	0.27 [0.11, 0.65]
Kwiecinski 1995	0 /62	2 /58		1.2	0.12 [0.01, 2.01]
Prins 1989	1 /30	2 /30		1.7	0.50 [0.05, 5.02]
Sandset 1990	2 /52	2 /51		2.3	0.98 [0.13, 7.17]
x Vissinger 1995	0 /20	0 /30		0.0	Not estimable
Subtotal (95% CI)	12 /902	21 /539		17.5	0.31 [0.15, 0.64]
Test for heterogeneity chi-square=2.15 df=4 p=0.7078					
Test for overall effect=-3.15 p=0.002					
04 Heparinoid (subcutaneous) vs control					
Cazzato 1989	1 /28	0 /29		0.6	7.66 [0.15, 386.19]
x Turpie 1987	0 /50	0 /25		0.0	Not estimable
Subtotal (95% CI)	1 /78	0 /54		0.6	7.66 [0.15, 386.19]
Test for heterogeneity chi-square=0.00 df=0					
Test for overall effect=1.02 p=0.3					
05 Heparinoid (intravenous) vs control					
TOAST 1998	0 /646	1 /635		0.6	0.13 [0.00, 6.70]
Subtotal (95% CI)	0 /646	1 /635		0.6	0.13 [0.00, 6.70]
Test for heterogeneity chi-square=0.00 df=0					
Test for overall effect=-1.01 p=0.3					
Total (95% CI)	69 /11470	104 /11074		100.0	0.60 [0.44, 0.81]
Test for heterogeneity chi-square=10.43 df=9 p=0.3165					
Test for overall effect=-3.31 p=0.0009					

.01   .1   1   10   100

Favours treatment   Favours control

Figure 9.8   Forest plot showing the effects of *any anticoagulant vs control* in acute ischaemic stroke on *symptomatic PE during the treatment period*. Reproduced from Gubitz *et al.* (2004), with permission from the authors and John Wiley & Sons Limited. Copyright Cochrane Library, reproduced with permission.

Symptomatic pulmonary embolism (PE)

Thirteen RCTs included data from 22,454 patients (95.8% of patients included in the overall review) in which fatal and non-fatal symptomatic PE were reported, but no

Table 9.1. Summary of the effects of anticoagulation vs control in acute ischaemic stroke.

Outcome	OR	95% CI	Absolute risk difference	95% CI
Death or dependency	0.99	0.93 to 1.04	Not significantly different	
Death	1.05	0.98 to 1.12	Not significantly different	
Recurrent ischaemic stroke	0.76	0.65 to 0.88	−0.9%	−0.4 to −1.3%
Symptomatic ICH (dose related)	2.52	1.92 to 3.30	+0.9%	+0.6 to +1.1%
Recurrent stroke of any type	0.97	0.85 to 1.11	Not significantly different	
Major ECH (dose related)	2.99	2.24 to 3.99	+0.9%	+0.7 to +1.2%
DVT (most asymptomatic)	0.21	0.15 to 0.29	−28.1%	−23.0% to −33.2%
PE	0.60	0.44 to 0.81	−0.4%	−0.1 to −0.6%

ECH: extracranial haemorrhage.

trial systematically sought asymptomatic PE by performing ventilation–perfusion scans in all patients at the end of the treatment period.

Anticoagulation was associated with a significant reduction in the odds of symptomatic PE (OR: 0.60, 95% CI: 0.44–0.81), from 1.0% (104/11,074) with control to 0.6% (69/11,470) with anticoagulants, which translated into about four pulmonary emboli avoided for every 1000 patients treated with anticoagulants (95% CI: one to six pulmonary emboli avoided), although this is likely to be an underestimate of the reduction in risk due to incomplete ascertainment of PE (Fig. 9.8).

Comment

Interpretation of the evidence
The data from RCTs indicate that routine immediate anticoagulation (with UFH, LMWH, heparinoid or a thrombin inhibitor) does not provide any net short- or long-term reduction in death or disability (Table 9.1).

In addition, the small amounts of (randomised) subgroup data evaluated do not provide any evidence to support the routine use of anticoagulants in any specific category of stroke patient, including those with: cardioembolic stroke, 'stroke in progression', vertebrobasilar territory stroke or following thrombolysis for acute ischaemic stroke to prevent re-thrombosis of the treated cerebral artery.

Although immediate anticoagulation leads to fewer recurrent ischaemic strokes, avoiding nine ischaemic strokes per 1000 patients treated (OR: 0.76, 95% CI: 0.65–0.88), it is also associated with a similar-sized additional nine symptomatic ICHs per 1000 patients treated (OR: 2.52, 95% CI: 1.92–3.30). The net result is no short- or long-term benefit in terms of preventing recurrent stroke.

There is a dose-dependent increase in both intra- and extracranial haemorrhage with heparins.

Immediate anticoagulation was associated with a highly significant 79% reduction in the odds of DVT during the treatment period, similar to that seen with the use of prophylactic heparin in patients undergoing different types of surgery. In absolute terms, the reduction in DVT with acute anticoagulation was substantial, with 281 DVT prevented per 1000 patients treated. However, most of these DVT were asymptomatic, and so their detection or prevention is of uncertain clinical relevance (i.e. it is symptomatic pulmonary emboli which are important to prevent).

The risk of symptomatic PE was reduced significantly with the use of anticoagulants (OR: 0.60, CI: 0.44–0.81). The absolute benefit was an additional four pulmonary emboli avoided per 1000 patients treated with anticoagulants. As the overall risk of symptomatic PE was low, and the absolute benefit small, the apparent reduction in DVT may have little clinical relevance if there is not a correspondingly large reduction in PE. However, there may well have been under-ascertainment of PE in all of the trials, since pulmonary emboli were not sought systematically. In addition, DVT can lead to morbidity (e.g. post-phlebitic leg and varicose ulcers), but data on these outcomes were not available from the trials. Nevertheless, although anticoagulations avoided at least 4 PE per 1000 patients treated (OR: 0.60, CI: 0.44–0.81) this benefit was offset by an extra nine major extracranial haemorrhages for every 1000 patients treated (OR: 2.99, 95% CI: 2.24–3.99).

Implications for practice

The data do not support the routine unselective use of immediate high-dose intravenous or subcutaneous anticoagulants in any form, including LMWHs and heparinoids, for any category of patient with acute ischaemic stroke. This is because the benefits of UFH, LMWHs and heparinoids in lowering the risk of arterial and venous thromboembolism are offset by a similar-sized risk of symptomatic ICH and ECH.

For patients at high risk of deep venous thrombosis, low-dose subcutaneous heparin may be worthwhile because it prevents DVT, but there is a small and definite increased risk of major haemorrhage. It may therefore be advisable to consider safer alternatives in immobile patients, such as aspirin, compression stockings, rehydration and early mobilisation (see Chapter 4).

Despite the lack of supporting data, anticoagulants are still given frequently, at least by North American neurologists (Al-Sadat et al., 2002). Clinicians who feel compelled to use immediate anticoagulants for specific categories of patients following acute ischaemic stroke should weigh any potential theoretical benefits with the risk of bleeding.

Implications for research

Further large-scale trials comparing immediate anticoagulation with control in patients with acute ischaemic stroke are probably not warranted unless they focus on patients with a specific aetiological subtype of ischaemic stroke or a particular intervention such as low-dose heparin combined with an antiplatelet agent (e.g. aspirin or clopidogrel).

The optimum antithrombotic regimen for the prevention of DVT and PE in stroke patients remains uncertain. Aspirin alone, fixed low-dose subcutaneous heparin, the combination of the two or the use of compression stockings are all promising possibilities. A very large-scale randomised trial with several tens of thousands of patients would be required to determine which has the most favourable balance of risk and benefit on overall clinical outcome.

LMWHs or heparinoids vs standard UFH for acute ischaemic stroke

Evidence

A systematic review identified five RCTs which direct compared the effects of LMWHs or heparinoids with those of standard UFH in a total of 705 patients with acute ischaemic stroke (Counsell and Sandercock, 2002; Sandercock *et al.*, 2005). Four trials compared a heparinoid (danaparoid), and one compared a LMWH (enoxaparin), with standard UFH.

Death

Overall, 72/414 (17.4%) of the patients allocated danaparoid or enoxaparin died during the scheduled follow-up period compared with 56/291 (19.2%) of those allocated UFH (OR: 0.94, 95% CI: 0.63–1.41) (Fig. 9.9).

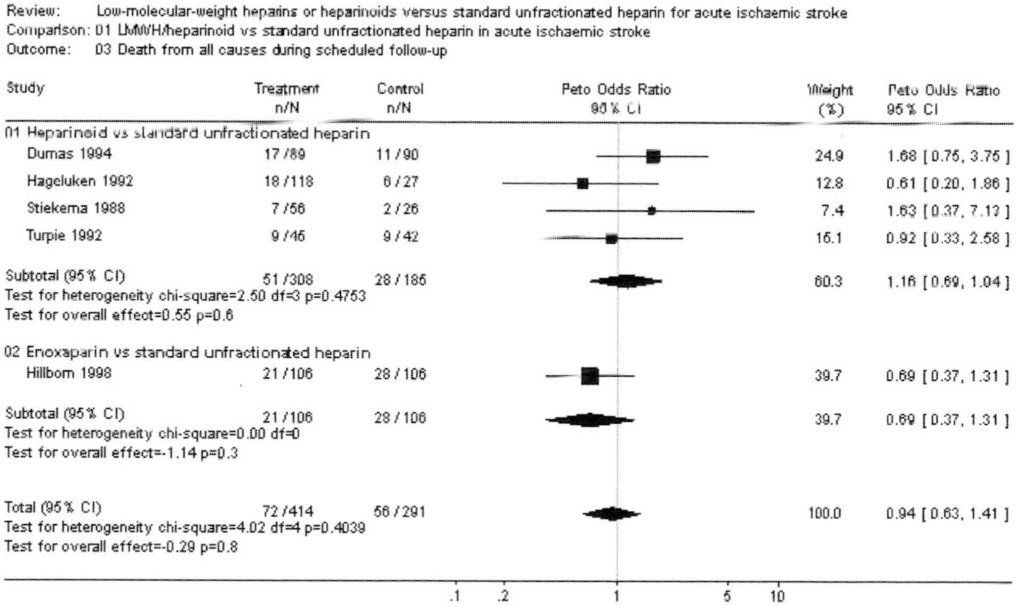

Review: Low-molecular-weight heparins or heparinoids versus standard unfractionated heparin for acute ischaemic stroke
Comparison: 01 LMWH/heparinoid vs standard unfractionated heparin in acute ischaemic stroke
Outcome: 03 Death from all causes during scheduled follow-up

Study	Treatment n/N	Control n/N	Peto Odds Ratio 95% CI	Weight (%)	Peto Odds Ratio 95% CI
01 Heparinoid vs standard unfractionated heparin					
Dumas 1994	17 /89	11 /90		24.9	1.68 [0.75, 3.75]
Hageluken 1992	18 /118	6 /27		12.8	0.61 [0.20, 1.86]
Stiekema 1988	7 /56	2 /26		7.4	1.63 [0.37, 7.12]
Turpie 1992	9 /46	9 /42		16.1	0.92 [0.33, 2.58]
Subtotal (95% CI)	51 /308	28 /185		60.3	1.16 [0.69, 1.04]
Test for heterogeneity chi-square=2.50 df=3 p=0.4753					
Test for overall effect=0.55 p=0.6					
02 Enoxaparin vs standard unfractionated heparin					
Hillbom 1998	21 /106	28 /106		39.7	0.69 [0.37, 1.31]
Subtotal (95% CI)	21 /106	28 /106		39.7	0.69 [0.37, 1.31]
Test for heterogeneity chi-square=0.00 df=0					
Test for overall effect=-1.14 p=0.3					
Total (95% CI)	72 /414	56 /291		100.0	0.94 [0.63, 1.41]
Test for heterogeneity chi-square=4.02 df=4 p=0.4039					
Test for overall effect=-0.29 p=0.8					

.1   .2   1   5   10

Figure 9.9   Forest plot showing the effects of *LMWH/heparinoid vs standard UFH* in acute ischaemic stroke on *death at the end of follow-up.* Reproduced from Sandercock *et al.* (2005), with permission from the authors and John Wiley & Sons Limited. Copyright Cochrane Library, reproduced with permission.

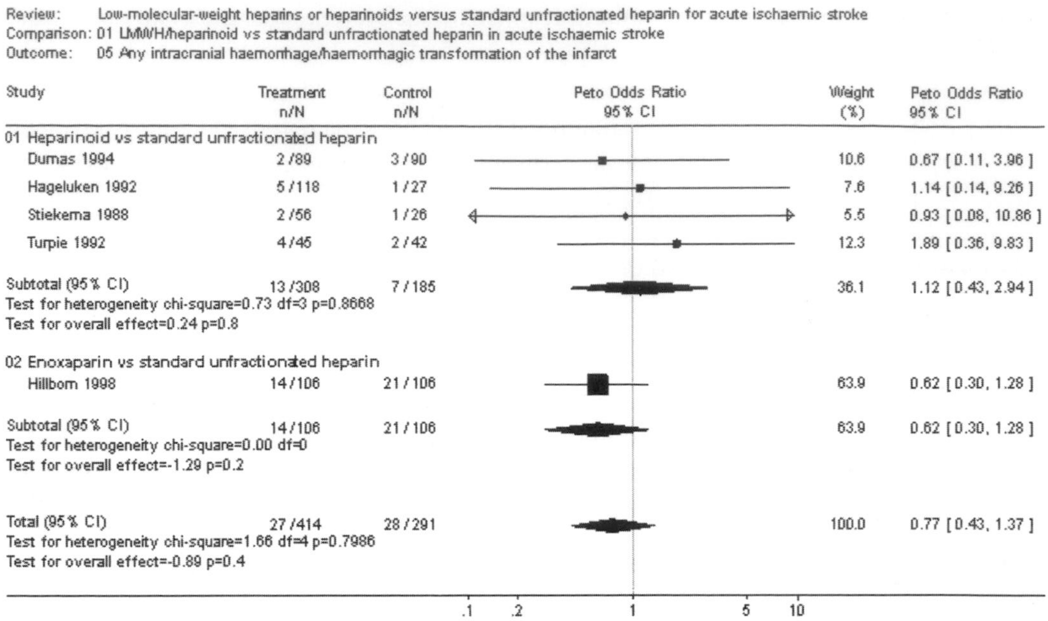

Review: Low-molecular-weight heparins or heparinoids versus standard unfractionated heparin for acute ischaemic stroke
Comparison: 01 LMWH/heparinoid vs standard unfractionated heparin in acute ischaemic stroke
Outcome: 05 Any intracranial haemorrhage/haemorrhagic transformation of the infarct

Study	Treatment n/N	Control n/N	Peto Odds Ratio 95% CI	Weight (%)	Peto Odds Ratio 95% CI
01 Heparinoid vs standard unfractionated heparin					
Dumas 1994	2 / 89	3 / 90		10.6	0.67 [0.11, 3.96]
Hageluken 1992	5 / 118	1 / 27		7.6	1.14 [0.14, 9.26]
Stiekema 1988	2 / 56	1 / 26		5.5	0.93 [0.08, 10.86]
Turpie 1992	4 / 45	2 / 42		12.3	1.89 [0.36, 9.83]
Subtotal (95% CI)	13 / 308	7 / 185		36.1	1.12 [0.43, 2.94]
Test for heterogeneity chi-square=0.73 df=3 p=0.8668					
Test for overall effect=0.24 p=0.8					
02 Enoxaparin vs standard unfractionated heparin					
Hillbom 1998	14 / 106	21 / 106		63.9	0.62 [0.30, 1.28]
Subtotal (95% CI)	14 / 106	21 / 106		63.9	0.62 [0.30, 1.28]
Test for heterogeneity chi-square=0.00 df=0					
Test for overall effect=-1.29 p=0.2					
Total (95% CI)	27 / 414	28 / 291		100.0	0.77 [0.43, 1.37]
Test for heterogeneity chi-square=1.66 df=4 p=0.7986					
Test for overall effect=-0.89 p=0.4					

.1   .2   1   5   10

Figure 9.10 Forest plot showing the effects of *LMWH/heparinoid vs standard UFH* in acute ischaemic stroke on *ICH at the end of follow-up*. Reproduced from Sandercock *et al.* (2005), with permission from the authors and John Wiley & Sons Limited. Copyright Cochrane Library, reproduced with permission.

Intracranial haemorrhage (ICH)

Direct comparisons of the effects of LMWHs or heparinoids with those of UFH showed no overall statistically significant difference in the rate of ICH (OR: 0.77, 95% CI: 0.43–1.37) (Fig. 9.10) (Counsell and Sandercock, 2002; Sandercock *et al.*, 2005). However, there was a non-significant trend towards less symptomatic ICH with enoxaparin compared with subcutaneous UFH in the one trial (OR: 0.62, 95% CI: 0.30–1.28) (Fig. 9.10).

Extracranial haemorrhage

Direct comparisons of the effects of LMWH or heparinoid compared with standard UFH show no significant different in the rate of minor extracranial haemorrhage during the treatment period (OR: 0.91, 95% CI: 0.56–12.48), and a non-significant trend towards an increase in major extracranial haemorrhage with LMWH or heparinoid compared with standard UFH during the treatment period (OR: 5.56, 95% CI: 0.68–45.6) (Counsell and Sandercock, 2002; Sandercock *et al.*, 2005) (Fig. 9.11).

Deep vein thrombosis (DVT)

Direct comparisons of the effects of LMWHs or heparinoids with those of UFH (Counsell and Sandercock, 2004) revealed that 55/414 (13%) patients allocated danaparoid or enoxaparin had DVT compared with 65/291 (22%) of those allocated

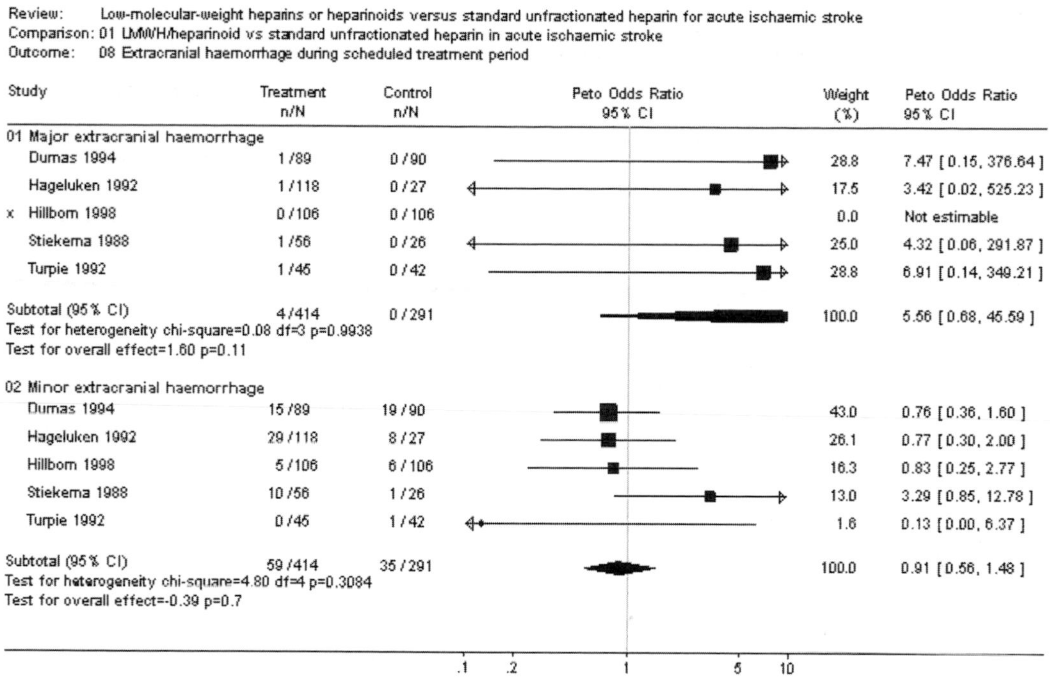

Review: Low-molecular-weight heparins or heparinoids versus standard unfractionated heparin for acute ischaemic stroke
Comparison: 01 LMWH/heparinoid vs standard unfractionated heparin in acute ischaemic stroke
Outcome: 08 Extracranial haemorrhage during scheduled treatment period

Study	Treatment n/N	Control n/N	Peto Odds Ratio 95% CI	Weight (%)	Peto Odds Ratio 95% CI
01 Major extracranial haemorrhage					
Dumas 1994	1/89	0/90		28.8	7.47 [0.15, 376.64]
Hageluken 1992	1/118	0/27		17.5	3.42 [0.02, 525.23]
x Hillbom 1998	0/106	0/106		0.0	Not estimable
Stiekema 1988	1/56	0/26		25.0	4.32 [0.06, 291.87]
Turpie 1992	1/45	0/42		28.8	6.91 [0.14, 349.21]
Subtotal (95% CI)	4/414	0/291		100.0	5.56 [0.68, 45.59]
Test for heterogeneity chi-square=0.08 df=3 p=0.9938					
Test for overall effect=1.60 p=0.11					
02 Minor extracranial haemorrhage					
Dumas 1994	15/89	19/90		43.0	0.76 [0.36, 1.60]
Hageluken 1992	29/118	8/27		26.1	0.77 [0.30, 2.00]
Hillbom 1998	5/106	6/106		16.3	0.83 [0.25, 2.77]
Stiekema 1988	10/56	1/26		13.0	3.29 [0.85, 12.78]
Turpie 1992	0/45	1/42		1.6	0.13 [0.00, 6.37]
Subtotal (95% CI)	59/414	35/291		100.0	0.91 [0.56, 1.48]
Test for heterogeneity chi-square=4.80 df=4 p=0.3084					
Test for overall effect=-0.39 p=0.7					

.1   .2   1   5   10

Figure 9.11   Forest plot showing the effects of *LMWH/heparinoid vs standard UFH* in acute ischaemic stroke on *extracranial haemorrhage during the treatment period*. Reproduced from Sandercock *et al.* (2005), with permission from the authors and John Wiley & Sons Limited. Copyright Cochrane Library, reproduced with permission.

UFH (Counsell and Sandercock, 2002; Sandercock *et al.*, 2005). This reduction was significant (OR: 0.52, 95% CI: 0.35–0.79), suggesting that LMWH or heparinoid decreases the occurrence of DVT compared to standard UFH (Fig. 9.12) (Counsell and Sandercock, 2002; Sandercock *et al.*, 2005).

Comment

Interpretation of the evidence

These data suggest that LMWH or heparinoids are more effective than UFH for preventing DVT. However, the number of major events (death, intra- and extra-cranial haemorrhage, and death) was too small to provide a reliable estimate of more important benefits and risks. No data on recurrent stroke or functional outcome in survivors was available.

Implications for practice

There is no evidence to support the routine use of anticoagulation in patients with acute ischaemic stroke because there is no overall net benefit. For clinicians who still wish to use some form of anticoagulant regimen in selected patients with acute ischaemic stroke, the criteria to identify those few patients who might benefit from

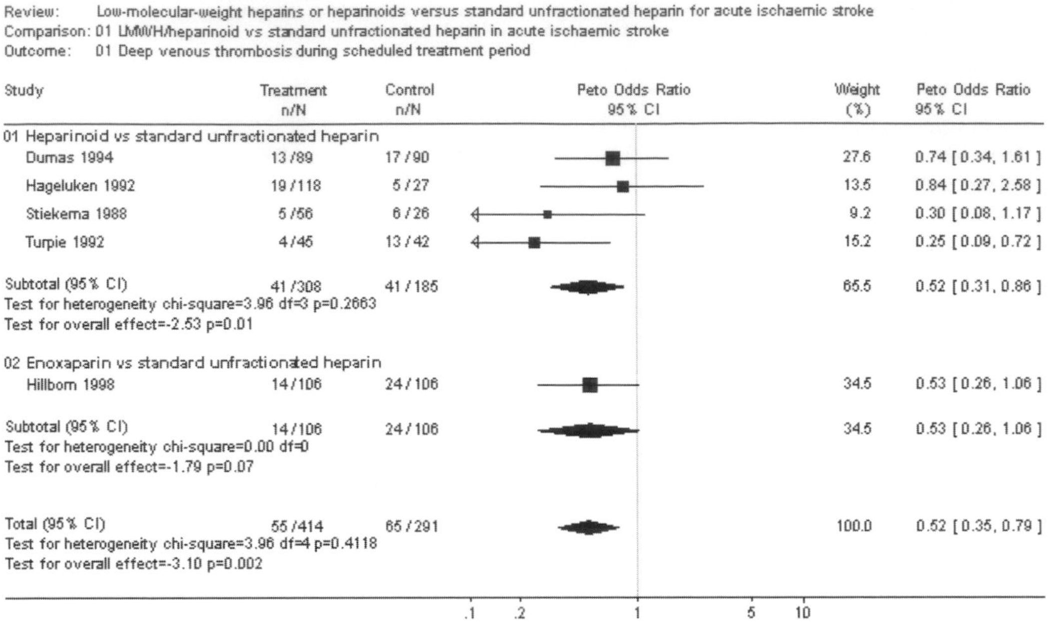

Review: Low-molecular-weight heparins or heparinoids versus standard unfractionated heparin for acute ischaemic stroke
Comparison: 01 LMWH/heparinoid vs standard unfractionated heparin in acute ischaemic stroke
Outcome: 01 Deep venous thrombosis during scheduled treatment period

Study	Treatment n/N	Control n/N	Peto Odds Ratio 95% CI	Weight (%)	Peto Odds Ratio 95% CI
01 Heparinoid vs standard unfractionated heparin					
Dumas 1994	13 /89	17 /90		27.6	0.74 [0.34, 1.61]
Hageluken 1992	19 /118	5 /27		13.5	0.84 [0.27, 2.58]
Stiekema 1988	5 /56	6 /26		9.2	0.30 [0.08, 1.17]
Turpie 1992	4 /45	13 /42		15.2	0.25 [0.09, 0.72]
Subtotal (95% CI)	41 /308	41 /185		65.5	0.52 [0.31, 0.86]
Test for heterogeneity chi-square=3.96 df=3 p=0.2663					
Test for overall effect=-2.53 p=0.01					
02 Enoxaparin vs standard unfractionated heparin					
Hillbom 1998	14 /106	24 /106		34.5	0.53 [0.26, 1.06]
Subtotal (95% CI)	14 /106	24 /106		34.5	0.53 [0.26, 1.06]
Test for heterogeneity chi-square=0.00 df=0					
Test for overall effect=-1.79 p=0.07					
Total (95% CI)	55 /414	65 /291		100.0	0.52 [0.35, 0.79]
Test for heterogeneity chi-square=3.96 df=4 p=0.4118					
Test for overall effect=-3.10 p=0.002					

.1   .2   1   5   10

Figure 9.12 *Forest plot showing the effects of* LMWH/heparinoid vs standard UFH *in acute ischaemic stroke on* DVT during the treatment period. Reproduced from Sandercock *et al.* (2005), with permission from the authors and John Wiley & Sons Limited. Copyright Cochrane Library, reproduced with permission.

UFH, LMWH or heparinoid have not been identified reliably. Although LMWH and heparinoids appear to be more effective at preventing DVT (and possibly also PE) than UFH, their relative safety and cost-effectiveness compared with UFH have not been established in patients with acute stroke.

Implications for research

Future large RCTs should compare the combination of low-dose LMWH (or heparinoid) plus aspirin, with aspirin alone (the current 'gold' standard), and perhaps also with a more aggressive LMWH (or heparinoid) regimen (as an optional third arm in the trial), during the first 2 weeks in patients with acute ischaemic stroke who are at high risk of DVT, PE and cardiogenic embolism, and low risk of haemorrhagic transformation of the cerebral infarct. A preliminary clinical trial of argatroban has been completed and the drug was considered safe (LaMonte *et al.*, 2004). Enoxaparin has been trialled in eight children with stroke (Burak *et al.*, 2003). Anticoagulants are also being explored as an adjunct to thrombolytic therapy (Schmulling *et al.*, 2003).

Anticoagulation for patients with acute ischaemic stroke who are in atrial fibrillation (AF)

Among patients with acute ischaemic stroke who are in AF, there is no evidence that early anticoagulation within the first few weeks improves outcome compared

Table 9.2. Effect of heparin in different doses on events within 14 days and outcome at 6 months in patients with atrial fibrillation (AF)[*].

	Heparin 12,500 U (n = 784)	Heparin 5000 U (n = 773)	No heparin (n = 1612)	P for trend
Events within 14 days	(%)	(%)	(%)	
Recurrent ischaemic stroke	2.3	3.4	4.9	0.001
Symptomatic ICH	2.8	1.3	0.4	<0.0001
Recurrent stroke of any type	5.0	4.7	5.3	0.6
Recurrent stroke or death	18.8	19.4	20.7	0.3
Outcome at 6 months	(%)	(%)	(%)	
Dead from any cause	38.9	37.8	39.1	0.8
Dead or dependent	78.1	78.8	78.5	0.8

[*]Within each of these groups, half of the patients were randomly assigned to aspirin 300 mg once daily.

with no heparin (Cerebral Embolism Study Group, 1983; Saxena *et al.*, 2001) or compared with aspirin (Berge *et al.*, 2000; Hart *et al.*, 2002) (see Chapter 15).

Evidence

Heparin vs no heparin

Among 18,451 patients who were randomised within 48 h of onset of acute ischaemic stroke in the IST to 14 days treatment with subcutaneous UFH or control, 3169 patients (17%) were in AF, of whom 784 were randomly allocated to UFH 12, 500 U s.c. bid, 773 to UFH 5000 U s.c. bid and 1612 to no heparin (Saxena *et al.*, 2001). Within each of these groups, half of the patients were randomly assigned to aspirin 300 mg once daily.

The proportion of AF patients with further events within 14 days allocated to UFH 12,500 U (n = 784), UFH 5000 U (n = 773) and to no-heparin (n = 1612) groups were as follows: ischaemic stroke, 2.3%, 3.4%, 4.9% (P = 0.001); haemorrhagic stroke, 2.8%, 1.3%, 0.4% (P < 0.0001); and any stroke or death, 18.8%, 19.4% and 20.7% (P − 0.3), respectively (Table 9.2). No effect of heparin on the proportion of patients dead or dependent at 6 months was apparent (Saxena *et al.*, 2001).

Heparin vs aspirin

The Heparin in Acute Embolic Stroke Trial (HAEST) was a multicentre, randomised, double-blind and double-dummy trial comparing the effect of LMWH (dalteparin 100 U/kg subcutaneously twice a day) started within 30 h of stroke onset, with aspirin (160 mg every day), on the prevention of recurrent stroke during the first 14 days among 449 patients with acute ischaemic stroke and AF (Berge *et al.*, 2000). The frequency of recurrent ischaemic stroke during the first 14 days was 19/244 (8.5%) in dalteparin-allocated patients vs 17/225 (7.5%) in aspirin-allocated patients (OR: 1.13, 95% CI: 0.57–2.24). There was also no benefit of dalteparin compared with aspirin on secondary events during the first 14 days: symptomatic cerebral haemorrhage 6/224 vs 4/225; symptomatic and asymptomatic cerebral haemorrhage 26/224 vs 32/225; progression of symptoms within the first 48 h 24/224 vs 17/225; and death 21/224 vs 16/225. There were no significant differences in functional outcome or death at 14 days or 3 months.

Comment

The present data do not provide any evidence that UFH or LMWH is superior to aspirin or no heparin for the treatment of acute ischaemic stroke in patients with AF. Whilst heparin reduces the risk of early recurrent ischaemic stroke, the benefits are offset by an increase in risk of symptomatic ICH, so that there is no change in the rate of early recurrent stroke or long-term death or dependency.

Whether selected subgroups would respond differently remains to be proven. Aspirin followed by early initiation of warfarin for long-term secondary prevention is reasonable antithrombotic management (see Chapters 10, 15) (Hart *et al.*, 2002).

Longer-term prevention in patients with non-cardioembolic ischaemic stroke or TIA

Anticoagulation vs control

Evidence

A systematic Review for the Cochrane Library identified 11 RCTs of long-term anti-coagulation vs control involving 2487 patients with non-cardioembolic ischaemic stroke or TIA (Sandercock *et al.*, 2002). The quality of the nine trials which predated routine CT scanning and the use of the International Normalised Ratio to monitor anticoagulation was poor.

Serious vascular events (non-fatal stroke including subarachnoid haemorrhage, non-fatal myocardial infarction (MI) or vascular death)
Only four trials provided data on this outcome (weighted mean follow-up 2.3 years). There was significant heterogeneity in the results of these trials (Chi-square 8.19 (d.f. = 3), $P < 0.05$), largely due to two trials (VA Study, 1961; Enger, 1965). In the Veterans Administration (VA) trial there was an excess of non-fatal recurrent ischaemic/unknown strokes and vascular deaths in the anticoagulated group. The reason for this may be chance.

Overall, random assignment to long-term anticoagulation was associated with no significant effect on the odds of non-fatal stroke, MI or vascular death compared with control (OR: 0.96, 95% CI: 0.68–1.37) (Fig. 9.13). Excluding the VA Cooperative study or the Enger study, or both, did not significantly change this result.

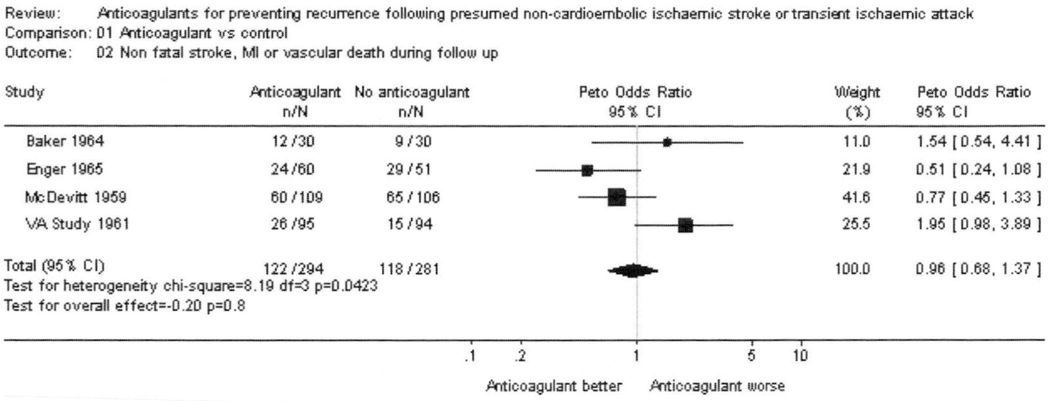

Review: Anticoagulants for preventing recurrence following presumed non-cardioembolic ischaemic stroke or transient ischaemic attack
Comparison: 01 Anticoagulant vs control
Outcome: 02 Non fatal stroke, MI or vascular death during follow up

Study	Anticoagulant n/N	No anticoagulant n/N	Peto Odds Ratio 95% CI	Weight (%)	Peto Odds Ratio 95% CI
Baker 1964	12 / 30	9 / 30		11.0	1.54 [0.54, 4.41]
Enger 1965	24 / 60	29 / 51		21.9	0.51 [0.24, 1.08]
McDevitt 1959	60 / 109	65 / 106		41.6	0.77 [0.45, 1.33]
VA Study 1961	26 / 95	15 / 94		25.5	1.95 [0.98, 3.89]
Total (95% CI)	122 / 294	118 / 281		100.0	0.96 [0.68, 1.37]

Test for heterogeneity chi-square=8.19 df=3 p=0.0423
Test for overall effect=-0.20 p=0.8

.1　.2　1　5　10
Anticoagulant better　　Anticoagulant worse

Figure 9.13　Forest plot showing the effects of *long-term anticoagulation vs control* in patients with previous presumed non-cardioembolic ischaemic stroke or TIA on *serious vascular events (non-fatal stroke, MI or vascular death) during the follow-up period.* Reproduced from Sandercock *et al.* (2002), with permission from the authors and John Wiley & Sons Limited. Copyright Cochrane Library, reproduced with permission.

Review: Anticoagulants for preventing recurrence following presumed non-cardioembolic ischaemic stroke or transient ischaemic attack
Comparison: 01 Anticoagulant vs control
Outcome: 03 Deaths from any cause during follow up

Study	Anticoagulant n/N	No anticoagulant n/N	Peto Odds Ratio 95% CI	Weight (%)	Peto Odds Ratio 95% CI
Baker 1964	9 / 30	5 / 30		4.9	2.00 [0.64, 6.82]
Bradshaw 1975	3 / 24	4 / 13		2.8	0.76 [0.16, 3.68]
Enger 1965	21 / 60	10 / 51		11.2	1.18 [0.53, 2.59]
Howard 1963	3 / 15	3 / 15		2.2	1.00 [0.17, 5.81]
McDevitt 1959	53 / 109	57 / 106		24.4	0.81 [0.48, 1.39]
Nat-Coop 1962	46 / 225	54 / 215		35.0	0.77 [0.49, 1.20]
SWAT 1998	3 / 61	2 / 58		2.2	1.44 [0.24, 8.55]
Thygesen 1964	4 / 33	3 / 35		2.9	1.46 [0.31, 6.90]
VA Study 1961	16 / 95	10 / 94		10.2	1.68 [0.74, 3.84]
Wallace 1964	5 / 27	7 / 25		4.2	0.59 [0.16, 2.13]
Total (95% CI)	163 / 679	161 / 654		100.0	0.95 [0.73, 1.24]

Test for heterogeneity chi-square=6.11 df=9 p=0.7286
Test for overall effect=-0.35 p=0.7

.1　.2　1　5　10
Anticoagulant better　　Anticoagulant worse

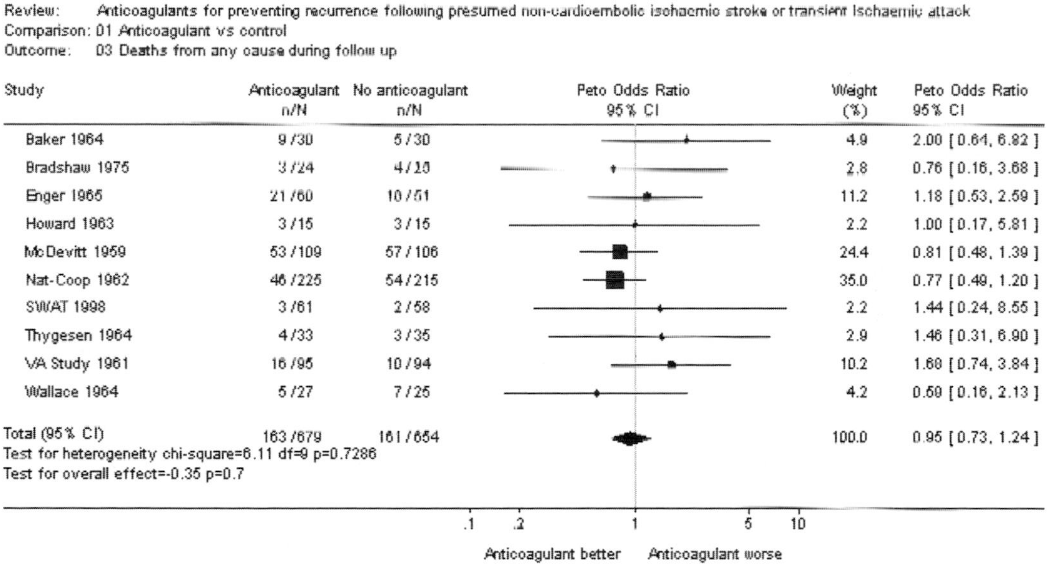

Figure 9.14　Forest plot showing the effects of *long-term anticoagulation vs control* in patients with previous presumed non-cardioembolic ischaemic stroke or TIA on *death during the follow-up period.* Reproduced from Sandercock *et al.* (2002), with permission from the authors and John Wiley & Sons Limited. Copyright Cochrane Library, reproduced with permission.

Death

Ten trials provided data on death from any cause during follow-up (weighted mean duration 1.8 years). The odds of any death in the anticoagulant treatment group were not significantly different from those in the control group (Fig. 9.14): 163/679

Review: Anticoagulants for preventing recurrence following presumed non-cardioembolic ischaemic stroke or transient ischaemic attack
Comparison: 01 Anticoagulant vs control
Outcome: 05 Recurrent ischaemic/unknown stroke during follow up

Study	Anticoagulant n/N	No anticoagulant n/N	Peto Odds Ratio 95% CI	Weight (%)	Peto Odds Ratio 95% CI
01 Fatal					
x Baker 1964	0 /30	0 /30		0.0	Not estimable
Bradshaw 1975	0 /24	1 /25		3.1	0.14 [0.00, 7.11]
Enger 1965	2 /60	3 /51		14.7	0.56 [0.09, 3.34]
McDevitt 1959	7 /109	8 /106		43.1	0.84 [0.30, 2.40]
Nat-Coop 1962	2 /225	9 /215		33.0	0.26 [0.08, 0.86]
Thygesen 1964	1 /33	0 /35		3.1	7.85 [0.16, 396.35]
VA Study 1961	0 /95	1 /94		3.1	0.13 [0.00, 6.75]
Subtotal (95% CI)	12 /576	22 /556		100.0	0.51 [0.26, 1.02]
Test for heterogeneity chi-square=4.84 df=5 p=0.4353					
Test for overall effect=-1.90 p=0.06					
02 Fatal and non fatal					
Baker 1964	5 /30	4 /30		3.3	1.29 [0.32, 5.27]
Bradshaw 1975	2 /24	2 /25		1.6	1.04 [0.14, 7.91]
Enger 1965	9 /60	15 /51		7.9	0.43 [0.17, 1.06]
LHSPS 1999	60 /550	64 /545		46.1	0.92 [0.63, 1.34]
McDevitt 1959	23 /109	23 /106		15.2	0.97 [0.50, 1.85]
Nat-Coop 1962	10 /225	17 /215		10.6	0.55 [0.25, 1.20]
SWAT 1998	2 /61	3 /58		2.0	0.63 [0.11, 3.73]
Thygesen 1964	7 /33	5 /35		4.2	1.60 [0.46, 5.52]
VA Study 1961	10 /95	4 /94		5.5	2.48 [0.84, 7.35]
Wallace 1964	2 /27	9 /25		3.7	0.19 [0.05, 0.70]
Subtotal (95% CI)	130 /1214	146 /1184		100.0	0.85 [0.66, 1.09]
Test for heterogeneity chi-square=14.05 df=9 p=0.1207					
Test for overall effect=-1.29 p=0.2					

.1   .2   1   5   10

Anticoagulant better   Anticoagulant worse

Figure 9.15 Forest plot showing the effects of *long-term anticoagulation vs control* in patients with previous presumed non-cardioembolic ischaemic stroke or TIA on *recurrent ischaemic/unknown stroke during the follow-up period.* Reproduced from Sandercock *et al.* (2002), with permission from the authors and John Wiley & Sons Limited. Copyright Cochrane Library, reproduced with permission.

(24%) patients died in the treatment group compared with 161/654 (24%) in control group (OR: 0.95, 95% CI: 0.73–1.24). There were slightly fewer vascular deaths (137/618 (22%)) in the treated group than in the control group (146/596 (24%)) but the reduction was not statistically significant (OR: 0.86, 95% CI: 0.66–1.13).

Recurrent ischaemic/unknown stroke
Seven trials reported fatal recurrent ischaemic strokes and 10 trials reported fatal and non-fatal recurrent ischaemic strokes (or recurrent stroke of unknown pathological type) over a weighted mean follow-up of 1.9 years. Given that CT scanning was not available for eight trials and that for the two trials where it was available

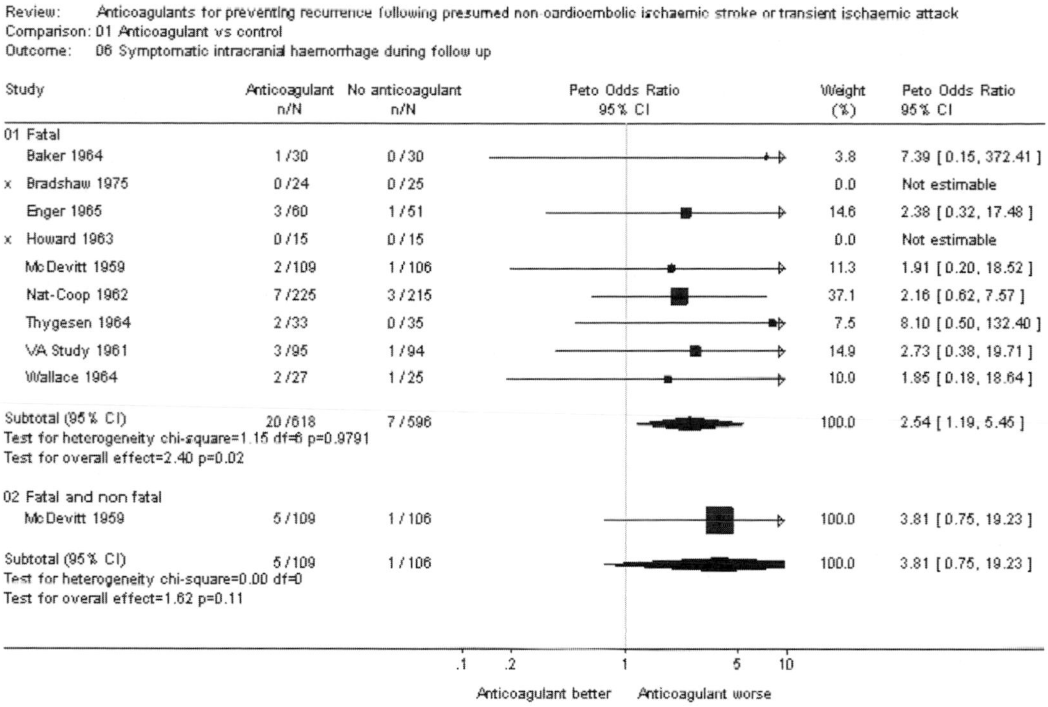

Review: Anticoagulants for preventing recurrence following presumed non-cardioembolic ischaemic stroke or transient ischaemic attack
Comparison: 01 Anticoagulant vs control
Outcome: 06 Symptomatic intracranial haemorrhage during follow up

Study	Anticoagulant n/N	No anticoagulant n/N	Peto Odds Ratio 95% CI	Weight (%)	Peto Odds Ratio 95% CI
01 Fatal					
Baker 1964	1/30	0/30		3.8	7.39 [0.15, 372.41]
x Bradshaw 1975	0/24	0/25		0.0	Not estimable
Enger 1965	3/60	1/51		14.6	2.38 [0.32, 17.48]
x Howard 1963	0/15	0/15		0.0	Not estimable
McDevitt 1959	2/109	1/106		11.3	1.91 [0.20, 18.52]
Nat-Coop 1962	7/225	3/215		37.1	2.16 [0.62, 7.57]
Thygesen 1964	2/33	0/35		7.5	8.10 [0.50, 132.40]
VA Study 1961	3/95	1/94		14.9	2.73 [0.38, 19.71]
Wallace 1964	2/27	1/25		10.0	1.85 [0.18, 18.64]
Subtotal (95% CI)	20/618	7/596		100.0	2.54 [1.19, 5.45]
Test for heterogeneity chi-square=1.15 df=6 p=0.9791					
Test for overall effect=2.40 p=0.02					
02 Fatal and non fatal					
McDevitt 1959	5/109	1/106		100.0	3.81 [0.75, 19.23]
Subtotal (95% CI)	5/109	1/106		100.0	3.81 [0.75, 19.23]
Test for heterogeneity chi-square=0.00 df=0					
Test for overall effect=1.62 p=0.11					

.1   .2   1   5   10
Anticoagulant better   Anticoagulant worse

Figure 9.16 Forest plot showing the effects of *long-term anticoagulation vs control* in patients with previous presumed non-cardioembolic ischaemic stroke or TIA on *symptomatic ICH during the follow-up period*. Reproduced from Sandercock *et al.* (2002), with permission from the authors and John Wiley & Sons Limited. Copyright Cochrane Library, reproduced with permission.

the numbers of recurrent strokes were not reported by pathological type, all non-fatal recurrences other than subarachnoid haemorrhages in these trials were classified as of unknown type. In trials which included patients with acute stroke, deaths due to the initial stroke were not included in this analysis.

Overall, there was a non-significant trend for fewer recurrent strokes in the anticoagulant group (Fig. 9.15). There were 130/1214 (10.7%) recurrent strokes in the treated group and 146/1184 (12.3%) in the control group (OR: 0.85, 95% CI: 0.66–1.09). There was a non-significant trend in favour of treatment for fatal recurrences alone (2% vs 4%, OR: 0.51, 95% CI: 0.26–1.02).

Symptomatic intracranial haemorrhage (ICH)

Data on fatal symptomatic ICH (most of which were confirmed at autopsy) were provided by nine trials and the results were remarkably consistent: anticoagulation more than doubled the odds of fatal intracranial bleeding (20/618 [3.2%] vs 7/596 [1.2%], OR: 2.54, 95% CI: 1.19–5.45) (Fig. 9.16) which was statistically significant ($2P = 0.02$). This was equivalent to anticoagulation causing about an extra 20 (95%

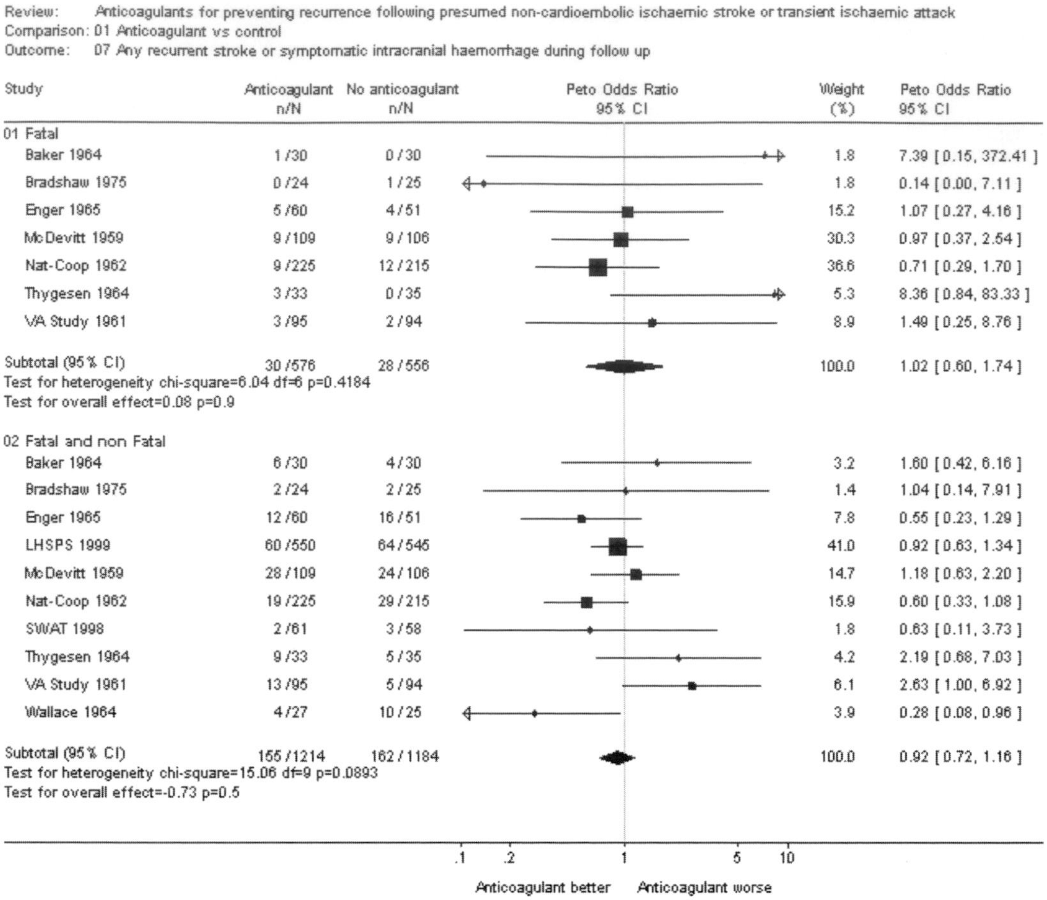

Review: Anticoagulants for preventing recurrence following presumed non-cardioembolic ischaemic stroke or transient ischaemic attack
Comparison: 01 Anticoagulant vs control
Outcome: 07 Any recurrent stroke or symptomatic intracranial haemorrhage during follow up

Study	Anticoagulant n/N	No anticoagulant n/N	Peto Odds Ratio 95% CI	Weight (%)	Peto Odds Ratio 95% CI
01 Fatal					
Baker 1964	1 /30	0 /30		1.8	7.39 [0.15, 372.41]
Bradshaw 1975	0 /24	1 /25		1.8	0.14 [0.00, 7.11]
Enger 1965	5 /60	4 /51		15.2	1.07 [0.27, 4.16]
McDevitt 1959	9 /109	9 /106		30.3	0.97 [0.37, 2.54]
Nat-Coop 1962	9 /225	12 /215		36.6	0.71 [0.29, 1.70]
Thygesen 1964	3 /33	0 /35		5.3	8.36 [0.84, 83.33]
VA Study 1961	3 /95	2 /94		8.9	1.49 [0.25, 8.76]
Subtotal (95% CI)	30 /576	28 /556		100.0	1.02 [0.60, 1.74]

Test for heterogeneity chi-square=6.04 df=6 p=0.4184
Test for overall effect=0.08 p=0.9

Study					
02 Fatal and non Fatal					
Baker 1964	6 /30	4 /30		3.2	1.60 [0.42, 6.16]
Bradshaw 1975	2 /24	2 /25		1.4	1.04 [0.14, 7.91]
Enger 1965	12 /60	16 /51		7.8	0.55 [0.23, 1.29]
LHSPS 1999	60 /550	64 /545		41.0	0.92 [0.63, 1.34]
McDevitt 1959	28 /109	24 /106		14.7	1.18 [0.63, 2.20]
Nat-Coop 1962	19 /225	29 /215		15.9	0.60 [0.33, 1.08]
SWAT 1998	2 /61	3 /58		1.8	0.63 [0.11, 3.73]
Thygesen 1964	9 /33	5 /35		4.2	2.19 [0.68, 7.03]
VA Study 1961	13 /95	5 /94		6.1	2.63 [1.00, 6.92]
Wallace 1964	4 /27	10 /25		3.9	0.28 [0.08, 0.96]
Subtotal (95% CI)	155 /1214	162 /1184		100.0	0.92 [0.72, 1.16]

Test for heterogeneity chi-square=15.06 df=9 p=0.0893
Test for overall effect=-0.73 p=0.5

.1   .2   1   5   10

Anticoagulant better   Anticoagulant worse

Figure 9.17 Forest plot showing the effects of *long-term anticoagulation vs control* in patients with previous presumed non-cardioembolic ischaemic stroke or TIA on *recurrent stroke of any type during the follow-up period.* Reproduced from Sandercock *et al.* (2002), with permission from the authors and John Wiley & Sons Limited. Copyright Cochrane Library, reproduced with permission.

CI: 3–38) fatal ICHs per 1000 patients treated during the whole of follow-up (weighted mean follow-up 1.8 years) and so about 11 extra per year per 1000 patients treated.

Any recurrent stroke or symptomatic ICH

Among the 10 trials that reported non-fatal and fatal recurrent stroke of any pathological type over a weighted mean follow-up 1.9 years, there was no evidence of a significant effect of anticoagulation. The rate of recurrent stroke was 155/1214 (12.8%) among patients assigned anticoagulation vs 162/1184 (13.7%) among patients assigned control (OR: 0.92, 95% CI: 0.72–1.16) (Fig. 9.17). The

Review: Anticoagulants for preventing recurrence following presumed non-cardioembolic ischaemic stroke or transient ischaemic attack
Comparison: 01 Anticoagulant vs control
Outcome: 08 Major extracranial haemorrhage during follow up

Study	Anticoagulant n/N	No anticoagulant n/N	Peto Odds Ratio 95% CI	Weight (%)	Peto Odds Ratio 95% CI
01 Fatal					
Baker 1964	1 /30	0 /30		10.1	7.39 [0.15, 372.41]
x Bradshaw 1975	0 /24	0 /25		0.0	Not estimable
x Enger 1965	0 /60	0 /51		0.0	Not estimable
x Howard 1963	0 /15	0 /15		0.0	Not estimable
McDevitt 1959	1 /109	0 /106		10.1	7.19 [0.14, 362.44]
Nat-Coop 1962	6 /225	1 /215		69.7	4.07 [0.91, 18.09]
VA Study 1961	1 /95	0 /94		10.1	7.31 [0.15, 368.53]
Subtotal (95% CI)	9 /558	1 /536		100.0	4.86 [1.40, 16.88]

Test for heterogeneity chi-square=0.18 df=3 p=0.981
Test for overall effect=2.49 p=0.01

02 Fatal and non Fatal					
Baker 1964	2 /30	0 /30		4.2	7.65 [0.47, 125.23]
x Bradshaw 1975	0 /24	0 /25		0.0	Not estimable
Enger 1965	1 /60	0 /51		2.1	6.36 [0.12, 324.72]
McDevitt 1959	3 /109	0 /106		0.3	7.32 [0.75, 71.18]
Nat-Coop 1962	22 /225	2 /215		48.4	5.54 [2.43, 12.60]
SWAT 1998	8 /61	6 /58		26.5	1.30 [0.43, 3.96]
VA Study 1961	4 /95	2 /94		12.4	1.06 [0.30, 0.01]
Subtotal (95% CI)	40 /604	10 /579		100.0	3.43 [1.94, 6.08]

Test for heterogeneity chi-square=5.51 df=5 p=0.3563
Test for overall effect=4.22 p=0.0000

```
          .1    .2         1         5    10
       Anticoagulant better   Anticoagulant worse
```

Figure 9.18 Forest plot showing the effects of *long-term anticoagulation vs control* in patients with previous presumed non-cardioembolic ischaemic stroke or TIA on *major extracranial haemorrhage the follow-up period.* Reproduced from Sandercock *et al.* (2002), with permission from the authors and John Wiley & Sons Limited. Copyright Cochrane Library, reproduced with permission.

95% CI for the effect on fatal events was equally wide (OR: 1.02, 95% CI: 0.60–1.74).

Major extracranial haemorrhage
Among the seven trials that reported extracranial haemorrhage, there was a large increase in the odds of fatal and non-fatal major extracranial haemorrhage in the anticoagulated group (40/604 [6.6%]) compared with the control group (10/579 [1.7%]) (Fig. 9.18). The OR was 3.43 (95% CI: 1.94–6.08, $2P < 0.0001$) and the absolute rates were an additional 49 (95% CI: 26–71) major extracranial haemorrhages per 1000 patients treated with anticoagulation during a mean weighted follow-up of 1.9 years (about 25 extra per year per 1000 patients) and an extra 14 (95% CI: 0–28) fatal extracranial haemorrhages per 1000 patients.

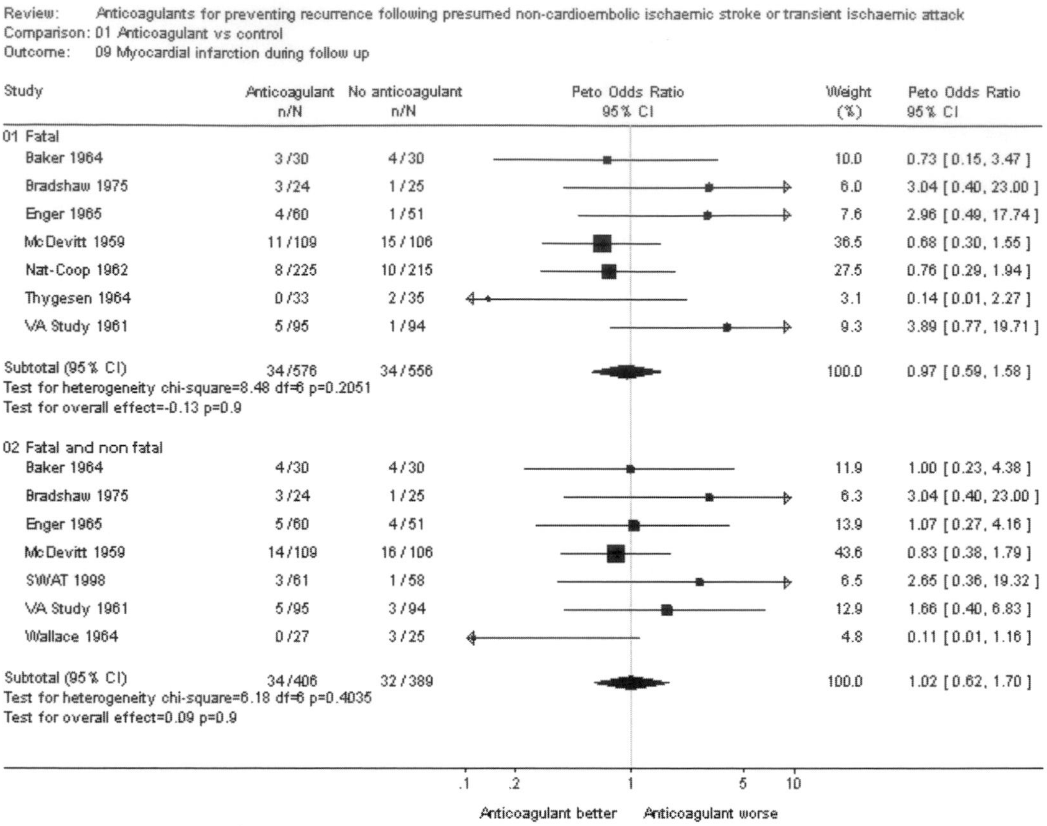

Review: Anticoagulants for preventing recurrence following presumed non-cardioembolic ischaemic stroke or transient ischaemic attack
Comparison: 01 Anticoagulant vs control
Outcome: 09 Myocardial infarction during follow up

Study	Anticoagulant n/N	No anticoagulant n/N	Peto Odds Ratio 95% CI	Weight (%)	Peto Odds Ratio 95% CI
01 Fatal					
Baker 1964	3 / 30	4 / 30		10.0	0.73 [0.15, 3.47]
Bradshaw 1975	3 / 24	1 / 25		6.0	3.04 [0.40, 23.00]
Enger 1965	4 / 60	1 / 51		7.6	2.96 [0.49, 17.74]
McDevitt 1959	11 / 109	15 / 106		36.5	0.68 [0.30, 1.55]
Nat-Coop 1962	8 / 225	10 / 215		27.5	0.76 [0.29, 1.94]
Thygesen 1964	0 / 33	2 / 35		3.1	0.14 [0.01, 2.27]
VA Study 1961	5 / 95	1 / 94		9.3	3.89 [0.77, 19.71]
Subtotal (95% CI)	34 / 576	34 / 556		100.0	0.97 [0.59, 1.58]

Test for heterogeneity chi-square=8.48 df=6 p=0.2051
Test for overall effect=-0.13 p=0.9

02 Fatal and non fatal					
Baker 1964	4 / 30	4 / 30		11.9	1.00 [0.23, 4.38]
Bradshaw 1975	3 / 24	1 / 25		6.3	3.04 [0.40, 23.00]
Enger 1965	5 / 60	4 / 51		13.9	1.07 [0.27, 4.16]
McDevitt 1959	14 / 109	16 / 106		43.6	0.83 [0.38, 1.79]
SWAT 1998	3 / 61	1 / 58		6.5	2.65 [0.36, 19.32]
VA Study 1961	5 / 95	3 / 94		12.9	1.66 [0.40, 6.83]
Wallace 1964	0 / 27	3 / 25		4.8	0.11 [0.01, 1.16]
Subtotal (95% CI)	34 / 406	32 / 389		100.0	1.02 [0.62, 1.70]

Test for heterogeneity chi-square=6.18 df=6 p=0.4035
Test for overall effect=0.09 p=0.9

.1   .2   1   5   10
Anticoagulant better   Anticoagulant worse

Figure 9.19   Forest plot showing the effects of *long-term anticoagulation vs control* in patients with previous presumed non-cardioembolic ischaemic stroke or TIA on *MI during the follow-up period.* Reproduced from Sandercock *et al.* (2002), with permission from the authors and John Wiley & Sons Limited. Copyright Cochrane Library, reproduced with permission.

Myocardial infarction (MI)

Seven trials reported fatal MI (weighted mean follow-up 1.8 years), and fatal and non-fatal MI (weighted mean follow-up 2.2 years). No significant differences were observed between the treated and control groups for either fatal MI alone (OR: 0.97, 95% CI: 0.59–1.58) or fatal and non-fatal MI combined (OR: 1.02, 95% CI: 0.62–1.70) (Fig. 9.19).

Other embolic events

Pulmonary embolism (PE) and peripheral arterial occlusion were reported by four trials but too few events occurred (16 fatal events, all of which were pulmonary emboli, 4 non-fatal pulmonary emboli, 9 non-fatal arterial occlusions) to give reliable estimates of the possible effects of long-term anticoagulation (fatal and non-fatal events: OR: 0.83, 95% CI: 0.38–1.78).

Review: Anticoagulants for preventing recurrence following presumed non-cardioembolic ischaemic stroke or transient ischaemic attack
Comparison: 01 Anticoagulant vs control
Outcome: 11 Non fatal stroke/intracranial haemorrhage or vascular death during follow up

Study	Anticoagulant n/N	No anticoagulant n/N	Peto Odds Ratio 95% CI	Weight (%)	Peto Odds Ratio 95% CI
Baker 1964	11 /30	9 /30		5.6	1.34 [0.46, 3.89]
Bradshaw 1975	5 /24	3 /25		2.8	1.88 [0.42, 8.44]
Enger 1965	23 /60	27 /51		11.4	0.56 [0.26, 1.18]
McDevitt 1959	57 /109	64 /106		21.9	0.72 [0.42, 1.23]
Nat-Coop 1962	53 /225	69 /215		36.4	0.65 [0.43, 0.99]
SWAT 1998	5 /61	5 /58		3.8	0.95 [0.26, 3.44]
Thygesen 1964	10 /33	7 /35		5.3	1.72 [0.58, 5.11]
VA Study 1961	26 /95	13 /94		12.8	2.28 [1.13, 4.60]
Total (95% CI)	190 /637	197 /614		100.0	0.88 [0.69, 1.13]

Test for heterogeneity chi-square=13.99 df=7 p=0.0513
Test for overall effect= 0.98 p=0.3

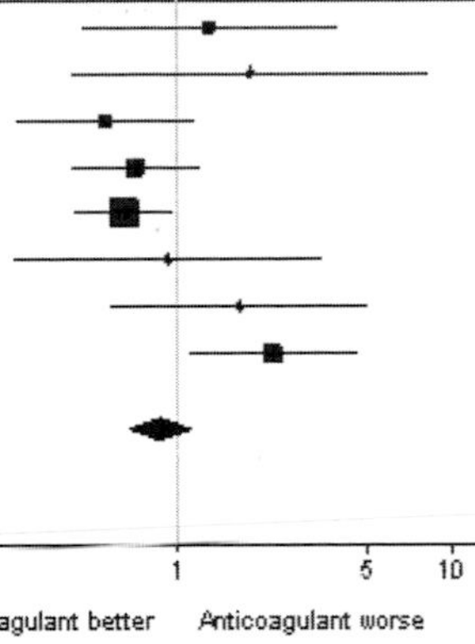

.1   .2   1   5   10

Anticoagulant better   Anticoagulant worse

Figure 9.20   Forest plot showing the effects of *long-term anticoagulation vs control* in patients with previous presumed non-cardioembolic ischaemic stroke or TIA on *non-fatal stroke or vascular death during the follow-up period*. Reproduced from Sandercock *et al.* (2002), with permission from the authors and John Wiley & Sons Limited. Copyright Cochrane Library, reproduced with permission.

Non-fatal stroke or vascular death

Eight trials (weighted mean follow-up 2.0 years) provided data on the composite outcome of non fatal stroke or vascular death, and there was no evidence of an effect of anticoagulation (OR: 0.88, 95% CI: 0.69–1.13) (Fig. 9.20).

Sensitivity analyses

For the three outcome events with most data (i.e. death from any cause, any recurrent stroke, and non-fatal stroke or vascular death) the overall results were consistent in the following:

1 Trials (SWAT, 1998; LHSPS, 1999) performed after 1980 which had access to CT and those published before 1980 which had no CT.

2 Trials in which follow-up was less than 1 year vs those in which it was more than 1 year.

3 Trials which excluded patients with AF vs those that did not.

4 The single small trial where anticoagulation was given with antiplatelet therapy and the trials where no antiplatelet therapy was given.

5 Analyses including only events that occurred whilst the allocated treatment was being taken vs intention-to-treat analyses.

6 Analyses that adjusted for differences in the duration of follow-up vs those that were unadjusted.

7 Trials in which anticoagulants were started within 14 days of the initial stroke in most patients vs those that started treatment later.

Comment

Interpretation of the evidence

There was no evidence of a benefit of long-term anticoagulant therapy in people with presumed non-cardioembolic ischaemic stroke or TIA, compared with control, on the risk of recurrent ischaemic stroke (OR: 0.85, 95% CI: 0.66–1.09), all serious vascular events (OR: 0.96, 95% CI: 0.68–1.37), death from any cause (OR: 0.95, 95% CI: 0.73–1.24) and death from vascular causes (OR: 0.86, 95% CI: 0.66–1.13). However, anticoagulants increased the risk of fatal ICH (OR: 2.54, 95% CI: 1.19–5.45), and major extracranial haemorrhage (OR: 3.43, 95% CI: 1.94–6.08), equivalent to 11 additional fatal ICHs and 25 additional major extracranial haemorrhages per year for every 1000 patients given anticoagulant therapy. It was not possible to determine whether the cerebral bleeding risks were related to the presence of white matter changes (leucoaraiosis) as has been suggested in some studies (The Stroke Prevention In Reversible Ischaemia Trial (SPIRIT) study group, 1997; Gorter *et al.*, 1999).

Implications for practice

There is no evidence to support the routine or widespread use of anticoagulant therapy for secondary prevention in patients with non-cardioembolic ischaemic stroke or TIA (i.e. who are not in AF). Anticoagulation in this type of patient carries a definite risk of major intra- and extracranial haemorrhage, without reducing the risk of ischaemic vascular events.

Implications for research

Further well designed randomised trials of long-term anticoagulation following non-cardioembolic ischaemic stroke or TIA are justified to define reliably whether there is an intensity of anticoagulation, a specific category of patient, or a type of new anticoagulant (e.g. direct thrombin inhibitor) where anticoagulants are more effective than the current 'gold standard' of antiplatelet therapy.

Oral anticoagulation vs antiplatelet therapy
(for more information refer to Chapter 10)

SUMMARY

Anticoagulation for patients with acute ischaemic stroke due to atherothrombo-embolism and cardiogenic embolism reduces recurrent ischaemic stroke compared with control during the treatment period but this benefit is offset by an increase in intracranial haemorrhage (ICH) and extracranial haemorrhage (ECH) so there is no net effect in reducing death and dependency after more than 1-month follow-up. The risks of anticoagulation, in causing intra- and extracranial haemorrhage, are dose-dependent.

Low-dose anticoagulation reduces the risk of DVT and PE compared with control, but the clinical relevance of this is unclear because many DVTs are asymptomatic, and the benefits appear to be offset by an increased risk of extracranial haemorrhage.

LMWH or heparinoids appear to decrease the occurrence of DVT compared with UFH but there are too few data to provide reliable information on their relative effects on other important outcomes such as death, functional independence, recurrent ischaemic stroke, and intra- and extracranial haemorrhage.

Aspirin is an effective antithrombotic alternative to anticoagulation and is safer when used in the acute phase of ischaemic stroke (see Chapter 10).

Further trials should aim to compare the combination of low-dose heparin and aspirin with aspirin alone in patients with acute ischaemic stroke who are at high risk of DVT, PE and cardiogenic embolism, and low risk of haemorrhagic transformation of the brain infarct.

Long-term oral anticoagulation is not more effective than control for patients with non-cardioembolic ischaemic stroke or TIA; it carries a definite risk of major haemorrhage without reducing the risk of ischaemic vascular events.

10

Antiplatelet therapy

The purpose of antiplatelet therapy, like that of anticoagulation (Chapter 9), in patients with acute ischaemic stroke or transient ischaemic attack (TIA) is to prevent recurrent ischaemic stroke and other serious vascular events (by preventing arterial thromboembolism and cardiogenic embolism) and to prevent venous thromboembolism.

Acute ischaemic stroke

Antiplatelet therapy vs control

Evidence

A systematic review of randomised trials comparing early antiplatelet therapy (started within 14 days of the stroke) with control in patients with definite or presumed ischaemic stroke identified nine trials involving 41,399 patients (Chen *et al.*, 2000; Sandercock *et al.*, 2003).

Antiplatelet regimens tested
Antiplatelet agents were broadly defined as any agents whose principal effects were to inhibit platelet adhesion and aggregation. These included:
- cyclo-oxygenase inhibitors (e.g. acetylsalicylic acid, ASA);
- thienopyridine derivatives (e.g. ticlopidine);
- phosphodiesterase inhibitors (e.g. dipyridamole);
- thromboxane A2 antagonists;
- agents with direct effects on platelet membrane receptors such as glycoprotein (Gp) IIb/III receptor and fibrinogen antagonists (e.g. defibrotide).

Two trials testing aspirin 160–300 mg once daily started within 48 h of onset contributed 98% of the data (CAST, 1997; IST, 1997).

Time window for inclusion

Trials included patients randomised within 6 h (MAST-I, 1995), 12 h (Ciufetti, 1990), 24 h (Abciximab, 2000), 48 h (CAST, 1997; IST, 1997) or 6 days (Pince, 1981; Ohtomo, 1991) of stroke onset.

Computed tomographical scanning

Four trials adequately excluded patients with intracerebral haemorrhage by computed tomographical (CT) scanning all patients before entry into the trial (Ciufetti, 1990; Ohtomo, 1991; MAST-I, 1995; Abciximab, 2000). Two trials (CAST, 1997; IST, 1997) performed a CT scan in almost all patients; in these trials, clinicians had to have a low threshold of suspicion of intracranial haemorrhage (ICH) prior to randomisation. In the Chinese Aspirin Stroke Trial (CAST), 87% had a CT prior to randomisation; by discharge, this number had risen to 94%. In the International Stroke Trial (IST), 67% were scanned before randomisation and 29% after randomisation, so that overall, 96% of patients were scanned. Two trials performed no CT scans (Pince, 1981; Turpie, 1983), and in one Japanese trial, the use of CT scanning was uncertain (Utsumi, 1988). As a result of the variable use of pre-randomisation CT scanning, some patients with intracerebral haemorrhage were inadvertently entered in the trials included in the main analyses of this review. This may have biased the results against antiplatelet agents, although this is unlikely given the relatively small numbers of patients involved. Furthermore, the inclusion of these patients may actually make the conclusions of the review more broadly applicable, since many hospitals admitting patients with acute stroke do not have immediate access to CT scanning and so acute treatment may have to be started without definite knowledge of the pathological type of stroke.

Stroke severity at entry

There appeared to be some variation in stroke severity among the included trials. For example, in the control group of the IST (1997), early death was recorded as 9%, but was only 4% in CAST (1997) even though patients in the CAST were assessed at 4 weeks, compared with 2 weeks in the IST. Early death was <1% in the Ohtomo trial (Ohtomo, 1991). Patients in the abciximab trial had to have a National Institute of Health (NIH) stroke scale score of at least 4 to qualify for trial entry (Abciximab, 2000).

Scheduled duration of trial treatment

The scheduled duration of treatment varied from 12 h (Abciximab, 2000) to 3 months (Utsumi, 1988). The scheduled follow-up period varied from 5 days (Abciximab, 2000) to 6 months (MAST-I, 1995; IST, 1997).

Randomisation

The method of randomisation provided adequate concealment of allocation in six trials (Turpie, 1983; Ohtomo, 1991; MAST-I, 1995; CAST, 1997; IST, 1997; Abciximab, 2000).

Baseline characteristics

The large numbers of patients randomised in the CAST (1997) and IST (1997) resulted in an equal distribution of baseline patient characteristics between the treatment and control groups. In two smaller trials (Utsumi, 1988; MAST-I, 1995), there were significant imbalances between the treatment and control groups in potentially important baseline factors (level of consciousness in the Utsumi trial and time to treatment in Multicentre Acute Stroke Trial – Italy (MAST-I)), but these differences cannot bias the overall results due to the small numbers of patients involved. In the abciximab trial, a higher proportion of placebo patients had cortical strokes (Abciximab, 2000).

Blinding

All trials except three used placebo as control. Two trials did not use placebo, but did use methods to obtain outcome data in a masked fashion (MAST-I, 1995; IST, 1997). In the IST, follow-up data were collected by self-completed questionnaire mailed to the patient 6 months after randomisation, or by telephone interview by a person blinded to treatment allocation. An analysis of 207 patients from the UK enrolled in the IST pilot study showed that at the 6-month follow-up, the majority of patients could not remember what they had been treated with, and so these patients were effectively 'blinded' (International Stroke Trial Pilot Study Collaborative Group, 1996). One trial (Utsumi, 1988) did not appear to use any form of blinded outcome assessment.

Follow-up

The maximum follow-up was 6 months. Four trials (Pince, 1981; Turpie, 1983; Utsumi, 1988; Ohtomo, 1991) excluded a total of 19 patients (9 antiplatelet, 10 control) after randomisation and, in addition, three trials (Ohtomo, 1991; CAST, 1997; IST, 1997) lost a total of 655 patients (323 antiplatelet, 332 control) to follow-up.

Death or dependency

Random allocation to antiplatelet therapy was associated with a significant decrease in death or dependency at the end of follow-up (odds ratio (OR): 0.94, 95% confidence interval (CI): 0.91–0.98) from 46.6% (9586/20,586) with control to 45.3% (9344/20,621) with antiplatelet therapy (Fig. 10.1) (Sandercock *et al.*, 2003). In absolute terms, 13 more patients were alive and independent at the end of follow-up for every 1000 patients treated with antiplatelet drugs.

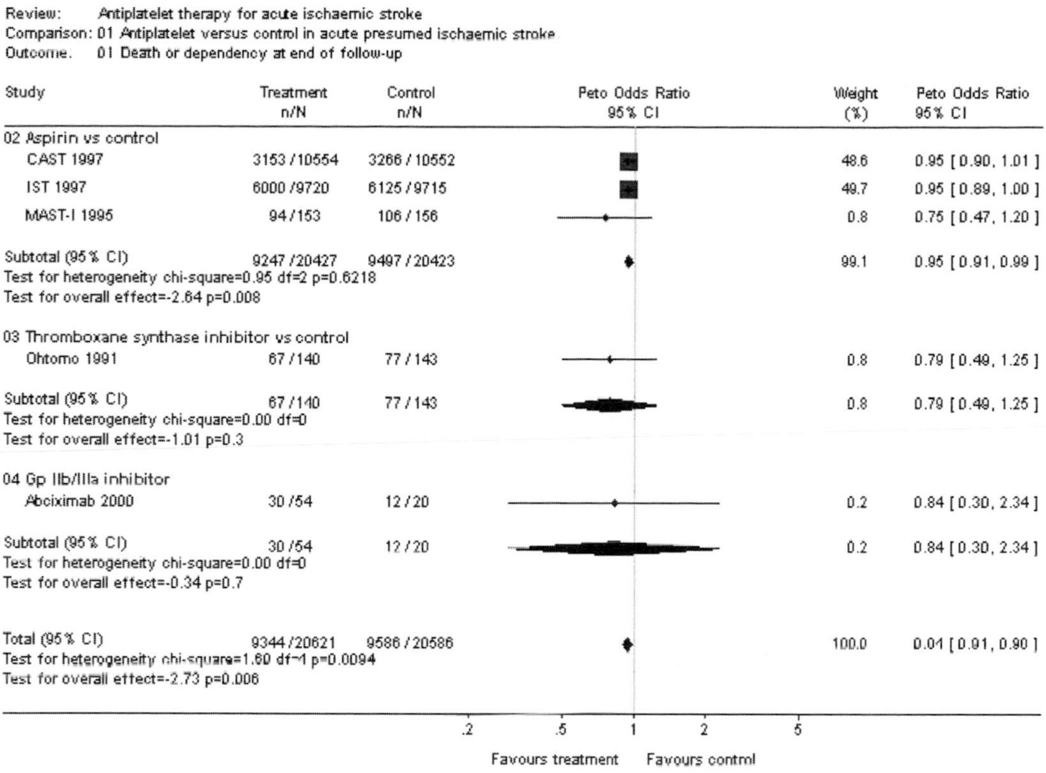

Review: Antiplatelet therapy for acute ischaemic stroke
Comparison: 01 Antiplatelet versus control in acute presumed ischaemic stroke
Outcome.   01 Death or dependency at end of follow-up

Study	Treatment n/N	Control n/N	Peto Odds Ratio 95% CI	Weight (%)	Peto Odds Ratio 95% CI
02 Aspirin vs control					
CAST 1997	3153 / 10554	3266 / 10552	■	48.6	0.95 [0.90, 1.01]
IST 1997	6000 / 9720	6125 / 9715	■	49.7	0.95 [0.89, 1.00]
MAST-I 1995	94 / 153	106 / 156	——◆——	0.8	0.75 [0.47, 1.20]
Subtotal (95% CI)	9247 / 20427	9497 / 20423	◆	99.1	0.95 [0.91, 0.99]
Test for heterogeneity chi-square=0.95 df=2 p=0.6218					
Test for overall effect=-2.64 p=0.008					
03 Thromboxane synthase inhibitor vs control					
Ohtomo 1991	67 / 140	77 / 143	——◆——	0.8	0.79 [0.49, 1.25]
Subtotal (95% CI)	67 / 140	77 / 143	◆	0.8	0.79 [0.49, 1.25]
Test for heterogeneity chi-square=0.00 df=0					
Test for overall effect=-1.01 p=0.3					
04 Gp IIb/IIIa inhibitor					
Abciximab 2000	30 / 54	12 / 20	——◆——	0.2	0.84 [0.30, 2.34]
Subtotal (95% CI)	30 / 54	12 / 20	◆	0.2	0.84 [0.30, 2.34]
Test for heterogeneity chi-square=0.00 df=0					
Test for overall effect=-0.34 p=0.7					
Total (95% CI)	9344 / 20621	9586 / 20586	◆	100.0	0.94 [0.91, 0.90]
Test for heterogeneity chi-square=1.60 df=1 p=0.0094					
Test for overall effect=-2.73 p=0.006					

.2   .5   1   2   5

Favours treatment   Favours control

Figure 10.1   Forest plot showing the effects of *any antiplatelet agent vs control* in acute ischaemic stroke on *death or dependency at the end of follow-up*. Reproduced from Sandercock *et al.* (2003), with permission from the authors and John Wiley & Sons Limited. Copyright Cochrane Library, reproduced with permission.

Pre-specified sensitivity analyses showed that the overall results (Fig. 10.1) were consistent if:

- trials were double blind (OR: 0.95, 95% CI: 0.89–1.00), or not (OR: 0.94, 95% CI: 0.89–1.00);
- patients with intracerebral haemorrhages were inadvertently randomised in the trials (597 in IST and 174 in CAST); the odds of a poor outcome were significantly lower among those allocated aspirin (OR: 0.68, 95% CI: 0.49–0.94), although the CI are wide. These data do not provide clear evidence of any harm to patients with haemorrhagic stroke inadvertently treated with aspirin.

Since this Cochrane Review, the results of the phase IIb Abciximab in Emergent Stroke Treatment Trial (AbESTT) have been published (AbESTT Investigators, 2003, 2005). The AbESTT study randomised 400 patients within 6 h of onset of ischaemic stroke to abciximab (a long-acting Gp IIb/IIIa antagonist) 0.25 mg/kg in bolus followed by a 12-h infusion of 0.125 μg/kg/min or placebo. A few patients were treated within 3 h, and about 50% of patients treated from 3 to 5 h after onset. A poor outcome at 3 months, defined as a modified Rankin Scale (mRS) of 2–6 (death or dependency), was achieved by 51.5% of patients assigned abciximab and by 60% of patients assigned placebo (OR: 0.71, 95% CI: 0.48–1.05, $P = 0.087$).

Another trial randomised 441 acute ischaemic stroke patients to aspirin (325 µg/day), $n = 220$, or placebo, $n = 221$, within 48 hours of stroke onset (Roden-Jullig et al., 2003). Patients were treated for 5 days and there were no significant differences in outcomes at 3 months in this underpowered study.

Complete recovery from stroke

Allocation to antiplatelet therapy significantly increased the odds of a complete recovery (OR: 1.06, 95% CI: 1.01–1.11, $2P = 0.01$). In absolute terms, 10 patients made a complete recovery for every 1000 patients treated (95% CI: 2–19 complete recoveries).

Death

During the scheduled treatment period, antiplatelet therapy was associated with a marginally significant reduction in death at the end of the treatment period (OR: 0.92, 95% CI: 0.85–1.00, $2P = 0.05$). In absolute terms, five fewer patients died during the treatment period for every 1000 patients treated with antiplatelet agents (95% CI: 0–9 fewer deaths).

At the end of follow-up, 1 month or more after randomisation, antiplatelet therapy was associated with a significant reduction in the odds of death (OR: 0.92, 95% CI: 0.87–0.98, $2P = 0.008$) from 12.9% (2662/20,681) of patients assigned control to 12.1% (2497/20,718) of patients assigned antiplatelet therapy (Fig. 10.2). In absolute terms, there were eight fewer deaths for every 1000 patients treated with antiplatelet agents (95% CI: 2–14 fewer deaths) (Sandercock et al., 2003).

Pre-specified sensitivity analysis showed no statistically significant difference in the effect of treatment on death at final follow-up between trials which were of a double-blind design (OR: 0.86, 95% CI: 0.75–0.99), or not (OR: 0.94, 95% CI: 0.87–1.00).

Recurrent ischaemic stroke

Antiplatelet therapy (chiefly aspirin) was associated with a statistically significant reduction in recurrent ischaemic strokes (OR: 0.77, 95% CI: 0.69–0.87, $2P = 0.00002$) from 3.1% (636/20,661) of patients assigned control to 2.4% (496/20,664) of patients assigned antiplatelet therapy (Fig. 10.3). In absolute terms, seven ischaemic strokes were avoided for every 1000 patients treated (95% CI: 4–10 ischaemic strokes avoided).

Symptomatic intracranial haemorrhage (ICH)

Antiplatelet therapy marginally but significantly increased the odds of symptomatic ICH (OR: 1.23, 95% CI: 1.00–1.50, $2P = 0.05$) from 0.8% (171/20,681) of patients assigned control to 1.0% (210/20,718) of patients assigned antiplatelet therapy

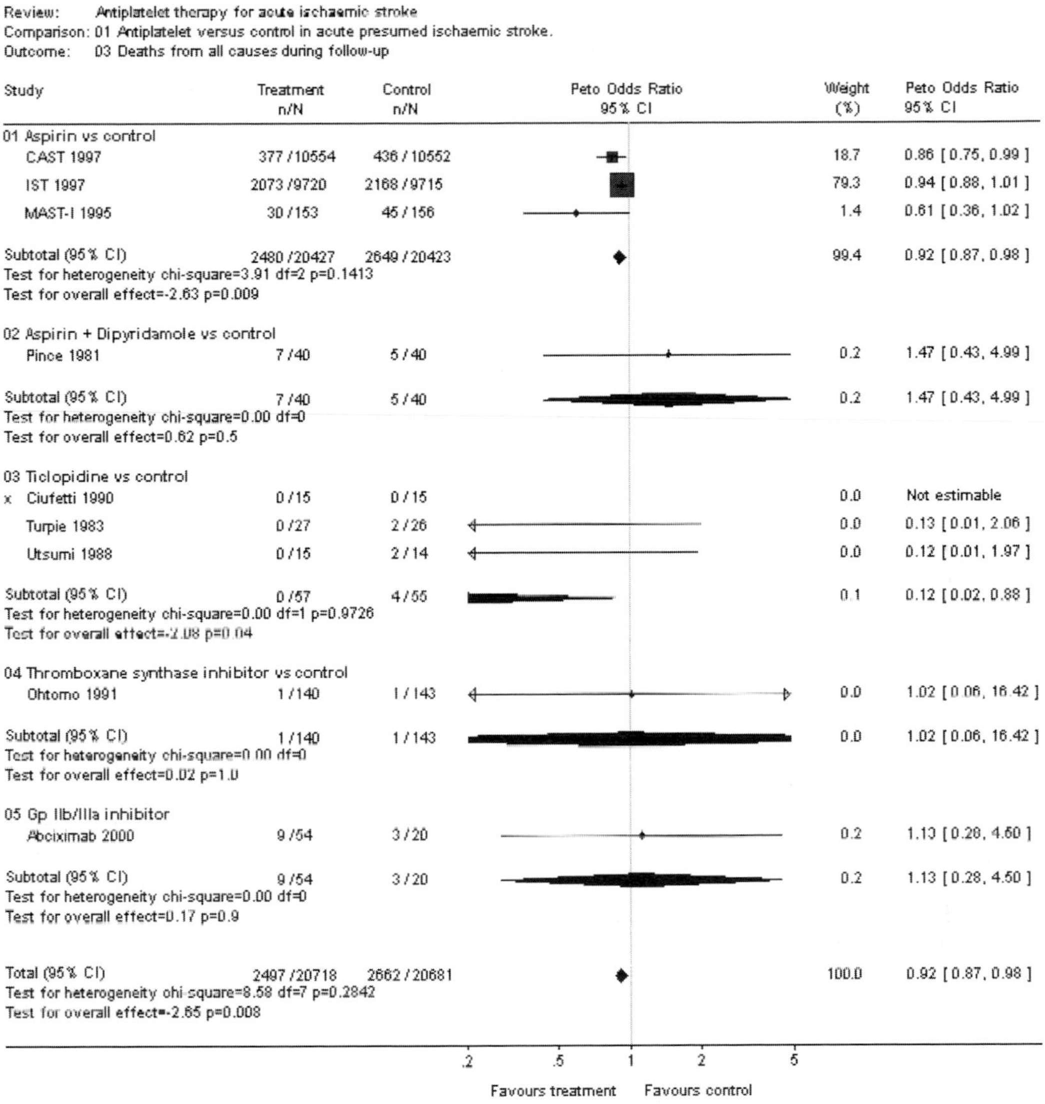

Review: Antiplatelet therapy for acute ischaemic stroke
Comparison: 01 Antiplatelet versus control in acute presumed ischaemic stroke.
Outcome: 03 Deaths from all causes during follow-up

Study	Treatment n/N	Control n/N	Peto Odds Ratio 95% CI	Weight (%)	Peto Odds Ratio 95% CI
01 Aspirin vs control					
CAST 1997	377 / 10554	436 / 10552		18.7	0.86 [0.75, 0.99]
IST 1997	2073 / 9720	2168 / 9715		79.3	0.94 [0.88, 1.01]
MAST-I 1995	30 / 153	45 / 156		1.4	0.61 [0.36, 1.02]
Subtotal (95% CI)	2480 / 20427	2649 / 20423		99.4	0.92 [0.87, 0.98]
Test for heterogeneity chi-square=3.91 df=2 p=0.1413					
Test for overall effect=-2.63 p=0.009					
02 Aspirin + Dipyridamole vs control					
Pince 1981	7 / 40	5 / 40		0.2	1.47 [0.43, 4.99]
Subtotal (95% CI)	7 / 40	5 / 40		0.2	1.47 [0.43, 4.99]
Test for heterogeneity chi-square=0.00 df=0					
Test for overall effect=0.62 p=0.5					
03 Ticlopidine vs control					
x Ciufetti 1990	0 / 15	0 / 15		0.0	Not estimable
Turpie 1983	0 / 27	2 / 26		0.0	0.13 [0.01, 2.06]
Utsumi 1988	0 / 15	2 / 14		0.0	0.12 [0.01, 1.97]
Subtotal (95% CI)	0 / 57	4 / 55		0.1	0.12 [0.02, 0.88]
Test for heterogeneity chi-square=0.00 df=1 p=0.9726					
Test for overall effect=-2.08 p=0.04					
04 Thromboxane synthase inhibitor vs control					
Ohtomo 1991	1 / 140	1 / 143		0.0	1.02 [0.06, 16.42]
Subtotal (95% CI)	1 / 140	1 / 143		0.0	1.02 [0.06, 16.42]
Test for heterogeneity chi-square=0.00 df=0					
Test for overall effect=0.02 p=1.0					
05 Gp IIb/IIIa inhibitor					
Abciximab 2000	9 / 54	3 / 20		0.2	1.13 [0.28, 4.60]
Subtotal (95% CI)	9 / 54	3 / 20		0.2	1.13 [0.28, 4.60]
Test for heterogeneity chi-square=0.00 df=0					
Test for overall effect=0.17 p=0.9					
Total (95% CI)	2497 / 20718	2662 / 20681		100.0	0.92 [0.87, 0.98]
Test for heterogeneity chi-square=8.58 df=7 p=0.2842					
Test for overall effect=-2.65 p=0.008					

.2   .5   1   2   5

Favours treatment   Favours control

Figure 10.2   Forest plot showing the effects of *any antiplatelet agent vs control* in acute ischaemic stroke on *death at the end of follow-up*. Reproduced from Sandercock *et al.* (2003), with permission from the authors and John Wiley & Sons Limited. Copyright Cochrane Library, reproduced with permission.

(Fig. 10.4). In absolute terms, there was an excess of two ICHs for every 1000 patients treated (95% CI: 0–4 additional ICHs).

     There is the possibility of some bias within these data, as there may have been a lower threshold for re-scanning patients who had deteriorated clinically if they were known to be receiving antithrombotic treatment (e.g. in the IST (1997)

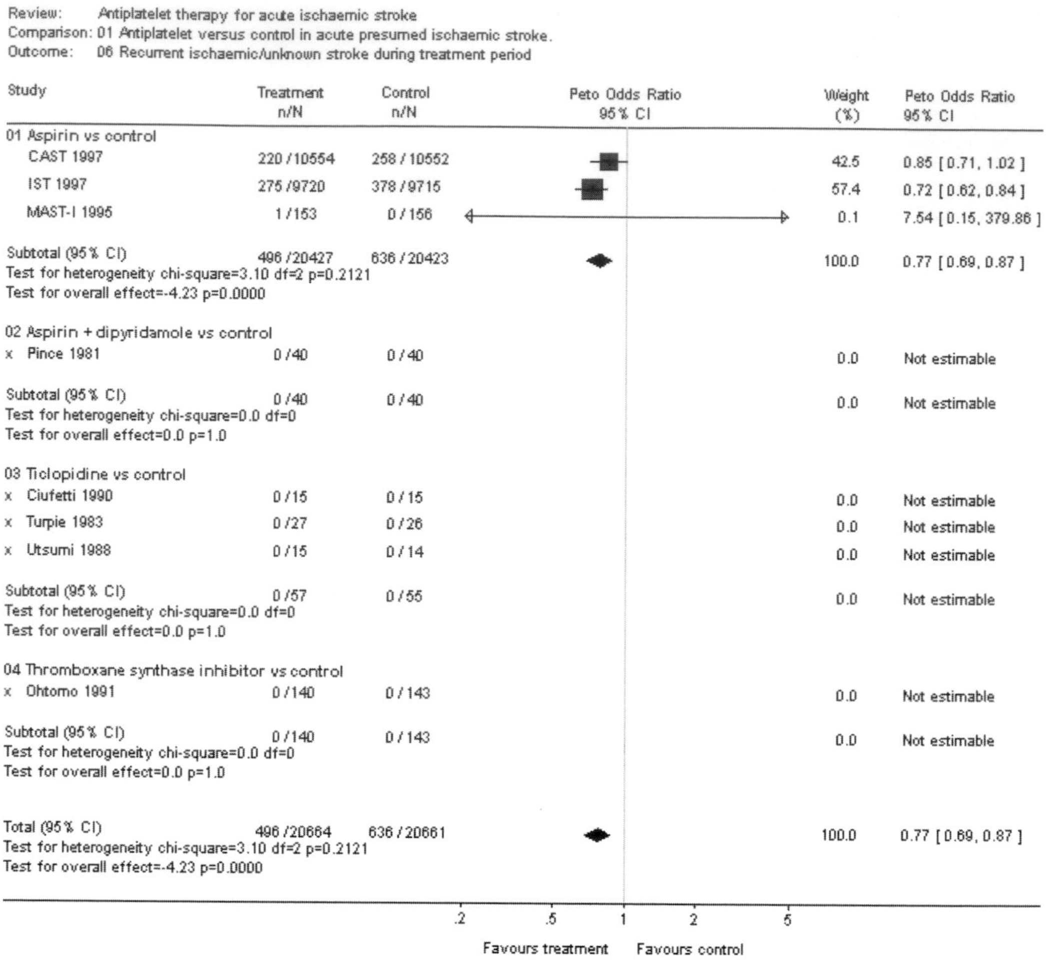

Review: Antiplatelet therapy for acute ischaemic stroke
Comparison: 01 Antiplatelet versus control in acute presumed ischaemic stroke.
Outcome: 06 Recurrent ischaemic/unknown stroke during treatment period

Study	Treatment n/N	Control n/N	Peto Odds Ratio 95% CI	Weight (%)	Peto Odds Ratio 95% CI
01 Aspirin vs control					
CAST 1997	220 / 10554	258 / 10552		42.5	0.85 [0.71, 1.02]
IST 1997	275 / 9720	378 / 9715		57.4	0.72 [0.62, 0.84]
MAST-I 1995	1 / 153	0 / 156		0.1	7.54 [0.15, 379.86]
Subtotal (95% CI)	496 / 20427	636 / 20423		100.0	0.77 [0.69, 0.87]

Test for heterogeneity chi-square=3.10 df=2 p=0.2121
Test for overall effect=-4.23 p=0.0000

02 Aspirin + dipyridamole vs control					
x Pince 1981	0 / 40	0 / 40		0.0	Not estimable
Subtotal (95% CI)	0 / 40	0 / 40		0.0	Not estimable

Test for heterogeneity chi-square=0.0 df=0
Test for overall effect=0.0 p=1.0

03 Ticlopidine vs control					
x Ciufetti 1990	0 / 15	0 / 15		0.0	Not estimable
x Turpie 1983	0 / 27	0 / 26		0.0	Not estimable
x Utsumi 1988	0 / 15	0 / 14		0.0	Not estimable
Subtotal (95% CI)	0 / 57	0 / 55		0.0	Not estimable

Test for heterogeneity chi-square=0.0 df=0
Test for overall effect=0.0 p=1.0

04 Thromboxane synthase inhibitor vs control					
x Ohtomo 1991	0 / 140	0 / 143		0.0	Not estimable
Subtotal (95% CI)	0 / 140	0 / 143		0.0	Not estimable

Test for heterogeneity chi-square=0.0 df=0
Test for overall effect=0.0 p=1.0

Total (95% CI)	496 / 20664	636 / 20661		100.0	0.77 [0.69, 0.87]

Test for heterogeneity chi-square=3.10 df=2 p=0.2121
Test for overall effect=-4.23 p=0.0000

.2   .5   1   2   5

Favours treatment   Favours control

Figure 10.3   Forest plot showing the effects of *any antiplatelet agent vs control* in acute ischaemic stroke on *recurrent ischaemic or unknown stroke at the end of follow-up*. Reproduced from Sandercock *et al.* (2003), with permission from the authors and John Wiley & Sons Limited. Copyright Cochrane Library, reproduced with permission.

in which treatment allocation was not blinded). The sensitivity analysis found no significant difference in the effect of treatment on symptomatic ICH during the treatment period between trials which were of a double-blind design (OR: 1.24, 95% CI: 0.95–1.63), or not (OR: 1.21, 95% CI: 0.89–1.64).

The phase IIb AbESTT trial (AbESTT Investigators, 2003, 2005) reported symptomatic incracranial haemorrhage within 5 days was experienced by 3.5% ($n = 7$) of the 200 patients assigned abciximab and by 1.0% ($n = 2$) of the 200 patients assigned placebo (OR: 3.11, 95% CI: 0.83–11.6) (AbESTT Investigators, 2003, 2005).

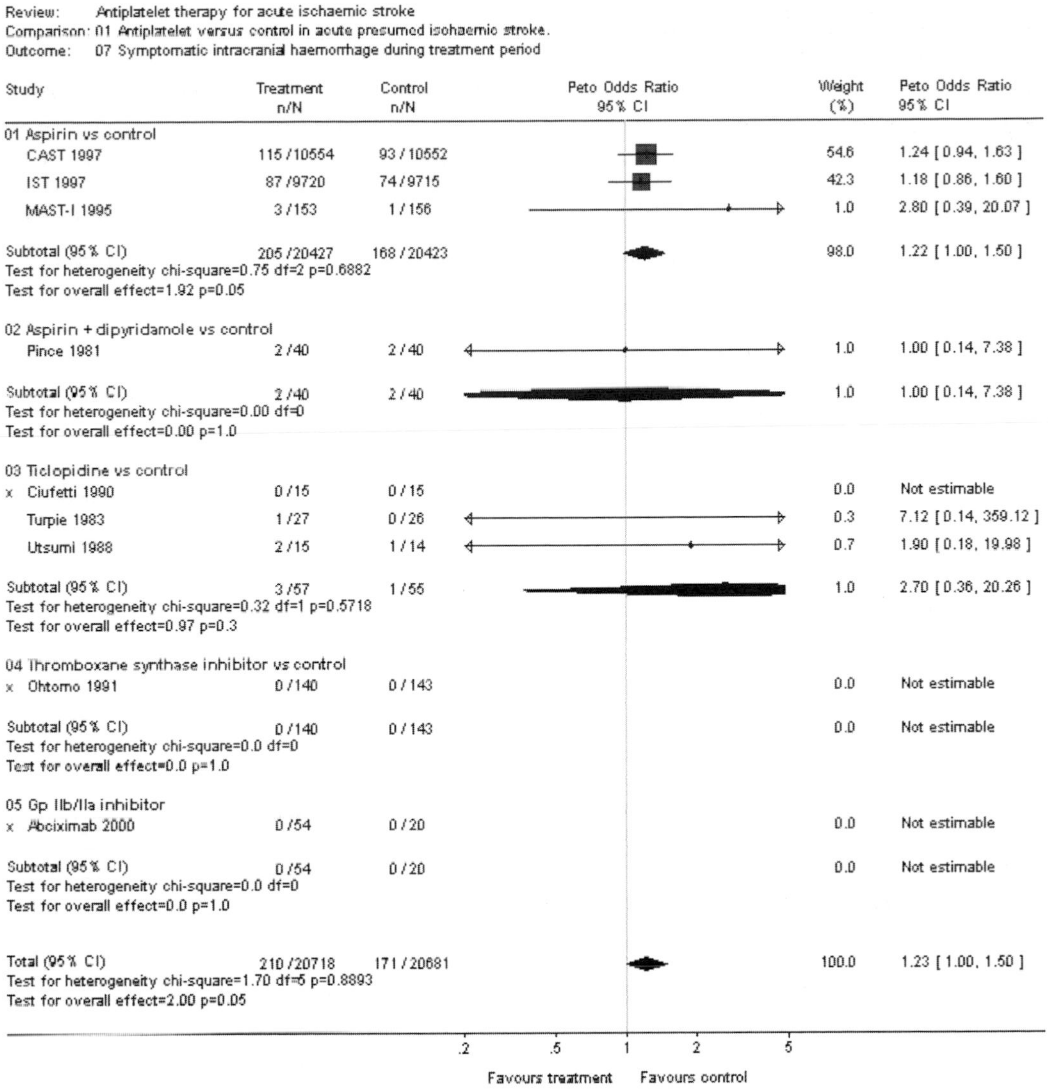

Review: Antiplatelet therapy for acute ischaemic stroke
Comparison: 01 Antiplatelet versus control in acute presumed ischaemic stroke.
Outcome: 07 Symptomatic intracranial haemorrhage during treatment period

Study	Treatment n/N	Control n/N	Peto Odds Ratio 95% CI	Weight (%)	Peto Odds Ratio 95% CI
01 Aspirin vs control					
CAST 1997	115 / 10554	93 / 10552		54.6	1.24 [0.94, 1.63]
IST 1997	87 / 9720	74 / 9715		42.3	1.18 [0.86, 1.60]
MAST-I 1995	3 / 153	1 / 156		1.0	2.80 [0.39, 20.07]
Subtotal (95% CI)	205 / 20427	168 / 20423		98.0	1.22 [1.00, 1.50]
Test for heterogeneity chi-square=0.75 df=2 p=0.6882					
Test for overall effect=1.92 p=0.05					
02 Aspirin + dipyridamole vs control					
Pince 1981	2 / 40	2 / 40		1.0	1.00 [0.14, 7.38]
Subtotal (95% CI)	2 / 40	2 / 40		1.0	1.00 [0.14, 7.38]
Test for heterogeneity chi-square=0.00 df=0					
Test for overall effect=0.00 p=1.0					
03 Ticlopidine vs control					
x Ciufetti 1990	0 / 15	0 / 15		0.0	Not estimable
Turpie 1983	1 / 27	0 / 26		0.3	7.12 [0.14, 359.12]
Utsumi 1988	2 / 15	1 / 14		0.7	1.90 [0.18, 19.98]
Subtotal (95% CI)	3 / 57	1 / 55		1.0	2.70 [0.36, 20.26]
Test for heterogeneity chi-square=0.32 df=1 p=0.5718					
Test for overall effect=0.97 p=0.3					
04 Thromboxane synthase inhibitor vs control					
x Ohtomo 1991	0 / 140	0 / 143		0.0	Not estimable
Subtotal (95% CI)	0 / 140	0 / 143		0.0	Not estimable
Test for heterogeneity chi-square=0.0 df=0					
Test for overall effect=0.0 p=1.0					
05 Gp IIb/IIIa inhibitor					
x Abciximab 2000	0 / 54	0 / 20		0.0	Not estimable
Subtotal (95% CI)	0 / 54	0 / 20		0.0	Not estimable
Test for heterogeneity chi-square=0.0 df=0					
Test for overall effect=0.0 p=1.0					
Total (95% CI)	210 / 20718	171 / 20681		100.0	1.23 [1.00, 1.50]
Test for heterogeneity chi-square=1.70 df=5 p=0.8893					
Test for overall effect=2.00 p=0.05					

.2   .5   1   2   5

Favours treatment   Favours control

Figure 10.4 Forest plot showing the effects of *any antiplatelet agent vs control* in acute ischaemic stroke on *symptomatic ICH at the end of follow-up*. Reproduced from Sandercock *et al.* (2003), with permission from the authors and John Wiley & Sons Limited. Copyright Cochrane Library, reproduced with permission.

Recurrent stroke of any type

Antiplatelet therapy was associated with a net reduction in the odds of recurrent stroke of any pathological type (OR: 0.88, 95% CI: 0.79–0.97, $2P = 0.01$) from 3.9% (802/20,681) of patients assigned control to 3.4% (712/20,718) of patients assigned antiplatelet therapy (Fig. 10.5).

In absolute terms, five recurrent ischaemic strokes or symptomatic ICHs were avoided for every 1000 patients treated (95% CI: 1–9 outcomes avoided).

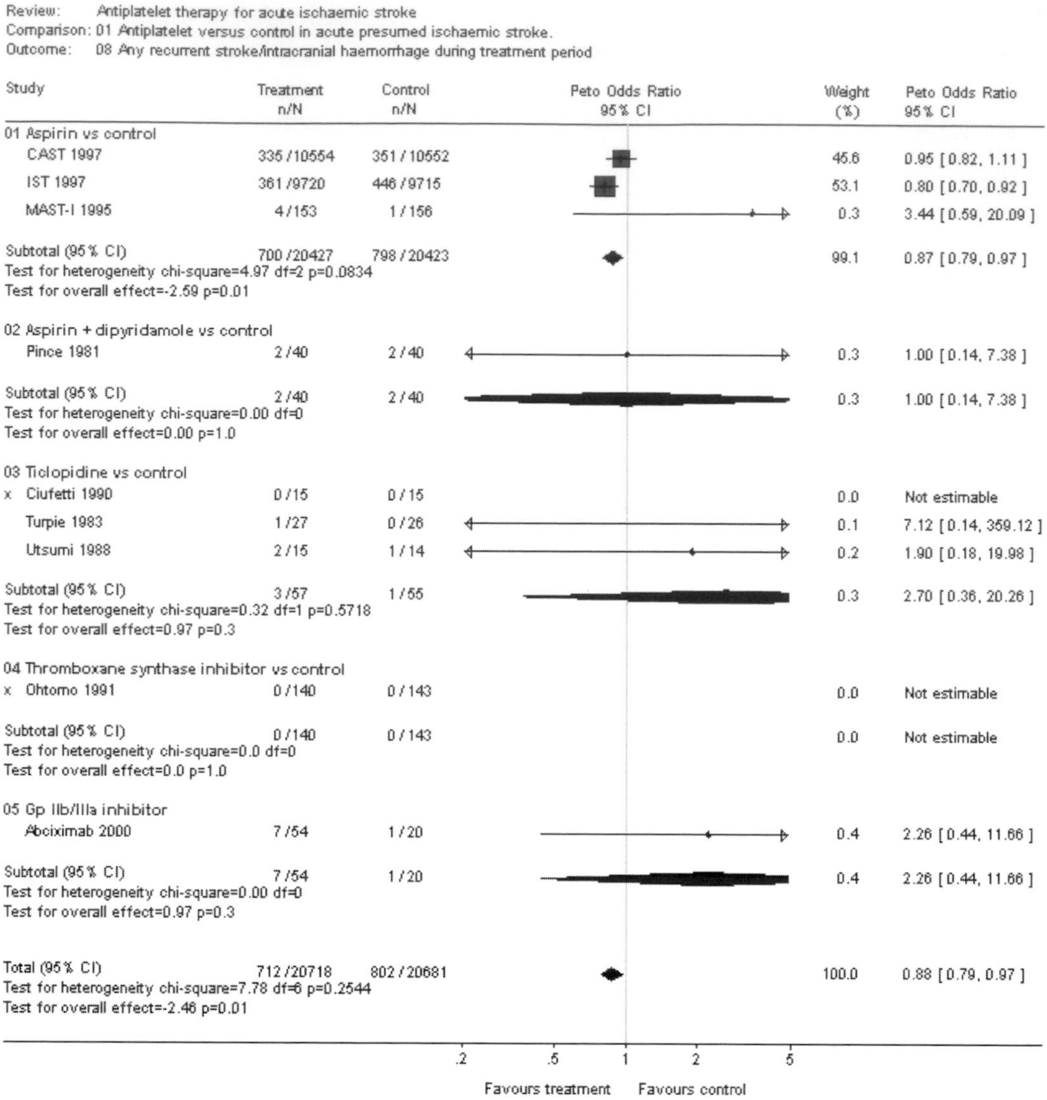

Review: Antiplatelet therapy for acute ischaemic stroke
Comparison: 01 Antiplatelet versus control in acute presumed ischaemic stroke.
Outcome: 08 Any recurrent stroke/intracranial haemorrhage during treatment period

Study	Treatment n/N	Control n/N	Peto Odds Ratio 95% CI	Weight (%)	Peto Odds Ratio 95% CI
01 Aspirin vs control					
CAST 1997	335 /10554	351 /10552		45.6	0.95 [0.82, 1.11]
IST 1997	361 /9720	446 /9715		53.1	0.80 [0.70, 0.92]
MAST-I 1995	4 /153	1 /156		0.3	3.44 [0.59, 20.09]
Subtotal (95% CI)	700 /20427	798 /20423		99.1	0.87 [0.79, 0.97]
Test for heterogeneity chi-square=4.97 df=2 p=0.0834					
Test for overall effect=-2.59 p=0.01					
02 Aspirin + dipyridamole vs control					
Pince 1981	2 /40	2 /40		0.3	1.00 [0.14, 7.38]
Subtotal (95% CI)	2 /40	2 /40		0.3	1.00 [0.14, 7.38]
Test for heterogeneity chi-square=0.00 df=0					
Test for overall effect=0.00 p=1.0					
03 Ticlopidine vs control					
x Ciufetti 1990	0 /15	0 /15		0.0	Not estimable
Turpie 1983	1 /27	0 /26		0.1	7.12 [0.14, 359.12]
Utsumi 1988	2 /15	1 /14		0.2	1.90 [0.18, 19.98]
Subtotal (95% CI)	3 /57	1 /55		0.3	2.70 [0.36, 20.26]
Test for heterogeneity chi-square=0.32 df=1 p=0.5718					
Test for overall effect=0.97 p=0.3					
04 Thromboxane synthase inhibitor vs control					
x Ohtomo 1991	0 /140	0 /143		0.0	Not estimable
Subtotal (95% CI)	0 /140	0 /143		0.0	Not estimable
Test for heterogeneity chi-square=0.0 df=0					
Test for overall effect=0.0 p=1.0					
05 Gp IIb/IIIa inhibitor					
Abciximab 2000	7 /54	1 /20		0.4	2.26 [0.44, 11.66]
Subtotal (95% CI)	7 /54	1 /20		0.4	2.26 [0.44, 11.66]
Test for heterogeneity chi-square=0.00 df=0					
Test for overall effect=0.97 p=0.3					
Total (95% CI)	712 /20718	802 /20681		100.0	0.88 [0.79, 0.97]
Test for heterogeneity chi-square=7.78 df=6 p=0.2544					
Test for overall effect=-2.46 p=0.01					

.2   .5   1   2   5

Favours treatment   Favours control

Figure 10.5 Forest plot showing the effects of *any antiplatelet agent vs control* in acute ischaemic stroke *on recurrent stroke of any type at the end of follow-up*. Reproduced from Sandercock *et al.* (2003), with permission from the authors and John Wiley & Sons Limited. Copyright Cochrane Library, reproduced with permission.

Major extracranial haemorrhage during the treatment period

Allocation to antiplatelet agents was associated with a significant increase in major extracranial haemorrhage (OR: 1.68, 95% CI: 1.34–2.09, $2P = 0.00001$) from 0.6% (116/20,681) of patients assigned control to 1.0% (196/20,718) of patients assigned antiplatelet therapy (Fig. 10.6).

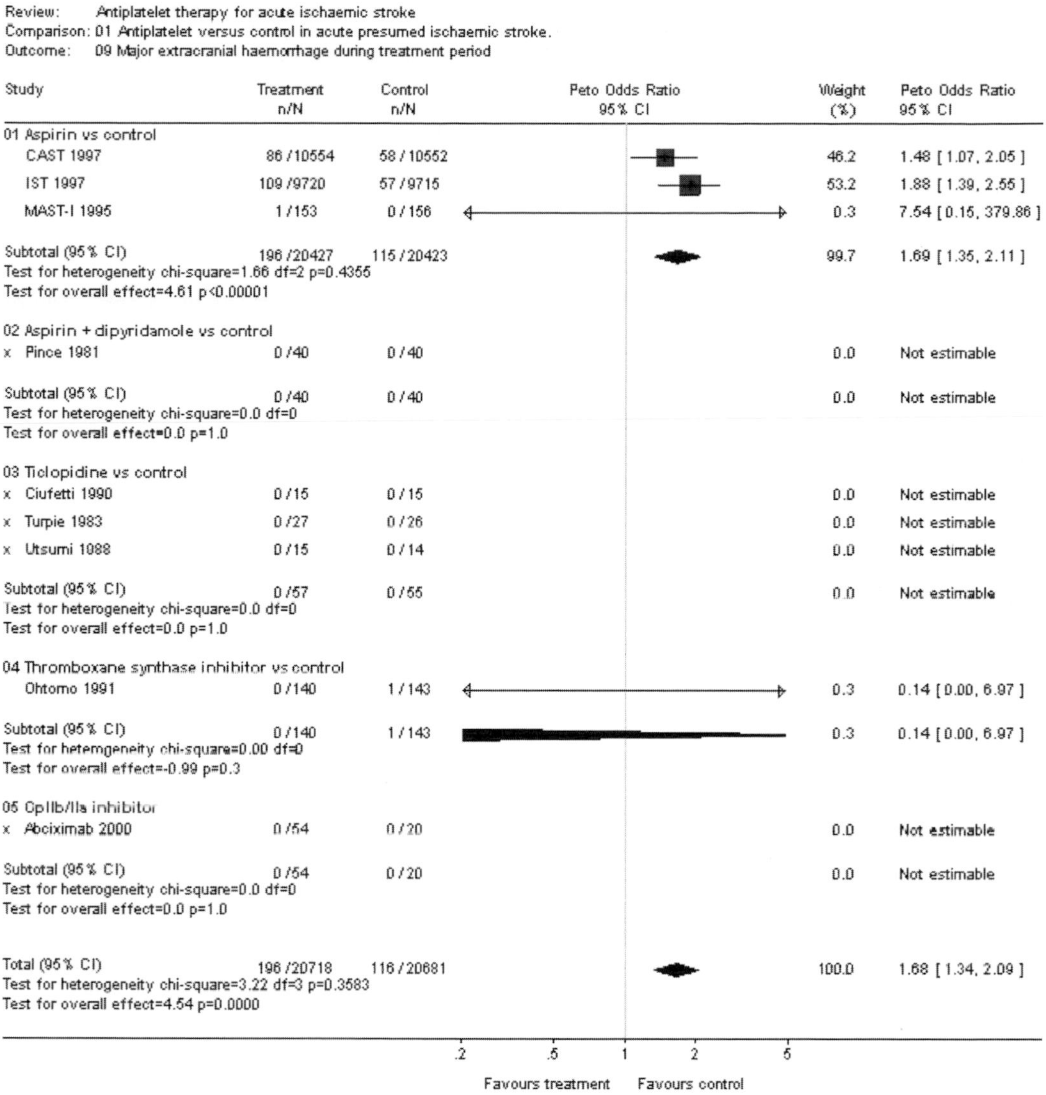

Review: Antiplatelet therapy for acute ischaemic stroke
Comparison: 01 Antiplatelet versus control in acute presumed ischaemic stroke.
Outcome: 09 Major extracranial haemorrhage during treatment period

Study	Treatment n/N	Control n/N	Peto Odds Ratio 95% CI	Weight (%)	Peto Odds Ratio 95% CI
01 Aspirin vs control					
CAST 1997	86 /10554	58 / 10552		46.2	1.48 [1.07, 2.05]
IST 1997	109 /9720	57 /9715		53.2	1.88 [1.39, 2.55]
MAST-I 1995	1 /153	0 / 156		0.3	7.54 [0.15, 379.86]
Subtotal (95% CI)	196 /20427	115 /20423		99.7	1.69 [1.35, 2.11]
Test for heterogeneity chi-square=1.66 df=2 p=0.4355					
Test for overall effect=4.61 p<0.00001					
02 Aspirin + dipyridamole vs control					
x Pince 1981	0 /40	0 /40		0.0	Not estimable
Subtotal (95% CI)	0 /40	0 /40		0.0	Not estimable
Test for heterogeneity chi-square=0.0 df=0					
Test for overall effect=0.0 p=1.0					
03 Ticlopidine vs control					
x Ciufetti 1990	0 /15	0 /15		0.0	Not estimable
x Turpie 1983	0 /27	0 /26		0.0	Not estimable
x Utsumi 1988	0 /15	0 /14		0.0	Not estimable
Subtotal (95% CI)	0 /57	0 /55		0.0	Not estimable
Test for heterogeneity chi-square=0.0 df=0					
Test for overall effect=0.0 p=1.0					
04 Thromboxane synthase inhibitor vs control					
Ohtomo 1991	0 /140	1 /143		0.3	0.14 [0.00, 6.97]
Subtotal (95% CI)	0 /140	1 /143		0.3	0.14 [0.00, 6.97]
Test for heterogeneity chi-square=0.00 df=0					
Test for overall effect=-0.99 p=0.3					
05 GpIIb/IIa inhibitor					
x Abciximab 2000	0 /54	0 /20		0.0	Not estimable
Subtotal (95% CI)	0 /54	0 /20		0.0	Not estimable
Test for heterogeneity chi-square=0.0 df=0					
Test for overall effect=0.0 p=1.0					
Total (95% CI)	196 /20718	116 /20681		100.0	1.68 [1.34, 2.09]
Test for heterogeneity chi-square=3.22 df=3 p=0.3583					
Test for overall effect=4.54 p=0.0000					

.2   .5   1   2   5

Favours treatment   Favours control

Figure 10.6 Forest plot showing the effects of *any antiplatelet agent vs control* in acute ischaemic stroke *on major extracranial haemorrhage during the treatment period*. Reproduced from Sandercock *et al.* (2003), with permission from the authors and John Wiley & Sons Limited. Copyright Cochrane Library, reproduced with permission.

In absolute terms, there were four additional major extracranial haemorrhages for every 1000 patients treated (95% CI: 2–6 additional extracranial haemorrhages).

Deep vein thrombosis during the treatment period

Two trials (Pince, 1981; Turpie, 1983) including data from 133 randomised patients (only 0.3% of patients included in the overall review) sought to systematically determine the effect of antiplatelet agents on the occurrence of 'symptomatic or asymptomatic deep vein thrombosis (DVT)' at the end of the treatment period, as detected by I-125 fibrinogen scanning.

Random allocation to antiplatelet treatment was associated with DVT in 16/67 (23.9%) patients, compared with 19/66 (28.8%) of those allocated to control (OR: 0.78, 95% CI: 0.36–1.67, $2P = 0.5$).

Symptomatic pulmonary embolism during the treatment period

Antiplatelet therapy was associated with a significant reduction in the odds of pulmonary embolism (OR: 0.71, 95% CI: 0.53–0.96, $2P = 0.03$) from 0.48%

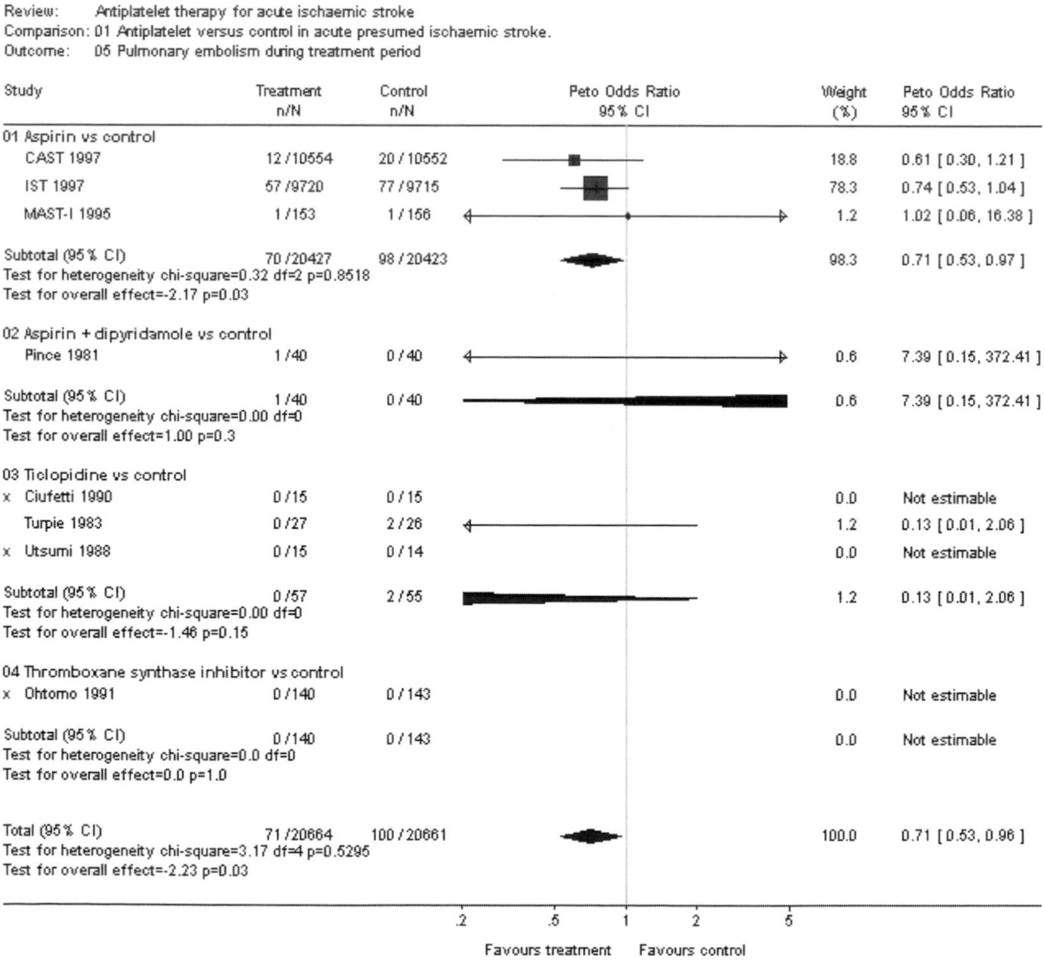

Review: Antiplatelet therapy for acute ischaemic stroke
Comparison: 01 Antiplatelet versus control in acute presumed ischaemic stroke.
Outcome: 05 Pulmonary embolism during treatment period

Study	Treatment n/N	Control n/N	Peto Odds Ratio 95% CI	Weight (%)	Peto Odds Ratio 95% CI
01 Aspirin vs control					
CAST 1997	12 /10554	20 / 10552		18.8	0.61 [0.30, 1.21]
IST 1997	57 /9720	77 /9715		78.3	0.74 [0.53, 1.04]
MAST-I 1995	1 /153	1 /156		1.2	1.02 [0.06, 16.38]
Subtotal (95% CI)	70 /20427	98 /20423		98.3	0.71 [0.53, 0.97]
Test for heterogeneity chi-square=0.32 df=2 p=0.8518					
Test for overall effect=-2.17 p=0.03					
02 Aspirin + dipyridamole vs control					
Pince 1981	1 /40	0 /40		0.6	7.39 [0.15, 372.41]
Subtotal (95% CI)	1 /40	0 /40		0.6	7.39 [0.15, 372.41]
Test for heterogeneity chi-square=0.00 df=0					
Test for overall effect=1.00 p=0.3					
03 Ticlopidine vs control					
x Ciufetti 1990	0 /15	0 /15		0.0	Not estimable
Turpie 1983	0 /27	2 /26		1.2	0.13 [0.01, 2.06]
x Utsumi 1988	0 /15	0 /14		0.0	Not estimable
Subtotal (95% CI)	0 /57	2 /55		1.2	0.13 [0.01, 2.06]
Test for heterogeneity chi-square=0.00 df=0					
Test for overall effect=-1.46 p=0.15					
04 Thromboxane synthase inhibitor vs control					
x Ohtomo 1991	0 /140	0 /143		0.0	Not estimable
Subtotal (95% CI)	0 /140	0 /143		0.0	Not estimable
Test for heterogeneity chi-square=0.0 df=0					
Test for overall effect=0.0 p=1.0					
Total (95% CI)	71 /20664	100 /20661		100.0	0.71 [0.53, 0.96]
Test for heterogeneity chi-square=3.17 df=4 p=0.5295					
Test for overall effect=-2.23 p=0.03					

.2   .5   1   2   5

Favours treatment   Favours control

Figure 10.7 Forest plot showing the effects of *any antiplatelet agent vs control* in acute ischaemic stroke *on pulmonary embolism during the treatment period.* Reproduced from Sandercock *et al.* (2003), with permission from the authors and John Wiley & Sons Limited. Copyright Cochrane Library, reproduced with permission.

(100/20,661) of patients assigned control to 0.34% (71/20,664) of patients assigned antiplatelet therapy (Fig. 10.7).

In absolute terms, one pulmonary embolism was avoided for every 1000 patients treated with antiplatelet agents (95% CI: 0–3 pulmonary emboli avoided). Since no trial sought pulmonary emboli systematically, the frequency of pulmonary embolism in treatment and control groups is likely to have been underestimated and the absolute benefit of antiplatelet therapy on pulmonary embolism underestimated.

Comment

Antiplatelet therapy with aspirin 160–300 mg daily, given orally (or per rectum in patients who cannot swallow), and started within 48 h of onset of presumed ischaemic stroke is associated with a small risk of bleeding (two extra symptomatic ICHs and four major extracranial haemorrhages for every 1000 patients treated), but the hazard is more than offset by the reduction in recurrent ischaemic stroke (7/1000) and pulmonary embolism (1/1000).

Overall, for every 1000 patients with acute ischaemic stroke who are treated early with aspirin, compared with no aspirin, there are 5 fewer early recurrent strokes of any type and, in the long term, 13 fewer patients who are dead or dependent. Among those who were alive and independent, an extra 10 make a complete recovery from their stroke, if they are given early aspirin rather than no aspirin (Table 10.1).

Indirect comparisons of different antiplatelet agents in this review showed no evidence of significant heterogeneity of effect among the different agents tested (aspirin alone, ticlopidine alone, the combination of aspirin and dipyridamole, and the Gp IIb/IIa inhibitor abciximab) but the data from the non-aspirin regimens were extremely limited, and such indirect comparisons are unreliable.

Table 10.1. Summary of the effects of antiplatelet therapy vs control in acute ischaemic stroke.

Outcome	OR	95% CI	Absolute risk difference (%)	95% CI
Death or dependency	**0.94**	0.91 to 0.98	**−1.3**	−0.4 to −2.2
Complete recovery	**1.06**	1.01 to 1.11	**+1.0**	+0.2 to +1.9
Death	**0.92**	0.87 to 0.98	**−0.8**	−0.2 to −1.4
Recurrent ischaemic stroke	**0.77**	0.69 to 0.87	**−0.7**	−0.4 to −1.0
Symptomatic ICH	**1.23**	1.0 to 1.5	**+0.2**	+0.0 to +0.4
Recurrent stroke of any type	**0.88**	0.79 to 0.97	**−0.5**	−0.1 to −0.9
Major ECH	**1.68**	1.34 to 2.09	**+0.4**	+0.2 to +0.6
DVT	**0.78**	0.36 to 1.67	**−4.9**	Not significant
PE	**0.71**	0.53 to 0.96	**−0.1**	−0.0 to −0.3

ICH: intracranial haemorrhage; ECH: extracranial haemorrhage; DVT: deep vein thrombosis;
PE: pulmonary embolism.

Nevertheless, the preliminary data from the first 200 patients with acute ischaemic stroke randomised to abciximab appear promising (AbESTT Investigators, 2005), and the results of the larger phase III trial of abciximab in acute ischaemic stroke are awaited (AbESTT-II) (see below; Adams, 2004).

Implications for practice

Aspirin 160–300 mg, should be given as soon as is possible (and continued as a once daily dose), in patients with suspected acute ischaemic stroke.

In patients who are unable to swallow safely, aspirin may be given per rectum as a suppository, or via a nasogastric tube, or intravenously (as 100 mg of the lysine salt of ASA).

For patients with known ICH or in whom ICH had not been ruled out by brain scanning before treatment was started, there is no evidence of net harm. Thus, if there is likely to be a delay before CT or magnetic resonance (MR) brain scanning can be performed to exclude ICH, it may be reasonable to give aspirin until the scan result is known. If the scan shows ICH, the aspirin should probably be discontinued. In patients with ICH who have a clear medical need to take aspirin (such as severe coronary heart disease), continuing aspirin may be justifiable.

In patients who cannot tolerate aspirin, an alternative antiplatelet agent should be considered, although the evidence for other agents is inadequate at present.

As the benefits of aspirin have been proven in the long-term secondary prevention of recurrent ischaemic stroke (see below), aspirin should be started even if a patient presents with stroke after 48 h. Treatment with aspirin should continue in hospital and after hospital discharge.

In view of the potential interaction, patients who have been treated with thrombolytic therapy should not be started on aspirin for 24–48 h.

Implications for research

The overall treatment effect of antiplatelet agents in acute ischaemic stroke is not large, and better acute therapies are therefore necessary. The question of whether any particular antiplatelet agent is superior to aspirin 160–300 mg in the treatment of acute ischaemic stroke remains to be determined, and would require a very large randomised trial to be answered reliably.

In patients with unstable coronary artery disease, trials have evaluated the addition of low-molecular-weight heparin or another antiplatelet agent (such as a Gp IIb/IIIa inhibitor or clopidogrel) to aspirin. There is a case for such trials to be undertaken in acute ischaemic stroke. A small study found that the combination of aspirin and a low-molecular-weight heparin (nadroparin) was not more effective than aspirin alone after stroke but it was underpowered to reliably identify or exclude a clinically important effect (Sarma and Roy, 2003).

The promising results of the phase IIb AbESTT trial (2003, 2005), in patients with a longer therapeutic window and a better safety profile than has been established with tissue plasminogen activator (tPA) within 3 h, has prompted a larger, currently ongoing, (phase III study of placebo vs abciximab 0.25 mg/kg bolus followed by a 12-h infusion of 0.125 µg/kg/min, 10 µg/min maximum), called the AbESTT-II trial, in a total of 1200 patients within 5 h, and another 600 patients between 5 and 6 h, of acute ischaemic stroke (Adams, 2004).

The results of the Management of AtheroThrombosis with Clopidogrel in High-risk patients with recent transient ischemic attack or ischemic stroke (MATCH) trial (Diener *et al.*, 2004; see below) have prompted researchers to call for a large randomised-controlled trial (RCT) testing the safety and efficacy of adding clopidogrel to aspirin immediately after TIA and ischaemic stroke (i.e. within 12–24 h, rather than 15 days), with a loading dose of clopidogrel (300 or 600 mg), in patients at high risk for early recurrent ischaemic stroke (e.g. with symptomatic large artery atherothromboembolism), and for a short period of about 3 months (when the benefits are likely to be greatest and the cumulative risks for bleeding lessened) (Hankey and Eikelboom, 2005).

There is also a case for further trials of low-dose subcutaneous heparin (or low-dose low-molecular-weight heparin) plus aspirin vs aspirin alone in the prevention of post-stroke DVT and pulmonary embolism (see Chapter 4), and in reducing neurological disability from the original or recurrent strokes. Such trials would need to include several tens of thousands of patients.

Anticoagulation vs antiplatelet therapy (in acute ischaemic stroke)

Evidence

A systematic review identified four RCTs involving a total of 16,558 patients which assessed (a) the effectiveness of anticoagulants compared with antiplatelet agents given within 14 days of onset of presumed or confirmed ischaemic stroke and (b) whether the addition of anticoagulants to antiplatelet agents offers any net advantage over antiplatelet agents alone (Berge and Sandercock, 2001, 2003).

The methodological quality was high in all four trials.

The anticoagulants tested were unfractionated heparin (UFH) and low-molecular-weight heparin. Aspirin was used as control in all trials.

Death or dependency

There was no evidence that anticoagulants were superior to aspirin in reducing death or dependency at long-term follow-up. Indeed, anticoagulation was associated

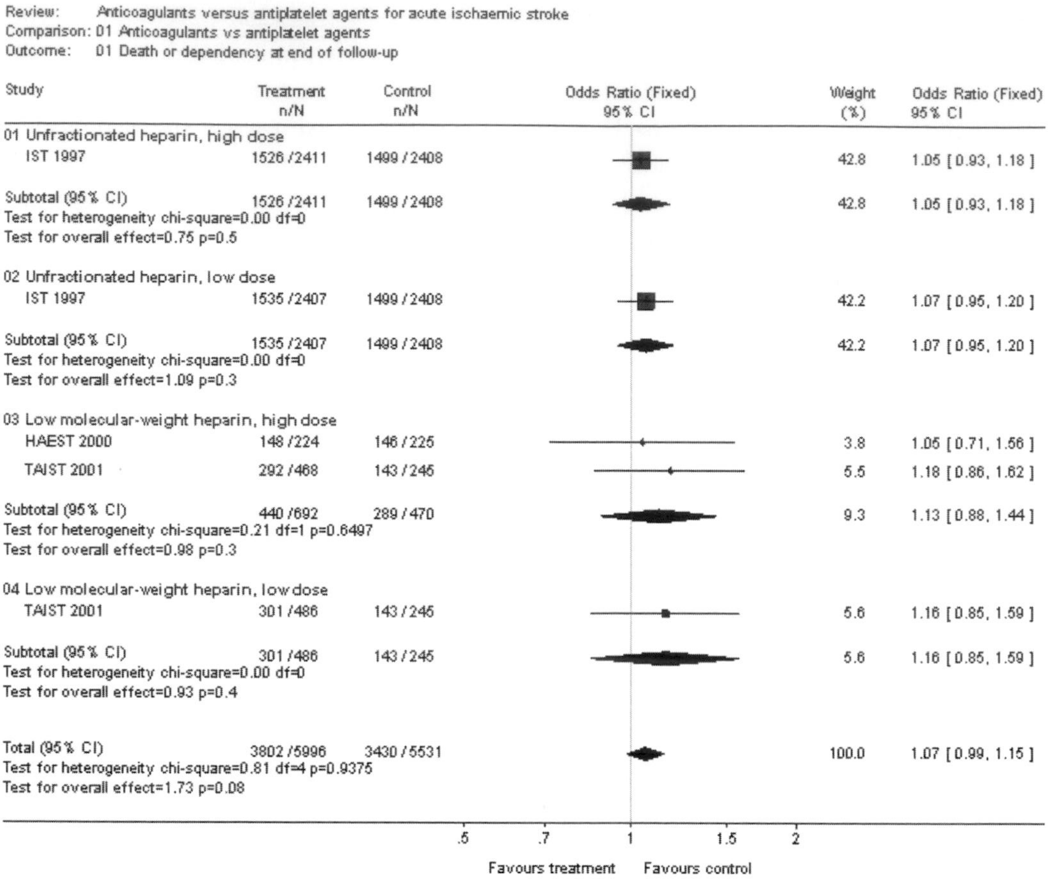

Review: Anticoagulants versus antiplatelet agents for acute ischaemic stroke
Comparison: 01 Anticoagulants vs antiplatelet agents
Outcome: 01 Death or dependency at end of follow-up

Study	Treatment n/N	Control n/N	Odds Ratio (Fixed) 95% CI	Weight (%)	Odds Ratio (Fixed) 95% CI
01 Unfractionated heparin, high dose					
IST 1997	1526 /2411	1499 /2408		42.8	1.05 [0.93, 1.18]
Subtotal (95% CI)	1526 /2411	1499 /2408		42.8	1.05 [0.93, 1.18]
Test for heterogeneity chi-square=0.00 df=0					
Test for overall effect=0.75 p=0.5					
02 Unfractionated heparin, low dose					
IST 1997	1535 /2407	1499 /2408		42.2	1.07 [0.95, 1.20]
Subtotal (95% CI)	1535 /2407	1499 /2408		42.2	1.07 [0.95, 1.20]
Test for heterogeneity chi-square=0.00 df=0					
Test for overall effect=1.09 p=0.3					
03 Low molecular-weight heparin, high dose					
HAEST 2000	148 /224	146 /225		3.8	1.05 [0.71, 1.56]
TAIST 2001	292 /468	143 /245		5.5	1.18 [0.86, 1.62]
Subtotal (95% CI)	440 /692	289 /470		9.3	1.13 [0.88, 1.44]
Test for heterogeneity chi-square=0.21 df=1 p=0.6497					
Test for overall effect=0.98 p=0.3					
04 Low molecular-weight heparin, low dose					
TAIST 2001	301 /486	143 /245		5.6	1.16 [0.85, 1.59]
Subtotal (95% CI)	301 /486	143 /245		5.6	1.16 [0.85, 1.59]
Test for heterogeneity chi-square=0.00 df=0					
Test for overall effect=0.93 p=0.4					
Total (95% CI)	3802 /5996	3430 /5531		100.0	1.07 [0.99, 1.15]
Test for heterogeneity chi-square=0.81 df=4 p=0.9375					
Test for overall effect=1.73 p=0.08					

.5   .7   1   1.5   2

Favours treatment   Favours control

Figure 10.8   Forest plot showing the effects of *anticoagulants vs antiplatelet agents* in acute ischaemic stroke *on death or dependency at the end of follow-up*. Reproduced from Berge and Sandercock (2001), with permission from the authors and John Wiley & Sons Limited. Copyright Cochrane Library, reproduced with permission.

with a non-significantly higher rate of death or dependency (63.4%; 3802/5996) compared with antiplatelet therapy (62.0%; 3430/5531); OR: 1.07, 95% CI: 0.99–1.15 (Fig. 10.8).

Death

Compared with aspirin, anticoagulants were associated with a small but significant increase in the number of deaths at the end of follow-up (OR: 1.10, 95% CI: 1.01–1.21), equivalent to 20 more deaths (95% CI: 0–30) per 1000 patients treated (Fig. 10.9).

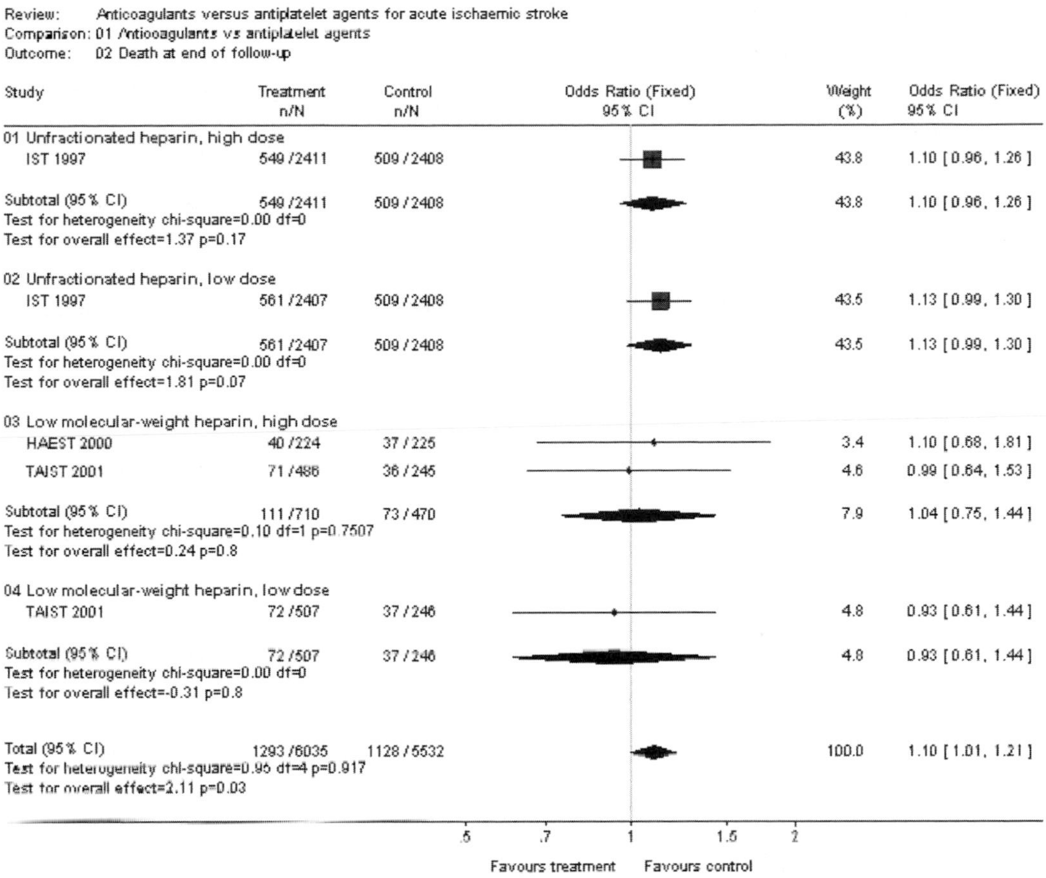

Review: Anticoagulants versus antiplatelet agents for acute ischaemic stroke
Comparison: 01 Anticoagulants vs antiplatelet agents
Outcome: 02 Death at end of follow-up

Study	Treatment n/N	Control n/N	Odds Ratio (Fixed) 95% CI	Weight (%)	Odds Ratio (Fixed) 95% CI
01 Unfractionated heparin, high dose					
IST 1997	549 /2411	509 / 2408		43.8	1.10 [0.96, 1.26]
Subtotal (95% CI)	549 /2411	509 / 2408		43.8	1.10 [0.96, 1.26]
Test for heterogeneity chi-square=0.00 df=0					
Test for overall effect=1.37 p=0.17					
02 Unfractionated heparin, low dose					
IST 1997	561 /2407	509 / 2408		43.5	1.13 [0.99, 1.30]
Subtotal (95% CI)	561 /2407	509 / 2408		43.5	1.13 [0.99, 1.30]
Test for heterogeneity chi-square=0.00 df=0					
Test for overall effect=1.81 p=0.07					
03 Low molecular-weight heparin, high dose					
HAEST 2000	40 /224	37 / 225		3.4	1.10 [0.68, 1.81]
TAIST 2001	71 /486	36 / 245		4.6	0.99 [0.64, 1.53]
Subtotal (95% CI)	111 /710	73 / 470		7.9	1.04 [0.75, 1.44]
Test for heterogeneity chi-square=0.10 df=1 p=0.7507					
Test for overall effect=0.24 p=0.8					
04 Low molecular-weight heparin, low dose					
TAIST 2001	72 /507	37 / 246		4.8	0.93 [0.61, 1.44]
Subtotal (95% CI)	72 /507	37 / 246		4.8	0.93 [0.61, 1.44]
Test for heterogeneity chi-square=0.00 df=0					
Test for overall effect=-0.31 p=0.8					
Total (95% CI)	1293 /6035	1128 / 5532		100.0	1.10 [1.01, 1.21]
Test for heterogeneity chi-square=0.95 df=4 p=0.917					
Test for overall effect=2.11 p=0.03					

| .5   .7   1   1.5   2 |

Favours treatment   Favours control

Figure 10.9   Forest plot showing the effects of *anticoagulants vs antiplatelet agents* in acute ischaemic stroke *on death at the end of follow-up*. Reproduced from Berge and Sandercock (2001), with permission from the authors and John Wiley & Sons Limited. Copyright Cochrane Library, reproduced with permission.

Recurrent ischaemic stroke

The risk of recurrent stroke of ischaemic or unknown type was not significantly different between patients randomly assigned anticoagulation and aspirin (OR: 1.09, 95% CI: 0.89–1.33) (Fig. 10.10).

Symptomatic intracranial haemorrhage (ICH)

Allocation to anticoagulation was associated with a significant increased risk of symptomatic ICH (1.2%) compared with aspirin (0.6%) (OR: 2.27, 95% CI: 1.49–3.46) (Fig. 10.11).

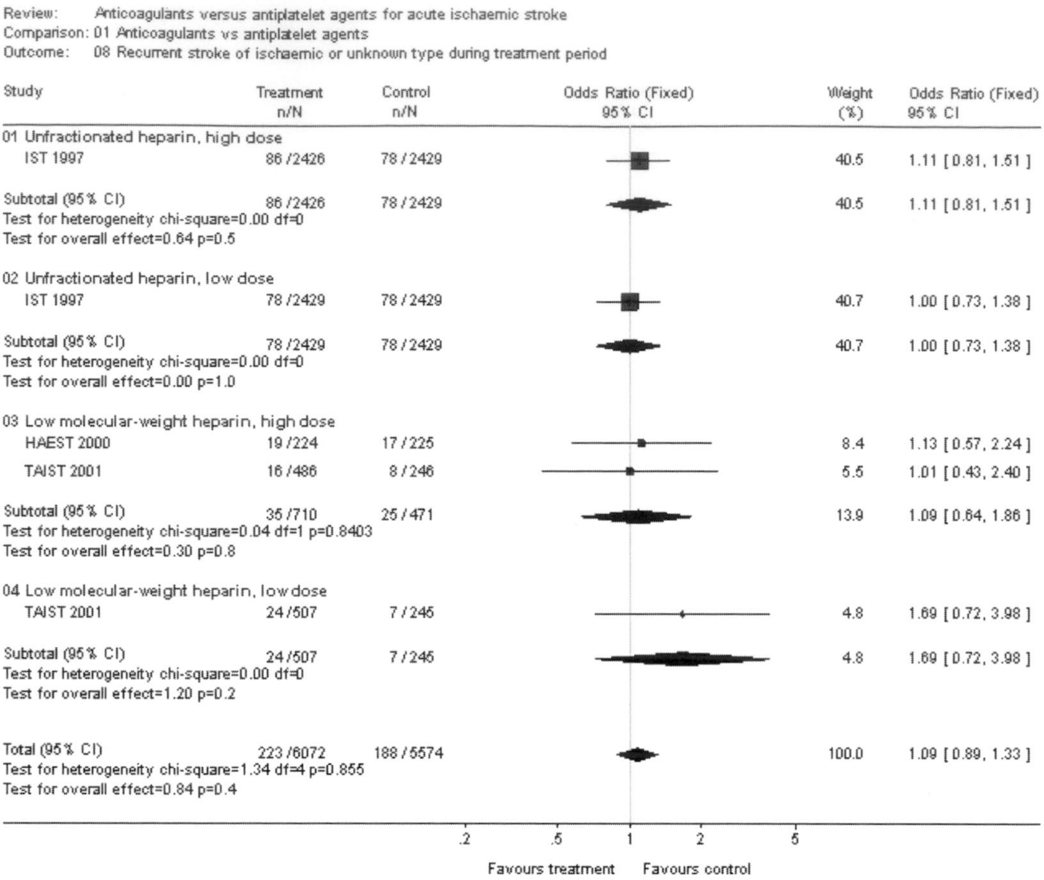

Review: Anticoagulants versus antiplatelet agents for acute ischaemic stroke
Comparison: 01 Anticoagulants vs antiplatelet agents
Outcome: 08 Recurrent stroke of ischaemic or unknown type during treatment period

Study	Treatment n/N	Control n/N	Odds Ratio (Fixed) 95% CI	Weight (%)	Odds Ratio (Fixed) 95% CI
01 Unfractionated heparin, high dose					
IST 1997	86 /2426	78 / 2429		40.5	1.11 [0.81, 1.51]
Subtotal (95% CI)	86 /2426	78 / 2429		40.5	1.11 [0.81, 1.51]
Test for heterogeneity chi-square=0.00 df=0					
Test for overall effect=0.64 p=0.5					
02 Unfractionated heparin, low dose					
IST 1997	78 /2429	78 / 2429		40.7	1.00 [0.73, 1.38]
Subtotal (95% CI)	78 /2429	78 / 2429		40.7	1.00 [0.73, 1.38]
Test for heterogeneity chi-square=0.00 df=0					
Test for overall effect=0.00 p=1.0					
03 Low molecular-weight heparin, high dose					
HAEST 2000	19 /224	17 / 225		8.4	1.13 [0.57, 2.24]
TAIST 2001	16 /486	8 / 246		5.5	1.01 [0.43, 2.40]
Subtotal (95% CI)	35 /710	25 / 471		13.9	1.09 [0.64, 1.86]
Test for heterogeneity chi-square=0.04 df=1 p=0.8403					
Test for overall effect=0.30 p=0.8					
04 Low molecular-weight heparin, low dose					
TAIST 2001	24 /507	7 / 246		4.8	1.69 [0.72, 3.98]
Subtotal (95% CI)	24 /507	7 / 246		4.8	1.69 [0.72, 3.98]
Test for heterogeneity chi-square=0.00 df=0					
Test for overall effect=1.20 p=0.2					
Total (95% CI)	223 /6072	188 / 5574		100.0	1.09 [0.89, 1.33]
Test for heterogeneity chi-square=1.34 df=4 p=0.855					
Test for overall effect=0.84 p=0.4					

```
        .2      .5       1       2       5
      Favours treatment    Favours control
```

Figure 10.10 Forest plot showing the effects of *anticoagulants vs antiplatelet agents* in acute ischaemic stroke *on recurrent stroke of ischaemic or unknown type at the end of follow-up*. Reproduced from Berge and Sandercock (2001), with permission from the authors and John Wiley & Sons Limited. Copyright Cochrane Library, reproduced with permission.

Recurrent stroke of any type (ischaemic or haemorrhagic)

Anticoagulation was associated with a non-significant increased odds of 'any recurrent stroke' during the treatment period (OR: 1.20, 95% CI: 0.99–1.46) (Fig. 10.12).

DVT and pulmonary embolism

Anticoagulants were associated with a significant reduction in DVT (OR: 0.19, 95% CI: 0.07–0.58) from 1.8% (13/716) with antiplatelet drugs to 0.3% (4/1217) with anticoagulation (Fig. 10.13), equivalent to 15 fewer (95% CI: 0–30) DVTs by 14 days per 1000 patients treated with anticoagulants instead of aspirin. However,

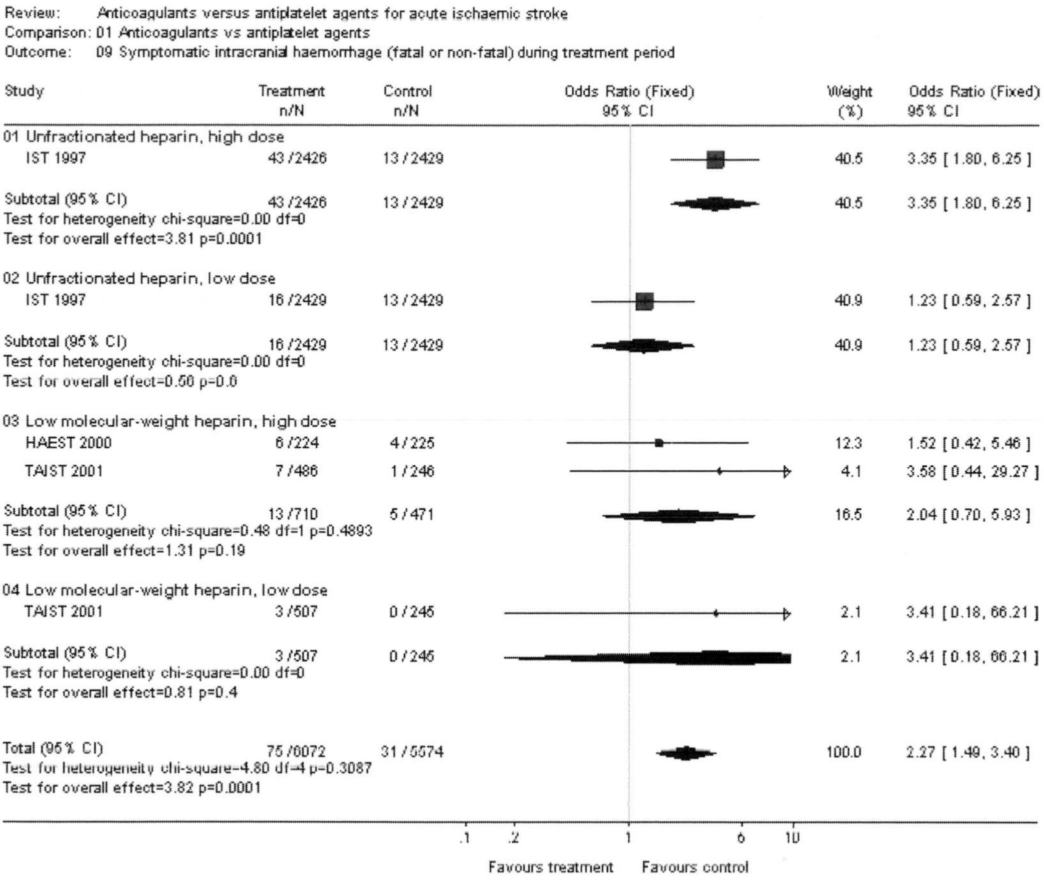

Review: Anticoagulants versus antiplatelet agents for acute ischaemic stroke
Comparison: 01 Anticoagulants vs antiplatelet agents
Outcome: 09 Symptomatic intracranial haemorrhage (fatal or non-fatal) during treatment period

Study	Treatment n/N	Control n/N	Odds Ratio (Fixed) 95% CI	Weight (%)	Odds Ratio (Fixed) 95% CI
01 Unfractionated heparin, high dose					
IST 1997	43 /2426	13 /2429		40.5	3.35 [1.80, 6.25]
Subtotal (95% CI)	43 /2426	13 /2429		40.5	3.35 [1.80, 6.25]
Test for heterogeneity chi-square=0.00 df=0					
Test for overall effect=3.81 p=0.0001					
02 Unfractionated heparin, low dose					
IST 1997	16 /2429	13 /2429		40.9	1.23 [0.59, 2.57]
Subtotal (95% CI)	16 /2429	13 /2429		40.9	1.23 [0.59, 2.57]
Test for heterogeneity chi-square=0.00 df=0					
Test for overall effect=0.50 p=0.6					
03 Low molecular-weight heparin, high dose					
HAEST 2000	6 /224	4 /225		12.3	1.52 [0.42, 5.46]
TAIST 2001	7 /486	1 /246		4.1	3.58 [0.44, 29.27]
Subtotal (95% CI)	13 /710	5 /471		16.5	2.04 [0.70, 5.93]
Test for heterogeneity chi-square=0.48 df=1 p=0.4893					
Test for overall effect=1.31 p=0.19					
04 Low molecular-weight heparin, low dose					
TAIST 2001	3 /507	0 /246		2.1	3.41 [0.18, 66.21]
Subtotal (95% CI)	3 /507	0 /246		2.1	3.41 [0.18, 66.21]
Test for heterogeneity chi-square=0.00 df=0					
Test for overall effect=0.81 p=0.4					
Total (95% CI)	75 /6072	31 /5574		100.0	2.27 [1.49, 3.40]
Test for heterogeneity chi-square=4.80 df=4 p=0.3087					
Test for overall effect=3.82 p=0.0001					

.1   .2   1   5   10

Favours treatment   Favours control

Figure 10.11 Forest plot showing the effects of *anticoagulants vs antiplatelet agents* in acute ischaemic stroke *on symptomatic ICH during the treatment period*. Reproduced from Berge and Sandercock (2004), with permission from the authors and John Wiley & Sons Limited. Copyright Cochrane Library, reproduced with permission.

there was no significant reduction in pulmonary embolism (OR: 0.85; 95% CI: 0.55–1.32)(Fig. 10.14).

Major extracranial haemorrhage
Anticoagulation was associated with a significant increase in major extracranial haemorrhagic during the treatment period (0.9%) compared with aspirin (0.4%) (OR: 1.94, 95% CI: 1.20–3.12) (Fig. 10.15).

Comment

Anticoagulants offer no net advantages over antiplatelet drugs in acute ischaemic stroke despite lower rates of DVT (Table 10.2).

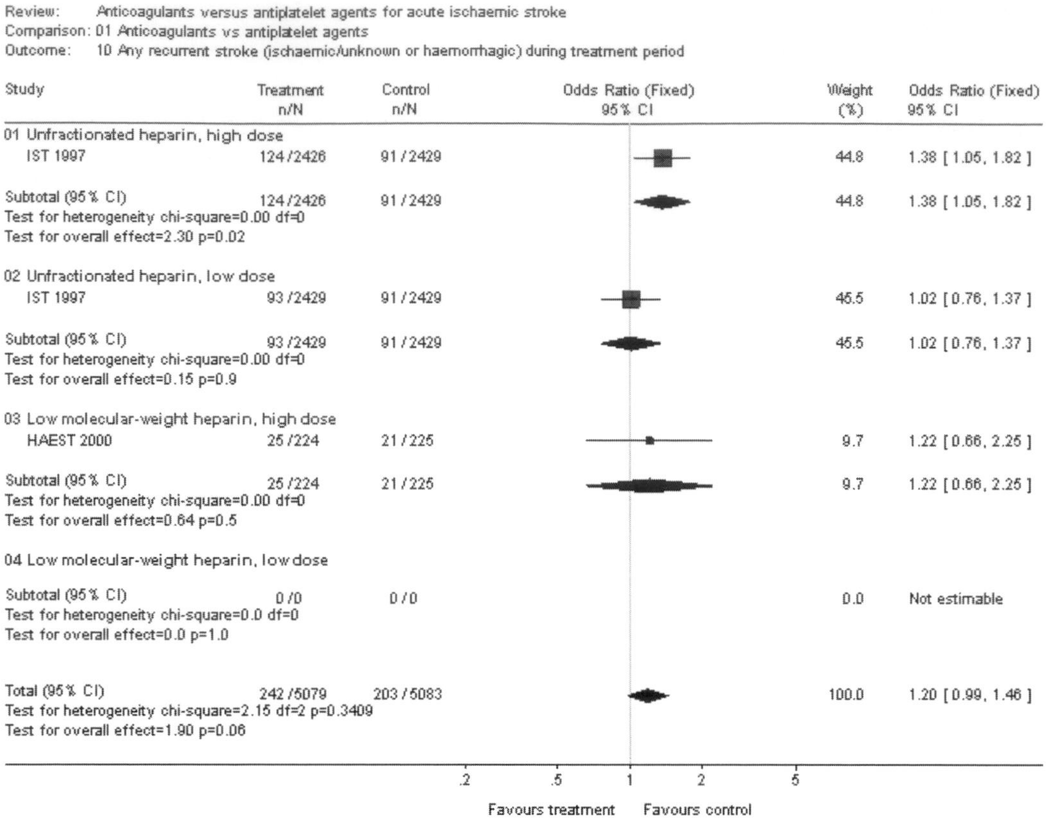

Review: Anticoagulants versus antiplatelet agents for acute ischaemic stroke
Comparison: 01 Anticoagulants vs antiplatelet agents
Outcome: 10 Any recurrent stroke (ischaemic/unknown or haemorrhagic) during treatment period

Study	Treatment n/N	Control n/N	Odds Ratio (Fixed) 95% CI	Weight (%)	Odds Ratio (Fixed) 95% CI
01 Unfractionated heparin, high dose					
IST 1997	124/2426	91/2429		44.8	1.38 [1.05, 1.82]
Subtotal (95% CI)	124/2426	91/2429		44.8	1.38 [1.05, 1.82]
Test for heterogeneity chi-square=0.00 df=0					
Test for overall effect=2.30 p=0.02					
02 Unfractionated heparin, low dose					
IST 1997	93/2429	91/2429		45.5	1.02 [0.76, 1.37]
Subtotal (95% CI)	93/2429	91/2429		45.5	1.02 [0.76, 1.37]
Test for heterogeneity chi-square=0.00 df=0					
Test for overall effect=0.15 p=0.9					
03 Low molecular-weight heparin, high dose					
HAEST 2000	25/224	21/225		9.7	1.22 [0.66, 2.25]
Subtotal (95% CI)	25/224	21/225		9.7	1.22 [0.66, 2.25]
Test for heterogeneity chi-square=0.00 df=0					
Test for overall effect=0.64 p=0.5					
04 Low molecular-weight heparin, low dose					
Subtotal (95% CI)	0/0	0/0		0.0	Not estimable
Test for heterogeneity chi-square=0.0 df=0					
Test for overall effect=0.0 p=1.0					
Total (95% CI)	242/5079	203/5083		100.0	1.20 [0.99, 1.46]
Test for heterogeneity chi-square=2.15 df=2 p=0.3409					
Test for overall effect=1.90 p=0.06					

```
          .2      .5      1       2       5
          Favours treatment   Favours control
```

Figure 10.12 Forest plot showing the effects of *anticoagulants vs antiplatelet agents* in acute ischaemic stroke *on any recurrent stroke during the treatment period*. Reproduced from Berge and Sandercock (2001), with permission from the authors and John Wiley & Sons Limited. Copyright Cochrane Library, reproduced with permission.

Low-dose unfractionated heparin (UFH) plus aspirin vs aspirin

Evidence

A subgroup analysis showed that, compared with aspirin, the combination of low-dose UFH and aspirin for patients with acute ischaemic stroke was associated with a non-significant trend towards a reduced risk of 'any recurrent stroke' at the end of the treatment period (OR: 0.75, 95% CI: 0.55–1.03) (Fig. 10.16) and early death at 14 days (OR: 0.84, 95% CI: 0.69–1.03) (Fig. 10.17), but no clear benefit on death at end of follow-up (OR: 0.98, 95% CI: 0.85–1.12) (Fig. 10.18) (Berge and Sandercock, 2001, 2003).

Indirect comparisons indicated that low-dose UFH is associated with lower rates of bleeding than high doses (Figs 10.19 and 10.20).

Since this review, a small trial of nadroparin plus aspirin, compared with aspirin alone, has been published but the trial was underpowered to reliably identify or

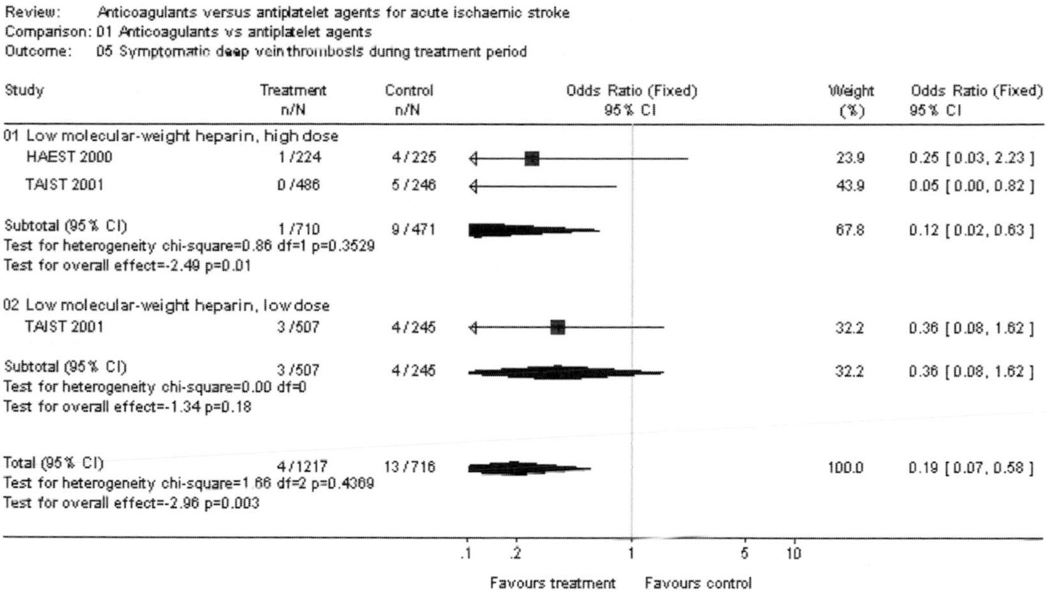

Review: Anticoagulants versus antiplatelet agents for acute ischaemic stroke
Comparison: 01 Anticoagulants vs antiplatelet agents
Outcome: 05 Symptomatic deep vein thrombosis during treatment period

Study	Treatment n/N	Control n/N	Odds Ratio (Fixed) 95% CI	Weight (%)	Odds Ratio (Fixed) 95% CI
01 Low molecular-weight heparin, high dose					
HAEST 2000	1 /224	4 /225		23.9	0.25 [0.03, 2.23]
TAIST 2001	0 /486	5 /246		43.9	0.05 [0.00, 0.82]
Subtotal (95% CI)	1 /710	9 /471		67.8	0.12 [0.02, 0.63]
Test for heterogeneity chi-square=0.86 df=1 p=0.3529					
Test for overall effect=-2.49 p=0.01					
02 Low molecular-weight heparin, low dose					
TAIST 2001	3 /507	4 /245		32.2	0.36 [0.08, 1.62]
Subtotal (95% CI)	3 /507	4 /245		32.2	0.36 [0.08, 1.62]
Test for heterogeneity chi-square=0.00 df=0					
Test for overall effect=-1.34 p=0.18					
Total (95% CI)	4 /1217	13 /716		100.0	0.19 [0.07, 0.58]
Test for heterogeneity chi-square=1.66 df=2 p=0.4369					
Test for overall effect=-2.96 p=0.003					

.1 .2 1 5 10
Favours treatment   Favours control

Figure 10.13 Forest plot showing the effects of *anticoagulants vs antiplatelet agents* in acute ischaemic stroke *on DVT during the treatment period*. Reproduced from Berge and Sandercock (2001), with permission from the authors and John Wiley & Sons Limited. Copyright Cochrane Library, reproduced with permission.

exclude a modest, but clinically important effect of treatment (Sarma and Roy, 2003).

Comment

The combination of low-dose UFH and aspirin appears to be associated with a trend towards net benefits compared with aspirin alone (Table 10.3), and this merits further research.

Longer-term secondary prevention

Aspirin vs control

Evidence

Efficacy
High vascular risk patients   Among patients at high vascular risk (past history of stroke, myocardial infarction (MI), peripheral arterial disease or diabetes), aspirin reduced the relative risk (RR) of the composite outcome of stroke, MI or death due to vascular causes (serious vascular events) by about 19% (95% CI: 15–23%) compared with placebo (Antithrombotic Trialists' Collaboration, 2002).

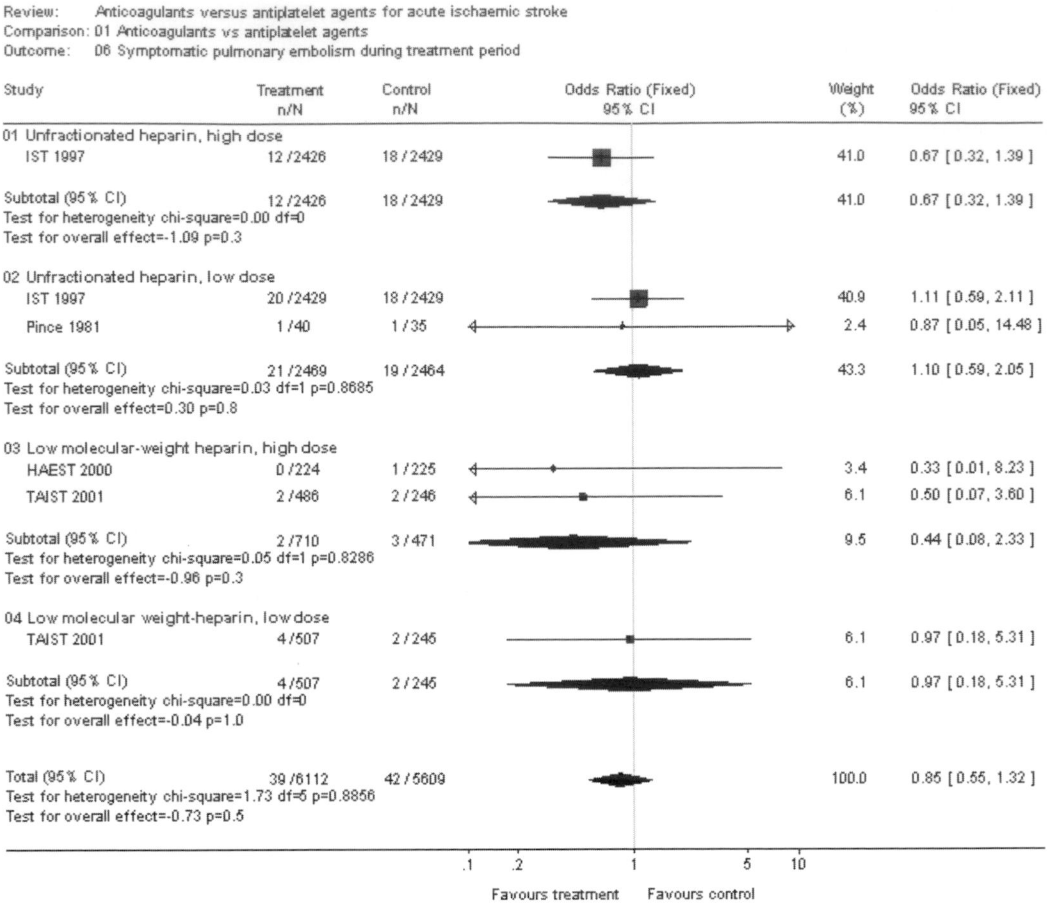

Review: Anticoagulants versus antiplatelet agents for acute ischaemic stroke
Comparison: 01 Anticoagulants vs antiplatelet agents
Outcome: 06 Symptomatic pulmonary embolism during treatment period

Study	Treatment n/N	Control n/N	Odds Ratio (Fixed) 95% CI	Weight (%)	Odds Ratio (Fixed) 95% CI
01 Unfractionated heparin, high dose					
IST 1997	12 /2426	18 /2429		41.0	0.67 [0.32, 1.39]
Subtotal (95% CI)	12 /2426	18 /2429		41.0	0.67 [0.32, 1.39]
Test for heterogeneity chi-square=0.00 df=0					
Test for overall effect=-1.09 p=0.3					
02 Unfractionated heparin, low dose					
IST 1997	20 /2429	18 /2429		40.9	1.11 [0.59, 2.11]
Pince 1981	1 /40	1 /35		2.4	0.87 [0.05, 14.48]
Subtotal (95% CI)	21 /2469	19 /2464		43.3	1.10 [0.59, 2.05]
Test for heterogeneity chi-square=0.03 df=1 p=0.8685					
Test for overall effect=0.30 p=0.8					
03 Low molecular-weight heparin, high dose					
HAEST 2000	0 /224	1 /225		3.4	0.33 [0.01, 8.23]
TAIST 2001	2 /486	2 /246		6.1	0.50 [0.07, 3.60]
Subtotal (95% CI)	2 /710	3 /471		9.5	0.44 [0.08, 2.33]
Test for heterogeneity chi-square=0.05 df=1 p=0.8286					
Test for overall effect=-0.96 p=0.3					
04 Low molecular weight-heparin, low dose					
TAIST 2001	4 /507	2 /245		6.1	0.97 [0.18, 5.31]
Subtotal (95% CI)	4 /507	2 /245		6.1	0.97 [0.18, 5.31]
Test for heterogeneity chi-square=0.00 df=0					
Test for overall effect=-0.04 p=1.0					
Total (95% CI)	39 /6112	42 /5609		100.0	0.85 [0.55, 1.32]
Test for heterogeneity chi-square=1.73 df=5 p=0.8856					
Test for overall effect=-0.73 p=0.5					

.1   .2   1   5   10

Favours treatment   Favours control

Figure 10.14 Forest plot showing the effects of *anticoagulants vs antiplatelet agents* in acute ischaemic stroke *on pulmonary embolism during the treatment period*. Reproduced from Berge and Sandercock (2004), with permission from the authors and John Wiley & Sons Limited. Copyright Cochrane Library, reproduced with permission.

TIA and ischaemic stroke patients   A systematic review of 11 RCTs of aspirin vs control in about 10,000 patients with previous stroke or TIA revealed that long-term aspirin therapy reduced the RR of recurrent serious vascular events by about 13% (95% CI: 6–19%) compared with placebo, from 22% (placebo) to 19% (aspirin) over 3 years (Fig. 10.21) (Algra and van Gijn, 1999). This corresponds to an absolute reduction in risk of serious vascular events of 30/1000 over about 3 years or about 10/1000 (1%) per year (Algra and van Gijn, 1999; Antithrombotic Trialists' Collaboration, 2002).

The more modest, but nevertheless consistent, relative effect of aspirin in patients with TIA and ischaemic stroke compared with all high-risk patients may

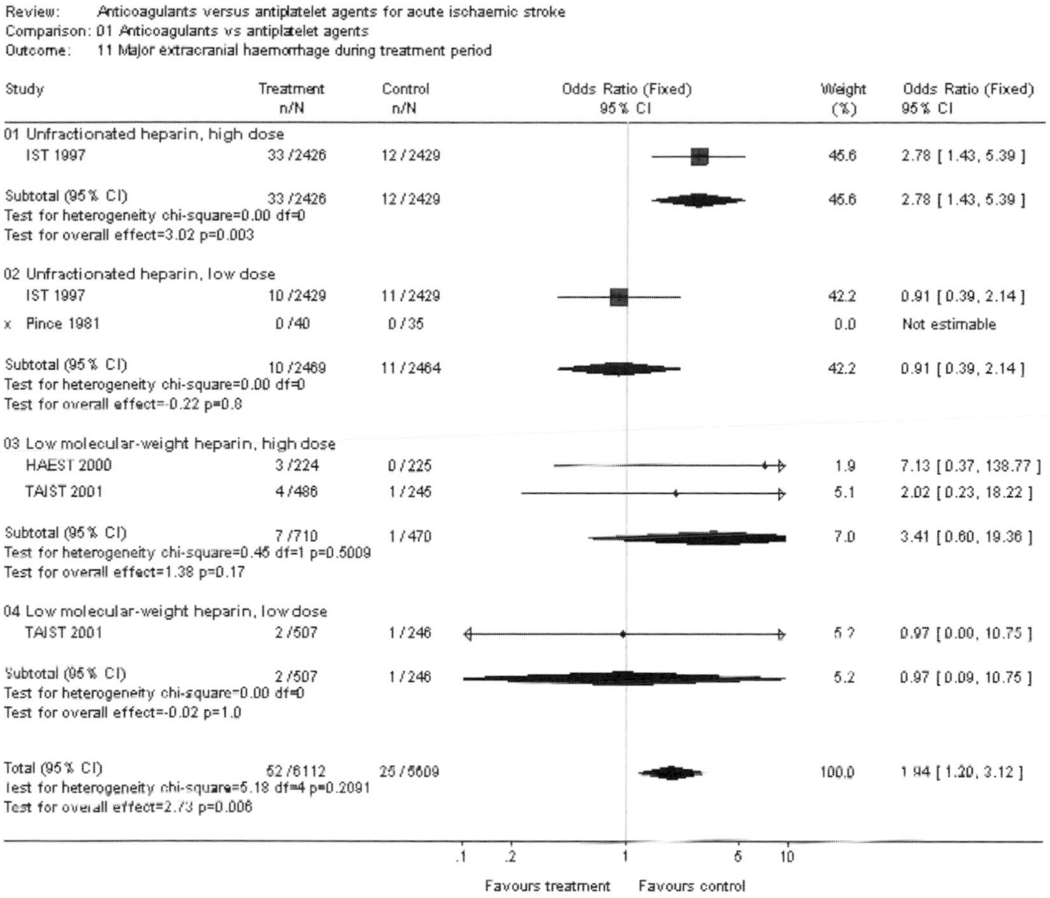

Review: Anticoagulants versus antiplatelet agents for acute ischaemic stroke
Comparison: 01 Anticoagulants vs antiplatelet agents
Outcome: 11 Major extracranial haemorrhage during treatment period

Study	Treatment n/N	Control n/N	Odds Ratio (Fixed) 95% CI	Weight (%)	Odds Ratio (Fixed) 95% CI
01 Unfractionated heparin, high dose					
IST 1997	33 /2426	12 /2429		45.6	2.78 [1.43, 5.39]
Subtotal (95% CI)	33 /2426	12 /2429		45.6	2.78 [1.43, 5.39]
Test for heterogeneity chi-square=0.00 df=0					
Test for overall effect=3.02 p=0.003					
02 Unfractionated heparin, low dose					
IST 1997	10 /2429	11 /2429		42.2	0.91 [0.39, 2.14]
x Pince 1981	0 /40	0 /35		0.0	Not estimable
Subtotal (95% CI)	10 /2469	11 /2464		42.2	0.91 [0.39, 2.14]
Test for heterogeneity chi-square=0.00 df=0					
Test for overall effect=-0.22 p=0.8					
03 Low molecular-weight heparin, high dose					
HAEST 2000	3 /224	0 /225		1.9	7.13 [0.37, 138.77]
TAIST 2001	4 /486	1 /245		5.1	2.02 [0.23, 18.22]
Subtotal (95% CI)	7 /710	1 /470		7.0	3.41 [0.60, 19.38]
Test for heterogeneity chi-square=0.45 df=1 p=0.5009					
Test for overall effect=1.38 p=0.17					
04 Low molecular-weight heparin, low dose					
TAIST 2001	2 /507	1 /246		5.2	0.97 [0.09, 10.75]
Subtotal (95% CI)	2 /507	1 /246		5.2	0.97 [0.09, 10.75]
Test for heterogeneity chi-square=0.00 df=0					
Test for overall effect=-0.02 p=1.0					
Total (95% CI)	52 /6112	25 /5609		100.0	1.94 [1.20, 3.12]
Test for heterogeneity chi-square=6.18 df=4 p=0.2091					
Test for overall effect=2.73 p=0.006					

```
        .1     .2          1          5    10
           Favours treatment    Favours control
```

Figure 10.15 Forest plot showing the effects of *anticoagulants vs antiplatelet agents* in acute ischaemic stroke *on major extracranial haemorrhage during the treatment period*. Reproduced from Berge and Sandercock (2001), with permission from the authors and John Wiley & Sons Limited. Copyright Cochrane Library, reproduced with permission.

reflect the aetiological heterogeneity of stroke (e.g. atherothrombosis, cardiogenic embolism, arterial dissection) or random error.

Adverse effects

Aspirin was associated with a dose-dependent excess of upper-gastrointestinal (GI) upset, and about a 60–70% relative excess of non-fatal extracranial haemorrhage (0.3%: no aspirin, 0.5%: aspirin, per year), which was mostly from the GI tract. This corresponds to an absolute excess risk of about 2/1000 patients treated per year and an increased risk of ICH of about 1/1000 patients treated for 3 years (He *et al.*, 1998; Derry and Loke, 2000; Antithrombotic Trialists' Collaboration, 2002; Serebruany *et al.*, 2004).

Table 10.2. Summary of the effects of anticoagulation vs antiplatelet therapy in acute ischaemic stroke.

Outcome	OR	95% CI	Absolute risk difference	95% CI
Death or dependency	**1.07**	0.99 to 1.15	**+1.4%**	+0.0 to 2.6
Death	**1.10**	1.01 to 1.29	**+2.0%**	+0.0 to 3.0
Recurrent ischaemic stroke	**1.09**	0.89 to 1.33	**No significant difference**	
Symptomatic ICH	**2.27**	1.49 to 3.46	**+0.6%**	
Recurrent stroke of any type	**1.20**	0.99 to 1.46	**No significant difference**	
Major ECH	**1.94**	1.20 to 3.12	**+0.5%**	
DVT	**0.19**	0.07 to 0.58	**−1.5%**	−0.0 to −3.0
PE	**0.85**	0.55 to 1.32	**No significant difference**	

ECH: extracranial haemorrhage; PE: pulmonary embolism.

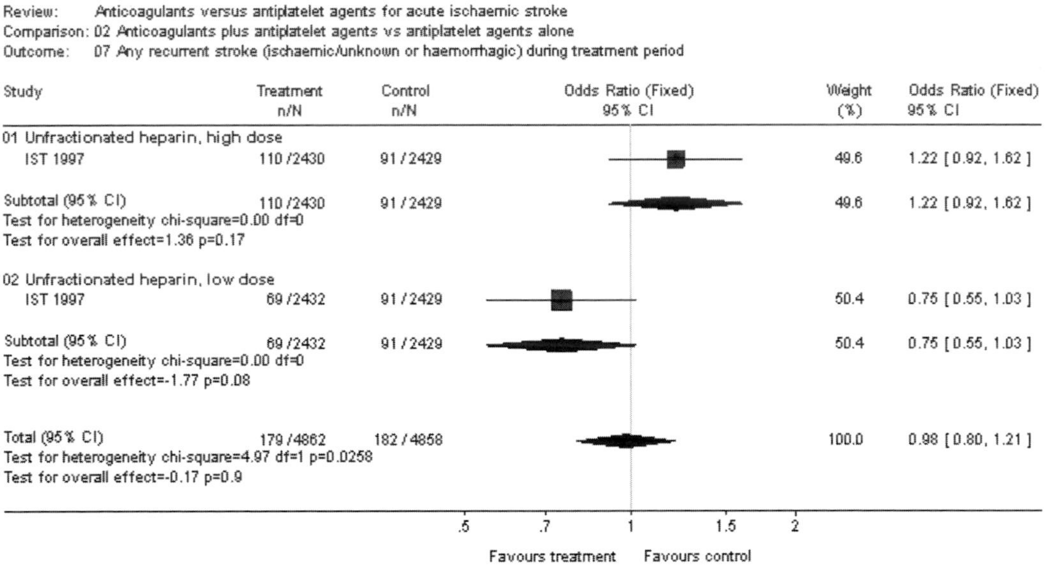

Figure 10.16   Forest plot showing the effects of *the combination of anticoagulation and aspirin vs aspirin* in acute ischaemic stroke *on stroke of any type during the treatment period.* Reproduced from Berge and Sandercock (2001), with permission from the authors and John Wiley & Sons Limited. Copyright Cochrane Library, reproduced with permission.

Dipyridamole vs control

Evidence

Efficacy
High vascular risk patients   Among high vascular risk patients, dipyridamole significantly reduced the RR of serious vascular events by about 10% (95% CI: 2–17%)

Review: Anticoagulants versus antiplatelet agents for acute ischaemic stroke
Comparison: 02 Anticoagulants plus antiplatelet agents vs antiplatelet agents alone
Outcome: 03 Death at end of treatment period

Study	Treatment n/N	Control n/N	Odds Ratio (Fixed) 95% CI	Weight (%)	Odds Ratio (Fixed) 95% CI
01 Unfractionated heparin, high dose					
IST 1997	226 /2430	226 /2429		49.6	1.00 [0.82, 1.21]
Subtotal (95% CI)	226 /2430	226 /2429		49.6	1.00 [0.82, 1.21]
Test for heterogeneity chi-square=0.00 df=0					
Test for overall effect=0.00 p=1.0					
02 Unfractionated heparin, low dose					
IST 1997	194 /2432	226 /2429		50.4	0.84 [0.69, 1.03]
Subtotal (95% CI)	194 /2432	226 /2429		50.4	0.84 [0.69, 1.03]
Test for heterogeneity chi-square=0.00 df=0					
Test for overall effect=-1.65 p=0.1					
Total (95% CI)	420 /4862	452 /4858		100.0	0.92 [0.80, 1.06]
Test for heterogeneity chi-square=1.39 df=1 p=0.2377					
Test for overall effect=-1.15 p=0.3					

```
        .5        .7        1        1.5        2
        Favours treatment    Favours control
```

Figure 10.17 Forest plot showing the effects of *the combination of anticoagulation and aspirin vs aspirin* in acute ischaemic stroke *on death at the end of the treatment period*. Reproduced from Berge and Sandercock (2001), with permission from the authors and John Wiley & Sons Limited. Copyright Cochrane Library, reproduced with permission.

Review: Anticoagulants versus antiplatelet agents for acute ischaemic stroke
Comparison: 02 Anticoagulants plus antiplatelet agents vs antiplatelet agents alone
Outcome: 02 Death at end of follow-up

Study	Treatment n/N	Control n/N	Odds Ratio (Fixed) 95% CI	Weight (%)	Odds Ratio (Fixed) 95% CI
01 Unfractionated heparin, high dose					
IST 1997	554 /2413	509 /2408		49.3	1.11 [0.97, 1.27]
Subtotal (95% CI)	554 /2413	509 /2408		49.3	1.11 [0.97, 1.27]
Test for heterogeneity chi-square=0.00 df=0					
Test for overall effect=1.52 p=0.13					
02 Unfractionated heparin, low dose					
IST 1997	501 /2410	509 /2408		50.7	0.98 [0.85, 1.12]
Subtotal (95% CI)	501 /2410	509 /2408		50.7	0.98 [0.85, 1.12]
Test for heterogeneity chi-square=0.00 df=0					
Test for overall effect=-0.30 p=0.8					
Total (95% CI)	1055 /4823	1018 /4816		100.0	1.04 [0.95, 1.15]
Test for heterogeneity chi-square=1.64 df=1 p=0.2002					
Test for overall effect=0.88 p=0.4					

```
        .5        .7        1        1.5        2
        Favours treatment    Favours control
```

Figure 10.18 Forest plot showing the effects of *the combination of anticoagulation and aspirin vs aspirin* in acute ischaemic stroke *on death at the end of follow-up*. Reproduced from Berge and Sandercock (2001), with permission from the authors and John Wiley & Sons Limited. Copyright Cochrane Library, reproduced with permission.

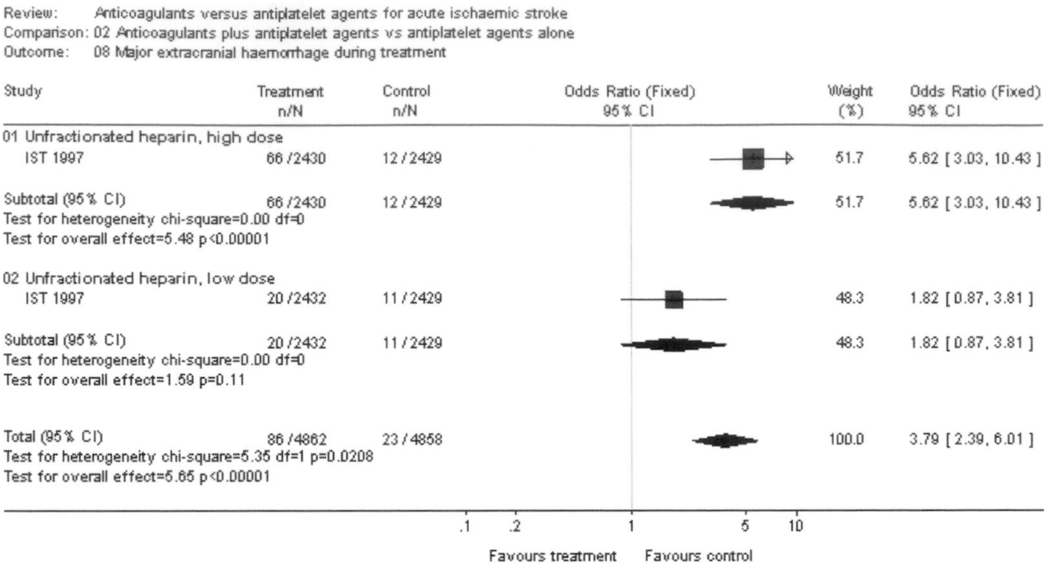

Review: Anticoagulants versus antiplatelet agents for acute ischaemic stroke
Comparison: 02 Anticoagulants plus antiplatelet agents vs antiplatelet agents alone
Outcome: 08 Major extracranial haemorrhage during treatment

Study	Treatment n/N	Control n/N	Odds Ratio (Fixed) 95% CI	Weight (%)	Odds Ratio (Fixed) 95% CI
01 Unfractionated heparin, high dose					
IST 1997	66 /2430	12 /2429		51.7	5.62 [3.03, 10.43]
Subtotal (95% CI)	66 /2430	12 /2429		51.7	5.62 [3.03, 10.43]
Test for heterogeneity chi-square=0.00 df=0					
Test for overall effect=5.48 p<0.00001					
02 Unfractionated heparin, low dose					
IST 1997	20 /2432	11 /2429		48.3	1.82 [0.87, 3.81]
Subtotal (95% CI)	20 /2432	11 /2429		48.3	1.82 [0.87, 3.81]
Test for heterogeneity chi-square=0.00 df=0					
Test for overall effect=1.59 p=0.11					
Total (95% CI)	86 /4862	23 /4858		100.0	3.79 [2.39, 6.01]
Test for heterogeneity chi-square=5.35 df=1 p=0.0208					
Test for overall effect=5.65 p<0.00001					

.1 .2 1 5 10
Favours treatment   Favours control

Figure 10.19 Forest plot showing the effects of *the combination of anticoagulation and aspirin vs aspirin* in acute ischaemic stroke *on major extracranial haemorrhage during the treatment period*. Reproduced from Berge and Sandercock (2001), with permission from the authors and John Wiley & Sons Limited. Copyright Cochrane Library, reproduced with permission.

Review: Anticoagulants versus antiplatelet agents for acute ischaemic stroke
Comparison: 02 Anticoagulants plus antiplatelet agents vs antiplatelet agents alone
Outcome: 06 Symptomatic intracranial haemorrhage (fatal or non-fatal) during treatment period

Study	Treatment n/N	Control n/N	Odds Ratio (Fixed) 95% CI	Weight (%)	Odds Ratio (Fixed) 95% CI
03 Unfractionated heparin, high dose					
IST 1997	42 /2430	13 /2429		49.7	3.27 [1.75, 6.10]
Subtotal (95% CI)	42 /2430	13 /2429		49.7	3.27 [1.75, 6.10]
Test for heterogeneity chi-square=0.00 df=0					
Test for overall effect=3.72 p=0.0002					
04 Unfractionated heparin, low dose					
IST 1997	19 /2432	13 /2429		50.3	1.46 [0.72, 2.97]
Subtotal (95% CI)	19 /2432	13 /2429		50.3	1.46 [0.72, 2.97]
Test for heterogeneity chi-square=0.00 df=0					
Test for overall effect=1.05 p=0.3					
Total (95% CI)	61 /4862	26 /4858		100.0	2.36 [1.49, 3.74]
Test for heterogeneity chi-square=2.80 df=1 p=0.0944					
Test for overall effect=3.66 p=0.0003					

.1 .2 1 5 10
Favours treatment   Favours control

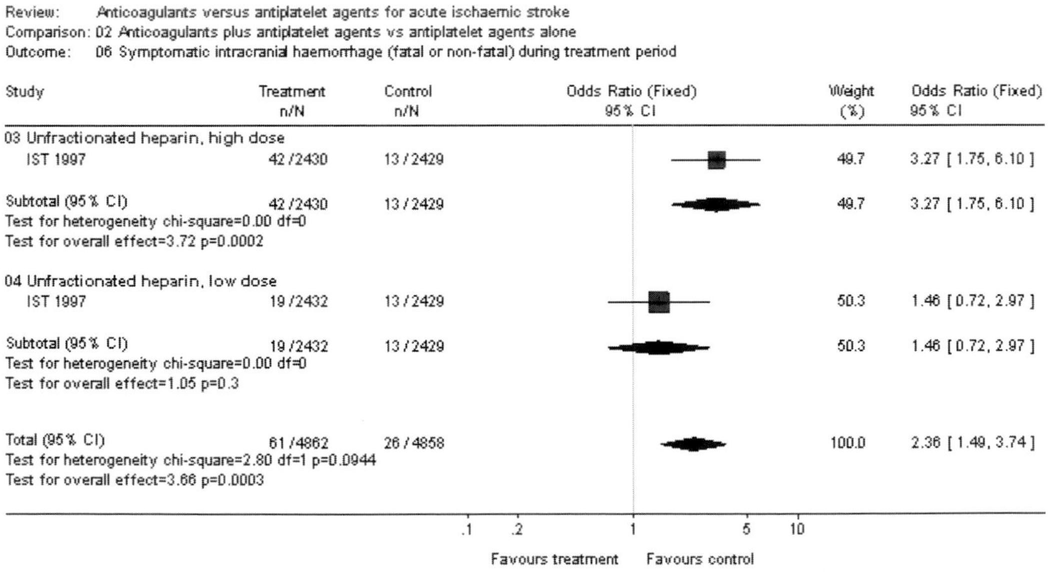

Figure 10.20 Forest plot showing the effects of *the combination of anticoagulation and aspirin vs aspirin* in acute ischaemic stroke *on symptomatic ICH during the treatment period*. Reproduced from Berge and Sandercock (2001), with permission from the authors and John Wiley & Sons Limited. Copyright Cochrane Library, reproduced with permission.

Table 10.3. Summary of the effects of low-dose UFH plus aspirin vs aspirin in acute ischaemic stroke.

Outcome	OR	95% CI	Absolute risk difference	95% CI
Death at end of treatment period (14 days)	0.84	0.69 to 1.01	No significant difference	
Death at end of follow-up	0.98	0.85 to 1.12	No significant difference	
Recurrent stroke	0.75	0.55 to 1.03	No significant difference	
Symptomatic ICH	1.46	0.72 to 2.97	No significant difference	
Major ECH	1.82	0.87 to 3.81	No significant difference	

ECH: extracranial haemorrhage.

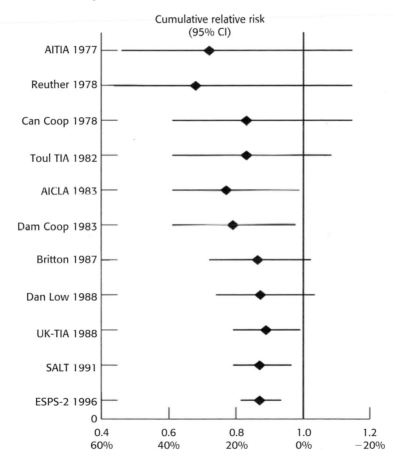

Figure 10.21 Cumulative meta-analysis of the 11 RCTs of aspirin vs control in about 10,000 patients with previous stroke or TIA showing that long-term aspirin therapy reduced the RR of recurrent serious vascular events by about 13% (95% CI: 6–19%) compared with placebo. Reproduced from Algra and van Gijn (1999), with permission from the British Medical Journal Publishing group and the authors.

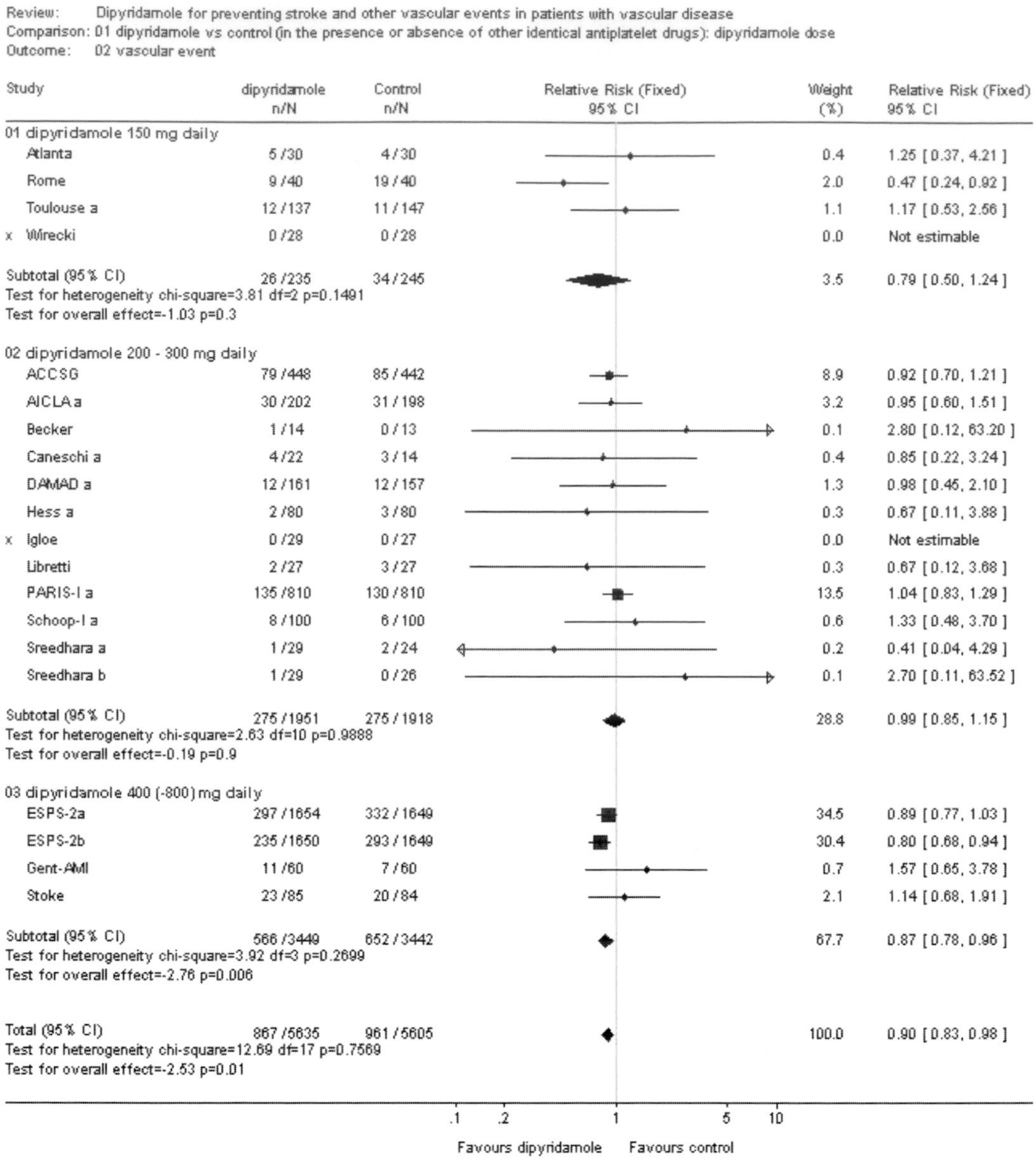

Review: Dipyridamole for preventing stroke and other vascular events in patients with vascular disease
Comparison: 01 dipyridamole vs control (in the presence or absence of other identical antiplatelet drugs): dipyridamole dose
Outcome: 02 vascular event

Study	dipyridamole n/N	Control n/N	Relative Risk (Fixed) 95% CI	Weight (%)	Relative Risk (Fixed) 95% CI
01 dipyridamole 150 mg daily					
Atlanta	5 / 30	4 / 30		0.4	1.25 [0.37, 4.21]
Rome	9 / 40	19 / 40		2.0	0.47 [0.24, 0.92]
Toulouse a	12 / 137	11 / 147		1.1	1.17 [0.53, 2.56]
x Wirecki	0 / 28	0 / 28		0.0	Not estimable
Subtotal (95% CI)	26 / 235	34 / 245		3.5	0.79 [0.50, 1.24]
Test for heterogeneity chi-square=3.81 df=2 p=0.1491					
Test for overall effect=-1.03 p=0.3					
02 dipyridamole 200 - 300 mg daily					
ACCSG	79 / 448	85 / 442		8.9	0.92 [0.70, 1.21]
AICLA a	30 / 202	31 / 198		3.2	0.95 [0.60, 1.51]
Becker	1 / 14	0 / 13		0.1	2.80 [0.12, 63.20]
Caneschi a	4 / 22	3 / 14		0.4	0.85 [0.22, 3.24]
DAMAD a	12 / 161	12 / 157		1.3	0.98 [0.45, 2.10]
Hess a	2 / 80	3 / 80		0.3	0.67 [0.11, 3.88]
x Igloe	0 / 29	0 / 27		0.0	Not estimable
Libretti	2 / 27	3 / 27		0.3	0.67 [0.12, 3.68]
PARIS-I a	135 / 810	130 / 810		13.5	1.04 [0.83, 1.29]
Schoop-I a	8 / 100	6 / 100		0.6	1.33 [0.48, 3.70]
Sreedhara a	1 / 29	2 / 24		0.2	0.41 [0.04, 4.29]
Sreedhara b	1 / 29	0 / 26		0.1	2.70 [0.11, 63.52]
Subtotal (95% CI)	275 / 1951	275 / 1918		28.8	0.99 [0.85, 1.15]
Test for heterogeneity chi-square=2.63 df=10 p=0.9888					
Test for overall effect=-0.19 p=0.9					
03 dipyridamole 400 (-800) mg daily					
ESPS-2a	297 / 1654	332 / 1649		34.5	0.89 [0.77, 1.03]
ESPS-2b	235 / 1650	293 / 1649		30.4	0.80 [0.68, 0.94]
Gent-AMI	11 / 60	7 / 60		0.7	1.57 [0.65, 3.78]
Stoke	23 / 85	20 / 84		2.1	1.14 [0.68, 1.91]
Subtotal (95% CI)	566 / 3449	652 / 3442		67.7	0.87 [0.78, 0.96]
Test for heterogeneity chi-square=3.92 df=3 p=0.2699					
Test for overall effect=-2.76 p=0.006					
Total (95% CI)	867 / 5635	961 / 5605		100.0	0.90 [0.83, 0.98]
Test for heterogeneity chi-square=12.69 df=17 p=0.7569					
Test for overall effect=-2.53 p=0.01					

.1   .2   1   5   10

Favours dipyridamole   Favours control

Figure 10.22   Forest plot showing the effects of *dipyridamole vs control* in high vascular risk patients *on serious vascular events (stroke, MI or death from vascular causes) at the end of follow-up.* Reproduced from De Schryver *et al.* (2002), with permission from the authors and John Wiley & Sons Limited. Copyright Cochrane Library, reproduced with permission.

compared with control (Fig. 10.22) (De Schryver *et al.*, 2002, 2003). The overall effect is consistent among different doses of dipyridamole. However, there was no evidence that dipyridamole is more effective in preventing vascular death compared with control (RR: 1.02, 95% CI: 0.90–1.17) (Fig. 10.23) (De Schryver *et al.*, 2002, 2003).

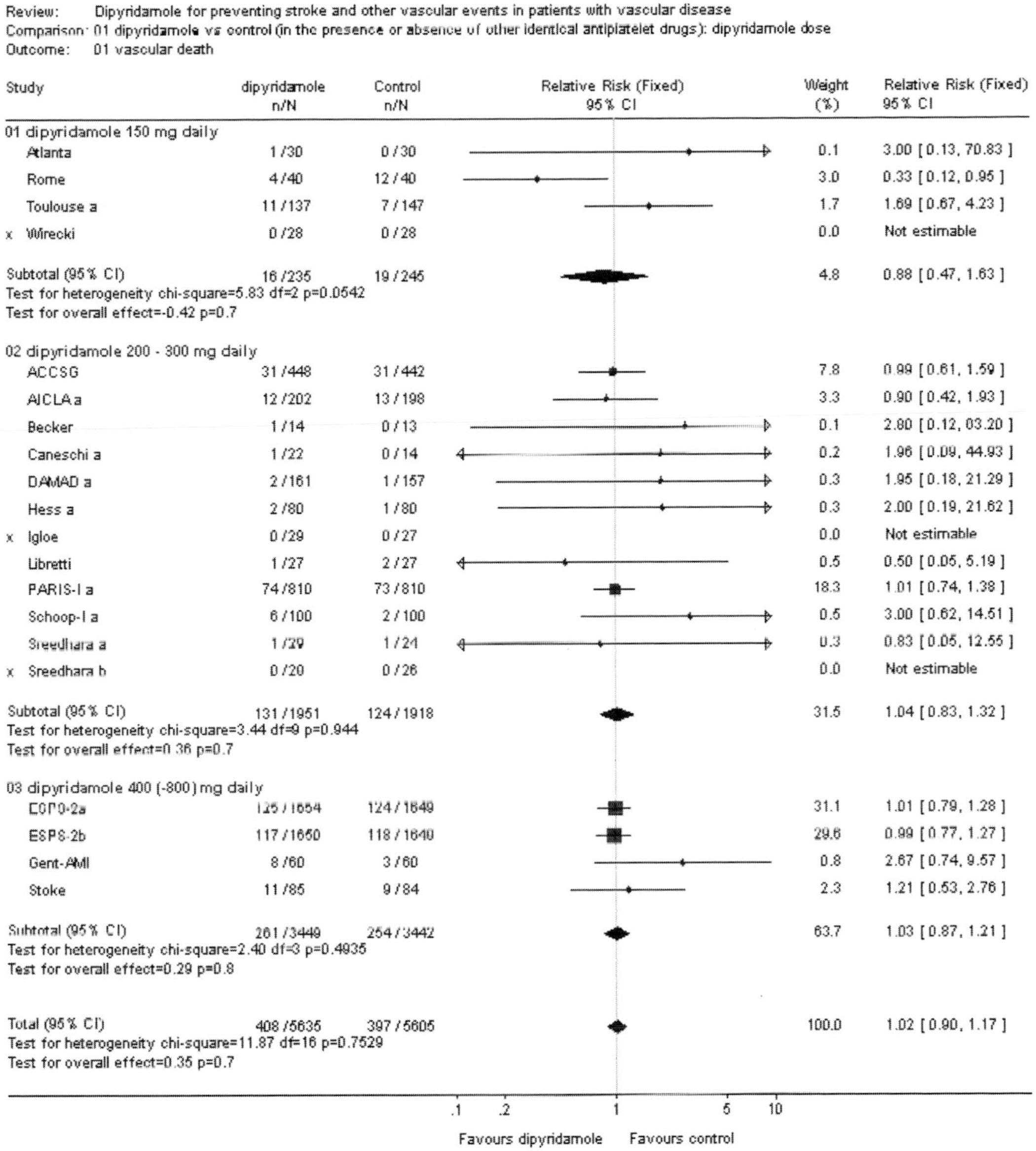

Review: Dipyridamole for preventing stroke and other vascular events in patients with vascular disease
Comparison: 01 dipyridamole vs control (in the presence or absence of other identical antiplatelet drugs): dipyridamole dose
Outcome: 01 vascular death

Study	dipyridamole n/N	Control n/N	Relative Risk (Fixed) 95% CI	Weight (%)	Relative Risk (Fixed) 95% CI
01 dipyridamole 150 mg daily					
Atlanta	1 /30	0 /30		0.1	3.00 [0.13, 70.83]
Rome	4 /40	12 /40		3.0	0.33 [0.12, 0.95]
Toulouse a	11 /137	7 /147		1.7	1.69 [0.67, 4.23]
x Wirecki	0 /28	0 /28		0.0	Not estimable
Subtotal (95% CI)	16 /235	19 /245		4.8	0.88 [0.47, 1.63]
Test for heterogeneity chi-square=5.83 df=2 p=0.0542					
Test for overall effect=-0.42 p=0.7					
02 dipyridamole 200 - 300 mg daily					
ACCSG	31 /448	31 /442		7.8	0.99 [0.61, 1.59]
AICLA a	12 /202	13 /198		3.3	0.90 [0.42, 1.93]
Becker	1 /14	0 /13		0.1	2.80 [0.12, 63.20]
Caneschi a	1 /22	0 /14		0.2	1.96 [0.09, 44.93]
DAMAD a	2 /161	1 /157		0.3	1.95 [0.18, 21.29]
Hess a	2 /80	1 /80		0.3	2.00 [0.19, 21.62]
x Igloe	0 /29	0 /27		0.0	Not estimable
Libretti	1 /27	2 /27		0.5	0.50 [0.05, 5.19]
PARIS-I a	74 /810	73 /810		18.3	1.01 [0.74, 1.38]
Schoop-I a	6 /100	2 /100		0.5	3.00 [0.62, 14.51]
Sreedhara a	1 /29	1 /24		0.3	0.83 [0.05, 12.55]
x Sreedhara b	0 /20	0 /26		0.0	Not estimable
Subtotal (95% CI)	131 /1951	124 /1918		31.5	1.04 [0.83, 1.32]
Test for heterogeneity chi-square=3.44 df=9 p=0.944					
Test for overall effect=0.36 p=0.7					
03 dipyridamole 400 (-800) mg daily					
ESPS-2a	125 /1654	124 /1649		31.1	1.01 [0.79, 1.28]
ESPS-2b	117 /1650	118 /1649		29.6	0.99 [0.77, 1.27]
Gent-AMI	8 /60	3 /60		0.8	2.67 [0.74, 9.57]
Stoke	11 /85	9 /84		2.3	1.21 [0.53, 2.76]
Subtotal (95% CI)	261 /3449	254 /3442		63.7	1.03 [0.87, 1.21]
Test for heterogeneity chi-square=2.40 df=3 p=0.4935					
Test for overall effect=0.29 p=0.8					
Total (95% CI)	408 /5635	397 /5605		100.0	1.02 [0.90, 1.17]
Test for heterogeneity chi-square=11.87 df=16 p=0.7529					
Test for overall effect=0.35 p=0.7					

.1   .2   1   5   10

Favours dipyridamole   Favours control

Figure 10.23 Forest plot showing the effects of *dipyridamole vs control* in high vascular risk patients *on death from vascular causes at the end of follow-up*. Reproduced from De Schryver *et al.* (2002), with permission from the authors and John Wiley & Sons Limited. Copyright Cochrane Library, reproduced with permission.

TIA and ischaemic stroke patients For patients with TIA or ischaemic stroke, dipyridamole reduced the RR of serious vascular events by about 13% (95% CI: 4–21%) compared with control (Fig. 10.24) (Diener *et al.*, 1996; De Schryver *et al.*, 2002, 2003).

Review: Dipyridamole for preventing stroke and other vascular events in patients with vascular disease
Comparison: 04 dipyridamole vs control (in presence or absence of other identical antiplatelet drugs): presenting disease
Outcome: 02 vascular event

Study	dipyridamole n/N	Control n/N	Relative Risk (Fixed) 95% CI	Weight (%)	Relative Risk (Fixed) 95% CI
01 cardiac disease					
Atlanta	5/30	4/30		0.4	1.25 [0.37, 4.21]
Becker	1/14	0/13		0.1	2.80 [0.12, 63.20]
Gent-AMI	11/60	7/60		0.7	1.57 [0.65, 3.78]
x Igloe	0/29	0/27		0.0	Not estimable
PARIS-I a	135/810	130/810		13.5	1.04 [0.83, 1.29]
Rome	9/40	19/40		2.0	0.47 [0.24, 0.92]
x Wirecki	0/28	0/28		0.0	Not estimable
Subtotal (95% CI)	161/1011	160/1008		16.6	1.01 [0.82, 1.23]

Test for heterogeneity chi-square=6.60 df=4 p=0.1588
Test for overall effect=0.06 p=1.0

Study	dipyridamole n/N	Control n/N		Weight (%)	Relative Risk (Fixed) 95% CI
02 (transient) cerebral ischaemia					
ACCSG	79/448	85/442		8.9	0.92 [0.70, 1.21]
AICLA a	30/202	31/198		3.2	0.95 [0.60, 1.51]
Caneschi a	4/22	3/14		0.4	0.85 [0.22, 3.24]
ESPS-2a	297/1654	332/1649		34.5	0.89 [0.77, 1.03]
ESPS-2b	235/1650	293/1649		30.4	0.80 [0.68, 0.94]
Stoke	23/85	20/84		2.1	1.14 [0.68, 1.91]
Toulouse a	12/137	11/147		1.1	1.17 [0.53, 2.56]
Subtotal (95% CI)	680/4198	775/4183		80.6	0.87 [0.79, 0.96]

Test for heterogeneity chi-square=3.00 df=6 p=0.8091
Test for overall effect=-2.85 p=0.004

Study	dipyridamole n/N	Control n/N		Weight (%)	Relative Risk (Fixed) 95% CI
03 arterial peripheral vascular disaease					
Hess a	2/80	3/80		0.3	0.67 [0.11, 3.88]
Libretti	2/27	3/27		0.3	0.67 [0.12, 3.68]
Schoop-I a	8/100	6/100		0.6	1.33 [0.48, 3.70]
Subtotal (95% CI)	12/207	12/207		1.2	1.00 [0.46, 2.17]

Test for heterogeneity chi-square=0.72 df=2 p=0.6961
Test for overall effect=0.00 p=1.0

Study	dipyridamole n/N	Control n/N		Weight (%)	Relative Risk (Fixed) 95% CI
04 diabetic retinopathy					
DAMAD a	12/161	12/157		1.3	0.98 [0.45, 2.10]
Subtotal (95% CI)	12/161	12/157		1.3	0.98 [0.45, 2.10]

Test for heterogeneity chi-square=0.00 df=0
Test for overall effect=-0.06 p=0.9

Study	dipyridamole n/N	Control n/N		Weight (%)	Relative Risk (Fixed) 95% CI
05 haemodialysis patients					
Sreedhara a	1/29	2/24		0.2	0.41 [0.04, 4.29]
Sreedhara b	1/29	0/26		0.1	2.70 [0.11, 63.52]
Subtotal (95% CI)	2/58	2/50		0.3	0.86 [0.16, 4.70]

Test for heterogeneity chi-square=0.88 df=1 p=0.3483
Test for overall effect=-0.18 p=0.9

Study	dipyridamole n/N	Control n/N		Weight (%)	Relative Risk (Fixed) 95% CI
Total (95% CI)	867/5635	961/5605		100.0	0.90 [0.83, 0.98]

Test for heterogeneity chi-square=12.69 df=17 p=0.7569
Test for overall effect=-2.53 p=0.01

.1   .2   1   5   10

Favours dipyridamole   Favours control

Figure 10.24 Forest plot showing the effects of *dipyridamole vs control* in high vascular risk patients *on serious vascular events at the end of follow-up according to the qualifying diagnosis of the enrolled patients*. Reproduced from De Schryver *et al.* (2002), with permission from the authors and John Wiley & Sons Limited. Copyright Cochrane Library, reproduced with permission.

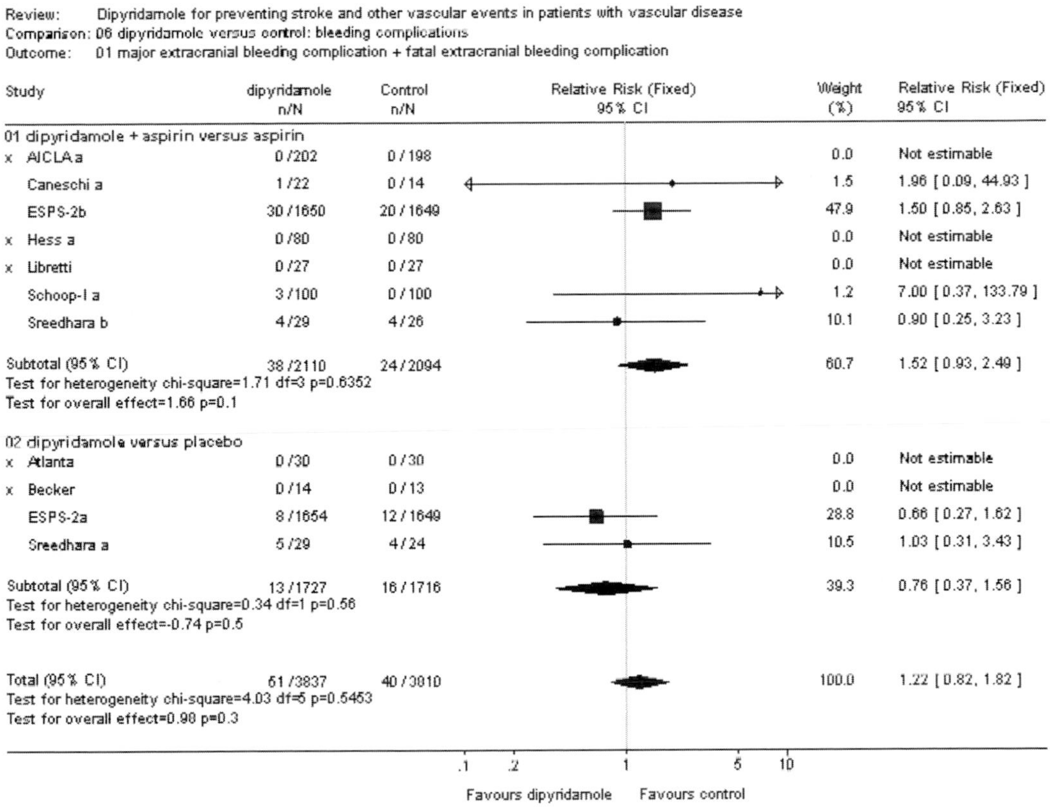

Review: Dipyridamole for preventing stroke and other vascular events in patients with vascular disease
Comparison: 06 dipyridamole versus control: bleeding complications
Outcome: 01 major extracranial bleeding complication + fatal extracranial bleeding complication

Study	dipyridamole n/N	Control n/N	Relative Risk (Fixed) 95% CI	Weight (%)	Relative Risk (Fixed) 95% CI
01 dipyridamole + aspirin versus aspirin					
x AICLA a	0 /202	0 / 198		0.0	Not estimable
Caneschi a	1 /22	0 / 14		1.5	1.96 [0.09, 44.93]
ESPS-2b	30 /1650	20 / 1649		47.9	1.50 [0.85, 2.63]
x Hess a	0 /80	0 / 80		0.0	Not estimable
x Libretti	0 /27	0 / 27		0.0	Not estimable
Schoop-I a	3 /100	0 / 100		1.2	7.00 [0.37, 133.79]
Sreedhara b	4 /29	4 / 26		10.1	0.90 [0.25, 3.23]
Subtotal (95% CI)	38 /2110	24 /2094		60.7	1.52 [0.93, 2.49]
Test for heterogeneity chi-square=1.71 df=3 p=0.6352					
Test for overall effect=1.66 p=0.1					
02 dipyridamole versus placebo					
x Atlanta	0 /30	0 / 30		0.0	Not estimable
x Becker	0 /14	0 / 13		0.0	Not estimable
ESPS-2a	8 /1654	12 / 1649		28.8	0.66 [0.27, 1.62]
Sreedhara a	5 /29	4 / 24		10.5	1.03 [0.31, 3.43]
Subtotal (95% CI)	13 /1727	16 / 1716		39.3	0.76 [0.37, 1.56]
Test for heterogeneity chi-square=0.34 df=1 p=0.56					
Test for overall effect=-0.74 p=0.5					
Total (95% CI)	61 /3837	40 /3810		100.0	1.22 [0.82, 1.82]
Test for heterogeneity chi-square=4.03 df=5 p=0.5453					
Test for overall effect=0.98 p=0.3					

.1   .2   1   5   10

Favours dipyridamole   Favours control

Figure 10.25 Forest plot showing the effects of *dipyridamole vs control* in high vascular risk patients on major and fatal extracranial bleeding complications at the end of follow-up. Reproduced from De Schryver *et al.* (2002), with permission from the authors and John Wiley & Sons Limited. Copyright Cochrane Library, reproduced with permission.

A meta-analysis of individual patient data from the RCTs indicated that among 4913 patients with TIA and ischaemic stroke randomised to dipyridamole vs control, assignment to dipyridamole was associated with an 18% (95% CI: 0–32%) reduction in odds of stroke, a 3% (95% CI: −42% to +34%) reduction in odds of MI, an 8% increase in odds of vascular death (95% CI: −18% to +42%) and a 14% (−3% to +27%) reduction in odds of serious vascular events, compared with control (Leonard-Bee *et al.*, 2005).

Adverse effects

Dipyridamole was not associated with an excess risk of *any* bleeding compared with control (4.7% dipyridamole, 4.2% control) (Leonard-Bee *et al.*, 2005), nor *major* or *fatal* extracranial bleeding complications, compared with control (RR: 0.76, 95% CI: 0.37–1.56) (Fig. 10.25) (De Schryver *et al.*, 2002, 2003).

However, dipyridamole was associated with an excess of headache, compared with control (37.2% dipyridamole vs 22.8% control) and was sufficiently severe to lead to discontinuation of study drug in the European Stroke Prevention Study (ESPS) 2 trial among 8.0% of patients assigned dipyridamole compared with 2.4% assigned placebo (RR: 3.20, 95% CI: 2.25–4.54) (Diener *et al.*, 1996). The headache is due to vasodilatation and is usually self-limited, but can occasionally last several weeks. Dipyridamole may also cause GI upset leading to discontinuation of study drug in some cases (placebo 3.6%, dipyridamole 6.2%; RR: 1.65, 95% CI: 1.21–2.26), and precipitate angina in patients with occlusive coronary artery disease by a steal effect (Keltz *et al.*, 1987; Virtanen *et al.*, 1989; Jain *et al.*, 1990; Akinboboye *et al.*, 2001).

Ticlopidine vs control

Evidence

Efficacy
High vascular risk patients   A meta-analysis of the 42 RCTs of ticlopidine vs control in a total of 6910 high vascular risk patients indicates that random allocation to long-term treatment over 2–3 years with oral ticlopidine 250 mg twice daily is associated with a 32% (standard error (SE): 7%) reduction in odds of subsequent major vascular events (stroke, MI or death due to vascular causes) over the course of treatment (2–3 years) compared with control (ticlopidine: 278/3435 [8.1%] vs control: 385/3475 [11.1%]) (Antithrombotic Trialists' Collaboration, 2002).

Ischaemic stroke patients   Among 1072 patients with atherothromboembolic ischaemic stroke in the preceding 1 week to 4 months, random allocation to (ticlopidine 250 mg twice daily) for up to 3 years (mean 24 months) was associated with a reduction in the risk of serious vascular events from 14.8% (placebo) to 11.3% per year (ticlopidine) in the intention-to-treat analysis, representing a relative risk reduction (RRR) with ticlopidine of 23.3% (95% CI: 1.0–40.5%, $P = 0.02$) (Gent *et al.*, 1989).

Adverse effects
Bleeding   Patients with ischaemic stroke assigned ticlopidine (250 mg twice daily) had a similar incidence of major bleeding as the placebo group (0.2% compared with 0.4%) over up to 3 years, but twice as many minor bleeding episodes (6.5% ticlopidine vs 3.0% placebo) (Gent *et al.*, 1989).

Neutropaenia   Ticlopidine increased the risk of neutropaenia (absolute neutrophil count $<$1200 cells/mm^3) in 2.1–2.4% of patients, and severe neutropaenia ($<$450 neutrophils/mm^3) in 0.8–0.9% of patients (Gent *et al.*, 1989; Dusitanond and Hankey, 2005). The neutropaenia typically occurs in the first few months after initiation of ticlopidine, and can be fatal because of the associated increased risk for serious infection. The neutropaenia resolves with cessation of drug administration.

Ticlopidine has also been associated with pancytopaenia.

Thrombotic thrombocytopaenic purpura   Ticlopidine is associated with an increased risk of thrombotic thrombocytopaenic purpura (TTP), affecting between 1 in 5000 patients and 1 in 6000 patients (Bennett *et al.*, 1998a, b, 1999; Steinhubl *et al.*, 1999).

TTP is a thrombotic microangiopathy characterised by intravascular platelet aggregation, which leads to profound thrombocytopaenia (usually $<$20,000/mm^3), mechanical haemolytic anaemia, fever and tissue ischaemia, commonly involving the brain and kidneys. It is thought to be immune mediated, in that the body responds to an antigenic stimulus, such as ticlopidine, by producing immunoglobulin G (IgG) autoantibodies which cross react with a metalloprotease that cleaves von Willebrand factor (vWF). Proteolysis of vWF is impaired, large vWF multimers bind to platelets, and platelet microthrombi form, particularly within the microcirculation of the brain, kidneys, heart, pancreas and adrenal glands.

In a review of 60 cases of ticlopidine-associated TTP, ticlopidine had been prescribed for less than 1 month in 80% of patients, and normal platelet counts had been found within 2 weeks of the onset of TTP (Bennett *et al.*, 1998a). The mortality rates in patients who underwent plasma exchange varied from 22% to 24% compared with mortality rates of 50–60% among patients who did not undergo this procedure. Limiting ticlopidine therapy to 2 weeks after stenting did not prevent the development of TTP (Bennett *et al.*, 1999).

GI upset   Diarrhoea occurs among about 20% of individuals taking ticlopidine, and usually during the first 2–3 weeks of ticlopidine administration, frequently related to failure to take the medication with food or with meals (Gent *et al.*, 1989; Dusitanond and Hankey, 2005).

Very rarely, chronic diarrhoea may occur after 1–2 months of ticlopidine therapy. It is usually a watery, mucus-containing diarrhoea without blood or fat, and is associated with microscopic lymphocytic colitis. The mechanism of diarrhoea is not fully understood. Changes in intestinal motility and malabsorption syndrome have been proposed as possible pathophysiological mechanisms.

Other GI adverse effects of ticlopidine include nausea, vomiting, dyspepsia and anorexia.

Skin rash   Skin rash occurs in about 10% of patients taking ticlopidine, and may be urticarial and pruritic (Gent *et al.*, 1989; Dusitanond and Hankey, 2005). It is usually mild and resolves with discontinuation of therapy. Ticlopidine may also cause a fixed drug eruption, toxic erythroderma and leucocytoclastic vasculitis (Dusitanond and Hankey, 2005).

Other less common adverse effects   Ticlopidine may be associated with the occurrence of thrombocytopaenia, aplastic anaemia, microangiopathy in myocardial small vessels, cholestasis and hepatitis, acute interstitial nephritis presenting with acute renal failure and deterioration of renal function, interstitial pulmonary disease, bronchiolitis obliterans-organising pneumonia (BOOP), diffuse alveolar damage, acute symmetrical polyarthritis or arthralgia, and typical features of drug-induced lupus: older age of onset, presence of pleurisy and arthritis, and no significant renal, haematological or central nervous system involvement (Gent *et al.*, 1989; Dusitanond and Hankey, 2005).

Cilostazol vs control

Evidence

Efficacy
Ischaemic stroke patients   Cilostazol is an antiplatelet drug that increases the cyclic adenosine monophosphate (AMP) levels in platelets via inhibition of cyclic AMP phosphodiesterase. It has been evaluated in one RCT involving 1095 patients with recent (1–6 months ago) ischaemic stroke, the Cilostazol Stroke Prevention Study (Gotoh *et al.*, 2000).

Compared with placebo, cilostazol 100 mg twice daily, reduced the risk of serious vascular events from 6.8% (placebo) to 4.2% per year (cilostazol); RRR: 38.8% (95% CI: 8.6–59.0), absolute risk reduction (ARR) 2.6% per year; number needed to treat (NNT): 38. Cilostazol also reduced the risk of recurrent ischaemic stroke (the primary outcome) by 41.7% (95% CI: 8.6–59.0) (Gotoh *et al.*, 2000).

Adverse effects
Adverse effects of cilostazol included headache, tachycardia and palpitations, which were probably related to its vasodilatory properties.

Aspirin and dipyridamole vs control

Evidence

Efficacy
High vascular risk patients Among high vascular risk patients, the combination of aspirin and dipyridamole significantly reduces the RR of serious vascular events (RRR: 26%, 95% CI: 20–32%) compared with control (Antithrombotic Trialists' Collaboration, 2002; De Schryver *et al.*, 2003).

TIA and ischaemic stroke patients Among 6946 patients with TIA and ischaemic stroke randomised to the combination of aspirin and dipyridamole vs control, a meta-analysis of individual patient data from the RCTs indicated that random assignment to the combination of aspirin and dipyridamole was associated with a 39% (95% CI: 29–49%) reduction in odds of stroke, a 33% (95% CI: 5–52%) reduction in odds of MI, a 9% reduction in odds of vascular death (95% CI: −12% to +27%) and a 34% (25–43%) reduction in odds of serious vascular events compared with control (Leonard-Bee *et al.*, 2005).

Adverse effects
The combination of aspirin and dipyridamole was associated with a greater incidence of headache (26.7% aspirin and dipyridamole vs 22.8% control) and any bleeding (8.1% aspirin and dipyridamole vs 4.2% control) compared with control in TIA and ischaemic stroke patients (Leonard-Bee *et al.*, 2005).

Dipyridamole vs aspirin

Evidence

Efficacy
High vascular risk patients Among high vascular risk patients, there is no evidence that dipyridamole is more effective in preventing vascular events compared with aspirin (RR: 1.02, 95% CI: 0.88–1.18) (Fig. 10.26) (De Schryver *et al.*, 2003).

Ticlopidine vs aspirin

Evidence

Efficacy
High vascular risk patients Among white patients at high vascular risk, ticlopidine does not significantly reduce the risk of serious vascular events compared with aspirin (RRR: 10%, 95% CI: −1% to 24%) (Fig. 10.27) (Hankey *et al.*, 2000).

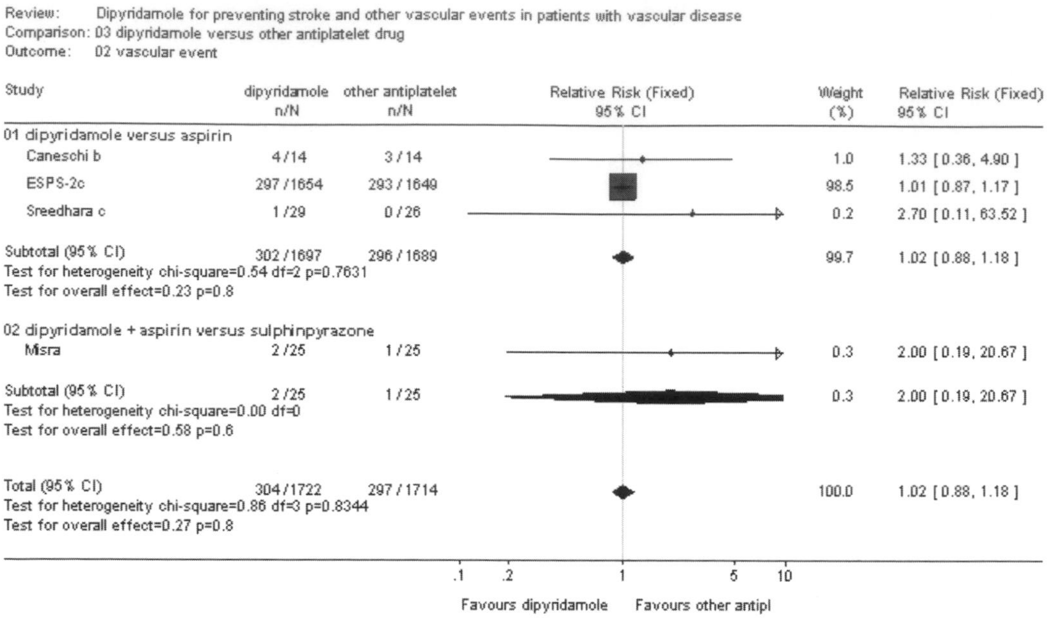

Review: Dipyridamole for preventing stroke and other vascular events in patients with vascular disease
Comparison: 03 dipyridamole versus other antiplatelet drug
Outcome: 02 vascular event

Study	dipyridamole n/N	other antiplatelet n/N	Relative Risk (Fixed) 95% CI	Weight (%)	Relative Risk (Fixed) 95% CI
01 dipyridamole versus aspirin					
Caneschi b	4/14	3/14		1.0	1.33 [0.36, 4.90]
ESPS-2c	297/1654	293/1649		98.5	1.01 [0.87, 1.17]
Sreedhara c	1/29	0/26		0.2	2.70 [0.11, 63.52]
Subtotal (95% CI)	302/1697	296/1689		99.7	1.02 [0.88, 1.18]
Test for heterogeneity chi-square=0.54 df=2 p=0.7631					
Test for overall effect=0.23 p=0.8					
02 dipyridamole + aspirin versus sulphinpyrazone					
Misra	2/25	1/25		0.3	2.00 [0.19, 20.67]
Subtotal (95% CI)	2/25	1/25		0.3	2.00 [0.19, 20.67]
Test for heterogeneity chi-square=0.00 df=0					
Test for overall effect=0.58 p=0.6					
Total (95% CI)	304/1722	297/1714		100.0	1.02 [0.88, 1.18]
Test for heterogeneity chi-square=0.86 df=3 p=0.8344					
Test for overall effect=0.27 p=0.8					

.1   .2   1   5   10

Favours dipyridamole   Favours other antipl

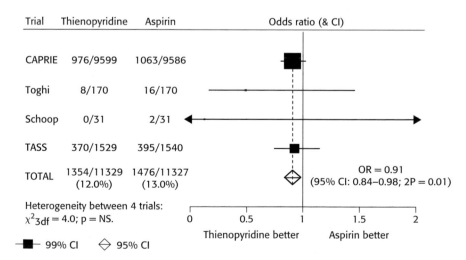

Figure 10.26 Forest plot showing the effects of *dipyridamole vs another antiplatelet drug* in high vascular risk patients *on serious vascular events* at the end of follow-up. Reproduced from De Schryver *et al.* (2002), with permission from the authors and John Wiley & Sons Limited. Copyright Cochrane Library, reproduced with permission.

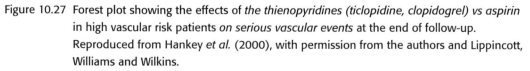

Trial	Thienopyridine	Aspirin	Odds ratio (& CI)
CAPRIE	976/9599	1063/9586	
Toghi	8/170	16/170	
Schoop	0/31	2/31	
TASS	370/1529	395/1540	
TOTAL	1354/11329 (12.0%)	1476/11327 (13.0%)	OR = 0.91 (95% CI: 0.84–0.98; 2P = 0.01)

Heterogeneity between 4 trials:
$\chi^2_{3df} = 4.0$; p = NS.

0   0.5   1   1.5   2

Thienopyridine better   Aspirin better

■— 99% CI   ◇ 95% CI

Figure 10.27 Forest plot showing the effects of *the thienopyridines (ticlopidine, clopidogrel) vs aspirin* in high vascular risk patients *on serious vascular events* at the end of follow-up. Reproduced from Hankey *et al.* (2000), with permission from the authors and Lippincott, Williams and Wilkins.

TIA and ischaemic stroke patients   Among 3069 patients with a TIA or mild ischaemic stroke in the preceding 3 months, randomly assigned to ticlopidine (250 mg twice daily) or aspirin (650 mg twice daily) for up to 2–6 years, allocation to ticlopidine was associated with a reduction in the odds of serious vascular events by 7% (95% CI: −9% to +21%) (Fig. 10.27) (Hass *et al.*, 1989).

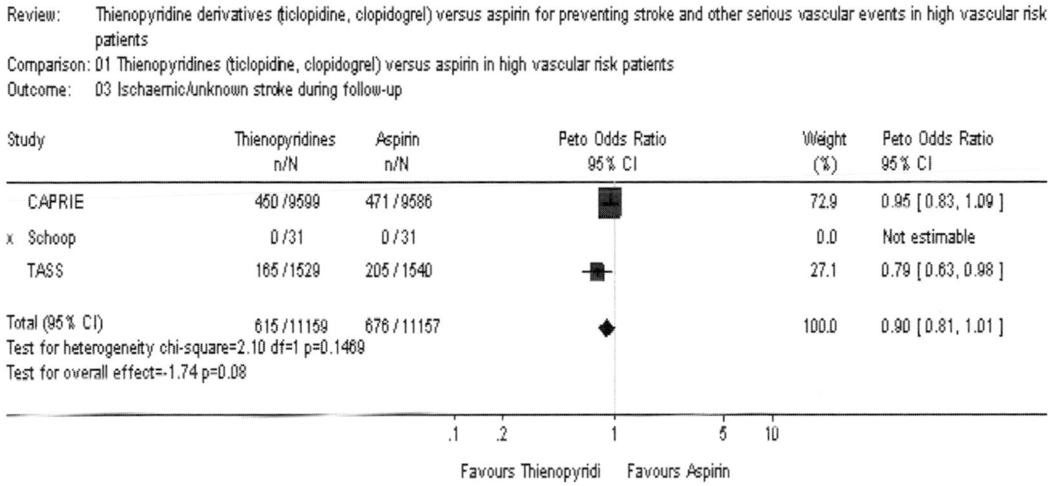

Review: Thienopyridine derivatives (ticlopidine, clopidogrel) versus aspirin for preventing stroke and other serious vascular events in high vascular risk
              patients
Comparison: 01 Thienopyridines (ticlopidine, clopidogrel) versus aspirin in high vascular risk patients
Outcome: 03 Ischaemic/unknown stroke during follow-up

Study	Thienopyridines n/N	Aspirin n/N	Peto Odds Ratio 95% CI	Weight (%)	Peto Odds Ratio 95% CI
CAPRIE	450 /9599	471 /9586		72.9	0.95 [0.83, 1.09]
x Schoop	0 /31	0 /31		0.0	Not estimable
TASS	165 /1529	205 / 1540		27.1	0.79 [0.63, 0.98]
Total (95% CI)	615/11159	676/11157		100.0	0.90 [0.81, 1.01]

Test for heterogeneity chi-square=2.10 df=1 p=0.1469
Test for overall effect=-1.74 p=0.08

.1   .2   1   5   10

Favours Thienopyridi   Favours Aspirin

Figure 10.28 Forest plot showing the effects of *the thienopyridines (ticlopidine, clopidogrel) vs another aspirin* in high vascular risk patients *on ischaemic or unknown stroke* at the end of follow-up. Reproduced from Hankey *et al.* (2000), with permission from the authors and John Wiley & Sons Limited. Copyright Cochrane Library, reproduced with permission.

Review: Thienopyridine derivatives (ticlopidine, clopidogrel) versus aspirin for preventing stroke and other serious vascular events in high vascular risk
              patients
Comparison: 01 Thienopyridines (ticlopidine, clopidogrel) versus aspirin in high vascular risk patients
Outcome: 04 Haemorrhagic stroke (symptomatic intracranial haemorrhage) during follow-up

Study	Thienopyridines n/N	Aspirin n/N	Peto Odds Ratio 95% CI	Weight (%)	Peto Odds Ratio 95% CI
CAPRIE	30 /9599	38 /9586		82.9	0.79 [0.49, 1.27]
x Japanese-B	0 /31	0 /31		0.0	Not estimable
TASS	7 /1529	7 /1540		17.1	1.01 [0.35, 2.88]
Total (95% CI)	37 /11159	45 /11157		100.0	0.82 [0.53, 1.27]

Test for heterogeneity chi-square=0.17 df=1 p=0.6774
Test for overall effect=-0.88 p=0.4

.1   .2   1   5   10

Favours Thienopyridi   Favours Aspirin

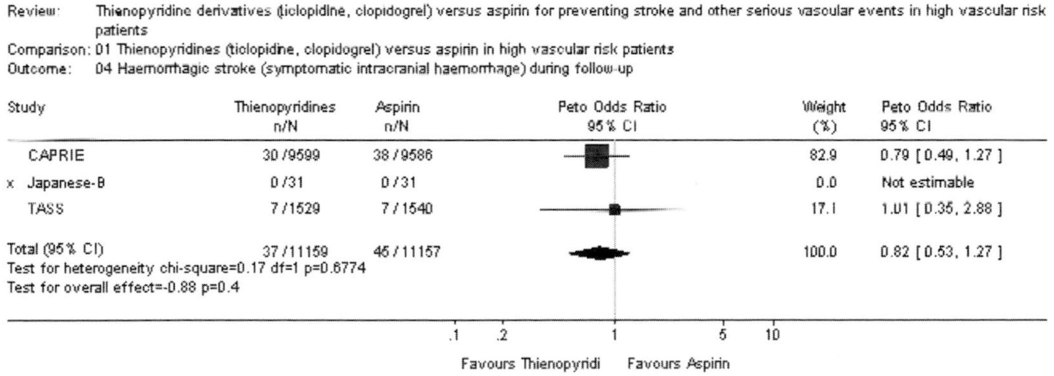

Figure 10.29 Forest plot showing the effects of *the thienopyridines (ticlopidine, clopidogrel) vs another aspirin* in high vascular risk patients *on haemorrhagic stroke* at the end of follow-up. Reproduced from Hankey *et al.* (2000), with permission from the authors and John Wiley & Sons Limited. Copyright Cochrane Library, reproduced with permission.

Ticlopidine significantly reduces the risk of ischaemic stroke compared with aspirin (OR: 0.79, 95% CI: 0.63–0.98) (Fig. 10.28) (Hankey *et al.*, 2000). As there is no excess of haemorrhagic stroke (Fig. 10.29), ticlopidine also significantly reduces the risk of all stroke compared with aspirin (OR: 0.79, 95% CI: 0.64–0.98) (Fig. 10.30).

There is no evidence from one RCT (TASS) that ticlopidine significantly reduces the odds of MI (OR: 1.19, 95% CI: 0.89–1.59) compared with aspirin (Fig. 10.31), but the 95% CI of the estimate of the OR are consistent with the overall result for MI and other serious vascular events, suggesting a marginal benefit compared with aspirin.

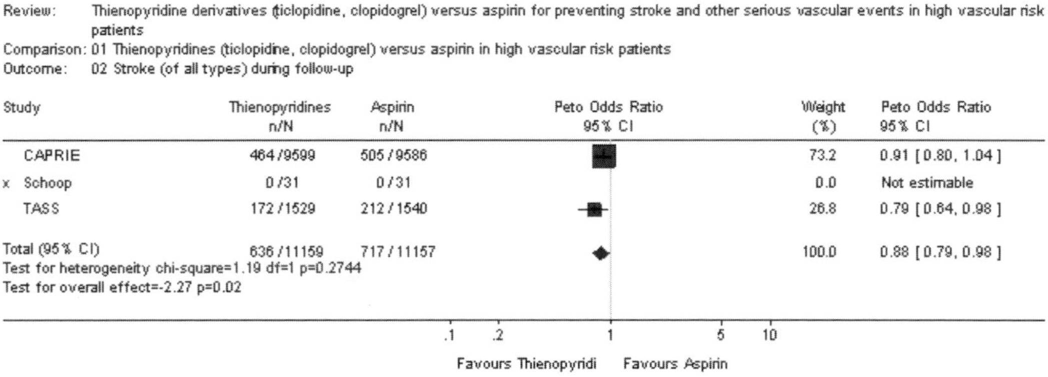

Figure 10.30 Forest plot showing the effects of *the thienopyridines (ticlopidine, clopidogrel) vs another aspirin* in high vascular risk patients *on stroke of all types* at the end of follow-up. Reproduced from Hankey *et al.* (2000), with permission from the authors and John Wiley & Sons Limited. Copyright Cochrane Library, reproduced with permission.

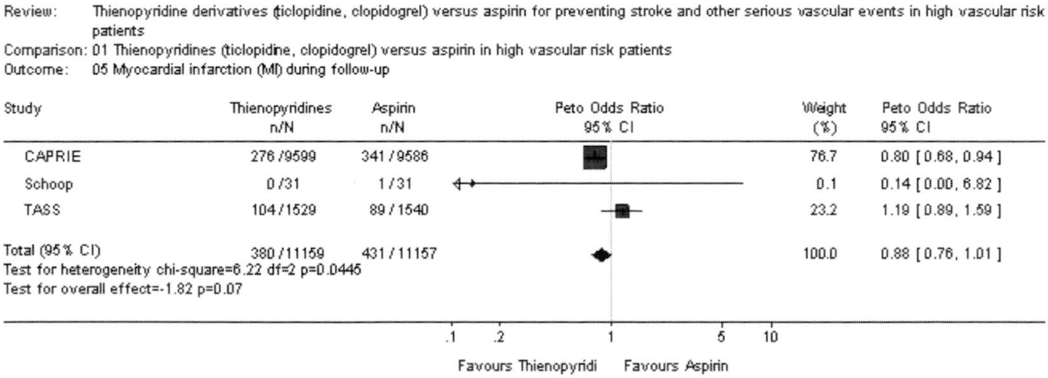

Figure 10.31 Forest plot showing the effects of *the thienopyridines (ticlopidine, clopidogrel) vs another aspirin* in high vascular risk patients on *MI* at the end of follow-up. Reproduced from Hankey *et al.* (2000), with permission from the authors and John Wiley & Sons Limited. Copyright Cochrane Library, reproduced with permission.

African-Americans with TIA or ischaemic stroke   Among African-Americans with TIA or ischaemic stroke ticlopidine is not more effective than aspirin (hazard ratio (HR): 1.22, 95% CI: 0.94–1.57) (Gorelick *et al.*, 2003).

Adverse effects

There was no clear difference between the thienopyridines (ticlopidine, clopidogrel) and aspirin in the odds of experiencing either intracranial or extracranial haemorrhage (Fig. 10.32).

However, compared with aspirin, the thienopyridines were associated with a lower risk of both GI haemorrhage and upper-GI upset, but with an increased risk of diarrhoea and of skin rash (Fig. 10.32).

There was substantial heterogeneity between the results for ticlopidine and clopidogrel, both for diarrhoea and for skin rash (Fig. 10.32). Compared with aspirin, ticlopidine is associated with a 2-fold increase in the odds of skin rash (11.8% ticlopidine vs 5.5% aspirin, OR: 2.2, 95% CI: 1.7–2.9) and diarrhoea (20.4% ticlopidine vs 9.9% aspirin, OR: 2.3, 95% CI: 1.9–2.8) (Hankey *et al.*, 2000).

Compared with aspirin, ticlopidine is associated with a 3-fold excess of neutropaenia ($<1.2 \times 10^9$/l) (2.3% ticlopidine vs 0.8% aspirin, OR: 2.7, 95% CI: 1.5–4.8) (Fig. 10.32).

There are no published trial data available for the frequency of thrombocytopaenia associated with ticlopidine compared with aspirin, but observational data have shown that ticlopidine is associated with a significant excess both of thrombocytopaenia and of TTP (see above, p. 229) (Bennett *et al.*, 1998a, b; 1999; Steinhubl *et al.*, 1999).

Clopidogrel vs aspirin

Evidence

Efficacy

High vascular risk patients   Among high vascular risk patients, clopidogrel significantly reduces the RR of stroke and all serious ischaemic vascular events by about 8.7% (95% CI: 0.3–16.3%) compared with aspirin (Fig. 10.27) (CAPRIE Steering Committee, 1996).

TIA and ischaemic stroke patients   For patients with previous TIA or ischaemic stroke, clopidogrel does not significantly reduce the risk of serious vascular events compared with aspirin (RRR: 7.3%, 95% CI: −5.7 to 18.7%), but the results are consistent with the significant effect of clopidogrel compared with aspirin in all high-risk patients (CAPRIE Steering Committee, 1996). These data are derived from one study, which was not designed to have the statistical power to reliably identify or exclude a modest but important treatment effect of clopidogrel in patient subgroups according

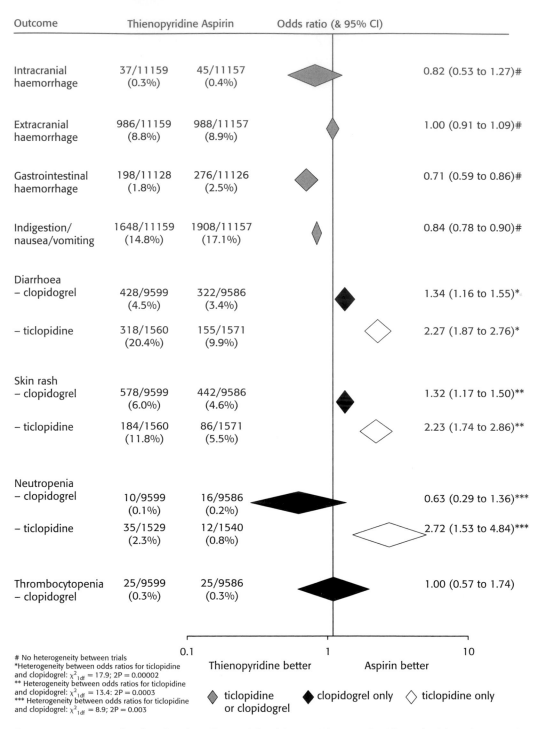

Outcome	Thienopyridine	Aspirin	Odds ratio (& 95% CI)
Intracranial haemorrhage	37/11159 (0.3%)	45/11157 (0.4%)	0.82 (0.53 to 1.27)#
Extracranial haemorrhage	986/11159 (8.8%)	988/11157 (8.9%)	1.00 (0.91 to 1.09)#
Gastrointestinal haemorrhage	198/11128 (1.8%)	276/11126 (2.5%)	0.71 (0.59 to 0.86)#
Indigestion/ nausea/vomiting	1648/11159 (14.8%)	1908/11157 (17.1%)	0.84 (0.78 to 0.90)#
Diarrhoea – clopidogrel	428/9599 (4.5%)	322/9586 (3.4%)	1.34 (1.16 to 1.55)*
– ticlopidine	318/1560 (20.4%)	155/1571 (9.9%)	2.27 (1.87 to 2.76)*
Skin rash – clopidogrel	578/9599 (6.0%)	442/9586 (4.6%)	1.32 (1.17 to 1.50)**
– ticlopidine	184/1560 (11.8%)	86/1571 (5.5%)	2.23 (1.74 to 2.86)**
Neutropenia – clopidogrel	10/9599 (0.1%)	16/9586 (0.2%)	0.63 (0.29 to 1.36)***
– ticlopidine	35/1529 (2.3%)	12/1540 (0.8%)	2.72 (1.53 to 4.84)***
Thrombocytopenia – clopidogrel	25/9599 (0.3%)	25/9586 (0.3%)	1.00 (0.57 to 1.74)

0.1　　　　　1　　　　　10

Thienopyridine better　　　Aspirin better

No heterogeneity between trials
*Heterogeneity between odds ratios for ticlopidine and clopidogrel: $\chi^2_{1df} = 17.9$; 2P = 0.00002
** Heterogeneity between odds ratios for ticlopidine and clopidogrel: $\chi^2_{1df} = 13.4$: 2P = 0.0003
*** Heterogeneity between odds ratios for ticlopidine and clopidogrel: $\chi^2_{1df} = 8.9$; 2P = 0.003

◆ ticlopidine or clopidogrel　　◆ clopidogrel only　　◇ ticlopidine only

Figure 10.32 Forest plot showing the effects of *the thienopyridines (ticlopidine, clopidogrel) vs another aspirin* in high vascular risk patients *on adverse effects* at the end of follow-up. Reproduced from Hankey *et al.* (2000), with permission from the authors and Lippincott, Williams and Wilkins.

to qualifying diagnoses (e.g. cerebrovascular disease) or outcome events (e.g. stroke) (CAPRIE Steering Committee, 1996). The trial was designed to have the statistical power to reliably identify or exclude a modest but important treatment effect of clopidogrel compared with aspirin in all high-risk patients combined.

Adverse effects

Clopidogrel is associated with significantly less GI haemorrhage (OR: 0.71, 95% CI: 0.6–0.9) and upper-GI symptoms (OR: 0.84, 95% CI: 0.8–0.9) compared with aspirin (Fig. 10.32) (CAPRIE Steering Committee, 1996; Hankey *et al.*, 2000). However, these data are derived from one trial where patients were pre-selected as being tolerant of aspirin, and the dose of aspirin was 325 mg daily (CAPRIE Steering Committee, 1996).

Clopidogrel is also associated with a significant one-third increased odds of skin rash (OR: 1.32, 95% CI: 1.2–1.5) and diarrhoea (OR: 1.34, 95% CI: 1.2–1.6) compared with aspirin (Fig. 10.32) (CAPRIE Steering Committee, 1996; Hankey *et al.*, 2000).

Triflusal vs aspirin

Evidence

Efficacy

A review of two recently published trials comparing triflusal with aspirin in a total of 2536 patients indicate that the combined end point of stroke, MI, vascular death and major haemorrhage occurred after more than 2 years of follow-up in 17.1% (217/1268) of patients assigned aspirin and 15.5% (197/1268) of patients assigned triflusal (RRR: 9.2%, 95% CI: −8.3% to +23.9%, $P = 0.31$) (Matiás-Guiu *et al.*, 2003; Anderson and Goldstein, 2004; Culebras *et al.*, 2004).

Adverse events

The only statistically significant result was for major haemorrhage, which occurred in 17.1% (49/1268) of patients assigned aspirin 325 mg/day and 15.5% (21/1268) of patients assigned triflusal (RRR: 57.1%, 95% CI: 29–74%, $P = 0.31$) (Matiás-Guiu *et al.*, 2003; Anderson and Goldstein, 2004; Culebras *et al.*, 2004).

Comment

These exploratory data suggest that triflusal may be associated with fewer major haemorrhages than aspirin 325 mg/day, but it is not certain whether such a difference in bleeding events would be seen with a dose of aspirin of 75–150 mg/day, as is recommended. Moreover, the possible safety benefits of triflusal are not accompanied by any benefits in terms of efficacy.

Aspirin plus oral Gp IIb/IIIa antagonists vs aspirin

Evidence

A meta-analysis of four large trials comparing the combination of aspirin and an oral Gp IIb/IIIa antagonist with aspirin alone in more than 33,000 patients undergoing percutaneous coronary intervention (PCI) or presenting with an acute coronary syndrome (ACS) demonstrated that the combination was associated with a highly significant increase in mortality and major bleeding, with no evidence for a reduction in the risk of a subsequent MI (Chew *et al.*, 2001). A further trial assessing the effects of adding the oral Gp IIb/IIIa receptor antagonist, lotrafiban, to aspirin among 9200 patients with a recent ischaemic stroke or TIA, MI, unstable angina or peripheral arterial disease was stopped early because of a trend towards similar adverse results (Topol *et al.*, 2000).

Aspirin plus dipyridamole vs aspirin

Evidence

Efficacy
High vascular risk patients   Among high vascular risk patients, the combination of aspirin and dipyridamole does not significantly reduce the RR of serious vascular events (RRR: 10%, 95% CI: 0–20%) compared with aspirin (Fig. 10.33) (Antithrombotic Trialists' Collaboration, 2002; De Schryver *et al.*, 2002, 2003).

TIA and ischaemic stroke patients   Among 6123 patients with TIA and ischaemic stroke randomised to the combination of aspirin and dipyridamole vs aspirin, a meta-analysis of individual patient data from the RCTs indicated that random assignment to the combination of aspirin and dipyridamole was associated with a 22% (95% CI: 7–35%) reduction in odds of stroke, an 5% (95% CI: −37% to +34%) reduction in odds of MI, an 2% increase in odds of vascular death (95% CI: −19% to +29%) and a 16% (3–28%) reduction in odds of serious vascular events, compared with control (Leonard-Bee *et al.*, 2005).

A statistically significant benefit of the combination of dipyridamole and aspirin was found only in the most recent and largest trial, in patients presenting after TIA or ischaemic stroke (Diener *et al.*, 1996). Most of the benefit was in preventing recurrent stroke, not coronary events (Diener *et al.*, 1996). Reasons for the significant effect on recurrent stroke in this single trial include the possibility that the newer, and more bioavailable, formulation of extended-release dipyridamole (as used in this trial) was more effective than the older preparation (as used in earlier trials). Extended-release dipyridamole yields continuous absorption and steady serum concentrations, whereas the older preparation is absorbed rapidly and only in a low-pH acidic milieu. This can lead to considerable variation in plasma

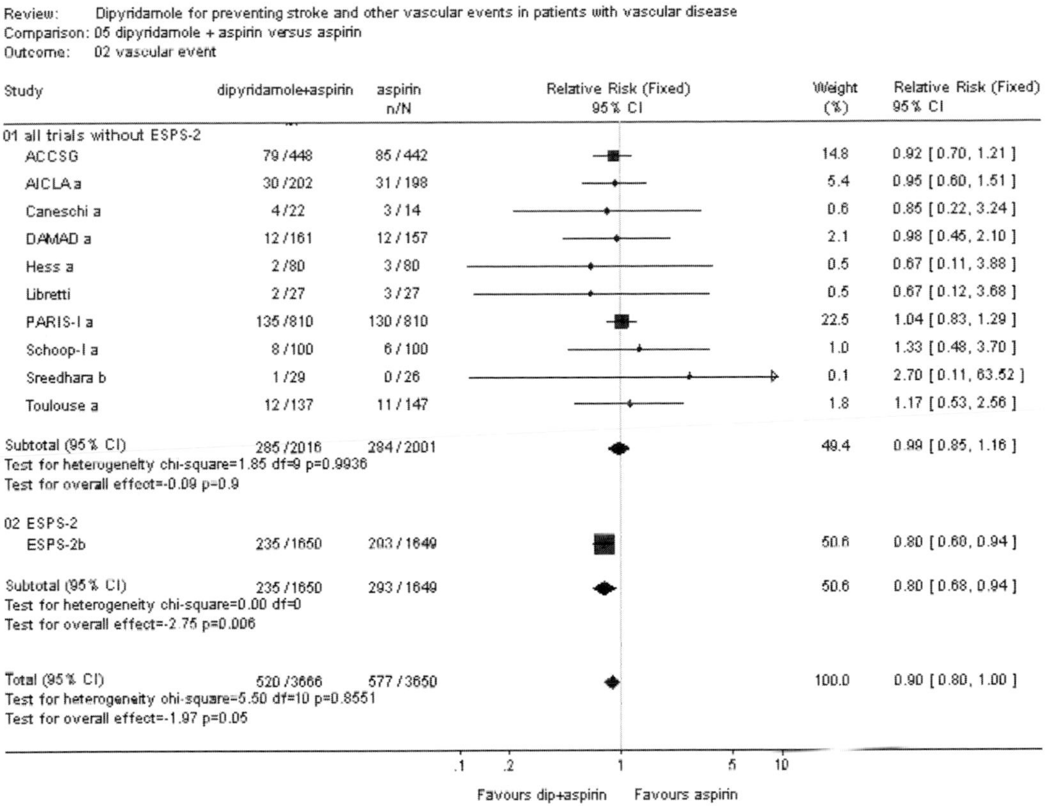

Review: Dipyridamole for preventing stroke and other vascular events in patients with vascular disease
Comparison: 05 dipyridamole + aspirin versus aspirin
Outcome: 02 vascular event

Study	dipyridamole+aspirin n/N	aspirin n/N	Relative Risk (Fixed) 95% CI	Weight (%)	Relative Risk (Fixed) 95% CI
01 all trials without ESPS-2					
ACCSG	79 /448	85 / 442		14.8	0.92 [0.70, 1.21]
AICLA a	30 /202	31 / 198		5.4	0.95 [0.60, 1.51]
Caneschi a	4 /22	3 / 14		0.6	0.85 [0.22, 3.24]
DAMAD a	12 /161	12 / 157		2.1	0.98 [0.45, 2.10]
Hess a	2 /80	3 / 80		0.5	0.67 [0.11, 3.88]
Libretti	2 /27	3 / 27		0.5	0.67 [0.12, 3.68]
PARIS-I a	135 /810	130 / 810		22.5	1.04 [0.83, 1.29]
Schoop-I a	8 /100	6 / 100		1.0	1.33 [0.48, 3.70]
Sreedhara b	1 /29	0 / 26		0.1	2.70 [0.11, 63.52]
Toulouse a	12 /137	11 / 147		1.8	1.17 [0.53, 2.56]
Subtotal (95% CI)	285 /2016	284 / 2001		49.4	0.99 [0.85, 1.16]

Test for heterogeneity chi-square=1.85 df=9 p=0.9936
Test for overall effect=-0.09 p=0.9

02 ESPS-2					
ESPS-2b	235 /1650	293 / 1649		50.6	0.80 [0.68, 0.94]
Subtotal (95% CI)	235 /1650	293 / 1649		50.6	0.80 [0.68, 0.94]

Test for heterogeneity chi-square=0.00 df=0
Test for overall effect=-2.75 p=0.006

| Total (95% CI) | 520 /3666 | 577 / 3650 | | 100.0 | 0.90 [0.80, 1.00] |

Test for heterogeneity chi-square=5.50 df=10 p=0.8551
Test for overall effect=-1.97 p=0.05

```
        .1      .2              1              5      10
```

Favours dip+aspirin   Favours aspirin

Figure 10.33 Forest plot showing the effects of *the combination of dipyridamole plus aspirin vs aspirin* in high vascular risk patients on *serious vascular events* at the end of follow-up. Reproduced from De Schryver *et al.* (2002), with permission from the authors and John Wiley & Sons Limited. Copyright Cochrane Library, reproduced with permission.

concentrations, particularly in older patients taking antacids or proton pump inhibitors. Dipyridamole also significantly, but modestly, lowers blood pressure (BP) by 1.1 mmHg systolic (0.7%) and 0.9 mmHg diastolic (0.6%), with or without aspirin ($P = 0.037$), and this may be a mechanism for the greater reduction in risk of stroke than MI (Leonard-Bee *et al.*, 2005). However, the reduction in stroke seen with dipyridamole in the meta-analysis was not statistically related to the fall in BP ($P = 0.37$) (Leonard-Bee *et al.*, 2005).

Adverse effects

The combination of dipyridamole and aspirin is associated with about a 6% absolute excess of headache sufficient to precipitate discontinuation of study drug, compared with aspirin alone (8.1% dipyridamole, 1.9% aspirin) (Diener *et al.*, 1996). Adding dipyridamole to aspirin does not significantly increase the risk of major or fatal extracranial bleeding, compared with aspirin alone (1.8%

dipyridamole plus aspirin, 1.1% aspirin; RR: 1.52, 95% CI: 0.93–2.49) (Fig. 10.25) (De Schryver *et al.*, 2003).

Aspirin plus clopidogrel vs aspirin

Evidence

Efficacy
Non-ST-segment elevation ACS patients   In patients with non-ST-segment elevation ACS, the combination of aspirin and clopidogrel reduces the RR of serious vascular events, compared with aspirin, by about 20% (95% CI: 10–28%) from 11.4% to 9.3% at 1 year (ARR: 2.1%) (The CURE Trial Investigators, 2001).

Adverse effects
The benefits of the combination of aspirin and clopidogrel, compared with aspirin, in patients with ACS are partially offset by a significant excess of major or life-threatening bleeding (3.7% vs 2.7%, RR: 1.38, 95% CI: 1.13–1.67, absolute risk increase (ARI): 1.0%) over 9 months, but not life-threatening haemorrhage (2.1% vs 1.8%, RR: 1.21, 95% CI: 0.95–1.56) or ICH (0.1% vs 0.1%) (The CURE Trial Investigators, 2001).

Symptomatic carotid stenosis   The Clopidogrel and Aspirin for Reduction of Emboli in Symptomatic Carotid Stenosis (CARESS) trial showed that in patients with recently symptomatic carotid stenosis combination therapy with clopidogrel and aspirin is more effective than aspirin alone in reducing asymptomatic embolisation (Markus *et al.*, 2005), see Chapter 11, page 276.

Aspirin plus clopidogrel vs clopidogrel

Evidence

Efficacy
TIA and ischaemic stroke patients   For patients with TIA or ischaemic stroke, the effectiveness and safety of the combination of aspirin 75 mg/day and clopidogrel 75 mg/day was compared with that of clopidogrel 75 mg/day in the recently published MATCH trial (Diener *et al.*, 2004). The MATCH study was a double-blind RCT in a total of 7599 patients with recent TIA (21%) or ischaemic stroke (79%) who were at high risk of recurrent vascular events (history of diabetes 68%, ischaemic stroke 26%, TIA 19%, MI 5%, angina 12% or symptomatic peripheral arterial disease 10%). The patients were randomised a median of 15 days (range 0–119 days) after TIA or ischaemic stroke, and treated for 18 months (Diener *et al.*, 2004). The trial was designed to have 80% power to reliably identify a reduction in the RR of ischaemic

stroke, MI, vascular death and rehospitalisation for acute ischaemic events (the primary outcome event) by 14%, from 13.3% with clopidogrel to 11.4% with clopidogrel plus aspirin (Diener *et al.*, 2004).

After 18 months, intention-to-treat analysis revealed that, compared with clopidogrel, the addition of aspirin to clopidogrel did not significantly reduce the primary outcome measure of efficacy (RRR: 6.4%, 95% CI: -4.6% to 16.3%, $P = 0.244$; ARR: 1.0%, from 16.7% (clopidogrel) to 15.7% (clopidogrel plus aspirin) at 18 months) (Diener *et al.*, 2004). The results were consistent among all subgroups examined, including aetiological subtypes of stroke and different vascular risk factors.

Adverse effects

Intention-to-treat analysis also revealed that, compared with clopidogrel alone, the addition of aspirin to clopidogrel was associated with a significant increase in life-threatening haemorrhage (the primary outcome measure of safety) from 1.3% (clopidogrel) to 2.6% (aspirin plus clopidogrel), which is 2-fold increase in RR, and an increase in absolute risk of 1.26% (95% CI: 0.64–1.88%) over 18 months ($P < 0.001$) (Diener *et al.*, 2004). Life-threatening haemorrhage was intracranial (0.7% clopidogrel, 1.1% clopidogrel plus aspirin) and GI (0.6% clopidogrel, 1.4% clopidogrel plus aspirin) (Diener *et al.*, 2004). Combination of antiplatelet therapy was also associated with a significant increase in major haemorrhage (0.6% clopidogrel, 1.9% clopidogrel plus aspirin, ARI: 1.36, 95% CI: 0.86–1.86) compared with clopidogrel alone (Diener *et al.*, 2004). The risk of bleeding was cumulative over time. The Kaplan–Meier survival curves for survival free of primary intracerebral haemorrhage for each treatment group did not separate until at 3–4 months after randomisation, suggesting that the benefit:risk ratio of clopidogrel plus aspirin vs clopidogrel may be greatest in the first few months after stroke. Multiple regression analysis failed to identify any key predictors of bleeding that were not also key predictors of ischaemic events.

Comment

Interpretation of the evidence

The results of the MATCH trial indicate that for every 1000 high-risk TIA or ischaemic stroke patients, the addition of aspirin to clopidogrel resulted in an estimated 10 fewer recurrent ischaemic events (not significant) and 13 more life-threatening haemorrhages (significant) after 18 months.

The effect of aspirin (when added to clopidogrel) on the risk of ischaemic events in the MATCH trial (RRR: 6.4%, 95% CI: -4.6% to 16.3%) is consistent with the known effect of aspirin, compared with placebo, in TIA and ischaemic stroke patients (RRR: 13%, 95% CI: 6–19%) (Algra and van Gijn, 1999).

The results of the MATCH trial are also consistent with the effects of the combination of aspirin and clopidogrel in patients with ACS (The CURE Trial Investigators,

2001). The MATCH trial compared the combination of aspirin plus clopidogrel with clopidogrel alone (Diener *et al.*, 2004), rather than aspirin alone, as was the case in the Clopidogrel in Unstable angina to prevent Recurrent Events (CURE) trial (2001). Statistical power for efficacy and safety was compromised by choosing clopidogrel as the comparitor because clopidogrel is more effective than aspirin (by about 9% in relative terms) and probably safer with respect to GI haemorrhage (CAPRIE Steering Committee, 1996; Hankey *et al.*, 2000). Furthermore, patients in the MATCH trial were not treated until a median of 15 days after their stroke, during which time at least 10% of patients could have had another stroke (Coull *et al.*, 2004); half of the patients had symptomatic small vessel disease, which is associated with a low risk of early recurrent stroke (Lovett *et al.*, 2004) and high risk of ICH (The SPIRIT Study Group, 1997); only a third of patients had symptomatic large artery atherothromboembolism, which is associated with a high risk for early recurrent stroke (Lovett *et al.*, 2004); and a loading dose of clopidogrel was not used (unlike in the CURE trial).

Implications for practice

1 If a patient presents with TIA or ischaemic stroke due to atherothromboembolism and is *not taking antiplatelet therapy*, then they should be considered for aspirin (Algra and van Gijn, 1999) if they are at low risk (Dippel *et al.*, 2004) of a recurrent ischaemic event, clopidogrel if allergic or intolerant of aspirin (The CAPRIE Steering Committee, 1996), and clopidogrel (The CAPRIE Steering Committee, 1996) or the combination of aspirin and dipyridamole (De Schryver *et al.*, 2003) if at high risk of a recurrent ischaemic event (Dippel *et al.*, 2004; Tran and Anand, 2004).

2 If a patient presents with atherothrombotic TIA or ischaemic stroke and is *taking aspirin* (i.e. an aspirin treatment failure), then consideration should be given to stopping the aspirin and starting clopidogrel (The CAPRIE Steering Committee, 1996), or adding dipyridamole to aspirin (De Schryver *et al.*, 2003), but not adding clopidogrel to aspirin (Diener *et al.*, 2004).

3 If a patient presents with atherothrombotic TIA or ischaemic stroke and is *taking clopidogrel*, then consideration should be given to staying on clopidogrel (The CAPRIE Steering Committee, 1996), or changing to aspirin (Algra and van Gijn, 1999) or the combination of dipyridamole and aspirin (De Schryver *et al.*, 2003), but not adding aspirin to the clopidogrel (Diener *et al.*, 2004).

4 If a patient presents with atherothrombotic TIA or ischaemic stroke and is *taking the combination of aspirin and clopidogrel*, then consideration should be given to aspirin monotherapy in patients at low risk of a recurrent ischaemic event (i.e. all vascular risk factors are well controlled) (Algra and van Gijn, 1999; Dippel *et al.*, 2004), clopidogrel monotherapy (The CAPRIE Steering Committee, 1996) or the combination of dipyridamole and aspirin (De Schryver *et al.*, 2003) in

patients at higher risk (Dippel *et al.*, 2004), and continuing aspirin and clopido-grel in patients who have had an ACS or coronary stent within 9 months or so (Mehta *et al.*, 2001; Steinhubl *et al.*, 2002).

Implications for research

Ongoing research aims to identify the independent risk factors for bleeding com-plications associated with combination antiplatelet therapy (e.g. old microbleeds on gradient-echo MR imaging (MRI) studies (Nighoghossian *et al.*, 2002)), and the optimal antiplatelet regimens.

A high priority is a dedication evaluation of the safety and efficacy of adding clopidogrel to aspirin immediately after TIA and ischaemic stroke (i.e. within 12–24 h, rather than 15 days), with a loading dose of clopidogrel (300 or 600 mg), in patients at high risk for early recurrent ischaemic stroke (e.g. with symptomatic large artery atherothromboembolism), and for a short period of about 3 months (when the benefits are likely to be greatest and the cumulative risks for bleeding lessened). This is the principle underlying the Fast Assessment of Stroke and Transient ischaemic attack (TIA) to prevent Early Recurrence (FASTER) trial (Hankey, 2004; Kennedy *et al.*, 2004; Hankey and Eikelboom, 2005).

Meanwhile, the safety and efficacy of adding clopidogrel to aspirin is also being studied in the longer term in stroke and other high-risk patients (Clopidogrel for High Atherothrombotic Risk and Ischemic Stabilization, Management and Avoidance, CHARISMA trial (Bhatt and Topol, 2004)), and in patients with TIA and ischaemic stroke caused by atrial fibrillation (Atrial fibrillation Clopidogrel Trial with Irbesartan for prevention of Vascular Events, ACTIVE trial), aortic arch atheroma (Arch-Related Cerebral Hazard, ARCH trial), carotid stenosis (Clopidogrel and Aspirin for Reduction of Emboli in Symptomatic carotid Stenosis, CARESS trial (Markus and Ringlestein, 2004), see Chapter 11) and intracranial small vessel disease (Secondary Prevention of Small Subcortical Strokes (SPS3) trial) (Benavente and Hart, 2004; Hankey, 2004).

The safety and efficacy of the combination of dipyridamole and aspirin compared with aspirin alone (ESPRIT trial (De Schryver *et al.*, 2000)) or clopidogrel alone (Prevention Regimen for Effectively avoiding Second Strokes (PRoFESS) trial (Sacco *et al.*, 2004)) in TIA and ischaemic stroke patients is currently also under evaluation in large randomised trials and should further clarify the role of dipyridamole in com-bination with aspirin for the treatment of acute cerebral ischaemia. The European/ Australasian Stroke Prevention in Reversible Ischaemia Trial (ESPRIT trial) has randomised 2578 TIA and ischaemic stroke patients of presumed arterial origin between aspirin and the combination of aspirin and dipyridamole as of 3 January 2005, yielding 7600 patient-years of follow-up. The trial should be complete in early 2006 when 9000 patient-years of follow-up have been achieved.

Table 10.4. Possible causes of recurrent ischaemic vascular events among TIA and stroke patients taking aspirin.

Non-atherothrombotic causes of vascular events
- Embolism from the heart (red, fibrin thrombi; vegetations; calcium; tumour; prostheses)
- Arteritis

Reduced bioavailability of aspirin
- Inadequate intake of aspirin (poor compliance)
- Inadequate dose of aspirin
- Concurrent intake of certain non-steroidal anti-inflammatory drugs (e.g. ibuprofen, indomethacin), possibly preventing the access of aspirin to cyclo-oxygenase-1-binding site

Alternative pathways of platelet activation
- Platelet activation by pathways that are not blocked by aspirin (e.g. red cell-induced platelet activation; stimulation of collagen, adenosine diphosphate, epinephrine and thrombin receptors on platelets)
- Increased platelet sensitivity to collagen and adenosine diphosphate
- Biosynthesis of thromboxane by pathways that are not blocked by aspirin (e.g. by cyclo-oxygenase-2 in monocytes and macrophages, and vascular endothelial cells)

Increased turnover of platelets
- Increased production of platelets by the bone marrow in response to stress (e.g. after coronary artery bypass surgery), introducing into blood stream newly formed platelets unexposed to aspirin during the 24-h dose interval (aspirin is given once daily and has only a 20-min half-life)

Genetic polymorphisms
- Polymorphisms involving platelet Gp Ia/IIa, Ib/V/IX and IIb/IIIa receptors, and collagen and vWF receptors
- Polymorphisms of cyclo-oxygenase-1, cyclo-oxygenase-2, thromboxane A_2-synthase or other arachidonate metabolism enzymes
- Factor XIII Val34Leu polymorphism, leading to variable inhibition of factor XIII activation by low-dose aspirin

Future research should continue to explore the independent clinical, imaging and laboratory (including genetic) factors associated with increased responsiveness, and also increased hazard, associated with antiplatelet therapy among *individual* patients (Caplan, 2004). For example, although aspirin reduces the odds of serious atherothrombotic vascular events in stroke patients by up to about one-quarter, it still fails to prevent most (at least 75%) serious vascular events. And, although recurrent vascular events in patients taking aspirin ('aspirin treatment failures') have many possible causes (Table 10.4), a potentially important cause is aspirin resistance, which requires further research (Eikelboom and Hankey, 2003; Bhatt, 2004; Hankey and Eikelboom, 2004).

Aspirin resistance has been used to describe several different phenomena. One is the inability of aspirin to protect patients from ischaemic vascular events. This has also been called *clinical aspirin resistance* (Bhatt and Topol, 2003; Patrono, 2003). However, this definition is retrospective and non-specific, and could apply to any of the conditions listed in Table 10.4. Furthermore, it is not realistic to expect that all vascular complications can be prevented by any single preventive strategy. Aspirin resistance has also been used to describe an inability of aspirin to produce an anticipated effect on one or more tests of platelet function, such as inhibiting biosynthesis of thromboxane, inhibiting platelet aggregation and causing a prolongation of the bleeding time (Patrono, 2003). This has been called *biochemical aspirin resistance*. However, the precise qualitative and quantitative abnormalities of platelet function which define biochemical aspirin resistance have not been established, let alone their clinical relevance. There are several different laboratory tests of platelet function which are being used to diagnose 'biochemical' aspirin resistance, and each has its own limitations.

For a laboratory measure of biochemical aspirin resistance to have clinical utility it must be associated independently and consistently with the occurrence of recurrent vascular events in patients taking aspirin; it must be standardised and valid; and clinical management should be altered on the basis of the results of testing: for example, it should be shown in RCTs that reversing the laboratory abnormality (with treatment) is followed by a reduction in the incidence of recurrent vascular events while taking aspirin. Finally, the overall benefits of testing should outweigh any adverse consequences and costs.

Two studies meet the first criterion, but no study meets the other three criteria. The first study showed an independent and significant association between increasing baseline urinary concentrations of 11-dehydrothromboxane B2 (a marker of *in vivo* thromboxane generation) and an increasing risk of future MI or cardiovascular death in patients at high vascular risk who were treated with aspirin (Eikelboom *et al.*, 2002). The second study showed an independent and significant association between the failure of aspirin to suppress agonist induced platelet aggregation and an increasing risk of serious vascular events in 326 patients with coronary or cerebral vascular disease who were treated with aspirin (HR: 4.1, 95% CI: 1.4–12.1) (Gum *et al.*, 2003). In this study, platelet aggregation was measured by optical platelet aggregometry. These data also show that up to 20% of future serious vascular events in high-risk vascular patients may be attributable to a failure of aspirin to suppress thromboxane production or platelet aggregation.

The therapeutic implications of a valid and reliable screening test for aspirin resistance, coupled with an effective treatment, are potentially noteworthy. However, before aspirin resistance can be accepted as a valid clinical entity worthy of screening and treatment, the other criteria mentioned above must be met. The first step is to develop a standardised definition and test of aspirin resistance. An appropriate definition of aspirin resistance may be: the lack of anticipated response to a therapeutic dose of aspirin (75–150 mg/day for at least 5 days in a compliant patient) that can be demonstrated by a specific, valid and reliable laboratory measure of the antiplatelet effects of aspirin and which correlates significantly, independently and consistently with an increased incidence of athero-thrombotic vascular events. The definition may be refined in the future to include proven genetic determinants (e.g. platelet polymorphisms), which mediate aspirin resistance and risk of ischaemic events. Further studies are required to externally validate the promise of urinary 11-dehydrothromboxane B2 and optical platelet aggregometry as laboratory measures of aspirin resistance.

Oral anticoagulation vs antiplatelet therapy

Evidence

Anticoagulation with high International Normalised Ratio (3.0–4.5) vs antiplatelet therapy

A systematic review identified four RCTs directly comparing oral anticoagulants *high* International Normalised Ratio (INR) (3.0–4.5) vs antiplatelet therapy in a total of 1870 patients with previous TIA or minor stroke of presumed arterial origin (Algra *et al.*, 2002, 2003).

Serious vascular events A meta-analysis of these trials showed that long-term oral anticoagulant therapy with a *high* INR (3.0–4.5) was associated with a significantly higher rate of recurrent serious vascular events (non-fatal stroke, non-fatal MI or vascular death) than antiplatelet therapy in the 1316 patients randomised (OR: 1.70, 95% CI: 1.12–2.59) (Fig. 10.34) (Algra *et al.*, 2002, 2003).

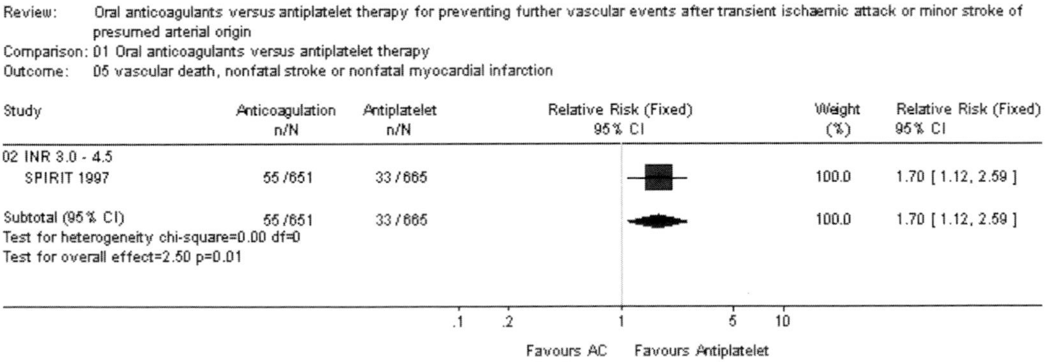

Review: Oral anticoagulants versus antiplatelet therapy for preventing further vascular events after transient ischaemic attack or minor stroke of presumed arterial origin
Comparison: 01 Oral anticoagulants versus antiplatelet therapy
Outcome: 05 vascular death, nonfatal stroke or nonfatal myocardial infarction

Study	Anticoagulation n/N	Antiplatelet n/N	Relative Risk (Fixed) 95% CI	Weight (%)	Relative Risk (Fixed) 95% CI
02 INR 3.0 - 4.5					
SPIRIT 1997	55 /651	33 /665		100.0	1.70 [1.12, 2.59]
Subtotal (95% CI)	55 /651	33 /665		100.0	1.70 [1.12, 2.59]

Test for heterogeneity chi-square=0.00 df=0
Test for overall effect=2.50 p=0.01

.1 .2   1   5 10
Favours AC   Favours Antiplatelet

Figure 10.34 Forest plot showing the effects of *anticoagulation with high INR (3.0–4.5) vs antiplatelet therapy* in patients with previous TIA or mild ischaemic stroke of presumed arterial origin on *serious vascular events* at the end of follow-up. Reproduced from Algra *et al.* (2002), with permission from the authors and John Wiley & Sons Limited. Copyright Cochrane Library, reproduced with permission.

Review: Oral anticoagulants versus antiplatelet therapy for preventing further vascular events after transient ischaemic attack or minor stroke of
presumed arterial origin
Comparison: 01 Oral anticoagulants versus antiplatelet therapy
Outcome: 09 major bleeding complication

Study	Anticoagulation n/N	Antiplatelet n/N	Relative Risk (Fixed) 95% CI	Weight (%)	Relative Risk (Fixed) 95% CI
01 INR 1.4 - 2.8					
WARSS 2001	38 / 1103	30 / 1103		100.0	1.27 [0.79, 2.03]
Subtotal (95% CI)	38 / 1103	30 / 1103		100.0	1.27 [0.79, 2.03]
Test for heterogeneity chi-square=0.00 df=0					
Test for overall effect=0.98 p=0.3					
02 INR 2.1 - 3.6					
Garde 1983	8 / 114	4 / 127		28.3	2.23 [0.69, 7.20]
Olsson 1980	7 / 68	3 / 67		22.6	2.30 [0.62, 8.52]
SWAT 1998	0 / 59	6 / 58		49.1	0.08 [0.00, 1.31]
Subtotal (95% CI)	15 / 241	13 / 252		100.0	1.19 [0.59, 2.41]
Test for heterogeneity chi-square=5.66 df=2 p=0.0591					
Test for overall effect=0.48 p=0.6					
03 INR 3.0 - 4.5					
SPIRIT 1997	53 / 651	6 / 665		100.0	9.02 [3.91, 20.84]
Subtotal (95% CI)	53 / 651	6 / 665		100.0	9.02 [3.91, 20.84]
Test for heterogeneity chi-square=0.00 df=0					
Test for overall effect=5.15 p<0.00001					

.01   .1   1   10   100

Favours AC   Favours Antiplatelet

Figure 10.35 Forest plot showing the effects of *oral anticoagulation vs antiplatelet therapy* in patients with previous TIA or mild ischaemic stroke of presumed arterial origin on *major bleeding complications* at the end of follow-up. Reproduced from Algra *et al.* (2002), with permission from the authors and John Wiley & Sons Limited. Copyright Cochrane Library, reproduced with permission.

Major bleeding complications   Oral anticoagulant therapy with a *high* INR (3.0–4.5) was associated with a highly significant excess of major bleeding complications compared with antiplatelet therapy (OR: 9.02, 95% CI: 3.91–20.84) (Fig. 10.35) (Algra *et al.*, 2002, 2003).

Serious vascular events or major bleeding complications   Oral anticoagulant therapy with a *high* INR (3.0–4.5) was associated with a significant excess of recurrent serious vascular events or major haemorrhage compared with antiplatelet therapy (OR: 2.30, 95% CI: 1.58–3.35) (Fig. 10.36) (Algra *et al.*, 2002, 2003).

Recurrent ischaemic stroke and recurrent stroke of any type   There was no difference between oral anticoagulants and antiplatelet therapy in the rate of recurrent ischaemic stroke (OR: 1.02, 95% CI: 0.49–2.13) (Fig. 10.37) but an excess of recurrent stroke of any type (OR: 2.04, 95% CI: 1.21–3.45) (Fig. 10.38) (Algra *et al.*, 2002).

Review: Oral anticoagulants versus antiplatelet therapy for preventing further vascular events after transient ischaemic attack or minor stroke of
            presumed arterial origin
Comparison: 01 Oral anticoagulants versus antiplatelet therapy
Outcome: 01 the composite vascular death, nonfatal stroke, nonfatal myocardial infarction or major bleeding complication

Study	Anticoagulation n/N	Antiplatelet n/N	Relative Risk (Fixed) 95% CI	Weight (%)	Relative Risk (Fixed) 95% CI
02 INR 3.0 - 4.5					
SPIRIT 1997	81 /651	36 /665		100.0	2.30 [1.58, 3.35]
Subtotal (95% CI)	81 /651	36 /665		100.0	2.30 [1.58, 3.35]

Test for heterogeneity chi-square=0.00 df=0
Test for overall effect=4.32 p=0.0000

```
        .1      .2            1         5    10
          Favours AC     Favours Antiplatelet
```

Figure 10.36 Forest plot showing the effects of *anticoagulation with high INR (3.0–4.5) vs antiplatelet therapy* in patients with previous TIA or mild ischaemic stroke of presumed arterial origin on *serious vascular events or major bleeding complication* at the end of follow-up. Reproduced from Algra *et al.* (2002), with permission from the authors and John Wiley & Sons Limited. Copyright Cochrane Library, reproduced with permission.

Review: Oral anticoagulants versus antiplatelet therapy for preventing further vascular events after transient ischaemic attack or minor stroke of
            presumed arterial origin
Comparison: 01 Oral anticoagulants versus antiplatelet therapy
Outcome: 06 recurrent ischaemic stroke

Study	Anticoagulation n/N	Antiplatelet n/N	Relative Risk (Fixed) 95% CI	Weight (%)	Relative Risk (Fixed) 95% CI
01 INR 2.1 - 3.6					
Garde 1983	7 /114	6 / 127		25.2	1.30 [0.45, 3.75]
Olsson 1980	1 /68	3 / 67		13.4	0.33 [0.04, 3.08]
Subtotal (95% CI)	8 /182	9 / 194		38.6	0.96 [0.38, 2.42]
02 INR 3.0 - 4.5					
SPIRIT 1997	14 /651	14 /665		61.4	1.02 [0.49, 2.13]
Subtotal (95% CI)	14 /651	14 /665		61.4	1.02 [0.49, 2.13]
Total (95% CI)	22 /833	23 /859		100.0	1.00 [0.56, 1.77]

Test for heterogeneity chi-square=1.19 df=1 p=0.2743
Test for overall effect=-0.08 p=0.9

Test for heterogeneity chi-square=0.00 df=0
Test for overall effect=0.06 p=1.0

Test for heterogeneity chi-square=1.19 df=2 p=0.5517
Test for overall effect=0.00 p=1.0

```
        .1      .2            1         5    10
          Favours AC     Favours Antiplatelet
```

Figure 10.37 Forest plot showing the effects of *oral anticoagulation vs antiplatelet therapy* in patients with previous TIA or mild ischaemic stroke of presumed arterial origin on *recurrent ischaemic stroke* at the end of follow-up. Reproduced from Algra *et al.* (2002), with permission from the authors and John Wiley & Sons Limited. Copyright Cochrane Library, reproduced with permission.

Death   Oral anticoagulant therapy with a high INR (3.0–4.5) was associated with a significant excess of death from any cause compared with antiplatelet therapy (RR: 2.38, 95% CI: 1.31–4.32) (Fig. 10.39) (Algra *et al.*, 2002, 2003).

Review: Oral anticoagulants versus antiplatelet therapy for preventing further vascular events after transient ischaemic attack or minor stroke of
           presumed arterial origin
Comparison: 01 Oral anticoagulants versus antiplatelet therapy
Outcome: 07 recurrent ischaemic stroke or intracranial haemorrhage

Study	Anticoagulation n/N	Antiplatelet n/N	Relative Risk (Fixed) 95% CI	Weight (%)	Relative Risk (Fixed) 95% CI
01 INR 2.1 - 3.6					
Garde 1983	7 / 114	7 / 127		52.3	1.11 [0.40, 3.08]
Olsson 1980	2 / 68	3 / 67		23.9	0.66 [0.11, 3.81]
SWAT 1998	1 / 59	3 / 58		23.9	0.33 [0.04, 3.06]
Subtotal (95% CI)	10 / 241	13 / 252		100.0	0.82 [0.37, 1.82]
Test for heterogeneity chi-square=1.06 df=2 p=0.5889					
Test for overall effect=-0.49 p=0.6					
02 INR 3. 0 - 4.5					
SPIRIT 1997	40 / 651	20 / 665		100.0	2.04 [1.21, 3.46]
Subtotal (95% CI)	40 / 651	20 / 665		100.0	2.04 [1.21, 3.46]
Test for heterogeneity chi-square=0.00 df=0					
Test for overall effect=2.66 p=0.008					

```
        .1    .2        1        5   10
           Favours AC    Favours Antiplatelet
```

Figure 10.38 Forest plot showing the effects of *oral anticoagulation vs antiplatelet therapy* in patients with previous TIA or mild ischaemic stroke of presumed arterial origin on *recurrent stroke of any type* at the end of follow-up. Reproduced from Algra *et al.* (2002), with permission from the authors and John Wiley & Sons Limited. Copyright Cochrane Library, reproduced with permission.

Fatal intracranial or extracranial haemorrhage   Oral anticoagulant therapy with a high INR (3.0–4.5) was associated with a significant excess of fatal haemorrhage compared with antiplatelet therapy (RR: 17.4, 95% CI: 2.3–130) (Fig. 10.40) (Algra *et al.*, 2002, 2003).

Anticoagulation with medium INR (2.1 to 3.6) vs antiplatelet therapy

Among the 493 patients randomised to long-term oral anticoagulant therapy with a *medium* INR (2.1–3.6) or antiplatelet therapy, there was no difference in the rate of recurrent ischaemic stroke (OR: 0.96, 95% CI: 0.38–2.42) (Fig. 10.37), recurrent stroke of any type (OR: 0.82, 95% CI: 0.37–1.82) (Fig. 10.38), recurrent stroke or vascular death (RR: 1.07, 95% CI: 0.54–2.12) or the rate of major bleeding complications (OR: 1.19, 95% CI: 0.59–2.41) (Fig. 10.35) (Algra *et al.*, 2002).

The Warfarin-Aspirin Symptomatic Intracranial Disease (WASID) trial showed that among 569 patients with TIA or ischaemic stroke caused by major intracranial artery stenosis (50–99%), random assignment to medium-intensity anticoagulation with warfarin (Target INR: 2.0–3.0) was associated with significantly higher rates of adverse events, and no benefit, compared with aspirin (1300 mg daily) (Chimowitz *et al.*, 2005). During a mean follow-up period of 1.8 years, the primary outcome of stroke or death from vascular causes occurred in 22.1% of patients

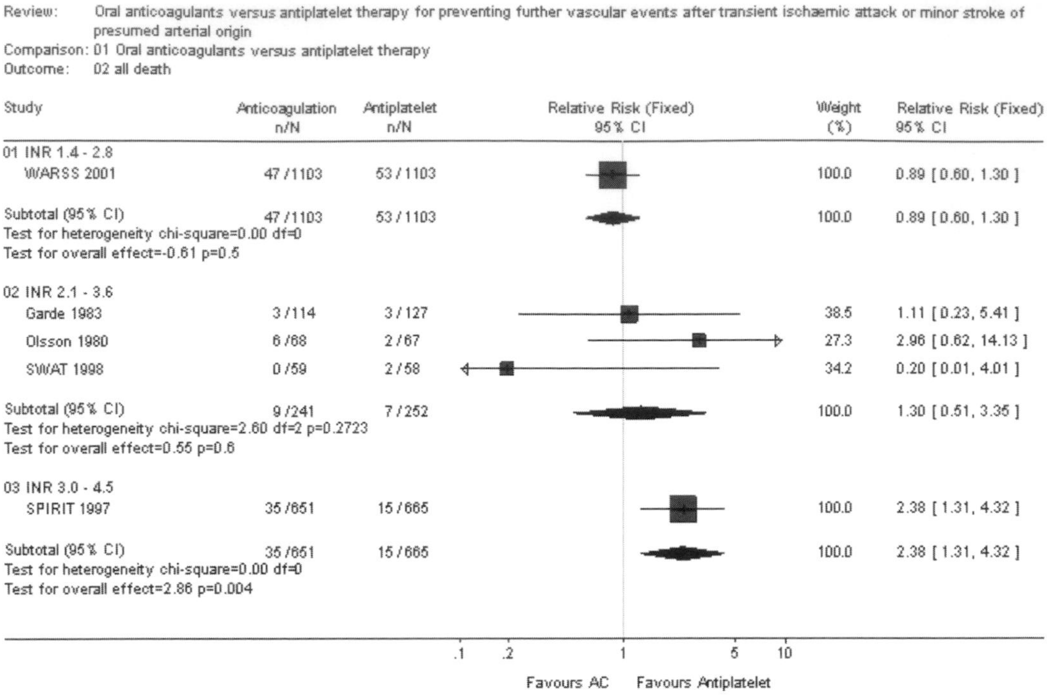

Review: Oral anticoagulants versus antiplatelet therapy for preventing further vascular events after transient ischæmic attack or minor stroke of
               presumed arterial origin
Comparison: 01 Oral anticoagulants versus antiplatelet therapy
Outcome: 02 all death

Study	Anticoagulation n/N	Antiplatelet n/N	Relative Risk (Fixed) 95% CI	Weight (%)	Relative Risk (Fixed) 95% CI
01 INR 1.4 - 2.8					
WARSS 2001	47 /1103	53 /1103		100.0	0.89 [0.60, 1.30]
Subtotal (95% CI)	47 /1103	53 /1103		100.0	0.89 [0.60, 1.30]
Test for heterogeneity chi-square=0.00 df=0					
Test for overall effect=-0.61 p=0.5					
02 INR 2.1 - 3.6					
Garde 1983	3 /114	3 /127		38.5	1.11 [0.23, 5.41]
Olsson 1980	6 /68	2 /67		27.3	2.96 [0.62, 14.13]
SWAT 1998	0 /59	2 /58		34.2	0.20 [0.01, 4.01]
Subtotal (95% CI)	9 /241	7 /252		100.0	1.30 [0.51, 3.35]
Test for heterogeneity chi-square=2.60 df=2 p=0.2723					
Test for overall effect=0.55 p=0.6					
03 INR 3.0 - 4.5					
SPIRIT 1997	35 /651	15 /665		100.0	2.38 [1.31, 4.32]
Subtotal (95% CI)	35 /651	15 /665		100.0	2.38 [1.31, 4.32]
Test for heterogeneity chi-square=0.00 df=0					
Test for overall effect=2.86 p=0.004					

.1   .2   1   5   10

Favours AC   Favours Antiplatelet

Figure 10.39 Forest plot showing the effects of *oral anticoagulation vs antiplatelet therapy* in patients with previous TIA or mild ischaemic stroke of presumed arterial origin on *death* at the end of follow-up. Reproduced from Algra *et al.* (2002), with permission from the authors and John Wiley & Sons Limited. Copyright Cochrane Library, reproduced with permission.

assigned aspirin and 21.8% assigned warfarin (HR: 1.04, 95% CI: 0.73–1.48). Warfarin was associated with higher rates of death (4.3% aspirin vs 9.7% warfarin, HR: 0.46, 95% CI: 0.23–0.90, for aspirin compared to warfarin), major haemorrhage (3.2% vs 8.3%, HR: 0.39, 0.18–0.84), and myocardial infarction or sudden death (2.9% vs 7.3%, HR: 0.40, 0.18–0.91) (Chimowitz *et al.*, 2005).

Low–medium-intensity oral anticoagulation (INR 1.4–2.8) vs antiplatelet therapy
The Warfarin–Aspirin Recurrent Stroke Study (WARSS, 2001) aimed to determine whether low- or medium-intensity oral anticoagulation (INR 1.4–2.8) was more effective than (i.e. superior to) aspirin 325 mg daily in a double-blind RCT involving 2206 patients with recent non-cardioembolic ischaemic strokes.

After 2 years of follow-up, patients randomly allocated warfarin experienced non-significantly more recurrent ischaemic strokes or deaths (17.8% warfarin, 16.0% aspirin, HR: 1.13, 95% CI: 0.92–1.38) and non-significantly more major haemorrhages (3.4% warfarin vs 2.7% aspirin, HR: 1.48, 95% CI: 0.93–2.44) compared with patients allocated aspirin (Figs 10.35, 10.39 and 10.40) (Mohr *et al.*, 2001).

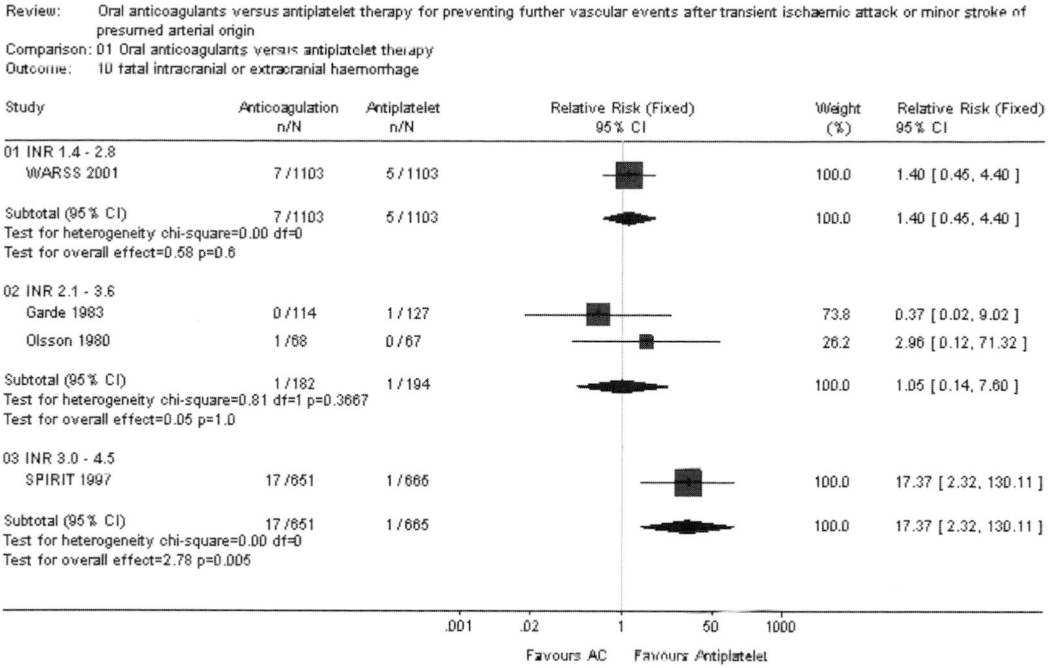

Review: Oral anticoagulants versus antiplatelet therapy for preventing further vascular events after transient ischaemic attack or minor stroke of presumed arterial origin
Comparison: 01 Oral anticoagulants versus antiplatelet therapy
Outcome: 10 fatal intracranial or extracranial haemorrhage

Study	Anticoagulation n/N	Antiplatelet n/N	Relative Risk (Fixed) 95% CI	Weight (%)	Relative Risk (Fixed) 95% CI
01 INR 1.4 - 2.8					
WARSS 2001	7 / 1103	5 / 1103		100.0	1.40 [0.45, 4.40]
Subtotal (95% CI)	7 / 1103	5 / 1103		100.0	1.40 [0.45, 4.40]
Test for heterogeneity chi-square=0.00 df=0					
Test for overall effect=0.58 p=0.6					
02 INR 2.1 - 3.6					
Garde 1983	0 / 114	1 / 127		73.8	0.37 [0.02, 9.02]
Olsson 1980	1 / 68	0 / 67		26.2	2.96 [0.12, 71.32]
Subtotal (95% CI)	1 / 182	1 / 194		100.0	1.05 [0.14, 7.60]
Test for heterogeneity chi-square=0.81 df=1 p=0.3667					
Test for overall effect=0.05 p=1.0					
03 INR 3.0 - 4.5					
SPIRIT 1997	17 / 651	1 / 665		100.0	17.37 [2.32, 130.11]
Subtotal (95% CI)	17 / 651	1 / 665		100.0	17.37 [2.32, 130.11]
Test for heterogeneity chi-square=0.00 df=0					
Test for overall effect=2.78 p=0.005					

.001   .02   1   50   1000

Favours AC   Favours Antiplatelet

Figure 10.40 Forest plot showing the effects of *oral anticoagulation vs antiplatelet therapy* in patients with previous TIA or mild ischaemic stroke of presumed arterial origin on *fatal intracranial or extracranial haemorrhage* at the end of follow-up. Reproduced from Algra *et al.* (2002), with permission from the authors and John Wiley & Sons Limited. Copyright Cochrane Library, reproduced with permission.

Comment

Interpretation of the evidence

The results of the Cochrane Review indicate that high-intensity anticoagulation (INR 3.0–4.5) is more hazardous than effective compared with antiplatelet therapy for patients with ischaemic stroke of presumed arterial origin.

Medium-intensity anticoagulation (INR 2.1 to 3.6) appears to be similar to antiplatelet therapy in efficacy and safety but the estimates are imprecise. More data are awaited from the ESPRIT trial (De Schryver *et al.*, 2000). The WASID trial shows that medium-intensity anticoagulation is associated with significantly higher rates of adverse events than aspirin in patients with symptomatic intracranial stenosis (Chimowitz *et al.*, 2005).

The data for low–medium-intensity oral anticoagulation can be interpreted in several different ways.

Low–medium-intensity warfarin is equally effective as aspirin The WARSS investigators interpreted their failure to reject the null hypothesis (of no significant difference in effectiveness between warfarin and aspirin) as indicating that 'both warfarin and aspirin (can be regarded) as reasonable therapeutic alternatives'. However, failure to reject the null hypothesis is not proof of the null hypothesis, or of equivalence. It may simply be the result of inadequate sample size to reliably detect, with 95% confidence, up to a 38% excess hazard of recurrent stroke or death (the primary outcome) for warfarin compared with aspirin, or up to an 8% excess hazard of recurrent stroke or death for aspirin compared with warfarin.

Low–medium-intensity warfarin is a potentially hazardous placebo   An interpretation that the effect of warfarin is equivalent to that of a placebo is based on an indirect comparison of the 13% (95% CI: −8% to 38%) excess relative hazard (11.25% excess RR) of recurrent ischaemic stroke or death among the WARSS patients randomised to warfarin, as opposed to aspirin, with the 13% (95% CI: 6–19%) excess RR of serious vascular events among the 10,000 TIA or ischaemic stroke patients randomised to placebo, as opposed to aspirin, in the 11 RCTs reviewed by Algra and van Gijn (1999). However, this indirect comparison is potentially flawed because it compares slightly different estimates (RR vs relative hazards), of slightly different outcome events, against the same control (aspirin), not each other. Such indirect comparisons are not reliable, in the same way that it is unreliable to compare two sporting teams by their respective performances against another team; it is more reliable to have them oppose each other directly.

Low–medium-intensity warfarin is not more effective than aspirin   The WARSS investigators aimed to determine whether warfarin would prove superior to aspirin in the prevention of recurrent ischaemic stroke in patients with a prior non-cardioembolic ischaemic stroke. They failed and the null hypothesis was rejected.

My interpretation of the evidence is that warfarin has not been proven to be superior to aspirin in patients with non-cardioembolic ischaemic stroke. It can be said with 95% confidence, that the results of the WARSS trial indicate that low–medium-intensity warfarin may be up to 8% more effective than aspirin, and it may up to 38% less effective. More trials are needed to refine these estimates (see below).

Implications for practice
For patients with recent non-cardioembolic ischaemic stroke who do not have a contraindication to warfarin therapy, warfarin should probably only be used in the context of an RCT, or perhaps if the patient is allergic to, intolerant of, or has failed effective antiplatelet therapies (aspirin, clopidogrel, dipyridamole) in isolation and combination, until the results of ongoing clinical trials (ESPRIT and ARCH) are known (see below).

Implications for research

It is possible that the WARSS trial failed to detect a favourable overall treatment effect of warfarin compared with aspirin (up to 8% less hazard of the primary outcome event) due to a lack of statistical power. In addition, such a favourable treatment effect may be even greater than 8% if warfarin is used at a higher INR of about 2.0–3.0 (ESPRIT, WASID and ARCH trials), and in patients with specific aetiological subtypes of ischaemic stroke such as those with aortic arch atherothromboembolism (ARCH trial), and the antiphospholipid antibody syndrome (Antiphospholipid Antibody Stroke Study). Finally, evaluating effectiveness by means of a more composite primary outcome event, which includes non-fatal intracranial and extracranial haemorrhage and MI, will not only yield more statistical power but may also provide a better perspective of the overall relative efficacy and safety of warfarin and antiplatelet therapies.

Ongoing clinical trials

- The ESPRIT trial is a randomised, single-blind trial which aims (in one arm of the trial) to compare the efficacy and safety of warfarin (INR 2.0–3.0) vs aspirin (in any dose between 30 and 325 mg daily) in patients after cerebral ischaemia due to presumed arterial causes (http://home.wxs.nl/~esprit) (De Schryver *et al.*, 2000). Treatment allocation is at random and open, but assessment of outcome is blind to the treatment allocation. The primary outcome is the composite event 'death from all vascular causes, non-fatal stroke, non-fatal MI or major bleeding complication'. As of January 2005, about 1200 of a planned 3000 patients have been randomised to warfarin vs aspirin (Ale Algra, Personal communication). An interim analysis of the incidence of ICH in the ESPRIT trial indicates that the overall rate of ICH is 0.31% (95% CI: 0.18–0.52%) per year, and 1.21% if all of them were included in the anticoagulation group (The European/Australasian Stroke Prevention in Reversible Ischaemia Trial (ESPRIT) Study Group, 2003). These interim data suggest that anticoagulation with achieved INR of 2.0–3.0 is reasonably safe in patients with cerebral ischaemia of arterial origin.

- The ARCH trial is an open RCT to test the null hypothesis that warfarin (INR 2.0–3.0) or clopidogrel 75 mg/day plus aspirin 75–325 mg/day in patients with a prior ischaemic stroke or peripheral embolism associated with proximal aortic plaque with complex ($\geqslant$4-mm thick and/or mobile) features are equally effective in preventing subsequent stroke or vascular events. All outcome events will be reviewed by an Endpoint Committee which is blinded to treatment allocation (Macleod *et al.*, 2004). A total of 1500 patients will be recruited and followed for 5 years.

SUMMARY

Apirin 160–300 mg daily and started within 48 h of onset of presumed ischaemic stroke is associated with a small risk of bleeding (two extra symptomatic ICHs and four major extracranial haemorrhages for every 1000 patients treated), but the hazard is more than offset by the reduction in recurrent ischaemic stroke (7/1000) and pulmonary embolism (1/1000). The net effects are that for every 1000 patients with acute ischaemic stroke who are treated early with aspirin, compared with no aspirin, there are 5 fewer early recurrent strokes of any type and, in the long term, 13 fewer patients who are dead or dependent. Among those who are alive and independent, an extra 10 make a complete recovery from their stroke if they are given early aspirin rather than no aspirin.

Gp IIb/IIIa receptor antagonists may be useful in the treatment of acute ischaemic stroke, and in strokes complicating endovascular procedures on the coronary and cerebral circulation. However, there is no indication to use these agents routinely whilst trials comparing these agents with placebo and with thrombolytic agents are in progress.

Anticoagulants (heparins) offer no net advantages over antiplatelet drugs in acute ischaemic stroke. The combination of low-dose UFH and aspirin appeared to be associated with net benefits over aspirin in a subgroup analysis, and this combination is worth testing in further large RCTs.

Long-term aspirin lowers the RR of stroke and other serious vascular events by about a sixth; 75–150 mg/day is the optimal dose. Higher doses are no more effective but cause more adverse events. Lower doses, as low as 30 mg/day, may be as effective, but there are not enough reliable data.

Clopidogrel is marginally but significantly better than aspirin alone in preventing recurrent serious vascular events, and has a definite role in patients who are intolerant of aspirin.

The addition of modified-release dipyridamole to aspirin seems to further lower stroke risk (but not risk of MI).

The combination of clopidogrel and aspirin is more effective than aspirin alone in unstable angina, but is not more effective (and is indeed more hazardous) than clopidogrel alone after TIA and ischaemic stroke.

Several trials are in progress comparing the combination of aspirin and clopidogrel with aspirin alone (FASTER, CHARISMA), the combination of dipyridamole and aspirin with aspirin alone (ESPRIT) and the combination of dipyridamole and aspirin with clopidogrel alone (PRoFESS) in patients with TIA and ischaemic stroke.

Long-term anticoagulation (INR 2.0–3.0) is not definitely more effective or hazardous than aspirin for patients with ischaemic stroke or TIA who are in sinus rhythm, and continues to be evaluated in an ongoing trial (ESPRIT).

Carotid artery revascularisation

Carotid stenosis is a cause of ischaemic stroke

Stenosis of the extracranial internal carotid artery (ICA) causes stroke, as proven by randomised trials which have shown that removing the extracranial ICA stenosis at its origin, by means of carotid endarterectomy (CEA), significantly reduces the risk of subsequent ipsilateral carotid territory ischaemic stroke (European Carotid Surgery Trial (ECST) Collaborative Group, 1991; North American Symptomatic Carotid Endarterectomy Trial (NASCET) Collaborators, 1991).

Observational studies in white populations suggest that about one-quarter of all first-ever ischaemic strokes and transient ischaemic attacks (TIAs) are caused by atherothromboembolism from the origin of the extracranial ICA (Sandercock *et al.*, 1989).

Mechanisms

The mechanisms by which extracranial ICA atherosclerosis causes ischaemic stroke are listed in Table 11.1.

Table 11.1. Mechanisms by which extracranial ICA atherosclerosis causes ischaemic stroke.

1 'Active' atherosclerotic plaque lesions may undergo endothelial erosion, fissuring or rupture, which exposes the subendothelial tissue to circulating blood, resulting in local thrombus formation, which may cause occlusion of the lumen of the ICA and infarction in the brain supplied by the ICA (Torvik *et al.*, 1989; Ogata *et al.*, 1990)

2 Plaque debris or thrombus may embolise and block a more distal vessel

3 Atherosclerotic plaque and/or thrombus may encroach upon the lumen of the ICA sufficiently to cause severe stenosis or occlusion, which may lead to hypoperfusion of distal brain regions, particularly in arterial border zones, and thus to 'watershed infarction'

Risk factors for ischaemic stroke caused by carotid stenosis

Degree of carotid stenosis

The risk of stroke ipsilateral to a carotid stenosis increases with the degree of symptomatic carotid stenosis until the artery distal to the stenosis begins to collapse (ECST Collaborative Group, 1991; NASCET Collaborators, 1991; Rothwell and Warlow, 2000; Rothwell *et al.*, 2000a). 'Collapse' or 'abnormal post-stenotic narrowing' of the ICA, resulting in near occlusion was initially identified in the NASCET, because it was not possible to measure the degree of stenosis using the NASCET method in cases in whom the post-stenotic ICA was narrowed or collapsed due to markedly reduced post-stenotic blood flow (Morgenstern *et al.*, 1997). The ECST subsequently also identified these patients, and both trials reported consistent results that these patients had a paradoxically low risk of stroke on best medical treatment alone (Morgenstern *et al.*, 1997; Rothwell and Warlow, 2000; Rothwell *et al.*, 2000a). The low risk of stroke was most probably due to the presence of a good collateral circulation, which is visible on angiography in the vast majority of the patients with narrowing of the ICA distal to a severe stenosis.

Recent neurological symptoms of carotid territory ischaemia

The risk of stroke ipsilateral to a carotid stenosis is also greater in patients with recent neurological symptoms of carotid territory ischaemia (Lovett *et al.*, 2003, 2004; Coull *et al.*, 2004). The risk is time dependent, being highest in the few weeks after the presenting event, reasonably high for the first year, and falling quickly over the next 2 years to that of neurologically asymptomatic carotid stenosis (ECST Collaborative Group, 1991; NASCET Collaborators, 1991; Rothwell *et al.*, 2000a; Coull *et al.*, 2004). The high early risk of recurrence probably represents the presence of an active unstable atherosclerotic plaque, and the rapid decline in risk over the subsequent year possibly reflects 'healing' of the unstable atheromatous plaque or an increase in collateral blood flow to the symptomatic hemisphere (ECST Collaborative Group, 1998; NASCET Collaborators, 1998; Rothwell and Warlow 2000; Rothwell *et al.*, 2000a).

Other factors

In addition to the severity of carotid stenosis, absence of near occlusion, the presence or absence of neurological symptoms, and the time since symptom onset, other factors have been associated with an increased risk of stroke in the presence of carotid stenosis. These include increasing age, multiple TIAs (suggesting an active, unstable plaque), an irregular and ulcerated plaque surface morphology (which are pathologically unstable), absence of angiographic collateral flow, impaired cerebral reactivity, a high frequency of transcranial Doppler (TCD)-detected emboli to the brain, hypertension and coronary heart disease (Table 11.2) (Rothwell and Warlow, 1999b; Rothwell *et al.*, 2000a, 2005).

Table 11.2. Independent prognostic factors for risk of ipsilateral ischaemic stroke in patients with recently symptomatic carotid stenosis who were randomised to best medical treatment alone in the ECST (Rothwell and Warlow, 1999b; Rothwell et al., 2005).

Risk factor	Hazard ratio	95% CI	P-value
Stenosis (per 10% increase)	1.18	1.10–1.25	<0.0001
Time since last event (per 7 days)	0.96	0.93–0.99	0.004
Presenting event			0.007
Ocular event	1.0		
Single TIA	1.41	0.75–2.66	
Multiple TIAs	2.05	1.16–3.60	
Minor stroke	1.82	0.99–3.34	
Major stroke	2.54	1.48–4.35	
Previous MI	1.57	1.01–2.45	0.047
Irregular/ulcerated plaque	2.03	1.31–3.14	0.0015
Diabetes	1.35	0.86–2.11	0.19
Near occlusion	0.49	0.19–1.24	0.14

The purpose of revascularisation of a symptomatic extracranial ICA stenosis is to reduce the risk of recurrent ipsilateral carotid territory ischaemic stroke by removing the source of carotid occlusion or thromboembolism. The two most commonly used strategies are CEA and carotid angioplasty with stenting.

Carotid endarterectomy

Evidence of overall risks and benefits

There have been five randomised-controlled trials (RCTs) comparing the effect of endarterectomy for symptomatic carotid stenosis combined with best medical therapy with the effect of best medical therapy alone (Fields et al., 1970; Shaw et al., 1984; Mayberg et al., 1991; ECST Collaborative Group, 1998; NASCET Collaborators, 1998).

The first two trials were small and more than 20 years ago, no longer reflecting current practice (Fields et al., 1970; Shaw et al., 1984). The larger Veterans Administration (VA) trial (VA#309) (Mayberg et al., 1991) showed a non-significant trend in favour of surgery, but was stopped prematurely when the initial results of the two largest trials were published (ECST Collaborative Group, 1991; NASCET Collaborators, 1991). The analyses of these trials were stratified by the severity of stenosis of the symptomatic carotid artery, but the degree of stenosis on pre-randomisation angiograms was measured using different methods.

Methods of measuring carotid stenosis

The NASCET method underestimated stenosis compared with the ECST method. Stenoses reported to be 70–99% in the NASCET were equivalent to 82–99% by the ECST method, and stenoses reported to be 70–99% by the ECST method were 55–99% by the NASCET method (Rothwell *et al.*, 1994).

Analysis of ECST using a common (NASCET) measurement of carotid stenosis

The ECST group re-measured the degree of carotid stenosis on their original angiograms using the method adopted by the NASCET group, and also redefined their outcome events to match those of NASCET, for comparability (Rothwell *et al.*, 2003a).

Re-analysis of the ECST showed that endarterectomy reduced the 5-year risk of *any stroke or surgical death* by 5.7% (95% confidence interval (CI): 0–11.6) in patients with [NASCET]50–69% stenosis ($n = 646$, $P = 0.05$) and by 21.2% (95% CI: 12.9–29.4) in patients with [NASCET]70–99% stenosis without 'near occlusion' ($n = 429$, $P < 0.0001$). Surgery was harmful in patients with <30% stenosis ($n = 1321$, $P = 0.007$) and of no benefit in patients with 30–49% stenosis ($n = 478$, $P = 0.6$). These results of ECST, when analysed in the same way as NASCET, were consistent with the NASCET results (Rothwell *et al.*, 2003a).

Analysis of pooled data from RCTs of endarterectomy for symptomatic carotid stenosis

A pooled analysis of data from the ECST, NASCET and VA#309 trials, which included over 95% of patients with symptomatic carotid stenosis ever randomised to endarterectomy vs medical treatment, showed that there was no statistically significant heterogeneity between the trials in the effect of the randomised treatment allocation on the relative risks (RRs) of any of the main outcomes in any of the stenosis groups (Rothwell *et al.* 2003b). Data were therefore merged on 6092 patients with 35,000 patient years of follow-up.

Risks

It is ironic that the precise purpose of CEA is to prevent stroke (and death), and paradoxically its major potential complication is peri-operative stroke (and death).

Peri-operative stroke or death

In the three trials of endarterectomy for symptomatic carotid stenosis, where post-operative complications were systematically reviewed, the overall pooled operative mortality was 1.1% (95% CI: 0.8–1.5), and the operative risk of stroke and death was 7.1% (95% CI: 6.3–8.1).

A systematic review of 57 surgical case series, involving a total of 13,285 CEAs, indicated that the *reported* peri-operative risk of stroke and death varied widely from <1% to more than 30%, but was usually about 3–8%, and was on average

5.1% (95% CI: 4.6–5.6%) (Rothwell *et al.*, 1996a, b; Goldstein *et al.*, 1997). The risk was higher in surgical case series in which patients were assessed post-operatively by a neurologist (7.7% (95% CI: 5.0–10.2%), odds ratio (OR): 1.62 (95% CI: 1.45–1.81)) (Rothwell, 1996a).

Based on the results from the trials, about one in 14 patients undergoing CEA for symptomatic carotid stenosis experiences a peri-operative stroke or dies in the peri-operative period. However, this risk cannot be generalised to one's own institution, surgeons or patients. A local prospective audit of a large number of patients undergoing CEA by each surgeon and centre is required, and referring doctors (and patients) should have access to the peri-operative stroke and death rate of their prospective surgeon(s) and centres, derived from such an independent and rigorous audit (Rothwell and Warlow, 1995; Goldstein *et al.*, 1997). However, interpretation of unusually high- or low-operative risks must take into account the effects of chance and case mix (Rothwell and Warlow, 1999a). Otherwise, over-simplistic interpretation of crude results may lead to unjustified criticism of individual surgeons, and not to improvements in patient care.

There are several other important prognostic factors for stroke, and peri-operative stroke and death associated with CEA which may influence the decision to operate.

Prognostic factors for peri-operative stroke or death

Patient factors   The risk of peri-operative stroke is greater in patients with *symptomatic* carotid stenosis than asymptomatic carotid stenosis. However, patients with *symptoms* of ocular ischaemia due to carotid stenosis (e.g. amaurosis fugax) have a *lower* risk of peri-operative stroke or death, and also a non-significantly *lower* risk of peri-operative stroke or death than patients undergoing CEA for *asymptomatic* carotid stenosis (Rothwell *et al.*, 1996b).

Other patient factors which have been associated with an increased risk of peri-operative stroke and death in trials of CEA for symptomatic carotid stenosis (Table 11.3) are as follows:

1 Female gender (perhaps because of smaller carotid arteries, perhaps more difficult to operate on).
2 Systolic blood pressure (SBP) >180 mmHg (perhaps increased risk of reperfusion injury and cerebral haemorrhage).
3 Peripheral arterial disease (a marker of atherosclerotic plaque burden).
4 Occlusion of the contralateral ICA (indicates poor collateral cerebral circulation).
5 Stenosis of the ipsilateral external carotid artery (poor collateral circulation) (Rothwell *et al.*, 1997). The risk of peri-operative stroke or death associated with CEA does not appear to be related to the degree of ipsilateral internal carotid stenosis (Table 11.4).

Table 11.3. Independent predictors of risk of peri-operative major stroke or death within 30 days of CEA in the ECST (Rothwell *et al.*, 1997; Rothwell and Warlow, 1999b).

Prognostic variable	Hazard ratio	95% CI	*P*-value
Female gender	2.05	1.29–3.24	0.002
SBP >180 mmHg	2.21	1.29–3.79	0.004
Peripheral arterial disease	2.48	1.51–4.13	0.0004

Table 11.4. Pooled peri-operative risks of stroke and death within 30 days of CEA according to degree of symptomatic carotid stenosis in patients who underwent CEA in the three RCTs of CEA.

Outcome	Carotid stenosis	Risk (%)	95% CI
Stroke or death	<50%	6.7	5.6–8.0
	50–69%	8.4	6.6–10.5
	≥70%	6.2	4.4–8.5
	Near occlusion	5.4	2.4–10.4
	Total	7.1	6.3–8.1
Death	<50%	1.0	0.6–1.6
	50–69%	1.4	0.8–2.5
	≥70%	0.9	0.3–2.0
	Near occlusion	0.7	0–3.7
	Total	1.1	0.8–1.5

Importantly, the operative risk of stroke and death is unrelated to the risk of stroke with best medical treatment alone (Rothwell *et al.*, 2003b, 2005) (Tables 11.2, 11.3, 11.4).

Surgical factors   The surgical factors which may be associated with an increased risk of peri-operative stroke or death are: (a) inexperience due to low surgeon and hospital case volumes (Feasby *et al.*, 2002); and (b) undertaking CEA in the very acute phase of stroke in evolution and crescendo TIAs, and during coronary artery surgery for patients with angina whose carotid stenosis was discovered during preparation for coronary artery surgery (Bond *et al.*, 2003a). For neurologically stable patients, such as those enrolled into the trials, there was no evidence of any increase in operative risk in patients operated within 2 weeks of their last event (Rothwell *et al.*, 2004). Moreover, in a systematic review of surgical case series, early surgery in neurologically stable patients was not associated with an increased operative risk (Bond *et al.*, 2003a).

Local adverse effects of CEA

Other specific adverse effects of CEA, besides those inherent in any operation, include:

1 lower cranial nerve palsy (about 5–9% of patients),
2 peripheral nerve palsy (about 1% of patients),
3 major neck haematoma requiring surgery or extended hospital stay (about 5–7% of patients),
4 wound infection (3%).

Prognostic factors for peri-operative cranial nerve palsy

Patients undergoing CEA for *recurrent* carotid stenosis have an increased risk of cranial nerve injury and wound haematoma (Bond *et al.*, 2003b).

The risk of functionally disabling bilateral vagal and hypoglossal nerve palsies is also increased in patients who have already had an endarterectomy on one side or are undergoing *bilateral* CEAs.

Net benefits and risks overall

Evidence from the Cochrane Library

The most recent systematic review for the Cochrane Library was completed in 1999 and only included data on death or disabling stroke from the 5950 patients enrolled in the NASCET and ECST. The two trials used different methods to measure stenosis, but a simple formula can be used to convert between the two methods.

Mild carotid stenosis (ECST < 70%; NASCET < 50%)   For patients with mild stenosis (ECST < 70% = NASCET < 50%), surgery increased the risk of disabling stroke or death by 20% (95% CI: 0–44%) from 11.4% (control) to 12.8% (surgery); absolute risk difference being 1.4% (Fig. 11.1). This is an odds increase of 23% (95% CI: 1.00–1.51). The number of patients needed to be operated on (number needed to treat, NNT) to cause one disabling stroke or death was 45 (95% CI: 22 to infinity) (Cina *et al.*, 1999).

Moderate carotid stenosis (ECST: 70–79%; NASCET: 50–69%)   For patients with moderate stenosis (ECST: 70–79% = NASCET: 50–69%), surgery reduced the RR of disabling stroke or death by 27% (95% CI: 15–44%), which is a reduction in odds of 31% (95% CI: 6–49%) (Fig. 11.2). The NNT to prevent one disabling stroke or death was 21 (95% CI: 11–125).

Severe carotid stenosis (ECST > 80%; NASCET > 70%)   For patients with severe stenosis (ECST > 80% = NASCET > 70%), surgery reduced the RR of disabling stroke or death by 48% (95% CI: 27–73%), which is an odds reduction of 52% (95% CI: 30–67%) (Fig. 11.3). The NNT to prevent one disabling stroke or death over 2–6 years follow-up was 15 (95% CI: 10–31) (Cina *et al.*, 1999).

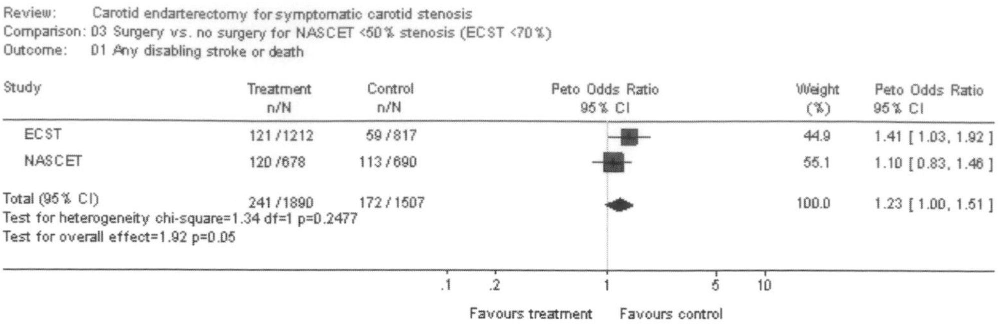

Review: Carotid endarterectomy for symptomatic carotid stenosis
Comparison: 03 Surgery vs. no surgery for NASCET <50% stenosis (ECST <70%)
Outcome: 01 Any disabling stroke or death

Study	Treatment n/N	Control n/N	Peto Odds Ratio 95% CI	Weight (%)	Peto Odds Ratio 95% CI
ECST	121 /1212	59 /817		44.9	1.41 [1.03, 1.92]
NASCET	120 /678	113 /690		55.1	1.10 [0.83, 1.46]
Total (95% CI)	241 /1890	172 / 1507		100.0	1.23 [1.00, 1.51]

Test for heterogeneity chi-square=1.34 df=1 p=0.2477
Test for overall effect=1.92 p=0.05

.1   .2   1   5   10
Favours treatment   Favours control

Figure 11.1   Forest plot showing the effects of *CEA* plus best medical therapy vs best medical therapy alone in patients with recently symptomatic carotid *stenosis of <50%* (NASCET method) on *any disabling stroke or death* at the end of the follow-up period. Reproduced from Cina *et al.* (1999), with permission from the authors and John Wiley & Sons Limited. Copyright Cochrane Library, reproduced with permission.

Review: Carotid endarterectomy for symptomatic carotid stenosis
Comparison: 02 Surgery vs. no surgery for NASCET 50-69% stenosis (ECST 70-79%)
Outcome: 01 Any disabling stroke or death

Study	Treatment n/N	Control n/N	Peto Odds Ratio 95% CI	Weight (%)	Peto Odds Ratio 95% CI
ECST	20 /231	21 / 170		22.5	0.67 [0.35, 1.29]
NASCET	64 /430	86 / 428		77.5	0.70 [0.49, 0.99]
Total (95% CI)	84 /661	107 / 598		100.0	0.69 [0.51, 0.94]

Test for heterogeneity chi-square=0.01 df=1 p=0.9141
Test for overall effect=-2.34 p=0.02

.1   .2   1   5   10
Favours treatment   Favours control

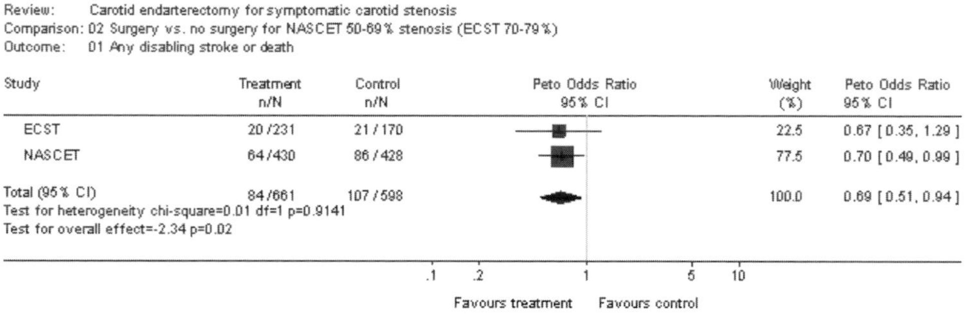

Figure 11.2   Forest plot showing the effects of *CEA* plus best medical therapy vs best medical therapy alone in patients with recently symptomatic carotid *stenosis of 50–69%* (NASCET method) on *any disabling stroke or death* at the end of the follow-up period. Reproduced from Cina *et al.* (1999), with permission from the authors and John Wiley & Sons Limited. Copyright Cochrane Library, reproduced with permission.

Evidence from a more recent analysis of pooled data from RCTs of endarterectomy for symptomatic carotid stenosis (Rothwell et al., 2003b)

Ipsilateral ischaemic stroke and any operative stroke or death   The more recent analysis of the pooled data from the three RCTs of endarterectomy for symptomatic carotid stenosis indicates that CEA increased the 5-year risk of ipsilateral ischaemic stroke in patients with less than 30% stenosis, as measured by the NASCET technique (absolute risk reduction (ARR): -2.2%, $P = 0.05$), had no net effect in those patients with 30–49% stenosis (ARR: 3.2%, $P = 0.6$), was of marginal benefit in those with 50–69% stenosis (ARR: 4.6%, $P = 0.04$), and was highly beneficial in

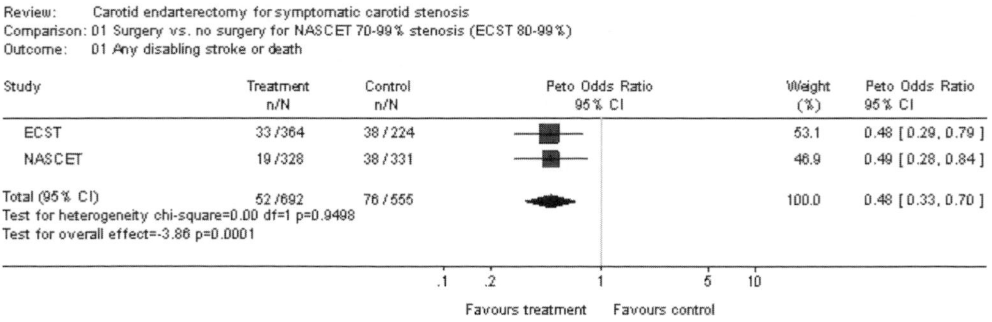

Review: Carotid endarterectomy for symptomatic carotid stenosis
Comparison: 01 Surgery vs. no surgery for NASCET 70-99% stenosis (ECST 80-99%)
Outcome: 01 Any disabling stroke or death

Study	Treatment n/N	Control n/N	Peto Odds Ratio 95% CI	Weight (%)	Peto Odds Ratio 95% CI
ECST	33 /364	38 / 224		53.1	0.48 [0.29, 0.79]
NASCET	19 /328	38 / 331		46.9	0.49 [0.28, 0.84]
Total (95% CI)	52 /692	76 / 555		100.0	0.48 [0.33, 0.70]

Test for heterogeneity chi-square=0.00 df=1 p=0.9498
Test for overall effect=-3.86 p=0.0001

.1   .2   1   5   10

Favours treatment   Favours control

Figure 11.3 Forest plot showing the effects of *CEA* plus best medical therapy vs best medical therapy alone in patients with recently symptomatic carotid *stenosis of 70–99%* (NASCET method) on *any disabling stroke or death* at the end of the follow-up period. Reproduced from Cina *et al.* (1999), with permission from the authors and John Wiley & Sons Limited. Copyright Cochrane Library, reproduced with permission.

those with 70% stenosis or greater without near occlusion (ARR: 15.9%, $P < 0.001$) (Fig. 11.4) (Rothwell *et al.*, 2003b). There was no long-term benefit for patients with near occlusion (ARR: -1.7%, $P = 0.9$).

Any stroke or operative death   For patients with recently symptomatic carotid stenosis of less than 50%, CEA was associated with an increase in absolute risk of *any stroke or death* at 5 years after randomisation (Fig. 11.4) (Rothwell *et al.*, 2003b).

For patients with recently symptomatic 50–69% stenosis, CEA was associated with a reduction in absolute risk of *any stroke or death* at 5 years after randomisation by 7.8% (95% CI: 3.1–12.5%), from about 27% (no surgery) to about 19% (with surgery); relative risk reduction (RRR): 28% (95% CI: 14–42%) (Fig. 11.4) (Rothwell *et al.*, 2003b).

For patients with recently symptomatic 70–99% stenosis, CEA was associated with a reduction in absolute risk of *any stroke or death* at 5 years after randomisation by 15.6% (95% CI: 9.8–20.7%), from about 33% (no surgery) to about 17% (with surgery); RRR: 48% (95% CI: 36–60%) (Fig. 11.4) (Rothwell *et al.*, 2003b).

For patients with near occlusion, CEA was associated with no reduction in absolute risk of *any stroke or death* at 5 years after randomisation (ARR: -0.1%; RRR: 2% (95% CI: -59% to 39%)) (Fig. 11.4). Although the CIs around the estimates of treatment effect in the near occlusions were wide, the difference in the effect of surgery between patients with near occlusion and patients with $\geqslant$70% stenosis without near occlusion was statistically highly significant for any stroke or death, and each of the other important outcomes. However, endarterectomy did reduce the risk of recurrent TIA (but not stroke) in patients with near occlusion (ARR: 15%, $P = 0.007$).

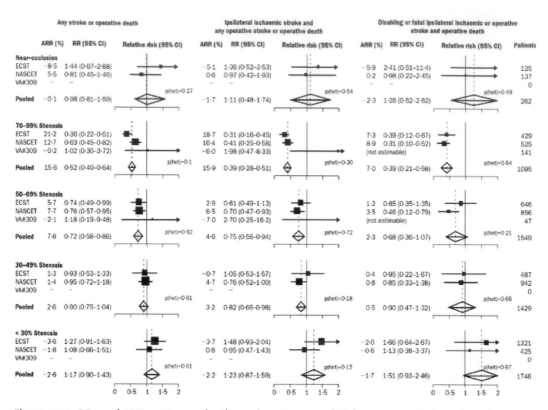

Figure 11.4 RRs and ARRs at 5 years for the main outcomes of trials among patients assigned CEA by degree of symptomatic carotid stenosis. Reproduced from Rothwell *et al.* (2003b), with permission from the authors and Elsevier Limited, publishers of the Lancet.

Disabling or fatal ipsilateral ischaemic stroke and/or surgical stroke or surgical death   Quantitatively similar results were seen for ipsilateral ischaemic stroke and surgical stroke or death, and qualitatively similar results were seen for disabling or fatal ipsilateral ischaemic stroke and/or surgical stroke or surgical death (Fig. 11.4).

Benefits in clinical subgroups and timing of surgery

Although endarterectomy reduces the RR of stroke by 48% (95% CI: 36–60%) over the next 5 years in patients with a recently symptomatic severe (70–99%) carotid stenosis, the ARR is relatively small (15.6%), because only 33% of these patients have a stroke on medical treatment alone (and 17% have a stroke after CEA).

The operation is therefore of no value for at least two-thirds (68%) of patients who, despite having a severe (70–99%) recently symptomatic carotid stenosis, are destined to remain stroke free for the next 5 years with best medical therapy alone (i.e. without surgery) and can only be harmed by surgery.

It would, therefore, be useful to be able to identify in advance, and operate on, only on the 15.6% of patients (one in six) with severe symptomatic carotid stenosis who are going to benefit over the next 5 years.

We therefore need to be able to more precisely identify those patients with severe symptomatic carotid stenosis who have a very high risk of stroke on medical treatment alone, coupled with a relatively low-operative risk. Simply relying on the presence or absence of recent carotid territory ischaemic symptoms and the degree of carotid stenosis is not good enough (although a good start).

When a systematic review of RCTs reveals a substantially significant overall treatment effect of several standard deviations, as is the case of CEA for severe symptomatic carotid stenosis reducing the RR of ipsilateral carotid territory ischaemic stroke and any operative stroke or death by 61% (95% CI: 0.49–0.72), there is sufficient statistical power to perform subgroup analyses with some confidence in the results (other than purely hypothesis-generating 'data dredging') (see 'Subgroup analyses', Chapter 2).

Subgroup analyses of pooled data from ECST and NASCET revealed that the effectiveness of CEA in patients with severe symptomatic carotid stenosis was modified significantly by three clinical variables: the patients' sex ($P = 0.003$), age ($P = 0.03$) and time from the last symptomatic event to randomisation ($P = 0.009$) (Rothwell et al., 2004). Benefit from surgery was greatest in men, patients aged ≥75 years, and patients randomised within 2 weeks after their last ischaemic event and fell rapidly with increasing delay. For patients with ≥50% stenosis, the number of patients needed to undergo surgery (NNT) to prevent one ipsilateral stroke in 5 years was 9 for men vs 36 for women, 5 for age ≥75 vs 18 for age <65 years, and 5 for patients randomised within 2 weeks after their last ischaemic event vs 125 for patients randomised >12 weeks (Rothwell, 2005). These observations were consistent across the 50–69% and ≥70% stenosis groups and similar trends were present in both ECST and NASCET (Fig. 11.5).

Sex

Women had a lower risk of ipsilateral ischaemic stroke on medical treatment and a higher-operative risk in comparison to men. For recently symptomatic carotid stenosis, surgery is very clearly beneficial in women with ≥70% stenosis, but not in women with 50–69% stenosis (Fig. 11.5). In contrast, surgery reduced the 5-year absolute risk of stroke by 8.0% (3.4–12.5) in men with 50–69% stenosis. This sex difference was statistically significant even when the analysis of the interaction was confined to the 50–69% stenosis group. These same patterns were also shown in both of the large published trials of endarterectomy for asymptomatic carotid stenosis

(Asymptomatic Carotid Atherosclerosis Study Group, 1995; MRC Asymptomatic Carotid Surgery Trial (ACST) Collaborative Group, 2004; Rothwell, 2004).

Age

Benefit from CEA increased with age in patients with recently symptomatic stenosis, particularly in patients aged over 75 years because of their high risk of stroke on medical treatment without a substantially increased risk of peri-operative stroke (Fig. 11.5). These findings are consistent with a recent systematic review of all published surgical case series which reported no increase in the operative risk of stroke and death in older age groups (Rothwell, 2005).

There is therefore no justification for withholding CEA in patients aged over 75 years who are deemed to be medically fit to undergo surgery.

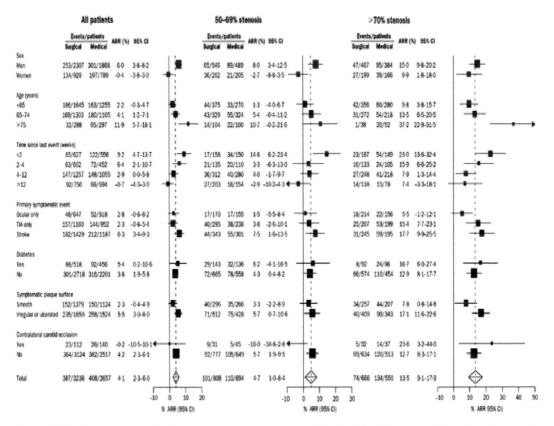

Figure 11.5 Absolute and relative reductions in 5-year actuarial risk of ipsilateral carotid territory ischaemic stroke and any stroke or death within 30 days after trial surgery according to pre-defined subgroups in all patients, individuals with 50–69% stenosis, and those with ⩾70% stenosis. Reproduced from Rothwell *et al.* (2004), with permission from the authors and Elsevier Limited, publishers of the Lancet.

Timing of CEA

Given the high early risk of stroke on medical treatment alone after a TIA or minor stroke in patients with carotid disease (Lovett *et al.*, 2003, 2004; Coull *et al.*, 2004) and the lack of an increased operative risk in neurologically stable patients (see above), early surgery is likely to be most effective. The pooled analysis of data from the trials shows that the benefit from endarterectomy is greatest in patients randomised within 2 weeks of their last event (Figs 11.5 and 11.6). This was particularly important in patients with 50–69% stenosis, where the reduction in the 5-year risk of stroke with surgery was considerable in those who were randomised within 2 weeks of their last event (14.8%, 95% CI: 6.2–23.4), but minimal in patients randomised later.

Other prognostic factors

Benefit from surgery is probably also greatest in patients presenting with stroke, intermediate in those with cerebral TIA and lowest in those with retinal events (Fig. 11.5). There was also a trend in the trials towards greater benefit in patients with irregular plaque than a smooth plaque.

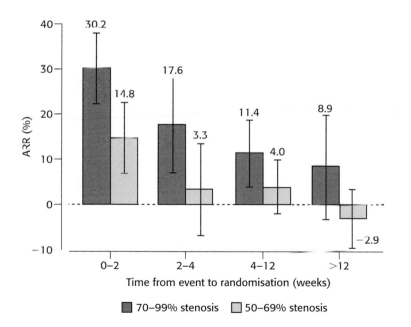

Figure 11.6 Absolute reductions in 5-year risk of ipsilateral carotid territory ischaemic stroke and any stroke or death within 30 days after trial surgery in patients with 50–69% stenosis and ≥70% stenosis without near occlusion stratified by the time from last symptomatic event to randomisation. Reproduced from Rothwell *et al.* (2004), with permission from the authors and Elsevier Limited, publishers of the Lancet.

These findings are consistent with the model for prediction of the risk of stroke on medical treatment in patients with recently symptomatic carotid stenosis, derived from the ECST, and validated externally in NASCET (Rothwell and Warlow, 1999b; Rothwell *et al.*, 2005) (Table 11.2, Figure 11.7).

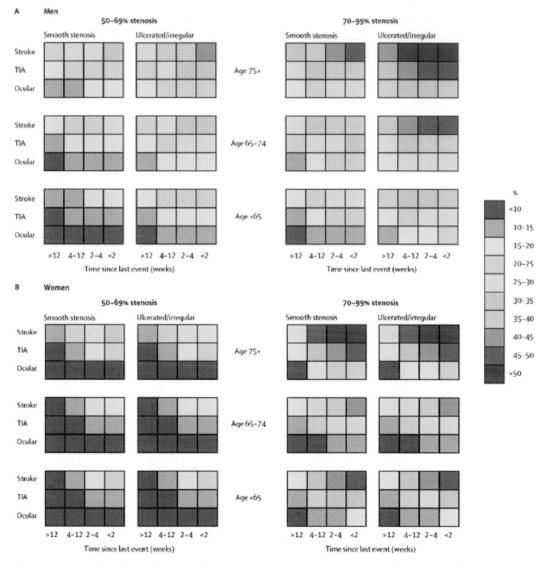

Figure 11.7 *Predicted absolute risk of ipsilateral ischaemic stroke at 5 years in patients with recently symptomatic carotid stenosis taking medical treatment.* This table was derived from a Cox regression model based on five clinically important patient characteristics in (A) men and (B) women. TIA = transient ischaemic attack. Stroke/TIA/Ocular refers to the most severe symptomatic ipsilateral ischaemic event in the past 6 months: Stroke > Cerebral TIA > Ocular Events only. Reproduced from Rothwell *et al.* (2005), with permission from the authors and Elsevier Limited, publishers of the Lancet.

Types of CEA

Local vs general anaesthetic for CEA

Although CEA dramatically reduces the risk of stroke in patients with recently symptomatic severe ICA stenosis, the benefit is dependent on maintaining a lower peri-operative stroke risk. This may depend, to some extent, on the type of anaesthetic used.

Evidence

A systematic review identified seven RCTs involving 554 operations which assessed the operative risks of CEA under local anaesthesia (LA) with CEA under general anaesthesia (GA) (Rerkasem et al., 2004, 2005). Meta-analysis of the seven RCTs revealed a non-significant trend towards reduced mortality within 30 days of operation with LA (pooled OR: 0.23, 95% CI: 0.05–1.02), but this estimate was based on a very small number of events (LA: 1 death, GA: 6 deaths) (Rerkasem et al., 2004, 2005). However, LA was associated with a more convincing reduction in local post-operative haemorrhage (OR: 0.31, 95% CI: 0.12–0.79) within 30 days of the operation. There was no evidence of a difference in the odds of operative stroke (OR: 1.01, 95% CI: 0.32–3.18), myocardial infarction (MI) (OR: 0.77, 95% CI: 0.21–2.88), or stroke or death within 30 days of the operation (OR: 0.63, 95% CI: 0.25–1.62) (Fig. 11.8).

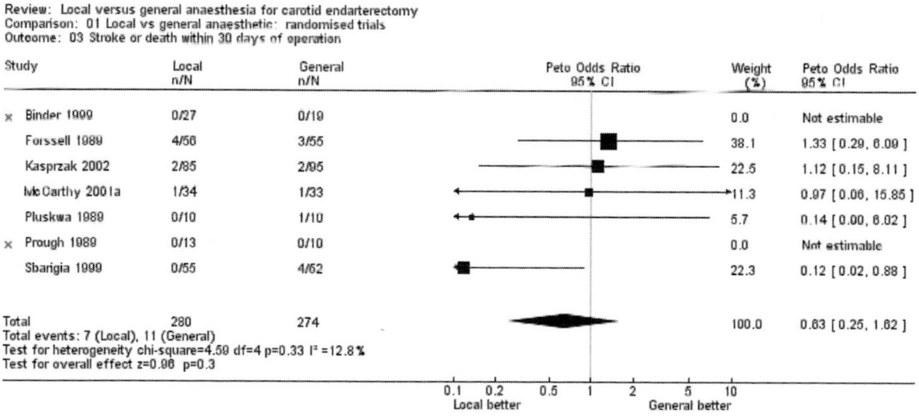

Review: Local versus general anaesthesia for carotid endarterectomy
Comparison: 01 Local vs general anaesthetic: randomised trials
Outcome: 03 Stroke or death within 30 days of operation

Study	Local n/N	General n/N	Peto Odds Ratio 95% CI	Weight (%)	Peto Odds Ratio 95% CI
x Binder 1999	0/27	0/19		0.0	Not estimable
Forssell 1989	4/56	3/55		38.1	1.33 [0.29, 6.09]
Kasprzak 2002	2/85	2/95		22.5	1.12 [0.15, 8.11]
McCarthy 2001a	1/34	1/33		11.3	0.97 [0.06, 15.85]
Pluskwa 1989	0/10	1/10		5.7	0.14 [0.00, 6.02]
x Prough 1989	0/13	0/10		0.0	Not estimable
Sbarigia 1999	0/55	4/62		22.3	0.12 [0.02, 0.88]
Total	280	274		100.0	0.63 [0.25, 1.62]

Total events: 7 (Local), 11 (General)
Test for heterogeneity chi-square=4.59 df=4 p=0.33 I² =12.8%
Test for overall effect z=0.96 p=0.3

0.1 0.2 0.5 1 2 5 10
Local better   General better

Figure 11.8 Forest plot showing the effects of *local anaesthetic vs general anaesthetic* for CEA in patients with carotid stenosis on any stroke or death within 30 days of operation. Reproduced from Rerkasem *et al.* (2004), with permission from the authors and John Wiley & Sons Limited. Copyright Cochrane Library, reproduced with permission.

Comment

There is insufficient reliable evidence comparing CEA under LA vs GA to allow informed conclusions.

A large randomised trial (General Anaesthetic vs Local Anaesthetic, GALA) is currently ongoing and has randomised more than 1000 patients so far (McCleary *et al.*, 2001).

Eversion vs conventional CEA

CEA is conventionally undertaken by a longitudinal arteriotomy. Eversion CEA, which employs a transverse arteriotomy and reimplantation of the carotid artery, has been reported to be associated with low peri-operative stroke and restenosis rates but an increased risk of complications associated with a distal intimal flap.

Evidence

A systematic review of five RCTs evaluating whether eversion CEA was safe and more effective than conventional CEA in a total of 2465 patients reported no significant differences between eversion and conventional CEA techniques in the rate of peri-operative stroke and/or death (1.7% eversion CEA vs 2.6% conventional CEA, OR: 0.44, 95% CI: 0.10–1.82), and stroke during follow-up (1.4% vs 1.7%; OR: 0.84, 95% CI: 0.43–1.64) (Cao *et al.*, 2000).

Although eversion CEA was associated with a significantly lower rate of restenosis >50% during follow-up than conventional CEA (2.5% eversion vs 5.2% conventional, Peto OR: 0.48, 95% CI: 0.32–0.72), there was no evidence that the eversion technique for CEA was associated with a lower rate of neurological events when compared to conventional CEA.

There were no statistically significant differences in local complications between the eversion and conventional group.

Comment

Interpretation of the evidence

There is insufficient evidence from randomised trials to reliably determine the RRs and benefits of eversion and conventional CEA. It is possible that carotid eversion is associated with a lower risk of long-term carotid occlusion and restenosis, but it is still unclear whether this is associated with a lower rate of subsequent neurological events.

Implications for practice

Until more reliable evidence is available, the choice of the surgical technique for CEA should depend on the experience and preference of the operating surgeon.

Implications for research

Further randomised trials are needed to more precisely define the relative and absolute benefits and risks of eversion and conventional CEA, and establish the clinically relevance (or not) of restenosis of the carotid artery (that was previously operated on) as a cause of subsequent stroke. Studies analysing the costs of eversion and conventional CEA are also needed.

Routine or selective carotid artery shunting for CEA (and different methods of monitoring in selective shunting)

One of the limitations of CEA is risk of peri-operative stroke, most of which are ipsilateral carotid territory ischaemic stroke, and some may result from temporary interruption of cerebral blood flow while the carotid artery is clamped during CEA. The duration of interrupted blood flow to the brain can be minimised by bridging the clamped section of the artery with a shunt. Potential disadvantages of shunting include complications such as air and plaque embolism and carotid artery dissection, and an increased risk of local complications such as nerve injury, haematoma, infection and long-term restenosis. However, reliable data on these risks and the potential benefits are limited. Consequently, some surgeons advocate routine shunting, whereas others prefer to use shunts selectively or avoid them altogether.

Evidence

A systematic review of the effect of routine vs selective, or never, shunting during CEA identified two trials involving 590 patients which compared routine shunting with no shunting, and one trial involving 131 patients which compared shunting with a combination of electroencephalographic (EEG) and carotid pressure measurement with shunting by carotid pressure measurement alone (Bond *et al.*, 2001, 2003b).

For routine vs no shunting, there was no significant difference in the rate of all stroke, ipsilateral stroke or death up to 30 days after surgery, although data were limited.

There was no significant difference between the risk of ipsilateral stroke in patients selected for shunting with the combination of EEG and carotid pressure assessment compared to pressure assessment alone, although again the data were limited.

Comment

Implications for practice

There is insufficient evidence from RCTs to support or refute the use of routine or selective shunting during CEA and there is little evidence to support the use of one form of monitoring over another in selecting patients requiring a shunt. The use of EEG monitoring combined with carotid pressure assessment may reduce the number of shunts required without increasing the stroke rate but more data are required to prove this.

Implications for research

A large multicentre randomised trial is required to assess whether shunting reduces the risk of peri-operative and long-term death and stroke. Even a modest 25% reduction in the RR of peri-operative stroke or death would result in approximately 15 fewer strokes and deaths per 1000 patients undergoing endarterectomy. However, to detect this reliably (80% power, 5% significance level) would require between 3000 and 5000 patients (Bond *et al.*, 2003b).

Two policies could be considered: routine shunting for all patients undergoing CEA or selective shunting in those at high risk of intra-operative cerebral ischaemia. The trial needs to be truly randomised, have long-term follow-up (several years) and have blinded outcome assessment preferably by neurologists. Patients should be stratified by age, sex, degree of ipsilateral and contralateral internal carotid stenosis, the experience of the surgeon, the use of patching and, in selective shunting, the method of monitoring of cerebral ischaemia.

As regards the method of monitoring in selective shunting, until the efficacy of shunting has been demonstrated, further trials of the method of monitoring are probably not merited. However, a systematic review of the sensitivity and specificity of the various methods of monitoring for cerebral ischaemia would be worthwhile to identify the best method of monitoring to be used in any trial of selective shunting.

Patch angioplasty vs primary closure for CEA

When undertaking a CEA, many surgeons use a patch of autologous vein, or synthetic material, to close the artery, enlarge the lumen and so they hope to reduce the risk of restenosis and stroke. However, it remains uncertain whether carotid patch angioplasty (with either a venous or a synthetic patch) reduced the risk of carotid artery restenosis and subsequent ischaemic stroke compared with primary closure of the ICA.

Evidence

A systematic review of RCTs assessing the safety and efficacy of routine or selective carotid patch angioplasty compared to CEA with primary closure identified seven trials involving 1127 patients undergoing 1307 operations (Bond *et al.*, 2003c). The quality of trials was generally poor. Follow-up varied from hospital discharge to 5 years.

Carotid patch angioplasty was associated with a reduction in the risk of stroke of any type (OR: 0.33, $P = 0.004$), ipsilateral stroke (OR: 0.31, $P = 0.0008$), and stroke or death during the peri-operative period (OR: 0.39, $P = 0.007$) and at long-term follow-up (OR: 0.59, $P = 0.004$) compared with CEA with primary closure.

Carotid patch angioplasty was also associated with a reduced risk of peri-operative arterial occlusion (OR: 0.15, 95% CI: 0.06–0.37, $P = 0.00004$), and decreased restenosis during long-term follow-up in five trials (OR: 0.20, 95% CI: 0.13–0.29, $P < 0.00001$).

Very few arterial complications, including haemorrhage, infection, cranial nerve palsies and pseudo-aneurysm formation were recorded with either patch or primary closure.

No significant correlation was found between use of patch angioplasty and the risk of either peri-operative or long-term all-cause death rates.

Comment

Interpretation of the evidence

Limited evidence suggests that carotid patch angioplasty may reduce the risk of peri-operative arterial occlusion and restenosis, and longer-term stroke or death.

Implications for practice

Although most vascular surgeons do not routinely use patching in patients undergoing CEA, the present data from RCTs (albeit based on small numbers) appear to support a recommendation in favour of routine patching.

The use of selective patching (e.g. for very narrow arteries) has not been studied in RCTs, so no evidence-based recommendations can be made.

Implications for research

The potential benefit of routine patching could be clinically important (up to 40 strokes prevented per 1000 patients treated) but in order to have reliable evidence on the risks and benefits of patching compared to primary closure, a large multicentre RCT will be required.

This trial should concentrate on clinical outcomes (deaths, all strokes, particularly fatal or disabling strokes and ipsilateral strokes) as opposed to restenosis and have long-term follow-up (perhaps 5 years).

Assuming a 30-day risk of stroke or death of 5%, the trial would need to recruit about 3000 patients to have an 90% chance of detecting a reduction in the absolute risk of death or stroke to 2.5% (this number would also give a >90% chance of detecting a reduction in the risk of stroke or death at 5 years from 25% to 20%). Such a trial should use a secure method of randomisation and be performed on a truly intention-to-treat basis with complete follow-up of all patients. Patients rather than arteries should be randomised so that the number of deaths and strokes are reported on a patient basis rather than an artery basis. Clinical follow-up should be blinded with independent assessment of strokes, preferably by neurologists. The results should be analysed according to the degree of narrowing of the artery and whether the patient had had a previous stroke or TIA or not. It would be possible to use a factorial design for such a trial so that some other procedure could be tested simultaneously, such as routine shunting. Until the benefit of carotid patching in terms of clinical outcomes for the patient is established, any future trials should include a control group of primary closure.

Patches of different types for carotid patch angioplasty during carotid endartectomy

Although CEA is effective in patients with symptomatic carotid stenosis, it is not clear whether different surgical techniques affect the outcome, and whether the use of carotid patch angioplasty is superior to primary closure in reducing the risk of restenosis and improving both short and long-term clinical outcome. Consequently, many vascular surgeons use carotid patching either routinely or selectively. Among those who do use carotid patching, however, there is debate over the choice of patch material. Vein patching (usually harvested from the saphenous vein and sometimes from the jugular vein) is favoured by some because it is easily available, easy to handle and possibly has a greater resistance to infection. Synthetic material, such as Dacron or polytetrafluoroethylene (PTFE), is favoured by others who feel that it offers a lower risk of patch rupture and aneurysmal dilatation, and also that it spares the morbidity associated with saphenous vein harvesting and leaves the vein which may be required for coronary bypass grafting at a later date. It is also possible that one type of synthetic material is better than the another. Furthermore, there are less commonly used materials such as bovine pericardium which have yet to be widely accepted.

Evidence

A systematic review of eight RCTs of the safety and efficacy of different materials for carotid patch angioplasty in 1480 operations identified four studies that had compared vein closure with PTFE closure, three compared vein to Dacron grafts, and one compared Dacron with PTFE (Bond *et al.*, 2003d, 2005).

There were too few operative events to determine whether there was any difference between the vein and Dacron patches for peri-operative stroke, death and arterial complications.

The one study that compared Dacron and PTFE patches found that, compared with PTFE, Dacron was associated with a significant increased risk of combined stroke, and TIA ($P = 0.03$) and restenosis at 30 days ($P = 0.01$), a borderline significant risk of peri-operative stroke ($P = 0.06$), and a non-significant increased risk of peri-operative carotid thrombosis ($P = 0.1$).

During follow-up for more than 1 year, there was no difference between the two types of patch for the risk of stroke, death or arterial restenosis, but the number of events was small.

There were significantly fewer pseudo-aneurysms associated with synthetic patches than vein (OR: 0.09, 95% CI: 0.02–0.49) but the numbers involved were small (15 events in 776 patients) and the clinical significance of this finding is uncertain.

Comment

Interpretation of the evidence

It is likely that the differences between different types of patch material are very small. Consequently, more data than are currently available will be required to establish whether any differences do exist.

Some evidence exists that PTFE patches may be superior to collagen impregnated Dacron grafts in terms of peri-operative stroke rates and restenosis. However the evidence is based upon data from a single, small trial and more studies that compare different types of synthetic graft are required to make firm conclusions.

Pseudo-aneurysm formation may be more common after use of a vein patch compared with a synthetic patch.

Implications for practice

There is no evidence to support the use of vein over synthetic patch material in CEA. The decision of which type of patch to use, if any, remains a matter of individual preference. However, if synthetic material is used, the currently available (limited) evidence from a single trial appears to show benefits from PTFE as opposed to Dacron material.

Implications for research

Further trials comparing one type of patch with another are required, but they will need large numbers of patients. Further, more trials are required which compare different types of synthetic graft material.

Adjunct medical therapies after carotid endartectomy

Antiplatelet therapy

Antiplatelet drugs are effective and safe for TIA and ischaemic stroke patients in preventing recurrent vascular events, and for patients undergoing vascular surgical procedures in reducing the risk of graft or native vessel occlusion (Chapter 10) (Antithrombotic Trialists' Collaboration, 2002). However, this does not necessarily mean they are effective and safe after CEA.

Evidence

Antiplatelet vs control

A systematic review of RCTs evaluating whether antiplatelet agents are safe and beneficial after CEA (Engelter and Lyrer, 2003, 2004) identified six trials of antiplatelet therapy administered for at least 30 days after CEA in a total of 907 patients who were followed up for at least 3 months. Most trials used high dose aspirin alone or in combination with other antiplatelet drugs.

Antiplatelet therapy was associated with a significant reduction in the odds of stroke of any type during follow-up (OR: 0.58, 95% CI: 0.34–0.98, $P = 0.04$) but not death (OR: 0.77, 95% CI: 0.48–1.24), intracranial haemorrhage (OR: 1.71, 95% CI: 0.73–4.03) or other serious vascular events.

Aspirin plus clopidogrel vs aspirin

In a recent study, 100 patients were assigned aspirin 150 mg per day for 4 weeks prior to CEA and then, on the night before CEA, they were randomised to placebo plus long-term aspirin 150 mg per day ($n = 54$) or clopidogrel 75 mg per day plus long-term aspirin 150 mg per day ($n = 46$) (Payne et al., 2004). Compared with placebo plus aspirin, assignment to clopidogrel plus aspirin was associated with a small (8.8%) but significant reduction in platelet response to adenosine diphosphate (ADP) ($P = 0.05$), a 10-fold reduction in the RR of patients having >20 emboli detected by TCD within 3 h of CE (OR: 10.23, 95% CI: 1.3–83.3, $P = 0.01$), and a significantly increased time from flow restoration to skin closure (an indirect marker of haemostasis) ($P = 0.04$). There was no increase in bleeding complications or blood transfusions.

These results are supported by the Clopidogrel and Aspirin for Reduction of Emboli in Symptomatic carotid Stenosis (CARESS) trial, which has shown that among patients with symptomatic carotid stenosis (before, not after, CEA), that the addition of clopidogrel to aspirin reduces the incidence of cerebral microemboli before (not after) CEA. The CARESS study was a randomised, double-blind, controlled trial comparing clopidogrel plus aspirin vs aspirin in 107 patients with recently (past 3 months) symptomatic carotid artery stenosis >50% and at least one characteristic microembolic signal (MES) detected during a 1-h TCD recording of the ipsilateral middle cerebral artery (MCA) before randomisation. At randomisation, patients were assigned either a 300 mg loading dose of clopidogrel (four tablets), followed by 75 mg clopidogrel once daily from day 2 to day 7 $\pm$ 1, or a matching placebo loading dose, and once daily placebo from day 2 to day 7 $\pm$ 1. Patients in both arms also received 75 mg aspirin (ASA) once daily from day 1 to day 7 $\pm$ 1 (on top of clopidogrel or placebo). All study drugs are administered orally. The primary efficacy endpoint was the occurrence of $\geqslant$1 MES vs none (MES positive or negative patient), detected by off-line analysis (by central reading centre) of the 1-h recording carried out on day 7 $\pm$ 1. Intention to treat analysis revealed a significant reduction in the primary endpoint: 43.8% of dual-therapy patients were MES positive on day 7, as compared with 72.7% of monotherapy patients (relative risk reduction 39.8%, 95% CI, 13.8 to 58.0; $P = 0.0046$) (Markus et al., 2005).

Comment

Interpretation of the evidence

Antiplatelet drugs reduce the odds of stroke after CEA, but not other major outcomes. However, a statistically significant hazardous effect of antiplatelet therapy may have been missed because of the relatively small sample size.

There is some evidence that the combination of clopidogrel and aspirin may be more effective than aspirin alone in reducing post-operative thromboemboli, as detected by TCD (Payne *et al.*, 2004). Data from several studies suggest that the presence of asymptomatic embolisation, as measured by TCD evidence of MESs, may predict future strokes or TIAs in patients with symptomatic stenosis; the risk is reported to be 8–31-fold higher in patients who are MES positive (or who have ⩾1 MES per TCD recording) than patients who are MES negative carriers of ICA stenosis (Valton *et al.*, 1998; Molloy and Markus, 1999).

Implications for practice

Antiplatelet therapy should be prescribed for all patients after CEA. Aspirin should probably be the first-line agent. Other antiplatelet agents such as clopidogrel and extended-release dipyridamole plus aspirin have also been shown to be effective in patients with TIA and ischaemic stroke not undergoing CEA (Chapter 10), and are likely (based on reasoning (Chapter 2), but not evidence) to also be effective after CEA.

Implications for research

Further research should focus on the effectiveness and safety of combinations of aspirin with other antiplatelet drugs.

There is preliminary evidence to suggest that a short period of treatment with aspirin and clopidogrel, for perhaps 1 month, might be more effective than aspirin during the acute phase of their event when patients with symptomatic carotid stenosis are at high risk of recurrent ischaemic events (Markus and Ringelstein, 2004; Payne *et al.*, 2004; Markus *et al.*, 2005). This requires a dedicated study in a large number of patients with the occurrence of recurrent stroke, other serious vascular events and bleeding complications as the primary outcome measure.

Anticoagulation

Evidence

There is no evidence to support the use of anticoagulation in patients with recently symptomatic carotid stenosis who are in sinus rhythm (Chapter 9). Warfarin with a target International Normalised Ratio (INR) of 3–4.5 was harmful in The Stroke

Prevention in Reversible Ischaemia Trial (SPIRIT) (The SPIRIT study group, 1997), and there was no additional benefit over aspirin from warfarin at a mean INR of 1.8 (target INR 1.4–2.8) in the WARSS trial (Warfarin Aspirin Recurrent Stroke Study Group, 2001) (Chapter 9).

No trials have evaluated warfarin vs aspirin specifically in patients with carotid disease (carotid stenosis (>50%) was an exclusion criterion in the WARSS trial).

Comment

Implications for practice

As the effect of warfarin in patients with symptomatic carotid stenosis undergoing CEA is likely to be qualitatively similar to that seen in other patients with TIA and ischaemic stroke due to arterial disease (based on reasoning (Chapter 2), not evidence), there is no indication to use oral anticoagulation after CEA.

However, an exception can be patients with TIA or ischaemic stroke who have both an apparently symptomatic carotid stenosis *and* atrial fibrillation (AF). Warfarin is effective and indicated in patients with TIA or ischaemic stroke who are in AF (Chapter 15). The decision to recommend anticoagulation and/or endarterectomy in these patients depends to some extent on whether the recent TIA or stroke is thought to be cardioembolic or due to carotid thromboembolism. This is can be difficult, if not impossible to determine sometimes. But if the computed tomography (CT) or magnetic resonance imaging (MRI) (diffusion-weighted image, DWI) brain scan shows multiple recent infarcts in multiple vascular territories, or echocardiography reveals apical thrombus or atrial enlargement, the source is likely to be the heart and anticoagulation is probably indicated. Alternatively, if echocardiography is normal and perhaps if any ischaemic lesions on brain imaging are confined to the ipsilateral carotid territory, it may be more appropriate to recommend endarterectomy and antiplatelet therapy.

Lowering blood pressure

Evidence

Lowering blood pressure effectively reduces the risk of recurrent stroke and other serious vascular events (Chapter 12) (PROGRESS Collaborative Group, 2001), but the effect in different aetiological subtypes of ischaemic stroke, such as symptomatic carotid stenosis, is unknown.

Among patients with bilateral severe, flow-limiting (≥70%) carotid stenosis who were randomised to best *medical* treatment alone in ECST and NASCET, the risk of subsequent stroke was significantly increased if their SBP at randomisation was <130 mmHg (hazard ratio (HR): 6.0, 95% CI: 2.4–14.7) or 130–149 mmHg

(HR: 2.5, 95% CI: 1.5 4.4) compared with patients with bilateral non-flow-limiting carotid stenosis <70% (Rothwell *et al.*, 2003a). There was no increase in stroke risk with higher SBP of 150 mmHg or more. The 5-year risk of stroke in patients with bilateral ⩾70% stenosis was 64.3% in those with SBP <150 mmHg (median value) vs 24.2% in those higher blood pressures ($P = 0.002$).

However, among patients with bilateral severe, flow-limiting (⩾70%) carotid stenosis who were randomised to CEA (plus best medical treatment) in ECST and NASCET, the 5-year risk of stroke in patients with bilateral ⩾70% stenosis was not significantly different in those with SBP <150 mmHg (median value) at randomisation compared with higher blood pressures (13.4% vs 18.3%, $P = 0.6$).

Comment

Interpretation of the evidence

The data from the ECST and NASCET suggest that aggressive lowering of SBP may be harmful in patients with bilateral severe carotid stenosis or severe symptomatic stenosis with contralateral occlusion if they have not undergone CEA. Otherwise, blood pressure lowering is likely to be safe and beneficial in patients with only unilateral ⩾70% stenosis (and following endarterectomy on one side in patients with bilateral severe carotid stenosis or severe symptomatic stenosis with contralateral occlusion) (Rothwell *et al.*, 2003a).

Implications for practice

It is likely that most patients with symptomatic carotid stenosis will benefit from gradual blood pressure lowering. However, the data from the ECST and NASCET suggest that aggressive lowering of SBP without endarterectomy may be harmful in patients with bilateral severe carotid stenosis or severe symptomatic stenosis with contralateral occlusion (Rothwell *et al.*, 2003a). These patients often also have disease of the vertebral arteries, the carotid siphon and the cerebral arteries (Thiele *et al.*, 1980; Gorelick, 1993); a loss of the normal autoregulatory capacity of the cerebral circulation, such that cerebral blood flow is directly dependent on perfusion pressure (Van der Grond *et al.*, 1995; Grubb *et al.*, 1998); and a high risk of recurrent stroke (Spence, 2000).

Lowering blood cholesterol

Evidence

Lowering blood cholesterol, by means of statin drugs, significantly reduces in the risk of all serious vascular events in patients with a history of symptomatic cerebrovascular disease a mean of 4.8 years ago, but there is no convincing evidence that they reduce the risk of recurrent stroke (Chapter 13) (Heart Protection Study Collaborative Group, 2004). However, statins also reduce the risk of patients undergoing CEA during follow-up by 50% and slow the progression of atheroma progression in patients with carotid plaque (Mercuri *et al.*, 1996).

Comment

Implications for practice

As it is likely (but not proven) that statins reduce the risk of recurrent stroke in the subgroup of patients with carotid disease, treatment with a statin is probably indicated in patients with symptomatic carotid stenosis after CEA.

The major reduction in stroke risk following intensive treatment with statins in the acute phase in patients with acute coronary syndromes (Waters *et al.*, 2002; Cannon *et al.*, 2004), suggests (but does not prove) that treatment should probably be initiated as soon as possible.

Carotid angioplasty and stenting

Transluminal angioplasty was initially undertaken in the 1960s in the limbs (Dotter *et al.*, 1967) and later in the renal, coronary and then cerebral arteries. Despite apprehension about the risks of plaque rupture and embolism causing stroke, angioplasty and/or stenting at the carotid bifurcation has increased in the past decade and is under investigation (and indeed being practised) as an alternative to endarterectomy. The main advantage is that carotid artery stenting is a less invasive revascularisation procedure than CEA.

Evidence

There have been five small RCTs of angioplasty and/or stenting vs endarterectomy in a total of 1269 patients (Naylor *et al.*, 1997; Alberts 2001; Carotid and Vertebral Transluminal Angioplasty Study (CAVATAS) Investigators, 2001; Brooks *et al.*, 2001, 2004; Higashida *et al.*, 2004; Yadav *et al.*, 2004; Coward *et al.*, 2004, 2005).

The largest of these small trials was the CAVATAS which randomly assigned 504 patients with carotid stenosis to endovascular treatment ($n = 251$) or CEA ($n = 253$) (CAVATAS Investigators, 2001). Among the patients assigned endovascular treatment, stents were used in 55 (26%) and balloon angioplasty alone in 158 (74%). The rates of major outcome events within 30 days of treatment did not differ significantly between endovascular treatment and surgery (6.4% vs 5.9%, respectively, for disabling stroke or death; 10.0% vs 9.9% for any stroke lasting more than 7 days, or death). Cranial neuropathy was reported in 22 (8.7%) surgery patients, but not after endovascular treatment ($P < 0.0001$). Major groin or neck haematoma occurred less often after endovascular treatment than after surgery (three (1.2%) vs 17 (6.7%), $P < 0.0015$). At 1 year after treatment, severe (70–99%) ipsilateral carotid stenosis was more usual after endovascular treatment (25 (14%) vs 7 (4%), $P < 0.001$). However, no substantial difference in the rate of ipsilateral stroke was noted with survival analysis up to 3 years after randomisation (adjusted HR: 1.04, 95% CI: 0.63–1.70, $P = 0.9$).

The Stenting and Angioplasty with Protection in Patients at High Risk for Endarterectomy (SAPPHIRE) trial aimed to determine whether a less invasive revascularisation strategy, carotid stenting, was not inferior to CEA, for patients with severe carotid artery stenosis and coexisting conditions that would have excluded them from previous trials of CEA (Yadav et al., 2004). The trial randomised 334 patients with neurologically symptomatic carotid stenosis of >50% or asymptomatic carotid stenosis of >80%, who had at least one coexisting condition that potentially increased the risk posed by CEA (e.g. cardiac or pulmonary disease, contralateral carotid occlusion, recurrent stenosis after endarterectomy, previous radiation therapy or radical surgery to the neck), to carotid stenting with the use of an emboli-protection device (167 patients, of whom 159 received the treatment) or to CEA (167 patients, of whom 151 received the assigned treatment). After 3 years of follow-up, the primary outcome event (the cumulative incidence of death, stroke or MI within 30 days after the procedure or death or ipsilateral stroke between 31 days and 1 year) occurred in 20 of the 167 patients randomly assigned to stenting (cumulative incidence: 12.2%) and in 32 of the 167 patients randomly assigned to endarterectomy (cumulative incidence: 20.1%). This is an absolute difference of 7.9% (95% CI: −0.7% to 16.4%, $P = 0.004$ for non-inferiority, $P = 0.053$ for superiority). At 1 year, carotid revascularisation was repeated in fewer patients who received stents that in those who had undergone endarterectomy (cumulative incidence: 0.6% vs 4.3%, $P = 0.04$).

Death or stroke within 30 days of the procedure

Overall, in the five RCTs, death or stroke occured within 30 days of PTA ± stent in 8.6% ($n = 50$) of 578 patients and within 30 days of CEA in 7.08% ($n = 41$) of 579 patients (OR: 1.26, 95% CI: 0.82–1.94) (Fig. 11.9) (Coward et al., 2004).

Death, stroke or MI within 30 days of the procedure

Death, stroke or MI occured within 30 days of PTA ± stent in 9.0% of patients, and in 9.1% patients assigned CEA (OR: 0.99, 95% CI: 0.66–1.48) (Fig. 11.10) (Coward et al., 2004).

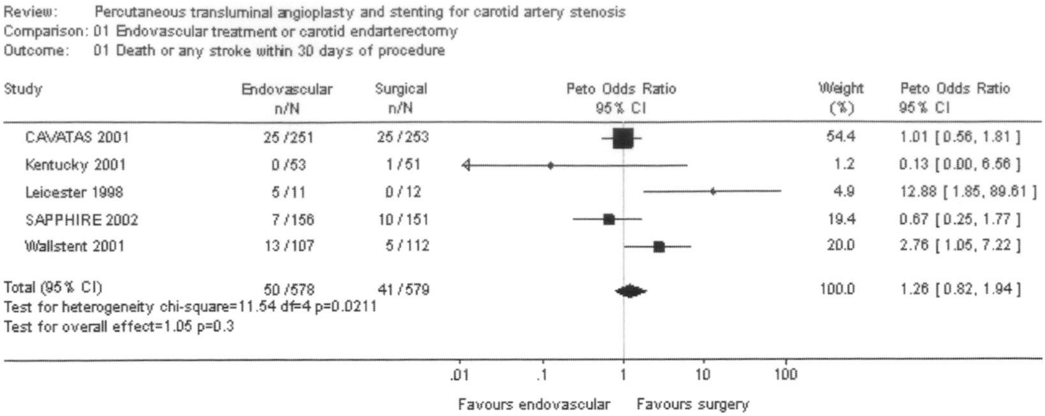

Review: Percutaneous transluminal angioplasty and stenting for carotid artery stenosis
Comparison: 01 Endovascular treatment or carotid endarterectomy
Outcome: 01 Death or any stroke within 30 days of procedure

Study	Endovascular n/N	Surgical n/N	Peto Odds Ratio 95% CI	Weight (%)	Peto Odds Ratio 95% CI
CAVATAS 2001	25 / 251	25 / 253		54.4	1.01 [0.56, 1.81]
Kentucky 2001	0 / 53	1 / 51		1.2	0.13 [0.00, 6.56]
Leicester 1998	5 / 11	0 / 12		4.9	12.88 [1.85, 89.61]
SAPPHIRE 2002	7 / 156	10 / 151		19.4	0.67 [0.25, 1.77]
Wallstent 2001	13 / 107	5 / 112		20.0	2.76 [1.05, 7.22]
Total (95% CI)	50 / 578	41 / 579		100.0	1.26 [0.82, 1.94]

Test for heterogeneity chi-square=11.54 df=4 p=0.0211
Test for overall effect=1.05 p=0.3

.01   .1   1   10   100
Favours endovascular   Favours surgery

Figure 11.9   Forest plot showing the effects of *endovascular treatment with percutaneous transluminal angioplasty ± stenting* + best medical therapy vs *CEA* plus best medical therapy in patients with carotid artery stenosis on *any stroke or death within 30 days of the procedure*. Reproduced from Coward *et al.* (2004), with permission from the authors and John Wiley & Sons Limited.

Review: Percutaneous transluminal angioplasty and stenting for carotid artery stenosis
Comparison: 01 Endovascular treatment or carotid endarterectomy
Outcome: 05 Death or stroke or myocardial infarction within 30 days of procedure

Study	Endovascular n/N	Surgery n/N	Peto Odds Ratio 95% CI	Weight (%)	Peto Odds Ratio 95% CI
CAVATAS 2001	25 / 251	28 / 253		50.2	0.89 [0.50, 1.57]
Kentucky 2001	0 / 53	1 / 51		1.1	0.13 [0.00, 6.56]
Leicester 1998	5 / 11	0 / 12		4.3	12.88 [1.85, 89.61]
SAPPHIRE 2002	9 / 156	19 / 151		26.9	0.44 [0.20, 0.96]
Wallstent 2001	13 / 107	5 / 112		17.5	2.76 [1.05, 7.22]
Total (95% CI)	52 / 578	53 / 579		100.0	0.99 [0.66, 1.48]

Test for heterogeneity chi-square=16.41 df=4 p=0.0025
Test for overall effect=-0.07 p=0.9

.01   .1   1   10   100
Favours endovascular   Favours surgery

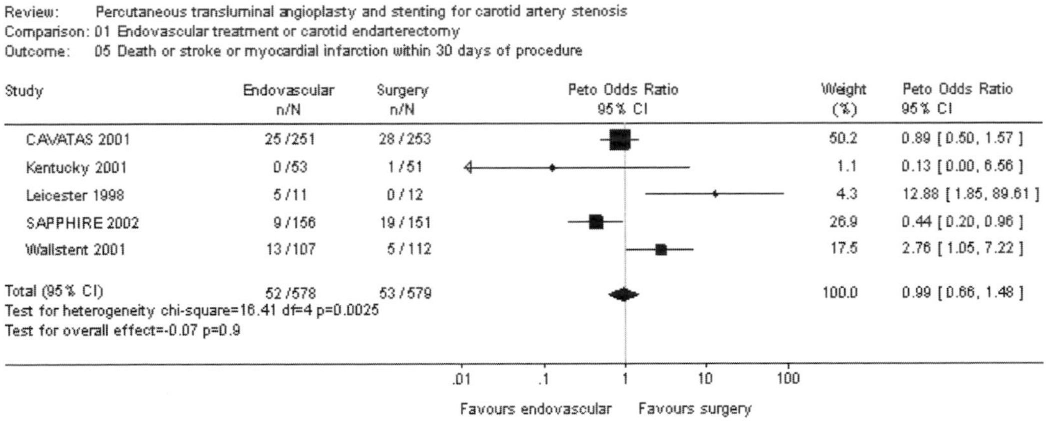

Figure 11.10   Forest plot showing the effects of *endovascular treatment with percutaneous transluminal angioplasty ± stenting* + best medical therapy vs *CEA* plus best medical therapy in patients with carotid artery stenosis on *any stroke, MI, or death within 30 days of the procedure*. Reproduced from Coward *et al.* (2004), with permission from the authors and John Wiley & Sons Limited.

Death or any stroke at 1 year after the procedure
Death or any stroke at one year after PTA ± stent occured in 13.7% of patients, compared with 10.4% of patients assigned CEA in the two trials with longer-term follow-up (OR: 1.36, 95% CI: 0.87–2.13) (Fig. 11.11) (Coward *et al.*, 2004).

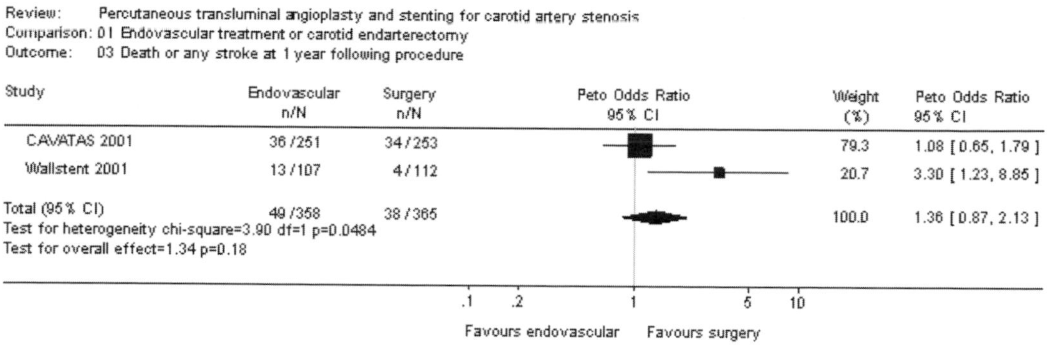

Review: Percutaneous transluminal angioplasty and stenting for carotid artery stenosis
Comparison: 01 Endovascular treatment or carotid endarterectomy
Outcome: 03 Death or any stroke at 1 year following procedure

Study	Endovascular n/N	Surgery n/N	Peto Odds Ratio 95% CI	Weight (%)	Peto Odds Ratio 95% CI
CAVATAS 2001	36 / 251	34 / 253		79.3	1.08 [0.65, 1.79]
Wallstent 2001	13 / 107	4 / 112		20.7	3.30 [1.23, 8.85]
Total (95% CI)	49 / 358	38 / 365		100.0	1.36 [0.87, 2.13]

Test for heterogeneity chi-square=3.90 df=1 p=0.0484
Test for overall effect=1.34 p=0.18

.1   .2   1   5   10

Favours endovascular   Favours surgery

Figure 11.11   Forest plot showing the effects of *endovascular treatment with percutaneous transluminal angioplasty ± stenting* + best medical therapy vs *CEA* plus best medical therapy in patients with carotid artery stenosis on *any stroke or death at one year after the procedure*. Reproduced from Coward *et al.* (2004), with permission from the authors and John Wiley & Sons Limited.

Review: Percutaneous transluminal angioplasty and stenting for carotid artery stenosis
Comparison: 01 Endovascular treatment or carotid endarterectomy
Outcome: 04 Cranial neuropathy within 30 days of procedure

Study	Endovascular n/N	Surgery n/N	Peto Odds Ratio 95% CI	Weight (%)	Peto Odds Ratio 95% CI
CAVATAS 2001	0 / 251	22 / 253		64.3	0.13 [0.05, 0.29]
Kentucky 2001	0 / 53	4 / 51		11.8	0.12 [0.02, 0.90]
× Leicester 1998	0 / 11	0 / 12		0.0	Not estimable
SAPPHIRE 2002	0 / 156	8 / 161		23.8	0.12 [0.03, 0.51]
Total (95% CI)	0 / 471	34 / 467		100.0	0.12 [0.06, 0.26]

Test for heterogeneity chi-square=0.00 df=2 p=0.9998
Test for overall effect=-5.96 p<0.00001

.01   .1   1   10   100

Favours endovascular   Favours surgery

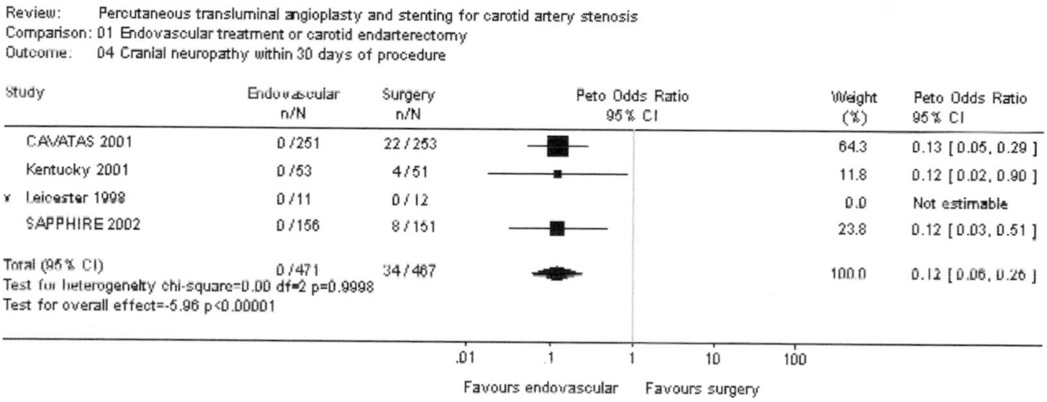

Figure 11.12   Forest plot showing the effects of *endovascular treatment with percutaneous transluminal angioplasty ± stenting* + best medical therapy vs *CEA* plus best medical therapy in patients with carotid artery stenosis on *cranial neuropathy within 30 days of the procedure*. Reproduced from Coward *et al.* (2004), with permission from the authors and John Wiley & Sons Limited.

Cranial neuropathy within 30 days of the procedure
Cranial neuropathy occured within 30 days of PTA ± stent in 0% of patients, compared with 7.3% of patients assigned CEA (OR: 0.12, 95% CI: 0.06–0.25) (Fig. 11.12) (Coward *et al.*, 2004).

Comment

Interpretation of the evidence

Taken together, these trials suggest that angioplasty ± stenting and carotid endarterectomy have similar early risks of death or stroke and similar long-term benefits, at least up to 1 year. However, the substantial heterogenetity among the trials renders the overall estimates of effect somewhat unreliable. Furthermore, two trials were stopped early because of safety concerns, so perhaps leading to an over-estimate of the risks of endovascular treatment. On the other hand, endovascular treatment appears to avoid completely the risk of cranial neuropathy. There is also uncertainty about the potential for restenosis to develop and cause recurrent stroke after endovascular treatment.

Implications for practice

The current evidence does not support a widespread change in clinical practice away from recommending CEA as the treatment of choice for suitable carotid artery stenosis.

The SAPPHIRE trials suggests that stenting with a protection device is an appropriate alternative to endarterectomy in patients at unacceptably increased risk for perioperative stroke or MI associated with CEA. However, the overall estimates of benefit and risk are imprecise due to the small sample size; further, the long-term effects of stenting beyond 1 year are not known. Moreover, the results of SAPPHIRE are not generalisable to patients at lower risk or to interventionalists who have not achieved comparable results following prospective and independent audit.

The use of carotid stenting is likely to increase but whether it will be confined to cases in which endarterectomy is technically difficult or risky will depend on the overall results of larger trials comparing the short and long-term benefits and risks of stenting vs endarterectomy (Internet Stroke Center, http://www.strokecenter.org/trials/(accessed May 11, 2005)). Hence, there is a strong case to continue recruitment in the current randomised trials comparing carotid stenting with endarterectomy.

Implications for research

Ongoing trials comparing the short and long-term benefits and risks of stenting vs endarterectomy need to be large enough to minimise random error in the estimates of the overall safety and effectiveness of stenting compared with endarterectomy, and to enable meaningful pre-specified analyses of subgroups (e.g. neurologically symptomatic and asymptomatic stenosis, severity of stenosis, time since symptoms, age, sex, and antiplatelet regimen). Several trials are currently in progress. These include the International Carotid Stenting Study (ICSS) which had recruited 527 patients by April 15, 2005 and aims to randomised 1500 patients over the subsequent 4 years (Featherstone *et al.*, 2004), the Carotid Revascularisation Endarterectomy vs Stenting Trial (CREST) which had recruited more than 1000 patients by July 2005 and aims to randomised 2500 patients by the end of 2006 (Howard *et al.*, 2004), and the Stent-supported Percutaneous Angioplasty of the

Carotid artery vs Endarterectomy (SPACE), trial which had recruited 860 patients by October 2004 and aims to randomise 1900 patients (Ringleb *et al.*, 2004; www.space.stroke-trial.com).

SUMMARY

Carotid endarterectomy

Interpretation of the evidence

With the exception of near-occlusion, CEA is of overall benefit in the long term for patients with recent symptomatic carotid stenosis above [NASCET]50% (equivalent to about [ECST]65% stenosis), provided that the surgical risk of stroke and death is less than about 7%.

The benefit is greater in patients with greater degrees of stenosis (until the artery distal to the stenosis begins to collapse), men, the elderly (aged 75 years or older) and those operated on early, within 2 weeks after the last ischaemic event, and falls rapidly with increasing delay.

For patients with $\geqslant$50% stenosis, the number of patients needed to undergo surgery to prevent one ipsilateral stroke in 5 years is nine for men vs 36 for women, five for patients aged 75 years or older vs 18 for patients younger than 65 years, and five for those treated within 2 weeks after their last ischaemic event vs 125 for patients randomised after more than 12 weeks.

Implications for practice

Patients with recent symptomatic carotid territory ischaemic events should be screened for the presence of carotid stenosis.

Colour Doppler ultrasonography, in experienced hands with modern equipment, is a quick, practical, inexpensive and reliable tool for identifying carotid, vertebral and subclavian disease. The available evidence, though not extensive, suggests that magnetic resonance (MR) angiography tends to overestimate the degree of stenosis, CT angiography tends to underestimate it, and colour Doppler ultrasonography is in the middle compared with the gold standard of catheter angiography (Rothwell and Warlow, 2000; Patel *et al.*, 2002).

Since the carotid surgery trials were all based on intra-arterial angiographic measurement of carotid stenosis, selective intra-arterial carotid angiography should continue to be used for assessing stenosis severity and selecting patients for endarterectomy (Johnston and Goldstein, 2001; Norris and Rothwell, 2001) unless non-invasive techniques such as carotid ultrasound, MR angiography and CT angiography, have been properly validated against catheter angiography within individual centres (Rothwell and Warlow, 2000). A particularly difficult area is the reliable detection and exclusion of near occlusion by non-invasive methods of carotid imaging (Bermann *et al.*, 1995; Ascher *et al.*, 2002).

However, because of delays due to waiting for a hospital bed, risks of invasive angiography in this predominantly older population with symptomatic vascular disease, and the substantial improvement in non-invasive vascular imaging have together meant that many centres have adopted alternative policies.

A reasonable alternative strategy is to undertake ultrasonography first and, if severe stenosis is suspected, arrange a further confirmatory non-invasive imaging test (MR or CT angiography or repeat ultrasonography) by an independent observer. If these two disagree, addition of a third non-invasive test would result in very few misclassified carotid stenoses. Furthermore, any minor loss of accuracy with the use of non-invasive tests probably more than offsets the complications of intra-arterial angiography.

Following the confusion generated by the use of different methods of measurement of stenosis in the original trials, it is recommended that the NASCET method be adopted as the standard in future (Rothwell *et al.*, 2003b).

For individual patients in whom symptomatic carotid stenosis has been detected, the net effectiveness of CEA is determined by the:

- Patient's absolute risk of an ipsilateral carotid territory ischaemic stroke (which can be prevented by CEA) – this is, on average, about 5–7% per year over 5 years, but is higher with more severe degrees of symptomatic stenosis, in men, in the elderly, within the first few weeks of symptom onset, and in the presence of irregular plaque surface morphology and impaired collateral flow and cerebral perfusion reserve.
- The surgical peri-operative stroke and death rate – this was about 7% on average in the RCTs, and is likely to be higher in women, and in patients with systolic hypertension, peripheral arterial disease, and occlusion of the contralateral ICA and ipsilateral external carotid artery. However, the experience of the surgeon and hospital are also crucial factors, and the results of a recent prospective audit of local surgical peri-operative stroke and death rates should be widely available.
- The patient's risk of other disabling and fatal events, and life-expectancy.
- The cost of the diagnostic assessment, CEA and post-operative care (Benade and Warlow, 2002a, b).
- The cost of the adverse outcomes of CEA (peri-operative stroke or death, cranial nerve palsy, wound infection or haematoma).
- The cost of the favourable outcomes of CEA (strokes (non-disabling, disabling, fatal) prevented).
- The generalisability of the results of the trials of CEA to all patients with symptomatic carotid stenosis and all surgeons performing CEA.

- The effectiveness compared with best medical therapy alone, and compared with best medical therapy combined with other alternative strategies of recanalising the carotid stenosis, such as carotid angioplasty and stenting.

Carotid stenting

Carotid stenting is less invasive than CEA and causes less local complications (cranial neuropathy and neck haematoma), but its long-term durability in preventing ipsilateral carotid ischaemic stroke, compared with CEA, remains to be determined reliably from the long-term follow-up of patients enrolled in ongoing large RCTs.

Lowering blood pressure

In the 1990s, it was established that there is a direct log-linear relationship between blood pressure (BP) levels and risk of stroke (MacMahon *et al.*, 1990). It was also established that increasing BP is a causal risk factor for stroke; a systematic review of randomised-controlled trials (RCTs) showed that lowering BP significantly reduced the risk of *first-ever* stroke (Collins *et al.*, 1990; Blood Pressure Lowering Treatment Trialists' Collaboration, 2000, 2003). Modest reductions in BP by about 10–12 mmHg systolic and 5–6 mmHg diastolic reduced the relative risk (RR) of stroke by about 38% and the RR of coronary heart disease by about 16% within a few years of beginning treatment. Larger (and smaller) reductions in BP produced larger (and smaller) reductions in risk of stroke. The five main classes of anti-hypertensive drugs (diuretics, β-blockers, calcium channel blockers, angiotensin-converting enzyme (ACE) inhibitors and angiotensin-receptor blockers (ARB)) were all effective in preventing stroke, and the magnitude of the effect was determined mainly by the magnitude of the BP lowering (Blood Pressure Lowering Treatment Trialists' Collaboration, 2000, 2003; Lawes *et al.*, 2004).

For individuals who have already experienced a symptomatic transient ischaemic attack (TIA) or mild ischaemic stroke, there was observational evidence from the UK TIA aspirin trial of a similar direct and continuous relationship between BP (both systolic and diastolic) and recurrent stroke, as there was between BP and first-ever stroke (Rodgers *et al.*, 1996). These data suggested that lowering diastolic BP by 5 mmHg was associated with a reduction in recurrent stroke by about a one-third (Rodgers *et al.*, 1996).

However, clinicians have long been concerned that actually lowering BP patients with known cerebrovascular disease, and especially those with significant occlusive cerebrovascular disease, may compromise cerebral perfusion and per-haps even increase the rate of recurrent ischaemic stroke due to haemodynamic insufficiency.

Evidence

A systematic review identified seven RCTs that investigated the effect of lowering BP on recurrent vascular events in 15,527 patients with prior ischaemic or haemorrhagic stroke or TIA (Rashid *et al.*, 2003). There were eight comparison groups.

Two-thirds of the data were derived from two studies: the Post-Stroke Antihypertensive Treatment Study (PATS) and Perindopril Protection Against Recurrent Stroke Study (PROGRESS) (PATS Collaborating Group, 1995; PROGRESS Collaborative Group, 2001).

The average time from stroke onset to randomisation ranged from 3 weeks to 14 months, and patients were followed for a period of 2–5 years.

Three RCTs limited recruitment to patients with high BP (Carter, 1970; Hypertension-Stroke Cooperative Study Group, 1974; Eriksson *et al.*, 1995) and the other trials enrolled patients irrespective of their baseline BP. Mean baseline BPs varied from 139 to 167 mmHg systolic and 79 to 100 mmHg diastolic.

Previous anti-hypertensive medications were discontinued before randomisation in two RCTs (Hypertension-Stroke Cooperative Study Group, 1974; PATS Collaborating Group, 1995).

Three classes of pharmacological agents were used to lower BP: β-receptor antagonists (atenolol), diuretics (indapamide, methyclothiazide) and ACE inhibitors (perindopril, ramipril); two earlier trials used mixed treatment including a centrally acting drug (methyldopa) or Rauwolfia alkaloid (deserpidine) (Carter, 1970; Hypertension-Stroke Cooperative Study Group, 1974). There were no relevant RCTs of non-pharmacological interventions (e.g. salt restriction), α-receptor antagonists, angiotensin II receptor antagonists or calcium channel blockers.

Blood pressure

Patients assigned active BP-lowering treatment experienced small reductions in systolic and diastolic BP (<10 mmHg systolic and <5 mmHg diastolic) compared with control, except in the Hypertension-Stroke Cooperative Study Group (HSCSG) which realised a reduction in BP in the treated group of 25 mmHg systolic and 12 mmHg diastolic compared with the control group (Hypertension-Stroke Cooperative Study Group, 1974).

The Heart Outcome Prevention Evaluation (HOPE) trial reported a reduction in daytime office BP of only 3.3 mmHg systolic and 1.4 mmHg diastolic (The Heart Outcomes Prevention Evaluation Study Investigators, 2000; Sleight *et al.*, 2001; Bosch *et al.*, 2002). This is likely to be an underestimate since treatment was given in the evening and BP was measured the next day in the office. Furthermore, a very small substudy of HOPE involving 38 patients with peripheral arterial disease who were randomised to ramipril (20 patients) or placebo (18 patients) taken at night,

Table 12.1. Effect of lowering BP on stroke, MI, all vascular events and death.

Outcome	Rate in control group (%)	OR	95% CI	P	P for heterogeneity
Stroke	11.5	0.76	0.63–0.92	0.005	0.01
MI	4.0	0.79	0.63–0.98	0.03	0.19
Vascular events	16.0	0.79	0.66–0.95	0.01	0.002
Vascular death	5.9	0.86	0.70–1.06	0.16	0.066
Death	9.6	0.91	0.79–1.05	0.18	0.17

OR and 95% CI determined using a random effects model.
Source: Rashid *et al.* (2003).

and followed up with 24 h ambulatory BP monitoring after 1 year, revealed that the 20 patients allocated ramipril had a reduction in *daytime* BP of 6 mmHg systolic and 2 mmHg diastolic, a reduction in *office* BP of 8 mmHg systolic and 2 mmHg diastolic, and a reduction in *24 h* BP of 17 mmHg systolic and 8 mmHg diastolic compared with the 18 patients allocated placebo (Svensson *et al.*, 2001).

Recurrent stroke

Among 15,527 patients with prior stroke or TIA who were randomised in seven RCTs to active anti-hypertensive treatment ($n = 7779$) or control ($n = 7748$), the rate of recurrent stroke was reduced from 11.5% (888/7748) with control to 8.7% (689/7779) with anti-hypertensive treatment (odds ratio (OR): 0.76, 95% confidence interval (CI): 0.63–0.92, absolute risk reduction (ARR): 2.7%) (Table 12.1) (Fig. 12.1).

Benefits were observed for all pathological and aetiological subtypes of stroke types and all major clinical groups studied (Chapman *et al.*, 2004), irrespective of the patients baseline level of BP, age, sex, race and time since stroke onset (the PROGRESS Collaborative Group, 2001).

There was significant heterogeneity among the trials ($P = 0.01$) which appeared to be related to varying effectiveness of the different drug classes (Table 12.2). Diuretics, which reduced the odds of stroke by 32% (95% CI: 8–50%), and the combination of a diuretic and ACE inhibitor, which reduced the odds of stroke by 45% (95% CI: 32–56%), appeared to be more effective than β-blockers and ACE inhibitors in indirect comparisons, but these differences could be confounded by other factors such as different magnitudes of BP reduction.

Myocardial infarction

Among 15,428 patients with prior stroke or TIA who were randomised in six RCTs to active anti-hypertensive treatment ($n = 7729$) or control ($n = 7699$), the rate of myocardial infarction (MI) was reduced from 4.0% (311/7699) with control to

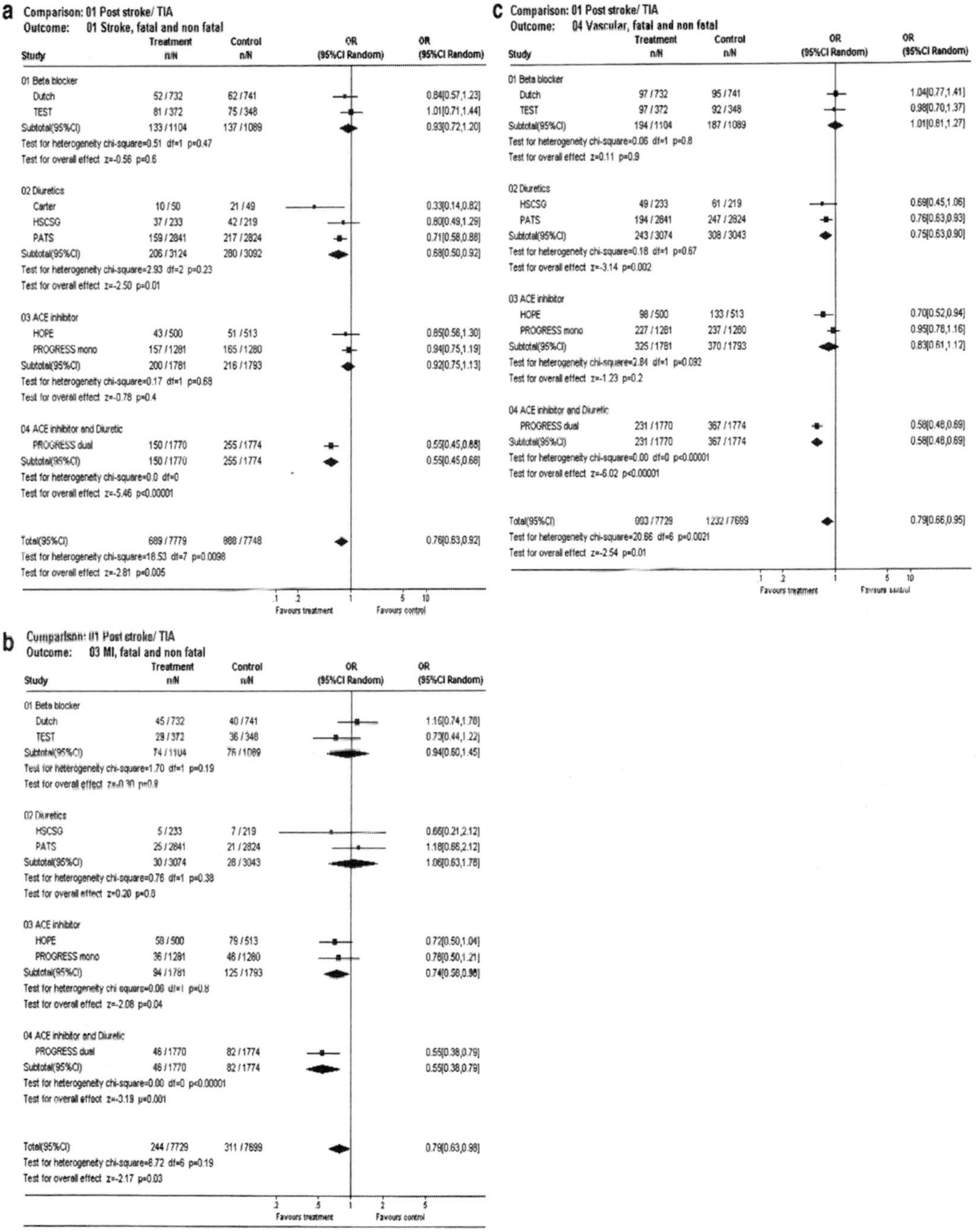

a Comparison: 01 Post stroke/ TIA
Outcome: 01 Stroke, fatal and non fatal

Study	Treatment n/N	Control n/N	OR (95%CI Random)	OR (95%CI Random)
01 Beta blocker				
Dutch	52 / 732	62 / 741		0.84[0.57,1.23]
TEST	81 / 372	75 / 348		1.01[0.71,1.44]
Subtotal(95%CI)	133 / 1104	137 / 1089		0.93[0.72,1.20]
Test for heterogeneity chi-square=0.51 df=1 p=0.47				
Test for overall effect z=-0.56 p=0.6				
02 Diuretics				
Carter	10 / 50	21 / 49		0.33[0.14,0.82]
HSCSG	37 / 233	42 / 219		0.80[0.49,1.29]
PATS	159 / 2841	217 / 2824		0.71[0.58,0.88]
Subtotal(95%CI)	206 / 3124	280 / 3092		0.68[0.50,0.92]
Test for heterogeneity chi-square=2.93 df=2 p=0.23				
Test for overall effect z=-2.50 p=0.01				
03 ACE inhibitor				
HOPE	43 / 500	51 / 513		0.85[0.56,1.30]
PROGRESS mono	157 / 1281	165 / 1280		0.94[0.75,1.19]
Subtotal(95%CI)	200 / 1781	216 / 1793		0.92[0.75,1.13]
Test for heterogeneity chi-square=0.17 df=1 p=0.68				
Test for overall effect z=-0.78 p=0.4				
04 ACE inhibitor and Diuretic				
PROGRESS dual	150 / 1770	255 / 1774		0.55[0.45,0.68]
Subtotal(95%CI)	150 / 1770	255 / 1774		0.55[0.45,0.68]
Test for heterogeneity chi-square=0.0 df=0				
Test for overall effect z=-5.46 p<0.00001				
Total(95%CI)	689 / 7779	888 / 7748		0.76[0.63,0.92]
Test for heterogeneity chi-square=18.53 df=7 p=0.0098				
Test for overall effect z=-2.81 p=0.005				

.1 .2   1   5 10
Favours treatment Favours control

b Comparison: 01 Post stroke/ TIA
Outcome: 03 MI, fatal and non fatal

Study	Treatment n/N	Control n/N	OR (95%CI Random)	OR (95%CI Random)
01 Beta blocker				
Dutch	45 / 732	40 / 741		1.15[0.74,1.78]
TEST	29 / 372	36 / 348		0.73[0.44,1.22]
Subtotal(95%CI)	74 / 1104	76 / 1089		0.94[0.60,1.45]
Test for heterogeneity chi-square=1.70 df=1 p=0.19				
Test for overall effect z=-0.30 p=0.8				
02 Diuretics				
HSCSG	5 / 233	7 / 219		0.66[0.21,2.12]
PATS	25 / 2841	21 / 2824		1.18[0.66,2.12]
Subtotal(95%CI)	30 / 3074	28 / 3043		1.06[0.63,1.78]
Test for heterogeneity chi-square=0.76 df=1 p=0.38				
Test for overall effect z=0.20 p=0.8				
03 ACE inhibitor				
HOPE	58 / 500	79 / 513		0.72[0.50,1.04]
PROGRESS mono	36 / 1281	46 / 1280		0.78[0.50,1.21]
Subtotal(95%CI)	94 / 1781	125 / 1793		0.74[0.56,0.98]
Test for heterogeneity chi-square=0.06 df=1 p=0.8				
Test for overall effect z=-2.08 p=0.04				
04 ACE inhibitor and Diuretic				
PROGRESS dual	46 / 1770	82 / 1774		0.55[0.38,0.79]
Subtotal(95%CI)	46 / 1770	82 / 1774		0.55[0.38,0.79]
Test for heterogeneity chi-square=0.00 df=0 p<0.00001				
Test for overall effect z=-3.19 p=0.001				
Total(95%CI)	244 / 7729	311 / 7699		0.79[0.63,0.98]
Test for heterogeneity chi-square=8.72 df=6 p=0.19				
Test for overall effect z=-2.17 p=0.03				

.2 .5   1   2   5
Favours treatment Favours control

c Comparison: 01 Post stroke/ TIA
Outcome: 04 Vascular, fatal and non fatal

Study	Treatment n/N	Control n/N	OR (95%CI Random)	OR (95%CI Random)
01 Beta blocker				
Dutch	97 / 732	95 / 741		1.04[0.77,1.41]
TEST	97 / 372	92 / 348		0.98[0.70,1.37]
Subtotal(95%CI)	194 / 1104	187 / 1089		1.01[0.81,1.27]
Test for heterogeneity chi-square=0.06 df=1 p=0.8				
Test for overall effect z=0.11 p=0.9				
02 Diuretics				
HSCSG	49 / 233	61 / 219		0.69[0.45,1.06]
PATS	194 / 2841	247 / 2824		0.76[0.63,0.93]
Subtotal(95%CI)	243 / 3074	308 / 3043		0.75[0.63,0.90]
Test for heterogeneity chi-square=0.18 df=1 p=0.67				
Test for overall effect z=-3.14 p=0.002				
03 ACE inhibitor				
HOPE	98 / 500	133 / 513		0.70[0.52,0.94]
PROGRESS mono	227 / 1281	237 / 1280		0.95[0.78,1.16]
Subtotal(95%CI)	325 / 1781	370 / 1793		0.83[0.61,1.12]
Test for heterogeneity chi-square=2.84 df=1 p=0.092				
Test for overall effect z=-1.23 p=0.2				
04 ACE inhibitor and Diuretic				
PROGRESS dual	231 / 1770	367 / 1774		0.58[0.48,0.69]
Subtotal(95%CI)	231 / 1770	367 / 1774		0.58[0.48,0.69]
Test for heterogeneity chi-square=0.00 df=0 p<0.00001				
Test for overall effect z=-6.02 p<0.00001				
Total(95%CI)	993 / 7729	1232 / 7699		0.79[0.66,0.95]
Test for heterogeneity chi-square=20.86 df=6 p=0.0021				
Test for overall effect z=-2.54 p=0.01				

.1 .2   1   5 10
Favours treatment Favours control

Figure 12.1   Forest plots of the effect of anti-hypertensive therapy in patients with prior stroke or TIA on subsequent stroke (a), MI (b), and all serious vascular events (stroke, MI or vascular death) (c). Reproduced from Rashid *et al.* (2003), with permission of the authors and Lippincott, Williams and Wilkins.

Table 12.2. Effect of drug class, prior BP status and stroke type on vascular outcome events.

Variable	Stroke		MI		All vascular events	
	OR	95% CI	OR	95% CI	OR	95% CI
All trials	0.76	0.63–0.92	0.79	0.63–0.98	0.79	0.66–0.95
Drug class						
Diuretic	0.68	0.50–0.92	1.06	0.63–1.78	0.75	0.63–0.90
β-blockers	0.93	0.72–1.20	0.94	0.60–1.45	1.01	0.81–1.27
ACE-I	0.93	0.75–1.14	0.74	0.56–0.98	0.83	0.61–1.13
Diuretic and ACE-I	0.55	0.44–0.68	0.55	0.38–0.79	0.57	0.48–0.68
Non-β-blocker	0.71	0.57–0.90	0.72	0.57–0.92	0.73	0.60–0.89
Baseline BP						
High BP	0.74	0.45–1.22			0.85	0.60–1.19
Any	0.75	0.60–0.94			0.78	0.63–0.97
Stroke type						
Ischaemic stroke	0.58	0.24–1.40			1.04	0.77–1.41
All stroke	0.78	0.63–0.96			0.76	0.63–0.92

Source: Rashid *et al.* (2003).

3.2% (244/7729) with anti-hypertensive treatment (OR: 0.79, 95% CI: 0.63–0.98, ARR: 0.8%) (Table 12.1).

MI events were almost 3-fold less frequent than stroke (control group rates: 4% (MI) vs 11.5% (stroke)) over the follow-up period of the studies (up to 5 years).

There was no significant heterogeneity among the trials ($P = 0.19$).

Stroke, MI or vascular death (all serious vascular events)

Among 15,428 patients with prior stroke or TIA who were randomised in six RCTs to active anti-hypertensive treatment ($n = 7729$) or control ($n = 7699$), the rate of serious vascular events was reduced from 16.0% (1232/7699) with control to 12.8% (993/7729) with anti-hypertensive treatment (OR: 0.79, 95% CI: 0.66–0.95, ARR: 3.2%) (Table 12.1).

There was significant heterogeneity among the trials ($P = 0.002$) which again appeared to be related to varying effectiveness of the different drug classes (Table 12.2). Diuretics, which reduced the odds of serious vascular events by 25% (95% CI: 10–37%), and the combination of a diuretic and ACE inhibitor, which reduced the odds of serious vascular events by 43% (95% CI: 32–52%), appeared to be more effective than β-blockers and ACE inhibitors alone in indirect comparisons. However, this may also be explained by greater BP reductions with diuretics and the combination of diuretics and ACE inhibitors.

Sensitivity analyses

Sensitivity analyses based on inclusion of studies of the highest quality alone did not result in any substantial change to the overall results. No publication bias was apparent on visual inspection of funnel plots or Egger's test for the outcomes of stroke and vascular events.

As the two trials involving a β-receptor antagonist recruited some patients during the acute phase of stroke (The Dutch TIA Study Group, 1993; Eriksson *et al.*, 1995), which may bias the results towards a poor outcome (Barer *et al.*, 1988), a *post hoc* analysis was undertaken of the effect of lowering BP with agents other than β-receptor antagonists (i.e. diuretics, ACE inhibitors or their combination) and the results are shown in Table 12.2. The positive effects of lowering BP on subsequent serious vascular events were greater in the trials which did not evaluate β-receptor antagonist trials.

The relative benefit of anti-hypertensive therapies in reducing the RR of stroke and all vascular events was statistically significant in trials which included all patients, irrespective of their BP status. It was statistically non-significant, but with comparable ORs and wider 95% CI, in trials that limited recruitment to patients with prior hypertension, because the numbers of patients and events in the latter studies were relatively small.

Outcome and BP

Reduction in stroke risk was related non-linearly (second-order quadratic function) to the difference in systolic BP between the active and control groups, irrespective of whether the HOPE ambulatory systolic BP data ($P = 0.004$) or office systolic BP data ($P = 0.002$) were used (Rashid *et al.*, 2003).

Comment

Interpretation of the evidence

Lowering BP or treating hypertension with a variety of anti-hypertensive agents in patients with prior TIA or stroke reduces the odds of recurrent stroke (OR: 0.76, 95% CI: 0.63–0.92), non-fatal stroke (OR: 0.79, 95% CI: 0.65–0.95), MI (OR: 0.79, 95% CI: 0.63–0.98), and total vascular events (OR: 0.79, 95% CI: 0.66–0.95) by about one-fifth to one-quarter. No significant effect was seen on vascular or all-cause mortality. Heterogeneity was present for several outcomes and was partly related to the class of anti-hypertensive drugs used; ACE inhibitors and diuretics separately, and especially together, reduced vascular events, while β-receptor antagonists had no significant effect. The reduction in stroke was related to the difference in systolic BP between treatment and control groups ($P = 0.002$).

Since this review, the Morbidity and mortality after Stroke Eprosartan compared with nitrendipine for Secondary prevention (MOSES) Trial compared the angiotensin receptor blocker (ARB) eprosartan with the calcium channel antagonist nitrendipine in a prospective, randomised, open, blinded end point (PROBE) design study among 1405 patients with hypertension and a previous stroke (mean one year ago) (Schrader *et al.*, 2005). Nitrendipine was chosen as the reference drug because it had been shown in the SYST-EUR trial to be significantly more effective than placebo in preventing first-ever stroke (Staessen *et al.*, 1997). Patients assigned eprosartan had no difference in blood pressure reduction but a significant reduction in the number of primary outcome events (death, cardiovascular or cerebrovascular events) after a mean 2.5 years follow-up (255 nitrendipine vs 206 eprosartan, $p = 0.014$) compared with nitrendipine (Schrader *et al.*, 2005).

Implications for practice

As some patients with previous stroke cannot tolerate much BP reduction, such as those who have severe occlusive arterial disease in the neck, care must be taken in lowering BP in individual patients.

BP lowering should probably wait until the acute phase of any stroke has resolved, perhaps for a week or two, because lowering BP, at least in theory, could reduce cerebral perfusion and worsen outcome because of impaired cerebral autoregulation in the ischaemic area (Chapter 4). Trials of very early BP lowering are in progress (Bath *et al.*, 2001, 2003; Blood Pressure In Acute Stroke Collaboration, 2001).

Thereafter, treatment should be introduced slowly and gently in all patients (or added to existing anti-hypertensive medication), irrespective of their baseline BP, pathological stroke type, age and race.

Treatment should probably begin with a diuretic (such as indapamide) and/or ACE inhibitor (such as perindopril or ramipril) rather than other drug classes for which there are less data. Drugs from other classes (e.g. the angiotensin receptor blocker [ARB], eprosartan) can then be added if BP remains high, for example, above levels such as 140/85 mmHg (or 130/80 mmHg in diabetics). However, the decision of which drugs should be used lies with the preferences of the responsible clinician and patient, and they are influenced by the presence of other diseases for which certain drug classes are specifically indicated (e.g. ACE inhibitors or ARBs in heart failure, β-receptor antagonists after MI) or contraindicated (e.g. the avoidance of ACE inhibitors and ARBs in renal artery stenosis and β-receptor antagonists in asthma).

If tolerated, the lower the target BP the better, down to perhaps 130/70 mmHg, provided any adverse effects are acceptable to the patient.

Treatment should be continued for several years, whilst the patient remains at increased risk, since the trials followed patients for up to 5 years.

Implications for research

A meta-analysis of individual patient data from the existing trials would allow the effect of lowering BP in subgroups to be studied, and update an earlier effort (Gueyffier *et al.*, 1997).

Further research in patients with previous stroke is also required for some of the major classes of anti-hypertensive agents, especially angiotensin receptor II antagonists and calcium channel blockers, because not all patients can take an ACE inhibitor and/or diuretic.

The Ongoing Telmisartan Alone and in combination with Ramipril Global Endpoint Trial (ONTARGET) aims to randomise 23,400 patients with symptomatic atherothrombosis of the heart, brain and limbs, or diabetes mellitus to an ACE-inhibitor (ramipril 10 mg daily), an ARB (telmisartan 80 mg daily), or the combination of ramipril 10 mg and telmisartan 80 mg daily, and follow up patients over a mean of 5.5 years for the occurrence of non-fatal stroke, non-fatal MI, death due to vascular causes, or hospitalisation for heart failure. Up to 5000 such patients who are unable to tolerate the ACE-inhibitor will be randomised to placebo or telmisartan 80 mg daily in the Telmisartan Randomisation AssessmeNt Study in aCE i – iNtolerant patients with cardiovascular Disease (TRANSCEND).

SUMMARY

Anti-hypertensive therapy for patients with prior stroke or TIA, which reduces BP modestly ($<10/<5$ mmHg), is associated with significant reductions in the RR of stroke, MI and all serious vascular events by about one-fifth to one-quarter, irrespective of the patients baseline BP, and pathological stroke type.

The absolute benefits of anti-hypertensive therapy are greater with greater reductions in BP. They are also greater for preventing recurrent stroke than for MI in the first few years after TIA or stroke, and for patients with higher absolute risk of serious events such as those with higher baseline BP.

The reductions in BP values and risks of stroke and serious vascular events are similar in magnitude to those predicted from epidemiological observations (Lawes *et al.*, 2004), they are consistent with the results of RCTs of BP lowering in the primary prevention of first-ever stroke (Blood Pressure Lowering Trialists Collaboration, 2003), and they are proportional to the degree of BP lowering. This suggests that it is likely that most, if not all, of the effect can be attributed to the lowering of BP. If so, this would suggest that other drugs which achieve similar BP reductions would achieve similar reductions in stroke risk, although extrapolation to β-blockers is perhaps less certain.

Lowering blood cholesterol concentrations

Evidence from observational studies

All stroke

A systematic review of 45 observational studies of about 450,000 people over 16 years identified no clear relation between plasma total cholesterol and the occurrence of any stroke (after adjusting for age, gender, ethnicity, blood pressure and history of cardiac disease), suggesting that cholesterol was not a risk factor for any stroke (Prospective Studies Collaboration, 1995). A more recent, but smaller meta-analysis of eight observational studies of 24,343 women found that increasing plasma cholesterol was a significant independent risk factor for death due to any stroke among black women less than 55 years of age (Horenstein *et al.*, 2002).

It is possible that the overall association between total cholesterol and all stroke dilutes real associations between cholesterol and pathological subtypes of stroke, and between cholesterol fractions and pathological and aetiological subtypes of stroke.

Subtypes of stroke

There is a weak (*positive*) association between increasing plasma cholesterol concentrations and increasing risk of *ischaemic* stroke which is partially offset by a weaker (*negative*) association between *decreasing* plasma cholesterol concentrations and increasing risk of *haemorrhagic* stroke (Iso *et al.*, 1989; Eastern Stroke and Coronary Heart Disease Collaborative Research Group, 1998; Koren-Morag *et al.*, 2002; Asia Pacific Cohort Studies Collaboration, 2003).

Fractions of cholesterol

Low-density lipoprotein-cholesterol

Increasing low-density lipoprotein-cholesterol (LDL-cholesterol) concentrations of 1.03 mmol/l (40 mg/dl) have been associated independently with a 14% (95% confidence interval (CI): 0–26%) increase in odds of ischaemic stroke or transient ischaemic attack (TIA) (Koran-Morag *et al.*, 2002).

Table 13.1. Hazard ratios for ischaemic stroke according to blood concentrations of lipid subfractions above or below the median value.

Lipid subfraction	Ischaemic stroke events per patient				Hazard ratio	95% CI
	Below median		Above median			
	Events	Patients	Events	Patients		
Apo B/apo A1	11	126	28	130	2.86	1.37–5.88
Apo B	13	130	27	131	2.27	1.14–4.50
Total cholesterol	17	138	28	146	1.79	0.95–3.35
LDL-cholesterol	18	134	26	140	1.49	0.83–2.77
LDL/HDL-cholesterol	20	135	24	138	1.28	0.70–2.38
Apo A1	22	140	22	141	1.16	0.62–2.16
HDL-cholesterol	22	143	23	143	1.01	0.55–1.87

Source: Bhatia *et al.* (2004).
Adjusted for age, sex, systolic blood pressure, smoking and diabetes.

High-density lipoprotein-cholesterol

A significant, independent (negative) association between decreasing plasma high-density lipoprotein (HDL) concentrations and increasing risk of ischaemic stroke has been identified in several studies (Tanne *et al.*, 1997; Simons *et al.*, 1998; Leppala *et al.*, 1999; Koran-Morag *et al.*, 2002).

Total cholesterol/HDL-cholesterol concentration ratio

A significant, independent, positive association exists between the ratio of total cholesterol/HDL-cholesterol concentrations and ischaemic stroke (Simons *et al.*, 2001).

Apolipoproteins

A recent small study has suggested that apolipoprotein B (apo B) and the ratio of a apo B/apolipoprotein A1 (apo A1) are stronger predictors of ischaemic stroke than total cholesterol, LDL-cholesterol or HDL cholesterol (Table 13.1) (Bhatia *et al.*, 2004). Among 290 patients with a history of TIA up to 3 years previously, 45 patients had a first-ever ischaemic stroke over the next 10 years, and the ratio of an apo B/ apo A1 was the lipid subfraction with the strongest adjusted association with ischaemic stroke (hazard ratio: 2.86, 95% CI: 1.37–5.88%) (Table 13.1).

Apolipoproteins make up the protein moiety of lipoproteins, with apo B being found mainly in LDL and apo A1 in HDL. Measurement of apo B and apo A1 provides information on the total number of atherogenic (apo B) and antiatherogenic (apo A1) particles.

Aetiological subtypes of ischaemic stroke

Increasing LDL-cholesterol concentrations have been associated independently with a 68% (95% CI: 23–230%) increase in odds of ischaemic stroke due to large artery atherothrombosis (Koran-Morag *et al.*, 2002).

Evidence from clinical trials

Prevention of all (first-ever and recurrent) stroke

A systematic review of the 33 randomised-controlled trials (RCTs) of cholesterol-lowering interventions published before 1998 found that among about 69,000 subjects (35,259 in intervention group, 33,523 in control group) who were followed for at least 6 months, and amongst whom a count of total strokes was available, there was about a 16% (95% CI: 7–25%) reduction in the odds of stroke over about 4 years, from 2.34% (784/33,523) among patients allocated control to 1.62% (570/35,259) among patients allocated a cholesterol-lowering intervention (Di Mascio *et al.*, 2000).

Since 1998, the effect of the cholesterol-lowering interventions lovastatin (AFCAPS/TexCAPS Research Group, 1998), gemfibrozil (Rubins *et al.*, 1999), bezafibrate (BIP Study Group, 2000), pravastatin (Arntz *et al.*, 2000), fluvastatin (Liem *et al.*, 2000), atorvastatin (Schwartz *et al.*, 2001) and simvastatin (Heart Protection Study, 2002, 2004) on initial and recurrent stroke has been studied in at least seven RCTs (Corvol *et al.*, 2003).

A subsequent systematic review and meta-analysis of 58 RCTs of cholesterol-lowering by any means indicated that lowering the concentration of LDL-cholesterol by 1.0 mmol/l decreased the risk of all stroke by 10% and lowering cholesterol by 1.8 mmol/l decreased the risk of stroke by 17% (95% CI: 9–25%) and the risk of coronary events by 61% (95% CI: 51–71%) (Law *et al.*, 2003).

Degree of plasma total cholesterol lowering (%) and stroke prevention

Regression analysis indicates that the degree of cholesterol lowering is related to the reduction in odds of stroke, and that cholesterol reductions of at least 14% are required to realise a reduction in total stroke incidence that is detectable as statistically significant (Di Mascio *et al.*, 2000).

Plasma total cholesterol (<10% reduction)

Among the eight trials of cholesterol-lowering interventions in 26,000 individuals (11,692 in intervention group, 14,927 in control group) in which total cholesterol was reduced by 8.8% (standard deviation (SD): 1.1), the odds of stroke was decreased by 4% (95% CI: −15 to +28%), from 1.77% (264/14,927) with control to 1.39% (163/11,692) with intervention (Di Mascio *et al.*, 2000).

Plasma total cholesterol (10–20% reduction)

Among the 13 trials of cholesterol-lowering interventions in 25,000 individuals (12,666 in intervention group and 12,621 in control group) in which total cholesterol was reduced by 15.2% (SD: 3.2), the odds of stroke was decreased by 23% (95% CI: 10–34%), from 3.0% (377/12,621) with control to 2.31% (293/12,666) with intervention (Di Mascio *et al.*, 2000).

Plasma total cholesterol (>20% reduction)

Among the 12 trials of cholesterol-lowering interventions in 16,000 individuals (10,901 in intervention group and 5975 in control group) in which total cholesterol was reduced by 23.9% (SD: 3.5), the odds of stroke was decreased by 25% (95% CI: 4–41%), from 3.0% (143/5975) with control to 2.31% (114/10,901) with intervention (Di Mascio *et al.*, 2000).

Type of cholesterol-lowering intervention and stroke prevention

The type of cholesterol-lowering intervention determines the degree of cholesterol reduction. Non-pharmacological (e.g. diets) and non-statin lipid-lowering interventions are less effective in reducing plasma cholesterol concentrations compared with statin drugs (3-hydroxy-3-methylglutaryl coenzyme A (HMG-CoA) reductase inhibitors). The mean reduction in cholesterol concentrations among trials of non statin interventions were half as great when compared to trials of statin drugs (Di Mascio *et al.*, 2000). Indeed, a significant decrease in stroke incidence has only been observed in trials of statin drugs.

Non-pharmacological interventions to lower plasma lipid concentrations

Among the five trials of non-pharmacological interventions to lower plasma lipid concentrations (diet, ileal bypass, LDL apheresis) in 2198 patients (1102 in intervention group and 1096 in control group), total cholesterol was reduced by 14.5% (SD: 3.7) and the odds of stroke was reduced by 28% (95% CI: −17% to +56%), from 3.6% (40/1096) in the control group to 2.6% (29/1102) in the intervention group; *P* for heterogeneity 0.7 (Di Mascio *et al.*, 2000).

Non-statin lipid-lowering drugs

Among the 12 trials of non-statin lipid-lowering drugs (clofibrate, niacin, colestipol, cholestyramine, gemfibrozil, probucol) in 27,519 patients (12,143 in intervention group, 15,376 in control group) published before 1998, total cholesterol was reduced by 12.6% (SD: 5.9) and stroke was decreased by 21%, from 1.76% (270/15,376) with control to 1.39% (169/12,143) with intervention (Di Mascio *et al.*, 2000).

Since 1998, the Veterans Affairs High-Density Lipoprotein Cholesterol Intervention Trial (VAHIT) showed that, compared with placebo, men with ischaemic heart disease (IHD) allocated to gemfibrozil 1200 mg for 5 years experienced no change in LDL-cholesterol levels (2.87 mmol/l), an increase in HDL levels by 6% (0.82–0.85 mmol/l), a reduction in triglyceride levels by 31% (1.81–1.25 mmol/l), and a reduction of stroke (as designated by the investigators) from 6.9% (88/1267) to 5.1% (64/1264); relative risk reduction (RRR): 27% (95% CI: 1–47%, $P = 0.04$) (Rubins et al., 1999). However, the rate of stroke (a secondary outcome event in this trial), as confirmed by the blinded adjudication committee of three neurologists, was not significantly different: 6% (76/1267) among patients allocated placebo vs 4.6% (58/1264) among patients allocated gemfibrozil; RRR: 24% (95% CI: -7% to $+45$%, $P = 0.1$). Furthermore, the BIP trial revealed that patients with known coronary heart disease (CHD) allocated to bezafibrate, compared to placebo, had a reduction in LDL-cholesterol levels by 6.5% (3.82 to 3.6 mmol/l) and TG levels by 21% (1.63 to 1.29 mmol/l), and an increase in HDL levels by 18% (0.89 to 1.03 mmol/l), but no significant difference in the rate of all stroke (placebo: 5.0%(77/1542), bezafibrate: 4.6% (72/1548); RRR: 7% (95% CI: -27% to $+32$%, $P = 0.66$)), or ischaemic stroke (placebo: 4.5% (69/1542), bezafibrate: 3.8% (59/1548); RRR: 15% (95% CI: -20% to $+39$%, $P = 0.36$)) (BIP Study Group, 2000).

Statin drugs

Until 1998, there had been 16 trials of HMG-CoA reductase inhibitors (statin drugs) in 39,000 non-elderly patients (22,014 in intervention group, 17,051 in control group). Among patients allocated to a statin, total cholesterol was reduced by 21.7% (SD: 4.3) and the odds of stroke was reduced by 23% (95% CI: 13–33%), from 2.78% (474/170510) with control to 1.69% (372/22,014) with a statin (Di Mascio et al., 2000). A reduction in the risk of stroke was apparent only among patients with a history of CHD who were allocated a statin, and most of the benefit was due to a reduction of non-fatal stroke; the effect on fatal stroke was unclear.

Since 1998, two small (Arntz et al., 2000) and three large (AFCAPS/TexCAPS Research Group, 1998; Schwartz et al., 2001; Heart Protection Study, 2002, 2004) controlled trials of statins have been published. In addition, there have been trials directly comparing different statins, such as the Pravastatin or Atorvastatin Evaluation and Infection Therapy (PROVE-IT) trial, in acute coronary syndrome (Cannon et al., 2004).

The AFCAPS/TexCAPS trial showed that asymptomatic individuals allocated to lovastatin 20–40 mg/day, compared to placebo, had a reduction in LDL-cholesterol by 25%, an increase in HDL-cholesterol by 6% and a significant reduction in the rate of stroke from 1.36% (45/3301) in the control group to 0.82% (27/3304) in the lovastatin group (odds reduction: 40%, 95% CI: 4–63% reduction) (AFCAPS/ TexCAPS Research Group, 1998).

The Myocardial Ischemia Reduction with Aggressive Cholesterol Lowering (MIRACL) study showed that allocation to atorvastatin 80 mg/day, compared to placebo, within 24–96 h of an acute coronary syndrome, and continued for 16 weeks, was associated with a reduction in total plasma cholesterol by 27% and in LDL-cholesterol by 40%, and a marginally significant reduction in all stroke from 1.6% (24/1548) in the placebo group to 0.8% (12/1538) in the atorvastatin group (RRR: 50%, 95% CI: 1–74%) (Schwartz *et al.*, 2001).

The Medical Research Council (MRC)/British Heart Foundation (BHF) Heart Protection Study (HPS) was a randomised, placebo-controlled trial of simvastatin 40 mg daily in 20,536 UK adults, aged 40–80 years, with a history of symptomatic occlusive vascular disease of the heart, brain or limbs, or diabetes mellitus, and a plasma total cholesterol >3.5 mmol/l (>135 mg/dl) (Heart Protection Study Collaborative Group, 2002). During the 5-year treatment period, about one-sixth (17%) of the patients allocated placebo subsequently 'crossed-over' to statin therapy, and about one-sixth (15%) of the patients allocated simvastatin were non-compliant and discontinued statin therapy. Therefore, 'intention-to-treat' comparisons assessed the effects of only about two-thirds (85% compliance minus 17% cross-over) taking simvastatin during the scheduled 5-year treatment period. This yielded an average LDL-cholesterol concentration of 1.0 mmol/l (standard error (SE): 0.02) lower (about two-thirds of the effect of actual use of 40 mg simvastatin daily) among patients allocated simvastatin compared with placebo. In addition, mean plasma total cholesterol was reduced by 1.2 mmol/l (0.02), and HDL-Cholesterol increased by 0.03 mmol/l (0.01), with simvastatin compared with placebo.

Among all 20,536 patients, random allocation to simvastatin 40 mg/day ($n = 10,269$) was associated with a significant and consistent proportional reduction in risk of all major coronary events (RRR: 27%, 95% CI: 21–33%), stroke (25%, 95% CI: 15–34%), and revascularisation procedures (24%, 95% CI: 17–30%) (Heart Protection Study Collaborative Group, 2002). The rate of all (non-fatal and fatal) stroke was reduced from 5.7% (585/10,267) with placebo to 4.3% (444/10,269) with simvastatin (RRR: 25%, 95% CI: 15–34%), which is an absolute risk reduction (ARR) of 14 strokes prevented per 1000 patients allocated simvastatin over 5 years ($2P < 0.0001$). This was chiefly due to a definite 30% (95% CI: 19–40%) proportional reduction in ischaemic stroke (placebo: 4.0%, simvastatin: 2.8%; $P < 0.0001$). There was no adverse effect of simvastatin on haemorrhagic stroke, although the number of haemorrhagic stroke events was very small (placebo: 0.5% ($n = 53$), simvastatin: 0.5% ($n = 51$); $P = 0.8$). Allocation to simvastatin was associated with a consistent, one-quarter proportional reduction in risk of mild, moderate, severe and fatal stroke (Heart Protection Study Collaborative Group, 2002, 2004).

The HPS showed that the proportional one-quarter reduction in serious vascular events was similar, and significant in each sub-category of baseline total plasma cholesterol and LDL-cholesterol, even among patients who presented with target LDL levels below 3.0 mmol/l (116 mg/dl) and total cholesterol levels below 5.0 mmol/l (<193 mg/dl). The results were also consistent in men and women, and in patients under and over 70 years of age at the time of randomisation.

Simvastatin was well tolerated. The annual excess risk of myopathy with simvastatin was about 0.01%. Abnormalities of liver function tests (>4 × upper limits of normal) were reported in 0.42% of the simvastatin group and 0.31% of the placebo group (Heart Protection Study Collaborative Group, 2002, 2004).

The statin drugs (simvastatin 40 mg/day, lovastatin 40 mg/day and atorvastatin 10 mg/day) lower LDL-cholesterol by about 37% from all pretreatment concentrations (Law et al., 2003).

Types of patients and stroke prevention

Primary prevention trials

Among eight primary prevention trials of cholesterol-lowering interventions in nearly 35,000 patients (20,280 in intervention group, 14,286 in control group), total cholesterol was reduced by 14.7% (SD: 5.6) and the odds of stroke was reduced by 4% (95% CI: −21% to +24%) (Di Mascio et al., 2000). Subsequent to this meta-analysis, the Colloborative Atorvastatin Diabetes Study (CARDS) randomised 2838 patients with type 2 diabetes, but without high concentrations of LDL-cholesterol (i.e. ⩾4.14 mmol/l) or a history of cardiovascular disease, to atorvastatin 10 mg daily or placebo for a median of 3.9 years (Colhoun et al., 2004). Assignment to atorvastatin was associated with a significant reduction in the rate of the compositive primary outcome event (stroke, coronary event or coronary revascularisation) (placebo: 2.46 per 100 person-years at risk, atorvastatin: 1.54 per 100 person-years at risk, rate reduction: 37%, 95% CI: 17–52, $P = 0.001$). Assessed separately, atorvastatin reduced the rate of stroke by 48% (11–69%), acute coronary events by 36% (9–55%) and death by 27% (1–48%). No excess of adverse events was recorded in the atorvastatin group.

Secondary prevention trials

Until 1998, there had been 25 secondary prevention trials in 33,000 patients (14,979 in intervention group, 18,237 in control group) (Di Mascio et al., 2000). The total cholesterol was reduced by 18.1% (SD: 6.6), and the odds of stroke was reduced by 20% (95% CI: 9–29%), from 3.53% (643/18,237) in the control group to 2.86% (428/14,979) in the intervention group (Di Mascio et al., 2000).

Patients with a history of CHD
Most strokes in the above trials occurred among patients with CHD who were randomised in the Scandinavian Simvastatin Survival Study (4S) (Scandinavian Simvastatin Survival Study Group, 1994), the Cholesterol and Recurrent Events (CARE) trial (Plehn *et al.*, 1999) and Long-Term Intervention with Pravastatin in Ischaemic Disease (LIPID) trials (White *et al.*, 2000; Byington *et al.*, 2001). These trials have established the effectiveness of statins in preventing stroke amongst patients with a history of CHD.

Patients with a history of stroke
Until the publication of the results of the Heart Protection Study in 2002, uncertainty had prevailed over the relative risks (RRs) and benefits of lipid-lowering therapies in patients with a history of stroke (and symptomatic atherosclerosis in other vascular beds, and diabetes) (Heart Protection Study Collaborative Group, 2002).

A systematic review of lipid-lowering interventions for preventing stroke recurrence had shown that among 627 patients with a history of stroke or TIA who were randomised in two trials (Acheson *et al.*, 1972; The Veterans Administration Cooperative Study Group, 1973) to clofibrate ($n = 315$) or control ($n = 312$), the odds of a recurrent stroke was non-significantly increased among patients allocated to clofibrate (14.4% control, 19.0% clofibrate; odds ratio: 1.48, 95% CI: 0.94–2.30%) (Fig. 13.1) (Manktelow *et al.*, 2002).

Among 821 patients with a history of stroke or TIA (and CHD) who were randomised in the CARE and LIPID trials (Plehn *et al.*, 1999; White *et al.*, 2000) to pravastatin ($n = 436$) or placebo ($n = 385$), the odds of a recurrent stroke was reduced by 33% (95% CI: -1% to $+56$%) from 15.1% (placebo) to 10.6% (pravastatin) (Fig. 13.1) (Manktelow *et al.*, 2002). The results were similar for patients with a history of stroke only.

The HPS subsequently showed that the proportional (one-quarter) reduction in event rate attributable to simvastatin (see page 301) was consistent (and significant) in each sub-category of patient studied, including those with CHD, cerebrovascular disease, peripheral artery disease and diabetes (Heart Protection Study Collaborative Group, 2002).

Among the 3289 people in HPS with a history of symptomatic ischaemic cerebrovascular disease a mean of 4.3 (SE: 0.1) years previously, 1820 patients had a past history of stroke only and 1460 patients had a past history of CHD *and* stroke. Random assignment to simvastatin 40 mg daily for 4.8 years (mean) was associated with a 20% (95% CI: 8–29%) reduction in the RR of any stroke, myocardial infarction (MI), vascular death or revascularisation procedure (major vascular events) compared with placebo (simvastatin: 24.7% vs placebo: 29.8%; $P = 0.001$) (Heart Protection

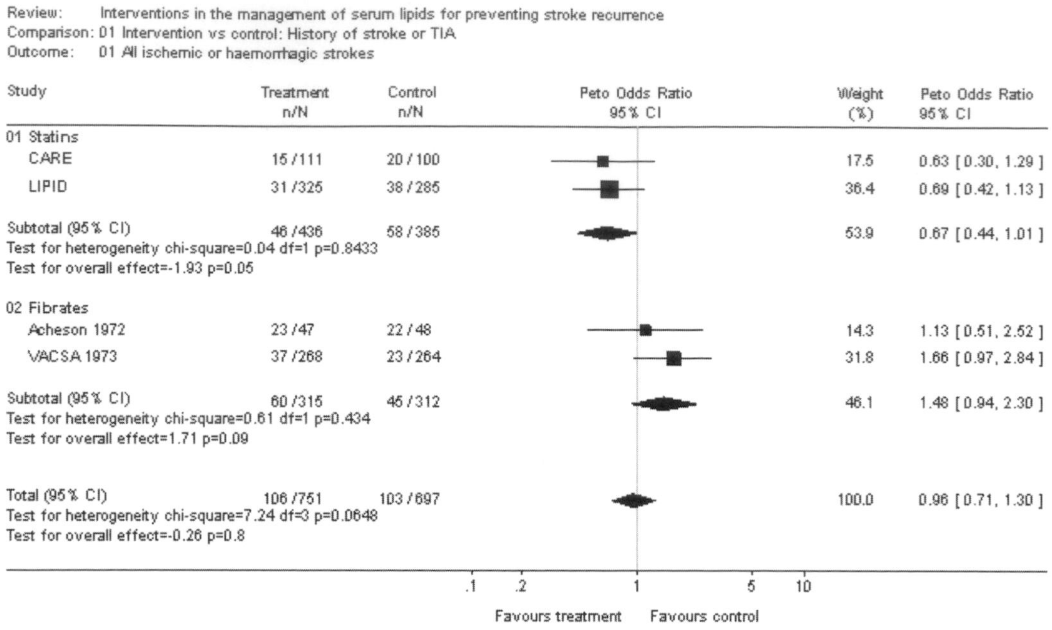

Review: Interventions in the management of serum lipids for preventing stroke recurrence
Comparison: 01 Intervention vs control: History of stroke or TIA
Outcome: 01 All ischemic or haemorrhagic strokes

Study	Treatment n/N	Control n/N	Peto Odds Ratio 95% CI	Weight (%)	Peto Odds Ratio 95% CI
01 Statins					
CARE	15 /111	20 / 100		17.5	0.63 [0.30, 1.29]
LIPID	31 /325	38 / 285		36.4	0.69 [0.42, 1.13]
Subtotal (95% CI)	46 /436	58 /385		53.9	0.67 [0.44, 1.01]
Test for heterogeneity chi-square=0.04 df=1 p=0.8433					
Test for overall effect=-1.93 p=0.05					
02 Fibrates					
Acheson 1972	23 /47	22 /48		14.3	1.13 [0.51, 2.52]
VACSA 1973	37 /268	23 /264		31.8	1.66 [0.97, 2.84]
Subtotal (95% CI)	60 /315	45 /312		46.1	1.48 [0.94, 2.30]
Test for heterogeneity chi-square=0.61 df=1 p=0.434					
Test for overall effect=1.71 p=0.09					
Total (95% CI)	106 /751	103 /697		100.0	0.96 [0.71, 1.30]
Test for heterogeneity chi-square=7.24 df=3 p=0.0648					
Test for overall effect=-0.26 p=0.8					

.1   .2   1   5   10

Favours treatment   Favours control

Figure 13.1 Forest plot showing the effect of lipid-lowering medications (statins, fibrates) compared with control for patients with a *history of stroke or TIA* on the incidence of subsequent *stroke* of any pathological type. Reproduced from Manktelow *et al.* (2002), with permission from the authors and John Wiley & Sons Limited. Copyright Cochrane Library, reproduced with permission.

Study Collaborative Group, 2004). The significant treatment effect of simvastatin emerged in the second year after randomisation and increased with time. The proportional reduction in risk (one-fifth) was consistent, irrespective of the individual's age, sex and baseline blood cholesterol when simvastatin treatment was initiated.

For the 1820 patients with previous stroke only, allocation to simvastatin was associated with a significant reduction in major vascular events from 23.6% (placebo) to 18.7% (simvastatin). This was an RRR of 21% (95% CI: 5–34%, $P < 0.001$), and ARR of 49 serious vascular events (4.9%) per 1000 stroke patients allocated simvastatin over 5 years. Among the 1460 patients with known CHD *and* a past history of stroke, allocation to simvastatin was associated with a similar reduction in any major vascular event from 37.4% (placebo) to 32.4% (simvastatin); RRR: 14% (95% CI: 0.5–25%), and ARR: 5% over 5 years.

A retrospective subgroup analysis of HPS data indicated that among patients with a history of cerebrovascular disease, simvastatin resulted in no reduction in recurrent stroke compared with placebo (simvastatin: 10.3%, placebo: 10.4%; RR: 0.98, 95% CI: 0.79–1.22), in contrast to other high-risk patients who had a highly significant reduction in stroke (simvastatin: 3.2%, placebo: 4.8%; heterogeneity $P = 0.002$).

Patients with a history of cerebrovascular disease who were assigned simvastatin experienced a 19% (SE: 12, $P = 0.1$) reduction in the RR of ischaemic stroke (simvastatin: 6.1%, placebo: 7.5%) but a near doubling in RR of haemorrhagic stroke (placebo: 0.7%, simvastatin: 1.3%). The latter contrasts with other high-risk patients who had a non-significantly lower risk of haemorrhagic stroke (heterogeneity $P = 0.03$).

Comments

Interpretation of the evidence

Population-based observational cohort studies show a variable weak (positive) relationship between increasing plasma total cholesterol concentrations and increasing risk of ischaemic stroke, which is partially offset by a weaker (negative) association between decreasing total cholesterol concentrations and increasing risk of haemorrhagic stroke.

RCTs show unequivocally that lowering plasma total cholesterol by about 1.2 mmol/l (and LDL-cholesterol by 1.0 mmol/l) decreases the risk of all stroke by about 10% overall (Law et al., 2003).

The reduction in risk of stroke with cholesterol lowering varies according to the presence or absence of a history of known vascular disease (i.e. primary vs secondary prevention studies). In people *without* known vascular disease, lowering the concentration of LDL cholesterol by 1.0 mmol/l decreased the risk of all stroke by 6% (95% CI. −14% to +22% reduction), similar to that expected from the observational cohort studies. In contrast, among people *with* known vascular disease, lowering the concentration of LDL-cholesterol by 1.0 mmol/l decreased the risk of all stroke by 22% (95% CI: 16–28%) (Law et al., 2003). And among people *with* known ischaemic stroke, lowering the concentration of LDL-cholesterol by 1.0 mmol/l decreased the risk of all stroke by 28% (95% CI: 20–35%), whereas for patients with haemorrhagic stroke, there was no significant effect (RRR: 3%, 95% CI: −47% to +35% reduction) (Law et al., 2003). The greater benefits among people with known vascular disease probably arises because ischaemic stroke due to atherothromboembolism is more common in people with known vascular disease and with known ischaemic stroke, so more of their strokes will be atherothromboembolic. Reduction in LDL-cholesterol concentration prevents atherothromboembolic ischaemic stroke but not haemorrhagic stroke (see below), accounting for the greater than expected effect of treatment in this group. This also explains the greater than expected reduction in RR of non-fatal stroke (23%, 95% CI: 16–29%) than fatal stroke (2%, 95% CI: −16% to +17%) with a reduction in LDL-cholesterol of 1.0 mmol/l, because a greater proportion of non-fatal strokes are ischaemic than fatal strokes (Law et al., 2003).

The proportional reduction in the risk of stroke and other serious vascular events for patients with a history of cerebrovascular disease (at least one-fifth, and up to one-third in compliant patients) is consistent, irrespective of the patient's age, sex, baseline plasma cholesterol concentration and absolute risk of stroke, but is increased in patients at highest risk of stroke, and with greater degrees of cholesterol lowering, and thus with statin medications, which are more potent than non-statin interventions in lowering cholesterol levels.

It remains uncertain why patients with a history of cerebrovascular disease, experience no reduction in RR of recurrent stroke with simvastatin compared with placebo (in contrast to other high-risk patients) and a near doubling in RR of haemorrhagic stroke (in contrast to other high-risk patients). These are the results of subgroup analyses which were not prespecified, and therefore they should be interpreted cautiously, and considered only hypothesis generating. However, the hypothesis that lowering cholesterol may increase the risk of haemorrhagic stroke existed before HPS (see above). Several non-randomised observational studies, and one underpowered randomised trial had reported that lower blood cholesterol concentrations might be associated with higher risks of haemorrhagic stroke (Iso *et al.*, 1989; Eastern Stroke and Coronary Heart Disease Collaborative Research Group, 1998; White *et al.*, 2000; Koren-Morag *et al.*, 2002). Current trials and a prospectively planned meta-analysis of all trials will provide further information about whether statins prevent recurrent stroke and increase the risk of haemorrhagic stroke (Cholesterol Treatment Trialists' Collaboration, 1995; The SPARCL investigators, 2003; Amarenco and Tonkin, 2004).

Implications for clinicians

These results suggest that adding a statin to existing stroke prevention treatments for stroke patients, is safe and effective in reducing the risk of serious vascular events, by at least one-quarter and, if compliance is maintained, by about one-third. The magnitude of the benefit depends on the individuals overall absolute risk of major vascular events, rather than their age, gender or plasma cholesterol concentration. If the baseline risk of a serious vascular event is about 5% per year, intention-to-treat with statin should reduce this risk to <4% per year; that is, treating 1000 such high-risk patients for 5 years should prevent at least 50 major vascular events and, if compliance is maintained and treatment continued over an even longer term, at least 100 major vascular events.

However, the results cannot necessarily be generalised to patients with acute ischaemic syndromes of the brain when the risk of recurrent stroke and haemorrhagic transformation of the cerebral infarct is higher (compared with 4.3 years (mean) after stroke when patients were randomised in HPS). Statins may be even more effective in preventing recurrent ischaemic events, but also more hazardous in causing or exacerbating haemorrhagic stroke, in the acute phase.

Whilst awaiting the results of ongoing trials, uncertainty about the safety and efficacy of statins in acute ischaemic stroke, and their long-term effects on recurrent stroke and haemorrhagic stroke, should not discourage widespread long-term use of statins in patients with atherothrombotic ischaemic stroke. Even if statins are associated with an excess of haemorrhagic strokes in patients with a history of previous ischaemic stroke and no reduction in stroke recurrence, the small absolute increase (about 2–6 haemorrhagic strokes per 1000 patients treated for 5 years) would be substantially offset by the large absolute reduction in major vascular events (about 51 per 1000 patients treated for 5 years). A similar situation exists with antiplatelet therapy for secondary stroke prevention.

Implications for research

The precision of the estimates of effectiveness and safety of statins in preventing recurrent stroke, amongst stroke patients, should be clarified further by the forthcoming results of the Stroke Prevention by Aggressive Reduction in Cholesterol Levels (SPARCL) trial, which compares atorvasatin 80 mg daily with placebo in 4300 adult men and women with recent (1–6 months prior to randomisation) non-disabling stroke or TIA, and LDL-cholesterol concentrations ≥2.6 mmol (100 mg/dl) and <4.9 mmol/l (190 mg/dl), but without a history of CHD (www.neuro.wustl.edu/stroke/trials) (The SPARCL investigators, 2003). The primary outcome measure is the time from randomisation to the first occurrence of any (fatal or non-fatal) stroke. Recruitment was completed in early 2001, and the 5-year follow-up continues

The Cholesterol Treatment Trialists' Collaboration is carrying out a meta-analysis of all randomised trials of cholesterol reduction that were of more than 2 years duration and included >1000 people, and the first cycle of the analyses, when combined with the BHF/MRC-HPS, will include data from 57,000 patients and 2200 strokes (Cholesterol Treatment Trialists' Collaboration, 1995).

SUMMARY

Although higher plasma cholesterol concentrations do not seem to be associated with increased risk of stroke risk, lowering the concentration decreases the risk.

The risk of stroke, and other serious vascular events, is reduced by about a quarter for a reduction of a fifth in cholesterol concentration.

This decrease can be achieved with statins, which are well-tolerated provided they are not given to patients with active liver or muscle disease.

The dose should be equivalent to 40 mg daily of simvastatin.

The RRRs are consistent irrespective of the baseline cholesterol concentration (above 3.5 mmol/l).

Modification of other vascular risk factors and lifestyle

Diabetes mellitus and glucose intolerance

Evidence

Risk factors for stroke

Diabetes mellitus and glucose intolerance are important risk factors for ischaemic stroke (Tuomilehto and Rastenye, 1999). Above a fasting blood glucose concentration of 4.9 mmol/l, there is a continuous association between fasting blood glucose levels and vascular disease; for every 1 mmol/l increase in fasting blood glucose there is a 21% (95% CI: 18–24%) increase in risk of stroke, 23% (95% CI: 19–27%) increase in risk of ischaemic heart disease events and 19% increase in cardiovascular deaths (Asia Pacific Cohort Studies Collaboration, 2004).

Effective strategies to reduce the risk of stroke in diabetics

Effective strategies to reduce the risk of stroke in diabetics include:

1 Preventing or delaying the onset of diabetes by appropriate lifestyle behaviours (to achieve target levels of risk factors) and perhaps use of the α-glucosidase inhibitor acarbose to improve insulin sensitivity (Chiasson *et al.*, 2002, 2003).

2 Preventing atherogenesis by optimally controlling risk factors such as high blood pressure (Heart Outcomes Prevention Evaluation (HOPE) Study Investigators, 2000a,c), high blood cholesterol (Heart Protection Study Collaborative Group, 2003; Colhoun *et al.*, 2004), high blood glucose (UK Prospective Diabetes Study (UKPDS) Group, 1998a,b) and smoking.

3 Preventing atherothrombosis, should an atherosclerotic plaque become eroded or rupture, with optimal antiplatelet therapy (Antithrombotic Trialists' Collaboration, 2002; Sacco *et al.*, 2003).

4 Recanalising any accessible arteries which are stenosed and symptomatic by means of carotid endarterectomy (Rothwell *et al.*, 2003).

Blood glucose control

Randomised trials have shown that more intensive treatment of hyperglycaemia results in fewer microvascular complications of diabetes (retinopathy and renal damage) and decreased progression of carotid artery intima–media thickness, but not necessarily fewer macrovascular complications (i.e. stroke and myocardial infarction (MI)) (UKPDS Group, 1998a,b; The Diabetes Control and Complications Trial/ Epidemiology of Diabetes Interventions and Complications Research Group, 2003).

Vascular risk factor control

There is no doubt from randomised-controlled trials (RCTs) that lowering blood pressure (by means of an angiotensin converting enzyme inhibitor) (HOPE Study Investigators, 2000) and blood cholesterol (by means of a statin drug) (Heart Protection Study Collaborative Group, 2003; Colhoun *et al.*, 2004) are effective in reducing the risk of stroke and other serious vascular events in diabetics by about one-quarter.

A small RCT of a long-term, intensive stepwise intervention targeted to multiple vascular risk factors (hyperglycaemia, hypertension, dyslipidaemia and microalbuminuria), together with aspirin, in 160 patients with type 2 diabetes showed that the 80 patients assigned intensive therapy had a significantly lower risk of cardiovascular disease (hazard ratio (HR): 0.47, 95% confidence interval (CI): 0.24–0.73) and microvascular events (Gaede *et al.*, 2003; Solomon, 2003).

Comment

Early detection of diabetes and glucose intolerance, followed by careful control of glycaemia and vascular risk factors to target levels (Table 14.1) are very likely to improve long-term outcome (Solomon, 2003). Rigorous control of blood pressure and blood cholesterol is likely to be at least, if not more, important than rigorous control of blood glucose in preventing serious vascular events.

Table 14.1. Target levels of risk factors in patients with diabetes.

- Blood pressure <130/80 mmHg
- Low-density lipoprotein cholesterol <2.6 mmol/l (100 mg/dl)
- Triglycerides <1.7 mmol/l (150 mg/dl)
- High-density lipoprotein cholesterol >1.1 mmol/l (40 mg/dl)[*]
- Glycosylated haemoglobin <7%

Source: Solomon, 2003.
To achieve targets, lifestyle interventions (diet and exercise) are recommended first, followed by pharmacological interventions, if necessary.
Recommendations from the American Diabetes Association (2003).
[*] In women, a level above 1.3 mmol/l (50 mg/dl) may be appropriate.

Hormone replacement therapy

Evidence

The Women's Health Initiative (WHI) was a RCT involving 16,608 women aged 50–79 years who were randomised to placebo ($n = 8102$) or 0.625 mg/day of conjugated equine oestrogen plus 2.5 mg/day of medroxyprogesterone acetate ($n = 8506$) and followed up for 5.6 years (Wassertheil-Smoller *et al.*, 2003). Stroke occurred in 151 (1.8% or 0.31%/year) patients assigned oestrogen plus progestin and 107 patients (1.3% or 0.24%/year) assigned placebo (HR: 1.31, 95% CI: 1.02–1.68). With adjustment for adherence, the HR was 1.50 (95% CI: 1.08–2.08). The absolute increase in risk was 0.5% over 5.6 years, indicating that treating 1000 patients with hormone replacement therapy (HRT) for 5.6 years may cause five strokes (Table 14.2). The number of patients who need to be treated with HRT to cause one stroke over 5.6 years (NNH, number needed to harm) is 220 (95% CI: 120–1265). For annualised event rates, HRT is associated with an absolute increase in risk of stroke of 0.07%/year, indicating that treating 10,000 patients with HRT for 1 year may cause seven strokes (NNH/year: 1429). Ischaemic stroke, which made up 79.8% of the strokes, occurred in 1.5% of patients assigned oestrogen plus progestin (0.26%/year) and 1.0% assigned placebo (0.18%/year) (HR: 1.44, 95% CI: 1.09–1.90; NNH: 213, 95% CI: 124–743). Haemorrhagic stroke occurred in 0.04% of patients assigned oestrogen plus progestin per year and 0.04% of patients assigned placebo per year (HR: 0.82, 95% CI: 0.43–1.56) (Wassertheil-Smoller *et al.*, 2003).

The results of the WHI (HR for stroke: 1.31, 95% CI: 1.02–1.68) are consistent with the 12% increase in the relative risk (RR) of stroke associated with HRT in a

Table 14.2. Absolute differences in the rates of stroke and other major disease outcomes among post-menopausal women receiving oestrogen/progestin therapy as compared with those receiving placebo.

Outcome	Number of events per 1000 women treated	
	First 2 years	5.6-year period
Stroke	1 more	5 more
Coronary events	3 more	4 more
Venous thromboembolism	6 more	9 more
Invasive breast cancer	No more (indeed fewer)	4 more
Hip fracture	1 fewer	2 fewer
Colorectal cancer	No difference	3 fewer
Death	No difference	No difference

preceding meta-analysis (Nelson *et al.*, 2002) and with known prothrombotic effects of HRT. Although the Heart and Estrogen/progestin Replacement Study (HERS) found the same regimen produced only a non-significant 9% increase stroke and transient ischaemic attacks (TIAs), 80% of patients were taking aspirin, and the CIs are consistent with those of the meta-analysis and WHI study (Grady *et al.*, 2002).

A systematic review of 28 RCTs assessing the effect of HRT on subsequent risk of stroke in a total of 39,769 subjects showed that random assignment to HRT was associated with a significant increase in total stroke (OR: 1.29, 95% CI: 1.13–1.47), non-fatal stroke (OR: 1.23, 1.06–1.44), stroke leading to death or disability (OR: 1.56, 1.11–2.20), and ischaemic stroke (OR: 1.29, 1.06–1.56). It was not associated with haemorrhagic stroke (OR: 1.07, 95% CI: 0.65–1.75) (Bath and Gray, 2005).

Comment

There is reasonably strong evidence from RCTs that in generally healthy post-menopausal women, with or without a history of vascular disease, hormone replacement therapy increases the risk of ischaemic stroke and of venous thromboembolism and may increase the risk of MI (Beral *et al.*, 2002).

Therefore, for women without menopausal symptoms, the harms of oestrogen plus progestin are likely to exceed the benefits, but the risks are small in absolute terms and with short duration therapy. HRT remains a suitable option for women with bothersome menopausal symptoms, but they should understand that there are some risks involved and should regularly re-assess their need for treatment with their clinician (Crawford and Langhorne, 2005). It is prudent to use the lowest effective dose for the shortest period.

Oral contraceptive use

Evidence

There have been no RCTs of oral contraceptive pill (OCP) use vs no OCP use on the risk of stroke. This is mainly because it would be unethical to randomly assign active oral contraceptive treatment or placebo to women. However there is a large body of evidence from observational studies, but these are prone to bias and confounding, as highlighted in Chapter 2 and above.

All stroke

A recent meta-analysis of cohort studies reported that oral contraceptives was not associated with an increased risk of all (ischaemic and haemorrhagic) stroke (odds ratio (OR): 0.95, 95% CI: 0.51–1.78) (Chan *et al.*, 2004).

Haemorrhagic stroke

Oral contraceptive use was not associated with an increased risk of haemorrhagic stroke (WHO Collaborative Study of Cardiovascular Disease and Steroid Hormone Contraception, 1996).

Ischaemic stroke

When the meta-analysis was restricted to the risk of *ischaemic* stroke, use of the low-dose oral contraceptive was associated with a 174% increased risk of ischaemic stroke (RR: 2.74).

These findings are consistent with those of an earlier systematic review of studies exploring the association between ischaemic stroke and use of the oral contraceptive in 16 population-based, cohort studies (Gillum *et al.*, 2000). The latter meta-analysis reported that (a) the risk of ischaemic stroke associated with current oral contraceptive use was increased (RR: 2.75, 95% CI: 2.24–3.38); (b) smaller oestrogen doses were associated with a lower risk of ischaemic stroke ($P = 0.01$ for trend), but risk was significantly elevated for all dosages and (c) for women taking low-dose oral contraceptives, the risk of ischaemic stroke was nearly doubled (RR: 1.93, 95% CI: 1.35–2.74) after controlling for smoking and hypertension. The upper 95% CI of this 93% relative increase includes the 174% increase reported by Chan *et al.* (2004).

In absolute terms, the 93% relative excess translated into an additional 4.1 ischaemic strokes per 100,000 non-smoking, normotensive women using low-oestrogen oral contraceptives or one additional ischaemic stroke per year per 24,000 such women (Gillum *et al.*, 2000; Chan *et al.*, 2004).

Comment

The available evidence suggests that the oral contraceptive is a risk factor for ischaemic stroke but not haemorrhagic stroke. The risk of ischaemic stroke is related to the dose of oestrogen in oral contraceptives. The relative increase in risk of ischaemic stroke among users of the low-dose oral contraceptive is about 2-fold. There is some imprecision in this estimate because older studies assessed higher doses of oestrogen, and in the past, women who took the OCP were more likely to smoke and drink alcohol. More recently, the OCP has been prescribed mostly for women who are less likely to smoke or to have other risk factors for stroke. Older and more recent studies, which failed to control for these factors, could have overestimated and underestimated the effect of OCP use on stroke risk, respectively. Irrespective, the absolute risk of ischaemic stroke associated with OCP is very small, particularly when the risks of pregnancy and termination (abortion), which are more common with routine use of other forms of contraception, are considered.

Furthermore, the increase in risk of ischaemic stroke associated with use of the OCP (RR: 1.93, 95% CI: 1.35–2.74) is consistent with the 44% increase in risk of ischaemic stroke associated with the combination of oestrogen and progestin reported in post menopausal women (see HRT above) (Wassertheil-Smoller *et al.*, 2003). These findings imply that combined oestrogen/progestin therapy increases the risk of ischaemic stroke regardless of whether women are pre- or post-menopausal. However, because the absolute risk of stroke is much greater in older (post-menopausal) women, and in those with a previous stroke or other vascular risk factors (e.g. hypertension, smoking), differences in prescribing oestrogen-containing compounds to pre- and post-menopausal women are likely to be justified (Seibert *et al.*, 2003).

Cigarette smoking

Evidence

Risk factor for stroke

Observational studies suggest that cigarette smoking (and passive smoking (Bonita *et al.*, 1999; Davey Smith, 2003; Whincup *et al.*, 2004)) is a causal risk factor for ischaemic stroke and subarachnoid haemorrhage because the association is independent of other risk factors, consistent among different studies, dose-related, strong and biologically plausible (Shinton and Beevers, 1989; Donnan *et al.*, 1993; Jamrozik *et al.*, 1994; Hankey, 1999). The effect of smoking on the risk of primary intracerebral haemorrhage is less clear but also probably adverse (Vessey *et al.*, 2003).

Quitting smoking

There have been no satisfactory RCTs where people have been randomised to 'continue smoking' or 'stop smoking', and observed for the risk of first-ever or recurrent stroke. And there probably never will be, as it would now be considered unethical given the strength of the observational evidence of the adverse health effects of smoking. Evidence from observational studies however, suggests that quitting smoking is associated with a decreased risk of stroke (Kawachi *et al.*, 1993).

Physician advice to quit smoking

A systematic review identified 29 randomised trials of smoking cessation advice from a medical practitioner, in which abstinence was assessed at least 6 months after advice was first provided, in over 31,000 smokers (Lancaster and Stead, 2004). In some trials, subjects were at risk of specified diseases (chest disease, diabetes, ischaemic heart disease), but most were from unselected populations. The most common setting for delivery of advice was primary care.

A meta-analysis of pooled data from 17 trials of brief advice vs no advice (or usual care) revealed a small but significant increase in the odds of quitting

(OR: 1.74, 95% CI: 1.48–2.05). This equates to an absolute difference in the cessation rate of about 2.5%. There was insufficient evidence, from indirect comparisons, to establish a significant difference in the effectiveness of physician advice according to the intensity of the intervention, the amount of follow-up provided, and whether or not various aids were used at the time of the consultation in addition to providing advice. Direct comparison of intensive vs minimal advice showed a small advantage of intensive advice (OR: 1.44, 95% CI: 1.24–1.67) and a small benefit of follow-up visits.

Only one study determined the effect of smoking advice on mortality and reported no statistically significant differences in death rates at 20-year follow-up.

Nicotine replacement therapy

Compared with control

A systematic review identified 103 randomised trials in which nicotine replacement therapy (NRT) was compared to placebo or to no treatment, and 20 which compared different doses of NRT (Silagy *et al.*, 2004). The odds of achieving abstinence from smoking was significantly increased with NRT compared to control (OR: 1.77, 95% CI: 1.66–1.88). The ORs for the different forms of NRT were 1.66 (95% CI: 1.52–1.81) for gum, 1.81 (95% CI: 1.63–2.02) for patches, 2.35 (95% CI: 1.63–3.38) for nasal spray, 2.14 (95% CI: 1.44–3.18) for inhaled nicotine and 2.05 (95% CI: 1.62–2.59) for nicotine sublingual tablet/lozenge. These odds ratios were largely independent of the duration of therapy, the intensity of additional support provided, or the setting in which the NRT was offered. In highly dependent smokers there was a significant benefit of 4 mg gum compared with 2 mg gum (OR: 2.20, 95% CI: 1.85–3.25). There was weak evidence that combinations of forms of NRT were more effective. Higher doses of nicotine patch may produce small increases in quit rates.

Compared with other pharmacotherapies

Only one study directly compared NRT to another pharmacotherapy. Quit rates with bupropion were higher than with nicotine patch or placebo (Silagey *et al.*, 2004).

Comment

All stroke patients who use tobacco in any form (cigarettes, pipe, cigars or chewing tobacco) should be advised to stop; the risks of stroke are likely to decline within 2–5 years of stopping (Kawachi *et al.*, 1993; Peto 1994; Foster *et al.*, 2004).

Simple advice from a clinician is modestly effective (and cost-effective) in facilitating smoking cessation (Lancaster and Stead, 2004).

All forms of NRT (nicotine gum, transdermal patch, nasal spray, inhaler and sublingual tablets) and bupropion are safe and effective for increasing smoking cessation rates in the short and long terms (Peters and Morgan, 2002; Silagy et al., 2004). They increase quit rates by about 1.5–2-fold. For patients who are particularly nicotine dependent, the 4 mg gum is significantly more effective than the lower dose. In less highly dependent smokers, the different preparations are comparable in their efficacy, but nicotine patches offer greater convenience and minimal need for instruction (Foster et al., 2004). Nicotine patches appear safe in people with coronary artery disease. Inhalers and nasal sprays are useful in patients with particularly severe nicotine craving. There are some specific contraindications to the use of bupropion, such as patients with a history of epilepsy. Conditions that might increase the risk of seizures, such as cortical stroke, are a relative contraindication. Other adverse reactions include hypersensitivity reactions such as facial oedema and serum-sickness-like illness.

The effectiveness of drug treatments is increased when associated with effective counselling or behavioural treatments (Peters and Morgan, 2002; Foster et al., 2004). Smoking cessation programmes delivered individually and regularly for several months via nurses can also be effective among smoker admitted to hospital with vascular disease (Quist-Paulsen and Gallefoss, 2003).

Encouraging stroke patients, and smoking partners of patients, to quit smoking may reduce the patient's exposure to environmental tobacco smoke and reduce the risk of stroke and other serious vascular events.

Alcohol

Evidence

Risk factor for stroke

A systematic review of 35 observational studies (cohort or case–control), in which stroke was recorded as an end point, indicated that heavy alcohol consumption (>60 g/day, equivalent to >5 standard drinks/day) increases the RR of all stroke (RR: 1.64, 95% CI: 1.4–1.9), ischaemic stroke (RR: 1.69, 95% CI: 1.3–2.1) and haemorrhagic stroke (RR: 2.18, 95% CI: 1.5–3.2), compared with abstainers (Reynolds et al., 2003).

In contrast, light or moderate alcohol consumption was associated with a lower risk of total and ischaemic stroke. Light consumption of alcohol <12 g/day (<1 standard drink/day) was associated with a lower risk of all stroke (RR: 0.83, 95% CI: 0.75–0.91) and ischaemic stroke (RR: 0.80, 95% CI: 0.67–0.96) compared with abstainers. Moderate consumption of alcohol of 12–24 g/day (1–2 standard drinks/day) was also associated with a lower risk of ischaemic stroke (RR: 0.72, 95% CI: 0.57–0.91) compared with abstainers (Reynolds et al., 2003).

The meta-regression analysis revealed a significant non-linear, U-shaped association between alcohol consumption and total-and-ischaemic stroke, and a linear relationship between alcohol consumption and haemorrhagic stroke (Reynolds *et al.*, 2003).

One mechanism by which high levels of alcohol consumption may increase the risk of stroke is that they are associated with high blood pressure (Hillbom *et al.*, 1999; Hommel and Jaillard, 1999).

Comment

Reducing heavy alcohol intake is advisable because it is likely to reduce blood pressure. Whether this will reduce the risk of stroke is not known, but the results of observational studies and RCTs suggest that a reduction of 2 mmHg in diastolic blood pressure is likely to decrease the risk of stroke by 15% and coronary heart disease by 6% (MacMahon *et al.*, 1990; Collins and MacMahon, 1994; MacMahon and Rodgers, 1994a,b; Cook *et al.*, 1995).

Exercise

Evidence

Risk factor for stroke

A systematic review of 23 studies (18 cohort and 5 case–control) found that moderate and high levels of physical activity are associated with a reduced risk of all stroke, ischaemic and haemorrhagic stroke compared with low-active individuals (Lee *et al.*, 2003).

Compared with low-active individuals, *highly* active individuals had a reduction in risk of all stroke (RR: 0.73, 95% CI: 0.67–0.79), ischaemic stroke (RR: 0.79, 95% CI: 0.69–0.91) and haemorrhagic stroke (RR: 0.66, 95% CI: 0.48–0.91) (Lee *et al.*, 2003).

Compared with low-active individuals, *moderately* active individuals had a statistically significant reduction in risk of all stroke (RR: 0.80, 95% CI: 0.74–0.86), and a non-significant reduction in ischaemic stroke (RR: 0.91, 95% CI: 0.80–1.05) and haemorrhagic stroke (RR: 0.85, 95% CI: 0.64–1.13) (Lee *et al.*, 2003).

The mechanisms by which physical activity might reduce stroke risk is by lowering body weight, blood pressure, blood viscosity, fibrinogen concentrations and platelet aggregability; enhancing fibrinolysis; and improving lipid profiles and endothelial function (Lee *et al.*, 2003).

However, the effects of physical activity and exercise programmes after stroke on the occurrence of further vascular events are unknown. They have not been evaluated by means of RCTs other than for functional recovery after stroke (Saunders *et al.*, 2004).

Comment

After a stroke, patients should probably be encouraged to return to normal physical activities, but the levels of physical activity likely to reduce the risk of further vascular events may not be achievable. However, exercise may bring other benefits (e.g. in the elderly, structured exercise programmes may reduce the risk of falls).

Weight reduction

Evidence

Risk factor for stroke

A prospective observational cohort study of 21,414 United States male physicians followed prospectively for 12.5 years recorded 747 incident cases of stroke (631 ischaemic strokes, 104 haemorrhagic strokes and 12 strokes of unknown type) (Kurth *et al.*, 2002). Compared with participants who had a body mass index (BMI) <23, those with a BMI of ⩾30 had an increased adjusted risk of all stroke (RR: 2.0, 95% CI: 1.5–2.7), ischaemic stroke (RR: 2.0, 95% CI: 1.4–2.7) and haemorrhagic stroke (RR: 2.2, 95% CI: 1.01–5.0) (Kurth *et al.*, 2002).

When BMI was evaluated as a continuous variable, each unit increase in BMI was associated with a significant increase in the adjusted risk of all stroke (RR: 6%, 95% CI: 4–8%), ischaemic stroke (RR: 6%, 95% CI: 3–8%) and haemorrhagic stroke (RR: 6%, 95% CI: 1–12%) (Kurth *et al.*, 2002).

Weight reduction effectively reduces blood pressure in hypertensive older people (Whelton *et al.*, 1998).

Comment

These data suggest that increasing BMI is a risk factor for stroke, independent of hypertension, cholesterol and diabetes.

The mechanism by which BMI increases the risk of stroke independent of hypertension and diabetes is uncertain, but may relate to an increase in prothrombotic factors (Kurth *et al.*, 2002).

Although it has not been shown in RCTs that lowering BMI prevents stroke, it would seem sensible to adopt a reduction of BMI in overweight individuals as another strategy to reduce the risk of stroke and other serious vascular events.

Dietary fat

Evidence

Risk factor for stroke

A population-based case–control study of 536 patients with stroke and 931 control subjects showed that consumption of meat more than four times weekly, compared with less, was associated independently and significantly with an increased odds of all stroke (OR: 2.17, 95% CI: 1.33–3.53); and use of reduced fat or skim milk, compared with full-strength milk, was associated with a reduced odds of all stroke (OR: 0.49, 95% CI: 0.31–0.76) (Jamrozik *et al.*, 1994). Use of reduced fat or skim milk was also associated with a significant reduction in odds of ischaemic stroke (OR: 0.43, 95% CI: 0.26–0.72).

A prospective observational cohort study of 43,732 United States male health professionals aged 40–75 years followed prospectively for 14 years recorded 725 incident cases of stroke (455 ischaemic strokes, 125 haemorrhagic strokes and 145 strokes of unknown type) (He *et al.*, 2003).

Compared with participants who had the lowest quintile of fat intake, those with the highest quintile of total fat intake had no increase in risk of ischaemic stroke (adjusted RR: 0.91, 95% CI: 0.65–1.28, $P = 0.77$ for trend) (He *et al.*, 2003). There was also a non-significant increase in risk of ischaemic stroke among individuals with the highest quintiles of intakes of animal fat (adjusted RR: 1.20, 95% CI: 0.84–1.70, $P = 0.47$ for trend), saturated fat (adjusted RR: 1.16, 95% CI: 0.81–1.65, $P = 0.59$ for trend), vegetable fat (adjusted RR: 1.07, 95% CI: 0.77–1.47, $P = 0.66$ for trend), and dietary cholesterol (adjusted RR: 1.02, 95% CI: 0.75–1.39, $P = 0.99$ for trend), and decrease in risk with higher quintiles of intake of monosaturated fat (adjusted RR: 0.88, 95% CI: 0.64–1.21, $P = 0.25$ for trend) or transunsaturated fat (adjusted RR: 0.87, 95% CI: 0.62–1.22, $P = 0.42$ for trend) compared with the lowest quintile of fat intake.

Comment

These data suggest that dietary fat intake is not a risk factor for stroke, but perhaps an increased intake of animal and saturated fat may be.

Dietary intake of whole grains

Evidence

Risk factor for stroke

A prospective observational cohort study of 75,521 United States nurses aged 36–83 years who completed a food frequency questionnaire in 1984, 1986, 1990 and 1994, detailing their intake of whole grain foods (whole grain breakfast cereal, brain, wheat germ, cooked oatmeal, couscous, dark bread and brown rice) were followed prospectively for 12 years (861, 900 person years) (Liu *et al.*, 2000, Fung *et al.*, 2004). There were 352 incident cases of ischaemic stroke recorded.

Compared with participants who had the lowest quintile of whole grain consumption, those with the highest quintile of whole grain intake had a significant risk of ischaemic stroke. The age-adjusted RRs from the lowest to the highest quin-tiles of whole grain intake were 1.00 (referent), 0.68 (95% CI: 0.49–0.94), 0.69 (95% CI: 0.51–0.95), 0.49 (95% CI: 0.35–0.69) and 0.57 (95% CI: 0.42–0.78, $P = 0.003$ for trend) (Liu et al., 2000, Fung et al., 2004).

Comment

These data suggest that higher intake of whole grain foods are associated with a lower risk of ischaemic stroke among women, independent of known vascular risk factors, and support the notion that a higher intake of whole grains may reduce the risk of ischaemic stroke. However, this has not been evaluated in RCTs.

Dietary fish

Evidence

Risk factor for stroke

A population-based case–control study of 536 patients with stroke and 931 control subjects showed that consumption of fish more than two times per month was associated independently with a reduced odds of first-ever stroke (OR: 0.60, 95% CI: 0.36–0.99) (Jamrozik et al., 1994), mainly because of a reduction in odds of haemorrhagic stroke (OR: 0.43, 95% CI: 0.20–0.96) rather than ischaemic stroke (OR: 0.90, 95% CI: 0.60–1.36).

A prospective observational cohort study of 43,671 United States male health professionals aged 40–75 years followed prospectively for 12 years recorded 608 incident cases of stroke (377 ischaemic strokes, 106 haemorrhagic strokes and 125 strokes of unknown type) (He et al., 2002).

Compared with men who consumed fish less than once per month, men who ate fish one to three times per month had a significantly lower risk of ischaemic stroke (adjusted RR: 0.57, 95% CI: 0.35–0.95) (He et al., 2002).

However, men who consumed fish five or more times per week did not have a further reduction in risk of stroke (RR: 0.54, 95% CI: 0.31–0.94).

By dichotomised fish intake, the risk for men who ate fish at least once per month compared with those who ate fish less than once per month as 0.56 (95% CI: 0.38–0.83) for ischaemic stroke and 1.36 (95% CI: 0.48–3.82) for haemor-rhagic stroke.

Effect of dietary supplement of *n*-3 polyunsaturated fats (a component of fish oil) of coronary events

In patients with previous MI, a dietary supplement of *n*-3 polyunsaturated fats (a component of fish oil) was associated with a reduction in death from cardiovascular causes, with no apparent effect on fatal or non-fatal stroke (GISSI-Prevenzione Investigators, 1999).

Comment

These data suggest that eating fish once per month or more may be associated with a lower risk of ischaemic stroke in men. There is also supporting evidence in women (Fung *et al.*, 2004).

The mechanisms by which fish consumption could protect against ischaemic stroke may be related to the overall favourable effects of long-chain ω-3 polyunsaturated fatty acids (PUFA), including eicosapentaenoic acid (EPA) and docosahexaenoic acid (DHA) on blood pressure, lipid profiles, platelet activity and endothelial function (He *et al.*, 2002; Kris-Etherton *et al.*, 2002).

However, the available evidence is insufficient to support the routine use of fish oil for stroke prevention.

Dietary intake of salt

Evidence

Risk of stroke

A population-based case–control study of 536 patients with stroke and 931 control subjects from the same community and matched for age and sex with the cases showed that adding salt to food was associated independently with an increased odds of all stroke (OR: 1.53, 95% CI: 1.01–2.31) (Jamrozik *et al.*, 1994), mainly because of an increase in odds of haemorrhagic stroke (OR: 3.46, 95% CI: 1.58–7.58) rather than ischaemic stroke (OR: 1.04, 95% CI: 0.72–1.51). These data suggested that about 20% (95% CI: 1–38%) of all primary intracerebral haemorrhages could be attributable to adding salt to food (presumably by increasing the risk of hypertensive intracerebral haemorrhage).

Short-term effect on blood pressure

A systematic review of randomised trials of a modest reduction in salt intake for a duration of 4 or more weeks identified 17 trials in individuals with elevated blood pressure ($n = 734$) and 11 trials in individuals with normal blood pressure ($n = 2220$) (Law *et al.*, 1991a,b; Midgley *et al.*, 1996; Cutler *et al.*, 1997; Graudal *et al.*, 1998; Alam and Johnson, 1999; He and Macgregor, 2004).

In individuals with *elevated* blood pressure the median reduction in 24-h urinary sodium excretion was 78 mmol (4.6 g/day of salt), the mean change (reduction) in systolic blood pressure was −4.97 (95% CI: −5.76 to −4.18) mmHg and the mean change (reduction) in diastolic blood pressure was -2.74 (95% CI: -3.22 to -2.26) mmHg (He and Macgregor, 2004).

In individuals with *normal* blood pressure the median reduction in 24-h urinary sodium excretion was 74 mmol (4.4 g/day of salt), the mean change (reduction) in systolic blood pressure was -2.03 (95% CI: -2.56 to -1.50) mmHg and the mean change (reduction) in diastolic blood pressure was -0.99 (95% CI: -1.40 to -0.57) mmHg. Weighted linear regression analyses showed a correlation between the reduction in urinary sodium and the reduction in blood pressure.

Longer-term effect on blood pressure

A systematic review and meta-analysis of all RCTs assessing the long-term effects (mortality, cardiovascular events, blood pressure, quality of life, weight, urinary sodium excretion, other nutrients and use of antihypertensive medications) of advice to restrict dietary sodium identified three trials in normotensives ($n = 2326$), five in untreated hypertensives ($n = 387$) and three in treated hypertensives ($n = 801$) with follow-up from 6 months to 7 years. The large, high quality (and therefore most informative) studies used intensive behavioural interventions.

Among a total of 3491 healthy adults, random assignment to intensive interventions that aimed to reduce sodium intake over 6 months to 7 years was associated with a reduction in sodium excretion of almost a quarter (35.5 mmol/24 h, 95% CI: 23.9–47.2 mmol/24 h) but this was associated with only small reductions in blood pressure by 1.1 (95% CI: 0.4–1.8) mmHg systolic and 0.6 (-0.3 to 1.5) mmHg diastolic at 13–60 months (Hooper *et al.*, 2002, 2004). The degree of reduction in sodium intake and change in blood pressure were not related. People on antihypertensive medications were able to stop their medication more often on a reduced sodium diet as compared with controls, while maintaining similar blood pressure control. The effect on death and cardiovascular events were unclear; there were 17 deaths, equally distributed between intervention and control groups. The interventions used were highly intensive and unsuited to primary care or population prevention programmes.

Comment

Adding salt to food appears to be a risk factor for stroke, particularly haemorrhagic stroke.

A modest reduction in salt intake for a duration of 4 or more weeks has a significant and, from a population viewpoint, potentially important effect on blood pressure in both individuals with normal and elevated blood pressure. The magnitude of salt reduction correlated with the magnitude of blood pressure reduction; within the daily intake range of 3–12 g/day, the lower the salt intake achieved, the lower the blood pressure.

Longer-term lower salt intake may help people on antihypertensive drugs to stop their medication while maintaining adequate control of blood pressure, but it remains uncertain whether sodium reduction reduces the risk of stroke and other serious vascular events.

Dietary intake of potassium

Evidence

Risk of stroke

An increased risk of stroke has been reported among elderly patients with atrial fibrillation who used diuretics and whose serum potassium concentrations were <4.0 mEq/l, but at least part of the increased risk may be explained by comorbid conditions and the renin/adlosterone profile rather than a direct effect of low serum potassium (Green et al., 2002; Hart and Pearce, 2003; Legge et al., 2003).

Effect on blood pressure

Systematic reviews of RCTs indicate that short-term increases in potassium intake by about 60–100 mmol/l (equivalent to five bananas) per day lowers blood pressure by about 4.4 (95% CI: 2.2–6.6) mmHg systolic and 2.5 (95% CI: 0.1–4.9) mmHg diastolic (Whelton et al., 1997).

Comment

Potassium supplementation lowers blood pressure, but it is not known if it lowers stroke risk. Adverse effects of potassium supplementation include gastrointestinal upset (belching, flatulence, diarrhoea) in 2–10% of cases. Special precautions are required in patients with renal failure and those taking drugs that increase serum potassium concentrations.

Dietary intake of fruit and vegetables

Evidence

Risk factor for stroke

A prospective observational cohort study of 40,349 Japanese men and women who completed a food frequency questionnaire in 1980 detailing their intake of fruit and vegetables were followed prospectively for 18 years (Sauvaget et al., 2003). There were 1926 stroke deaths identified during the follow-up period (48% cerebral infarction, 24% intracerebral haemorrhage, 8% subarachnoid haemorrhage and 21% from other cerebrovascular diseases). Compared with participants whose intake of fruit and green yellow vegetables was once or less per week, men and women whose intake was daily had a significant 20–40% reduction in death from total stroke, and ischaemic and haemorrhagic stroke.

Effect on blood pressure

A 6-month RCT of a brief negotiation method to encourage an increase in consumption of fruit and vegetables to at least five daily portions in 690 healthy participants aged 25–64 years showed that increased fruit and vegetable intake was associated with a decrease in systolic blood pressure by 4.0 (95% CI: 2.0–6.0) mmHg and diastolic blood pressure by 1.5 (95% CI: 0.2–2.7) mmHg (John *et al.*, 2002).

The Dietary Approaches to Stop Hypertension (DASH) trial also reported that an increase in dietary fruit and vegetables for 8 weeks reduced systolic blood pressure by 2.8 mmHg and diastolic blood pressure by 1.1 mmHg more than a control diet (Appel *et al.*, 1997). The DASH investigators reported a larger lowering of blood pressure in participants assigned a combination diet (low in dairy products with reduced saturated and total fat in addition to being enriched with fruit and vegetables).

Comment

Fruit and vegetables reduce blood pressure, probably by increasing potassium intake (Whelton *et al.*, 1997), and may reduce the risk of stroke (Fung *et al.*, 2004).

Dietary intake of antioxidants

Laboratory evidence suggests that oxidative modification of low-density lipoprotein (LDL) cholesterol may be an important stage in the formation and rupture of atherosclerotic plaques (Witzum, 1994). A number of dietary constituents have antioxidant properties, such as certain minerals (e.g. selenium, copper, zinc, manganese), vitamins (C and E), pro-vitamins (β-carotene) and flavonoids.

Evidence

Risk factor for stroke

Observational studies of intake of antioxidants and stroke risk suggest that low antioxidant intake (chiefly β-carotene and vitamin C) are associated with an increased risk of stroke (Manson *et al.*, 1993; Keli *et al.*, 1996; Daviglus *et al.*, 1997; Ness and Powles, 1999; Vokó *et al.*, 2003). The most recent was a prospective population-based cohort study of 5197 residents of Rotterdam, the Netherlands who were free of stroke, of mean age 68 years, and followed prospectively for 6.4 years (Vokó *et al.*, 2003). There were 277 incident cases of ischaemic stroke recorded. Compared with participants who had the lowest tertile of vitamin C consumption, those with the second and third tertile of vitamin C intake had a significantly lower risk of ischaemic stroke. The adjusted RRs from the lowest to the highest tertiles of vitamin C intake were 1.00 (referent), 0.69 (95% CI: 0.49–0.98) and 0.66 (95% CI: 0.46–0.93) (Vokó *et al.*, 2003). Regression models, which included vitamin C intake as a continuous variable, show that the RR of ischaemic stroke was 0.85 (95% CI: 0.72–0.99) per increase in vitamin C intake of 1 SD.

Effect of vitamin E supplementation on stroke and other vascular events

A systematic review identified seven RCTs of vitamin E (α-tocopherol) in a dose range of 50–800 U and eight RCTs of β-carotene treatment in a dose range of 15–50 mg, in which 1000 or more patients were followed up for 1.4–12.0 years (Heart Protection Study Collaborative Group, 2002; Vivekananthan *et al.*, 2003; Lawlor *et al.*, 2004).

A meta-analysis of the seven RCTs of vitamin E (α-tocopherol), in a total of 81,788 patients, showed that random assignment to vitamin E was associated with no reduction in stroke (3.6% vitamin E vs 3.5% control, OR: 1.02, 95% CI: 0.92–1.12, $P = 0.71$), cardiovascular death (6.0% vitamin E vs 6.0% control, OR: 1.0, 95% CI: 0.94–1.06, $P = 0.94$), death from all causes (11.3% vitamin E vs 11.1% control, OR: 1.02, 95% CI: 0.98–1.06, $P = 0.42$), or the composite end point of cardiovascular death or non-fatal MI (9.8% vitamin E vs 9.8% control, OR: 1.0, 95% CI: 0.94–1.07, $P = 0.93$) compared with control treatment (Vivekananthan *et al.*, 2003).

Effect of β-carotene supplementation on stroke and other vascular events

Among the eight RCTs of β-carotene treatment, in a total of 138,113 patients, random assignment to β-carotene was associated with no reduction in stroke (2.3% β-carotene vs 2.3% control, OR: 1.0, 95% CI: 0.91–1.09, $P = 0.92$), but a small, yet significant, increase in cardiovascular death (3.4% β-carotene vs 3.1% control, OR: 1.10, 95% CI: 1.03–1.17, $P = 0.003$) and death from all causes (7.4% β-carotene vs 7.0% control, OR: 1.07, 95% CI: 1.02–1.11, $P = 0.003$) compared with control treatment (Vivekananthan *et al.*, 2003).

Comment

Observational studies suggest that administering antioxidant compounds, by protecting cholesterol from oxidation, may reduce the risk of ischaemic stroke. However, RCTs provide good evidence that β-carotene or vitamin E supplementation is of no benefit, and that in heavy smokers β-carotene increases the risk of lung cancer and all-cause mortality (Morris and Carson, 2003; US Preventive Services Task Force, 2003; Vivekananthan *et al.*, 2003).

There is insufficient evidence to recommend for or against antioxidant combinations, and supplements of vitamin A or C (Morris and Carson, 2003; US Preventive Services Task Force, 2003; Vivekananthan *et al.*, 2003).

The above data also highlight the importance of not relying on evidence from observational studies to establish causality because bias and confounding cannot be eliminated; RCTs are needed to show that lowering the prevalence and level of the risk factor independently reduces the incidence of the disease (Lawlor *et al.*, 2004; Vandenbroucke, 2004).

Dietary intake of B-vitamins

Evidence

Risk factor for stroke

Systematic reviews of non-genetic observational studies (cohort and case–control studies) indicate that the association between serum total homocysteine (tHcy) concentration and the risk of ischaemic stroke is positive, strong, dose-related, reasonably consistent among studies and independent of other recorded vascular risk factors (The Homocysteine Studies Collaboration, 2002; Wald *et al.*, 2002, 2004). After adjusting for confounding caused by known vascular risk factors and correction for regression dilution caused by random variation in Hcy measurements, a 25% increase in tHcy (about 3 µmol/l (0.41 mg/l)) is associated with about a 19% increase in odds of stroke (OR: 0.81, 95% CI: 0.69–0.95) (The homocysteine studies collaboration, 2002). Although the association is also biologically plausible (Faraci and Lentz, 2004), it is not known whether it is causal because bias and confounding cannot be eliminated (Lawlor *et al.*, 2004; Vandenbroucke, 2004). For example, reverse causality bias may account for the stronger association found in retrospective case–control studies, in which tHcy was measured in blood collected after the onset of stroke, than in prospective studies (The Homocysteine Studies Collaboration, 2002; Wald *et al.*, 2002). And, the association may be confounded by other factors (such as smoking, lower socioeconomic class, existing atherosclerosis and renal impairment) that increase both tHcy and stroke risk, and were not measured, and adjusted for, in these studies. Resolving the issue of causality is important because tHcy can be lowered effectively, safely and affordably by B-vitamins (folic acid, vitamins B12 and B6) (Homocysteine Lowering Trialists' Collaboration, 1998; He *et al.*, 2004).

Effect of B-vitamin supplementation on risk of recurrent ischaemic stroke

The Vitamins in Stroke Prevention (VISP) trial was the first (and only published) large RCT to evaluate the effect of lowering Hcy by B-vitamin supplementation on 'hard' clinical outcomes such as recurrent stroke (Toole *et al.*, 2004). It compared high-dose vitamins (folic acid: 2.5 mg, vitamin B12: 0.4 mg, vitamin B6: 25 mg) with low-dose vitamins (folic acid: 0.02 mg, vitamin B12: 0.006 mg, vitamin B6: 0.2 mg). Both treatment groups received the same daily dose of nine other vitamins, according to the recommendation of the Food and Drug Administration (FDA). An absolute difference in mean tHcy of 2 μmol/l was achieved; 13 μmol/l in the low-dose group vs 11 μmol/l in the high-dose group. After 2 years of follow up, the cumulative incidence of recurrent cerebral infarction was 8.4% among 1814 patients allocated high-dose vitamins compared with 8.1% among 1835 patients allocated low-dose vitamins (risk ratio (RR): 1.0, 95% CI: 0.8–1.3, $P = 0.80$) (Toole *et al.*, 2004). The cumulative incidence of death was 5.4% in the high-dose group vs 6.3% in the low-dose group (RR: 0.9, 95% CI: 0.7–1.1).

Comment

Although the VISP trial did not identify a significant benefit of high-dose compared with low-dose therapy, it did not reliably exclude a modest but important reduction in the RR of stroke of ≤20%, and perhaps an even greater reduction with greater reductions in tHcy. The unexpectedly small difference in tHcy between the high- and low-dose groups may reflect the fortification of grains and staple foods with folate and widespread use of vitamin supplements in North America. These factors are likely to have reduced the mean concentrations of tHcy in the population and the number of people with severe folate deficiency (Jacques *et al.*, 1999). It may also reflect the fact that, in the presence of folate repletion, blood concentrations of tHcy are highly dependent on vitamin B12 (Quinlivan *et al.*, 2002) and in the VISP trial: (a) the low-dose group received the recommended daily intake of vitamin B12 (raising their tHcy); (b) the high-dose group received a dose of vitamin B12 that may have been too low for adequate absorption in elderly patients (and therefore too low to reduce their tHcy) (Rajan *et al.*, 2002) and (c) in both treatment groups patients who had low blood concentrations of vitamin B12 (<150 pmol/l) were treated with B12 injections (thus reducing statistical power). The lower-than-anticipated rates of recurrent strokes in both treatment groups, and the short duration of follow up (2 years) also limited the statistical power of the VISP trial to reliably identify or exclude a modest but important benefit of B-vitamin therapy.

More data are needed to refine the estimates of effectiveness of B-vitamins and to provide placebo-controlled estimates of their effectiveness in other populations with different prevalences of genetic and environmental factors that influence tHcy.

The VITAmins TO Prevent Stroke (VITATOPS) trial is an international, multi-centre, randomised, double-blind, placebo-controlled trial which aims to determine whether B-vitamin supplements (folic acid: 2 mg, B6: 25 mg, B12: 500 μg) reduce the risk of stroke, other serious vascular events and revascularisation procedures, dementia and depression, compared with placebo, in patients with recent stroke or TIAs of the brain or eye. To reliably identify a 15% reduction in RR of the primary outcome event (stroke and other serious vascular events) from 8% to 6.8%/year with an α of 0.05 and power of 80%, 8000 patients need to be randomised and followed up for an average of 2 years. As of January 2005, 4600 patients had been randomised in 73 centres, 19 countries and five continents (http://vitatops.highway1.com.au) (The VITATOPS Trial Study Group, 2002).

Whilst awaiting the results of the ongoing clinical trials of B-vitamin therapy in stroke and other patient groups, insufficient evidence exists to recommend routine screening and treatment of high tHcy with B-vitamins to prevent atherothrombotic vascular disease (Hankey and Eikelboom, 2004, 2005; B-vitamin Treatment Trialists' Collaboration, 2005).

Mediterranean diet

Evidence

Risk factor for stroke

A prospective population-based cohort of 22,043 adults in Greece completed a food frequency questionnaire at baseline which included a 10-point traditional Mediterranean diet scale that incorporated the salient characteristics of this diet: cereals, fruit and nuts, vegetables, potatoes, legumes/beans, olive oil, dairy products (cheese, yoghurt), fish, eggs, meat (poultry weekly, other monthly) (Trichopoulou et al., 2003). The individuals were followed prospectively for 44 months during which time 275 deaths were recorded.

A higher degree of adherence to the Mediterranean diet was associated with a reduction in total mortality (adjusted HR associated with a 2-point increment in the Mediterranean diet score: 0.75, 95% CI: 0.64–0.87), death due to coronary heart disease (HR: 0.76, 95% CI: 0.47–0.94) and death due to cancer (HR: 0.76, 95% CI: 0.59–0.98).

Effect of an Indo-Mediterranean diet on coronary events

A randomised, blinded, controlled trial in 1000 high vascular risk patients showed the 499 patients assigned an Indo-Mediterranean diet consumed more fruits, vegetables, nuts, legumes and n-3 fatty acids, and had lower serum cholesterol concentrations and lower rates of non-fatal MI (4.2% vs 8.6%, relative risk reduction (RRR): 53%, 95% CI: 21–72%), sudden cardiac death (1.2% vs 3.2%, RRR: 67%, 95% CI: 14–87%), and total cardiac end points (7.8% vs 15.2%, RRR: 52%, 95% CI: 29–67%), at 2 years follow-up than the 501 patients assigned a control diet similar to the step 1 National Cholesterol Education Program (NCEP) prudent diet (Singh et al., 2002).

Comment

Greater adherence to the traditional Mediterranean diet or Indo-Mediterranean diet may be associated with a significant reduction in total mortality.

The Indo-Mediterranean diet differs from the Mediterranean diet because fish, rapeseed and olive oils are replaced by mustard or soybean oils, green leafy vegetables, certain nuts and whole grains.

There are no data on the effect of these diets on risk of stroke.

SUMMARY

There is no reliable evidence from RCTs that quitting smoking, controlling blood glucose, losing weight, taking regular exercise, abandoning heavy alcohol consumption and improving diet (less salt and saturated fat) reduce the risk of recurrent stroke or other serious vascular events. However, such evidence is very difficult to obtain, and these changes probably do all help to reduce the risk of stroke.

It would therefore seem appropriate for survivors of atherothrombotic and cardioembolic ischaemic stroke to endeavour to reduce their risk of recurrent stroke and other serious vascular events by the modifications to their lifestyle as listed in Table 14.3. If these measures do reduce the risk of stroke, they probably do so by reducing causal risk factors such as blood pressure, cholesterol and diabetes (Table 14.4) (Diabetes Prevention Program Research Group, 2002; Appel *et al.*, 2003). If a reduction of 2 mmHg in diastolic blood pressure decreases the risk of stroke by 15% and coronary heart disease by 6% (MacMahon *et al.*, 1990; Collins and MacMahon, 1994; MacMahon and Rodgers, 1994; Cook *et al.*, 1995), it is likely that these

Table 14.3. Optimal lifestyle to prevent stroke.

Smoking: avoid
Alcohol: restrict to 1–2 standard drinks daily
Physical activity: regular (daily or second daily)
Body weight and waist/hip ratio: ideal (minimise intra-abdominal/visceral obesity)

Diet
Fat: <30% of caloric intake; predominantly non-hydrogenated unsaturated vegetable fats and ω-3 fatty acids instead of saturated animal fats
Carbohydrates: whole grains
Fruit and vegetables
Salt: decrease from 9–12 g/day to 5–6 g/day

Avoid: β-carotene, vitamin E, long-term HRT.

Table 14.4. Effect of lifestyle modifications on blood pressure.

Lifestyle change	Effect on blood pressure (systolic/diastolic) (mmHg)
• ↓ Salt to 12 mmol/day	↓ 3.9/1.9
• ↑ Potassium to 80 mmol/day	↓ 4.4/2.5
• ↑ Fruit and vegetables by 1.4 portions/day	↓ 4.0/1.5
• ↑ Fish to 3 g/day	↓ 4.5/2.5
• ↓ Alcohol by 20 g/day	↓ 4.0/2.0
• ↑ Aerobic exercise to 30 min/day	↓ 4.7/3.1
• ↓ Body weight by 3–9%	↓ 3.0/2.0

simple measures could have a dramatic effect on reducing the risk of stroke and the burden of stroke on the individual patient, their carer(s) and the community.

In order to achieve these lifestyle changes, both the individual and the community must share responsibility. Governments have a responsibility to improve public education, recreational and educational facilities; work with the food, tobacco and alcohol industries; and legislate and impose taxes against hazardous lifestyle behaviours (e.g. smoking and perhaps salt in foods). A cultural change is also required among some individuals and communities to promote the incorporation of regular physical activity, a healthy diet and minimal exposure to smoking into everyday life.

Antithrombotic therapy for preventing recurrent cardiogenic embolism

About 20% of first ever and recurrent ischaemic strokes are due to embolism from the heart. The most common source of embolism from the heart is a dilated, fibrillating, left atrium (non-rheumatic atrial fibrillation (NRAF)) causing stasis of blood in the left atrial appendage. Other major sources of thrombus include a dilated left atrium caused by rheumatic atrial fibrillation (RAF); valvular heart disease due to prosthetic heart valves, rheumatic mitral stenosis and infective endocarditis; thrombus overlying an akinetic or dyskinetic left ventricle due to recent myocardial infarction or a dilated cardiomyopathy and intracardiac tumours (Table 15.1).

Atrial fibrillation

Atrial fibrillation (AF) is a common dysrhythmia. Its prevalence increases with age, from about 2% in the general population to 5% in people older than 65 years, and

Table 15.1. Prevalence of potential cardiac sources (values in %) of embolism in patients with first-ever ischaemic stroke.

Any AF	13
Without RHD	11
With RHD	1
Mitral regurgitation	6
Recent (<6 weeks) myocardial infarction	5
Prosthetic valve	1
Mitral stenosis	1
Paradoxical embolism	1
Any of the above	20
Other sources of uncertain significance	11
(aortic stenosis/sclerosis; mitral annulus calcification, mitral valve prolapse, etc.)	

Source: Sandercock *et al.,* (1989); Oxfordshire Community Stroke Project.

Table 15.2. Risk stratification and prophylaxis in AF.

High risk (6–12% per year risk of stroke)
- Age >65 years and hypertension or diabetes
- Previous TIA or stroke
- Valvular heart disease
- Heart failure
- Recent myocardial infarction
- Impaired left ventricular function on echocardiography
- Thyroid disease
- Left atrial thrombus or left atrial spontaneous echo contrast (TOE done on basis of clinical suspicion)

Treatment: Warfarin (target INR: 2.0–3.0) if possible and not contraindicated

Moderate risk (3–5% per year risk of stroke)
- Age <65 years and hypertension or diabetes
- Age >65 years and not in high-risk group

Treatment: Warfarin (target INR: 2.0–3.0) or aspirin 75–300 mg/day, depending on individual case and echocardiography findings

Low risk (≤1% per year risk of stroke)
- Age <65 and no hypertension, diabetes, TIA, stroke or other clinical risk factors

Treatment: Nil or aspirin 75–300 mg/day

10% in people older than 75 years (Kannel *et al.*, 1982, 1998; Wolf *et al.*, 1991). It may occur as a single episode, a series of recurrent episodes ('paroxysmal' AF), or continuously ('permanent' or 'chronic' AF).

AF is an important dysrhythmia because it may signify underlying heart disease, it may cause symptoms of decreased cardiac output (e.g. malaise, effort intolerance) or palpitations, and it is associated with an increased risk of systemic thromboembolism and stroke (Peters *et al.*, 2002).

Risk of stroke

This risk of stroke averages about 5% per year among all individuals in non-valvular AF, which is about 5–6 times greater than for people of the same age who are in sinus rhythm (Wolf *et al.*, 1983, 1991; Kannel *et al.*, 1998). Following an initial stroke, the stroke recurrence rate varies in different studies between 2% and 15% in the first year following stroke, and is 5% yearly thereafter. The mortality rate is also 5% yearly (CETF, 1986; Sherman, 1986). The risk of recurrence is dependent on the type of cardiac abnormality (CETF, 1986) and also on the presence of a previous history of transient ischaemic attack (TIA) or ischaemic stroke, hypertension, diabetes, age greater than 75 years and echocardiographic evidence of left ventricular dysfunction (Table 15.2) (Atrial Fibrillation Investigators, 1994;

Gage *et al.*, 2004). Patients with combined rheumatic heart disease (RHD) and AF show the highest recurrence rate. The incidence of RHD, however, has declined in Western societies and the most common cardioembolic source is NRAF (CETF, 1986). AF becomes increasingly important as a risk factor for stroke with increasing age, with an attributable risk that rises from 1.5% for patients in their 50s, to 23.5% for those in their 80s (Kannel *et al.*, 1998; Hart and Halperin, 2001).

Causes of stroke associated with AF

AF is present in about 15% of all patients with ischaemic stroke and TIA, but is causal in about two-thirds of these strokes (or 10% of all ischaemic strokes) (Sandercock *et al.*, 1992; Whisnant *et al.*, 1999). AF causes ischaemic stroke by giving rise to embolism of thrombus from the left atrium, and left atrial appendage in particular, to the brain. The three components of Virchow's 'triad' of thrombogenesis are likely to be important. Firstly, there is stasis of blood due to the loss of atrial contraction that accompanies AF. Stasis is most marked in the left atrial appendage, the most common site for thrombus formation in these patients (Hart and Halperin, 2001). The stasis is accompanied by, secondly, hypercoagulability, as evidence by increased concentrations of fibrin D-dimer and β-thromboglobulin (Lip *et al.*, 1996); and thirdly, by endothelial dysfunction, as shown by direct evidence of atrial endocardial abnormalities in autopsy studies (Shirani and Alaeddini, 2000), and increased concentrations of circulating surrogate markers of endothelial damage or dysfunction, most notably von Willebrand factor (Heppell *et al.*, 1997). All three factors probably contribute to the development of the prothrombotic state that accompanies AF.

Other causes of stroke in patients with AF, accounting for about one-third of cases of stroke in AF patients, are embolism from the heart affected by other diseases (e.g. valvular heart disease), atherothromboembolism from the aortic arch or large arteries of extra- and intracranial carotid and vertebrobasilar circulations, and intracranial small vessel disease (Sandercock *et al.*, 1989, 1992).

Acute ischaemic stroke (see Chapter 9)

Evidence

Anticoagulation (heparin) vs control

The International Stroke Trial included a large subgroup of patients with acute ischaemic stroke who were in AF (*n* = 3169 patients) and randomised to subcutaneous unfractionated heparin or control. Although heparin reduced the 14-day risk of ischaemic stroke by more than 50%, the benefit was offset by an increase in brain haemorrhage (Table 15.3) (Saxena, 2001; Hart *et al.*, 2002).

Table 15.3. Effects of subcutaneous unfractionated heparin in different doses given with 48 h of acute ischaemic stroke and continued for 14 days after stroke onset, compared to no heparin, on events within 14 days and outcome at 6 months in patients with AF and acute ischaemic stroke.

	Heparin 12,500 U ($n = 784$)	Heparin 5000 U ($n = 773$)	No heparin ($n = 1612$)	P, overall Chi-square
Events within 14 days				
• Recurrent ischaemic/ unknown stroke	18(2.3%)	26(3.4%)	79(4.9%)	0.006
• Symptomatic ICH	22(2.8%)	10(1.3%)	7(0.4%)	<0.0001
• Recurrent stroke of any pathological type	39(5.0%)	36(4.7%)	86(5.3%)	0.8
Outcome at 6 months				
• Dead	305(38.9%)	292(37.8%)	630(39.1%)	0.8
• Dead or dependent	612(78.1%)	609(78.8%)	1266(78.5%)	0.9

Source: Saxena *et al.* (2001). ICH: intracranial haemorrhage.

Anticoagulation (heparin) vs antiplatelet (aspirin) therapy

The Heparin in Acute Embolic Stroke Trial (HAEST) trial randomised 449 patients with acute ischaemic stroke and AF to a low-molecular-weight heparin or aspirin. Heparin did not reduce the risk of recurrent stroke during the first 14 days after stroke that was attributed to AF (Berge, 2000; Hart *et al.*, 2002).

Comment

Randomised trials comparing heparin with control (Saxena *et al.*, 2001) and with aspirin (Berge *et al.*, 2000) during the first 2 weeks of acute ischaemic stroke among patients in AF showed no benefit from early anticoagulation, because any net gains from reduction in recurrent ischaemic stroke were offset by the excess hazards of haemorrhagic stroke (Table 15.3) (see Chapter 9) (Berge *et al.*, 2000; Saxena *et al.*, 2001).

The timing of anticoagulation after recent ischaemic stroke depends on the risk of recurrent thromboembolism (Atrial Fibrillation Investigators, 1994) (Table 15.2) and the risk of symptomatic haemorrhagic transformation of the brain infarct. The risk of haemorrhagic transformation is higher within the first 2 weeks and in patients with large brain infarcts and uncontrolled hypertension (Hart *et al.*, 1995).

Common empirical practice is to treat acute ischaemic stroke patients who are in AF immediately with aspirin 300 mg/day and then, depending on the above factors, begin warfarin 5 mg/day between days 3 and 14 after stroke onset (depending on the balance of risks of re-embolisation vs haemorrhage), aiming to achieve an International Normalised Ratio (INR) of 2.0–3.0 (Gallus *et al.*, 2000; Hart *et al.*, 2002).

Longer-term prevention of recurrent cardiogenic ischaemic stroke

Anticoagulation (warfarin) vs control

Evidence

Until the end of the 1980s, the management of patients with NRAF was based entirely on evidence from uncontrolled, non-randomised studies. Around 1990, five large clinical trials investigated the value of anticoagulation in the (primary) prevention of first-ever stroke and other vascular events in patients with NRAF (AFASAK, 1989; BAATAF, 1990; CAFA, 1991; SPAF, 1991; VA-SPINAF, 1992). A systematic review of these five randomised trials concluded that warfarin consistently decreased the risk of first-ever stroke in patients with AF (a 68% reduction in relative risk) with virtually no increase in the frequency of major bleeding (AFI, 1994; Hart *et al.*, 1999; McNamara *et al.*, 2003).

A systematic review for the Cochrane Library identified two randomised-controlled trials (RCTs) comparing the long-term effect of oral anticoagulation with control for (secondary) prevention of recurrent stroke and other serious vascular events, in 485 patients with NRAF and a previous TIA or minor ischaemic stroke (VA-SPINAF, 1992; EAFT, 1993; Saxena and Koudstaal, 2004a, b). The two RCTs were the European Atrial Fibrillation Trial (EAFT) (EAFT, 1993) and the Veterans Affairs Stroke Prevention In Nonrheumatic Atrial Fibrillation (VA-SPINAF) study (VA-SPINAF, 1992).

In the EAFT, 1007 NRAF patients with a TIA or minor stroke within the preceding 3 months were divided into two groups, those without (group 1) or with (group 2) contraindications to anticoagulants. Patients in group 1 ($n = 669$) were randomised to treatment with open-label anticoagulants (target INR range: 2.5–4.0), or double-blind treatment with 300 mg aspirin or matching placebo. Group 2 patients ($n = 338$) were randomised to double-blind treatment with aspirin or placebo (see below). Forty-three per cent were randomised within 2 weeks of stroke onset. The mean duration of follow-up was of 2.3 years, and follow-up visits were planned 4 monthly (EAFT, 1993).

In the VA-SPINAF study, which was primarily a primary prevention study, only 46 NRAF patients with a history of stroke were entered. The time since the cerebral ischaemic event was unknown. Patients were randomised to double-blind treatment with warfarin (prothrombin-time ratio, 1.2–1.5; estimated INR 1.4–2.8) or matching placebo. All patients were followed for 3 years or until the study was terminated. The mean duration of follow-up was of 1.7 years (VA-SPINAF, 1992).

In both studies, an intention-to-treat analysis was performed, and the outcome events were adjudicated by committees blinded to the treatment allocation.

Stroke In the group of patients in the EAFT without contraindication to anti-coagulants, the annual rate of stroke was 4% in patients assigned to anticoagulants ($n = 225$) vs 12% in patients assigned to placebo ($n = 214$). In absolute terms, 80 strokes were prevented per 1000 patients treated with anticoagulants per year.

In the VA-SPINAF study, four patients in the placebo group ($n = 25$) against two in the anticoagulant group ($n = 21$) suffered a recurrent stroke (VA-SPINAF, 1992).

The results of the two trials combined show that anticoagulants are highly effective: they reduce the odds of recurrent stroke, disabling as well as non-disabling, by two-thirds (odds ratio (OR): 0.36, 95% confidence interval (CI): 0.22–0.58) (Fig. 15.1) (Saxena and Koudstaal, 2004a, b).

Serious vascular events In the group of patients in the EAFT without contraindi-cation to anticoagulants, the annual rate of all vascular events (vascular death, recur-rent stroke (ischaemic or haemorrhagic), myocardial infarction and systemic embolism) was 8% in patients assigned to anticoagulants ($n = 225$) vs 17% in patients assigned to placebo ($n = 214$). In absolute terms, 90 vascular events (mainly strokes) were prevented per 1000 patients treated with anticoagulants per year.

In the VA-SPINAF study, the number of all vascular events was 8/21 in the war-farin group vs 11/25 in the placebo group (OR: 0.78, 95% CI: 0.20–2.9).

The results of the two trials combined show that anticoagulants reduce the odds of all vascular events by nearly half (OR: 0.55, 95% CI: 0.37–0.82) (Fig. 15.2) (Saxena and Koudstaal, 2004a, b).

Bleeding In the EAFT the incidence of bleeding events (major or minor, intra- or extracranial) on anticoagulation was low (2.8% per year vs 0.7 per year in the placebo group). Despite a mean age of 71 years, the absolute annual excess of

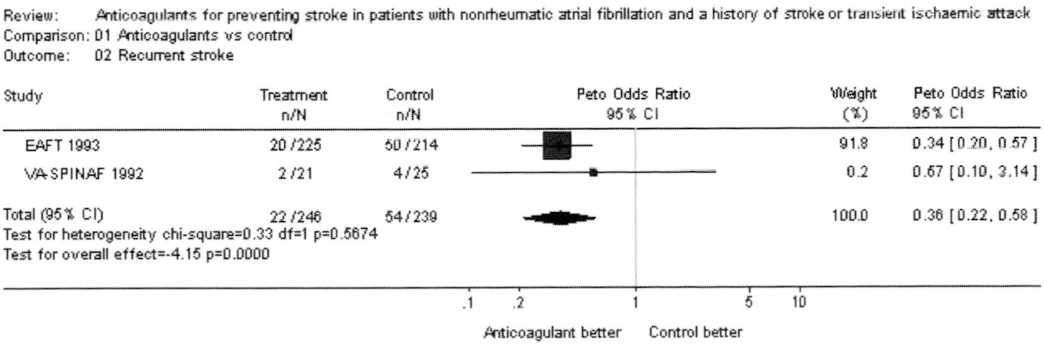

Review: Anticoagulants for preventing stroke in patients with nonrheumatic atrial fibrillation and a history of stroke or transient ischaemic attack
Comparison: 01 Anticoagulants vs control
Outcome: 02 Recurrent stroke

Study	Treatment n/N	Control n/N	Peto Odds Ratio 95% CI	Weight (%)	Peto Odds Ratio 95% CI
EAFT 1993	20 /225	50 /214		91.8	0.34 [0.20, 0.57]
VA-SPINAF 1992	2 /21	4 /25		0.2	0.67 [0.10, 3.14]
Total (95% CI)	22 /246	54/239		100.0	0.36 [0.22, 0.58]

Test for heterogeneity chi-square=0.33 df=1 p=0.5674
Test for overall effect=-4.15 p=0.0000

.1   .2   1   5   10

Anticoagulant better   Control better

Figure 15.1 Forest plot showing the effects of *oral anticoagulants vs control* in patients with NRAF and a history of stroke or TIA on *recurrent stroke* at the end of follow-up. Reproduced from Saxena and Koudstaal (2004a), with permission from the authors and John Wiley & Sons Limited. Copyright Cochrane Library, reproduced with permission.

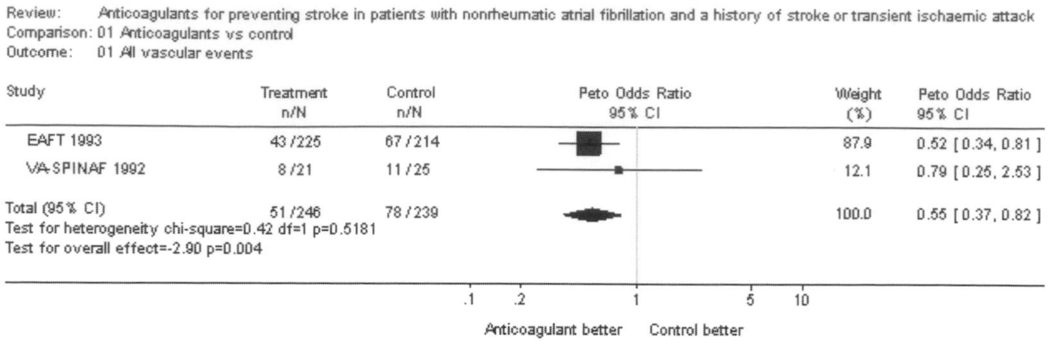

Review: Anticoagulants for preventing stroke in patients with nonrheumatic atrial fibrillation and a history of stroke or transient ischaemic attack
Comparison: 01 Anticoagulants vs control
Outcome: 01 All vascular events

Study	Treatment n/N	Control n/N	Peto Odds Ratio 95% CI	Weight (%)	Peto Odds Ratio 95% CI
EAFT 1993	43 /225	67 /214		87.9	0.52 [0.34, 0.81]
VA-SPINAF 1992	8 /21	11 /25		12.1	0.79 [0.25, 2.53]
Total (95% CI)	51 /246	78 /239		100.0	0.55 [0.37, 0.82]

Test for heterogeneity chi-square=0.42 df=1 p=0.5181
Test for overall effect=-2.90 p=0.004

.1 .2 1 5 10
Anticoagulant better   Control better

Figure 15.2 Forest plot showing the effects of *oral anticoagulants vs control* in patients with NRAF and a history of stroke or TIA on *serious vascular events* at the end of follow-up. Reproduced from Saxena and Koudstaal (2004a), with permission from the authors and John Wiley & Sons Limited. Copyright Cochrane Library, reproduced with permission.

Review: Anticoagulants for preventing stroke in patients with nonrheumatic atrial fibrillation and a history of stroke or transient ischaemic attack
Comparison: 01 Anticoagulants vs control
Outcome: 04 Major extracranial bleed

Study	Treatment n/N	Control n/N	Peto Odds Ratio 95% CI	Weight (%)	Peto Odds Ratio 95% CI
EAFT 1993	13 /225	2 /214		100.0	4.32 [1.55, 12.10]
Total (95% CI)	13 /225	2 /214		100.0	4.32 [1.55, 12.10]

Test for heterogeneity chi-square=0.00 df=0
Test for overall effect=2.79 p=0.005

.1 .2 1 5 10
Anticoagulant better   Control better

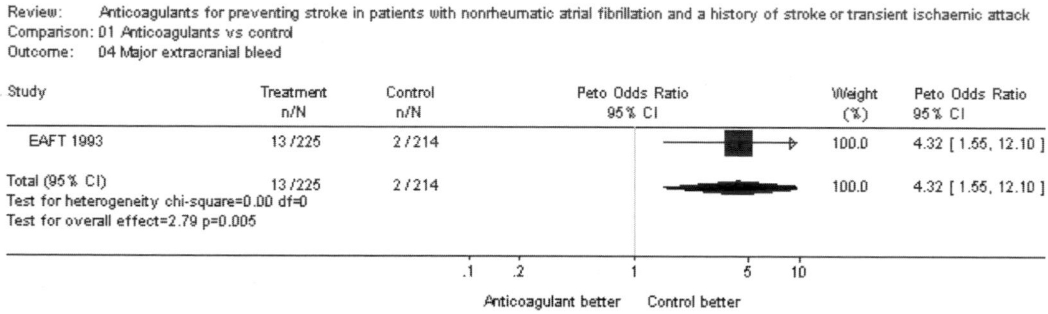

Figure 15.3 Forest plot showing the effects of *oral anticoagulants vs control* in patients with NRAF and a history of stroke or TIA on *major extracranial haemorrhages* at the end of follow-up. Reproduced from Saxena and Koudstaal (2004a), with permission from the authors and John Wiley & Sons Limited. Copyright Cochrane Library, reproduced with permission.

major bleeds was 21 per 1000 patients treated, and there was no documented intracerebral bleeding.

In the VA-SPINAF study, no intracranial bleeds occurred.

The results of the two trials combined show that anticoagulants were associated with a significant increase in major extracranial bleeding complications (2.8% per year (oral anticoagulants) vs 0.7% per year (placebo); OR: 4.32, 95% CI: 1.55–12.1, absolute excess 2.1% per year) (Fig. 15.3) but there was no excess of intracranial bleeds among patients using anticoagulants (OR: 0.13, 95% CI: 0.00–6.49); indeed there were no intracranial bleeds at all (Fig. 15.4).

Intensity of oral anticoagulation The EAFT Study Group performed an analysis to determine the intensity of oral anticoagulant therapy that provided the best

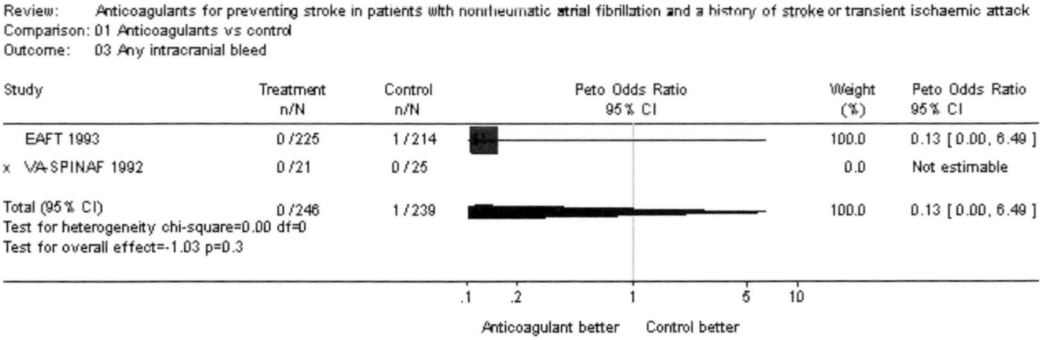

Review: Anticoagulants for preventing stroke in patients with nonrheumatic atrial fibrillation and a history of stroke or transient ischaemic attack
Comparison: 01 Anticoagulants vs control
Outcome: 03 Any intracranial bleed

Study	Treatment n/N	Control n/N	Peto Odds Ratio 95% CI	Weight (%)	Peto Odds Ratio 95% CI
EAFT 1993	0 /225	1 /214		100.0	0.13 [0.00, 6.49]
x VA-SPINAF 1992	0 /21	0 /25		0.0	Not estimable
Total (95% CI)	0 /246	1 /239		100.0	0.13 [0.00, 6.49]

Test for heterogeneity chi-square=0.00 df=0
Test for overall effect=-1.03 p=0.3

.1   .2   1   5   10

Anticoagulant better   Control better

Figure 15.4   Forest plot showing the effects of *oral anticoagulants vs control* in patients with NRAF and a history of stroke or TIA on *major intracranial haemorrhages* at the end of follow-up. Reproduced from Saxena and Koudstaal (2004), with permission from the authors and John Wiley & Sons Limited. Copyright Cochrane Library, reproduced with permission.

balance between the prevention of thromboembolism and the occurrence of bleeding complications. They found that the target value for the INR should be set at 3.0, and values below 2.0 and above 5.0 should be avoided (EAFT, 1995). A case–control study that analysed the lowest effective intensity of prophylactic anti-coagulation in patients with NRAF also found that the risk of stroke (Hylek, 1996) and its severity rises steeply at INRs below 1.8–2.0 (Hylek, 2003).

Comment

Interpretation of the evidence   The results of the two studies indicate that in patients with NRAF and a recent TIA or minor ischaemic stroke, oral anticoagulant treatment decreases the odds of recurrent stroke (disabling and non-disabling) by two-thirds, from about 12% per year (control) to 4% per year (oral anticoagulants; absolute risk reduction (ARR) 8% per year) and almost halves the odds of serious vascular events.

Although there was a 4-fold increase in serious bleeding complications, the absolute excess was 2.1% per 1000 patients treated, so the benefit was not negated.

These results for the (secondary) prevention of recurrent stroke are highly consistent with those for the (primary) prevention of first-ever stroke with oral anticoagulation in patients with NRAF in terms of the proportional risk reduction (about two-thirds). However, because of the much higher absolute incidence of recurrent stroke than first-ever stroke, oral anticoagulation for patients with TIA and ischaemic stroke who are in AF realises greater absolute benefits of 90 vascular events (mainly strokes) prevented for every 1000 patients treated for 1 year, at the cost of 21 serious bleeding complications. Although there were no intracranial bleeds in the patients treated with warfarin, there was a definite increase in major extracranial bleeding complications (2.8% per year vs 0.7% per year in the placebo group; OR: 4.32, 95% CI: 1.55–12.1).

Implications for practice   These results indicate that anticoagulants should be prescribed to patients with NRAF and a recent TIA or minor ischaemic stroke, unless there is a major contraindication, particularly those related to poor adherence and bleeding risk.

The target value for the INR should be set between 2.0 and 3.0 for safe and effective stroke prevention.

There remains uncertainty about the ideal timing of initiating anticoagulant therapy. Acute therapy with low-molecular-weight-heparin or unfractionated heparin does not appear to be beneficial, the modest benefits being outweighed by the modest risks. It is generally recommended that oral anticoagulation be initiated after the first 1–2 weeks of stroke onset.

Implications for research   The main issues to resolve relate to the timing of when to start oral anticoagulant therapy after a stroke, and how long to continue anticoagulant treatment for, and the quest for safer and more acceptable antithrombotic agents.

Although data for 3169 patients with AF from the International Stroke Trial show that treatment with heparin should not be started within the first 2 weeks after stroke, as the risk of bleeding complications in this phase is so high that it completely offsets the benefits (see Chapter 9) (Saxena, 2001), it is not known whether this also holds true for treatment with warfarin. The EAFT findings do not definitively answer this question since only 43% of the patients were randomised within 2 weeks after onset of neurological symptoms.

It is also uncertain how long antithrombotic treatment should be continued. However, because the risk of both recurrent embolic ischaemic events and anticoagulant-associated haemorrhages remained fairly constant and cumulative during the relatively short period of follow-up (mean follow-up 2.3 years), and not confined to the early period after the initial event, it is suggested (but not proven) that anticoagulant treatment should be given for as long as possible, unless a contraindication occurs.

Antiplatelet (aspirin) therapy vs control

Among individuals in AF but no previous stroke, aspirin reduces the risk of first-ever stroke by about 22% (95% CI: 2–38%), from 5.2% (placebo) to 3.7% (aspirin) per year without any significant excess of intracranial haemorrhage (aspirin 0.16%, control 0.13%) or major extracranial bleeding (aspirin 0.5%, control 0.6%) (Antithrombotic Trialists' Collaboration, 2002).

Evidence

A systematic review identified one RCT which evaluated the effect of antiplatelet therapy compared with control for (secondary) prevention of recurrent stroke in people with NRAF and a previous TIA or ischaemic stroke (Koudstaal, 1996). A total 404 patients were randomly assigned aspirin (300 mg/day) and 378 placebo, and followed for a mean follow-up of 2.3 years.

Stroke   Random assignment to aspirin was not associated with any significant reduction in the risk of recurrent stroke (12% (placebo) vs 10% (aspirin) per year; OR: 0.89, 95% CI: 0.64–1.24) (Fig. 15.5).

Serious vascular events   Random assignment to aspirin was not associated with any significant reduction in the annual rate of all vascular events, including vascular death, recurrent stroke (ischaemic or haemorrhagic), myocardial infarction and systemic embolism (19% (placebo) vs 15% (aspirin) per year; OR: 0.84, 95% CI: 0.63–1.14) (Fig. 15.6).

These estimates suggest that aspirin may prevent about 40 vascular events (of all types) per 1000 patients treated for 1 year.

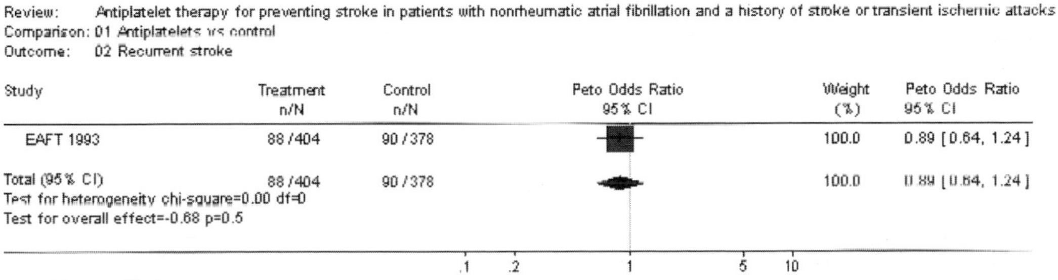

Review: Antiplatelet therapy for preventing stroke in patients with nonrheumatic atrial fibrillation and a history of stroke or transient ischemic attacks
Comparison: 01 Antiplatelets vs control
Outcome: 02 Recurrent stroke

Study	Treatment n/N	Control n/N	Peto Odds Ratio 95% CI	Weight (%)	Peto Odds Ratio 95% CI
EAFT 1993	88 /404	90 /378		100.0	0.89 [0.64, 1.24]
Total (95% CI)	88 /404	90 /378		100.0	0.89 [0.64, 1.24]

Test for heterogeneity chi-square=0.00 df=0
Test for overall effect=-0.68 p=0.5

.1   .2   1   5   10

Figure 15.5   Forest plot showing the effects of *antiplatelet therapy vs control* in patients with NRAF and a history of stroke or TIA on *stroke* at the end of follow-up. Reproduced from Koudstaal (1996), with permission from the authors and John Wiley & Sons Limited. Copyright Cochrane Library, reproduced with permission.

Review: Antiplatelet therapy for preventing stroke in patients with nonrheumatic atrial fibrillation and a history of stroke or transient ischemic attacks
Comparison: 01 Antiplatelets vs control
Outcome: 01 All vascular events

Study	Treatment n/N	Control n/N	Peto Odds Ratio 95% CI	Weight (%)	Peto Odds Ratio 95% CI
EAFT 1993	130 /404	136 /378		100.0	0.84 [0.63, 1.14]
Total (95% CI)	130 /404	136 /378		100.0	0.84 [0.63, 1.14]

Test for heterogeneity chi-square=0.00 df=0
Test for overall effect=-1.12 p=0.3

.1   .2   1   5   10

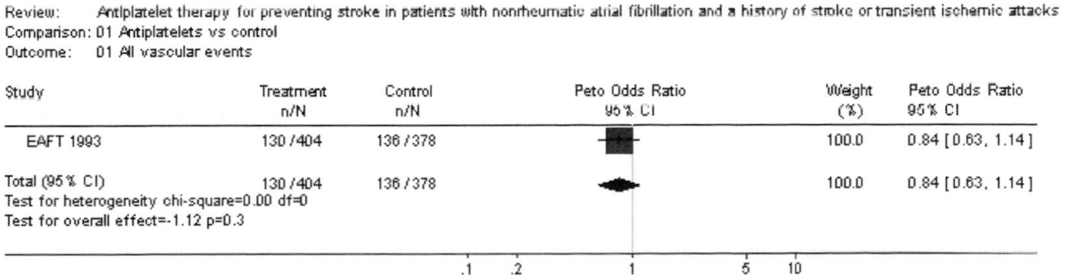

Figure 15.6   Forest plot showing the effects of *antiplatelet therapy vs control* in patients with NRAF and a history of stroke or TIA on *serious vascular events* at the end of follow-up. Reproduced from Koudstaal (1996), with permission from the authors and John Wiley & Sons Limited. Copyright Cochrane Library, reproduced with permission.

Bleeding   The incidence of major bleeding events, requiring hospitalisation, blood transfusion or surgical treatment, was low (0.9% per year for aspirin vs 0.7% for placebo) (Figs 15.7–15.8).

Comment

Aspirin may modestly reduce the risk of vascular events in people with NRAF, but the effect shown in the single trial was not statistically significant.

Anticoagulation (warfarin) vs antiplatelet (aspirin) therapy

Evidence

A systematic review identified two RCTs comparing the effect of anticoagulants with antiplatelet agents, for secondary prevention, in people with NRAF and previous TIA or minor ischaemic stroke (Van Walraven *et al.*, 2002; Saxena and Koudstaal, 2003, 2005).

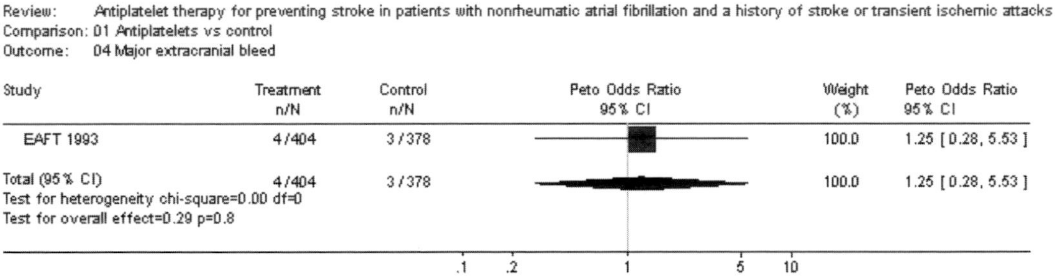

Review: Antiplatelet therapy for preventing stroke in patients with nonrheumatic atrial fibrillation and a history of stroke or transient ischemic attacks
Comparison: 01 Antiplatelets vs control
Outcome: 04 Major extracranial bleed

Study	Treatment n/N	Control n/N	Peto Odds Ratio 95% CI	Weight (%)	Peto Odds Ratio 95% CI
EAFT 1993	4 / 404	3 / 378		100.0	1.25 [0.28, 5.53]
Total (95% CI)	4 / 404	3 / 378		100.0	1.25 [0.28, 5.53]

Test for heterogeneity chi-square=0.00 df=0
Test for overall effect=0.29 p=0.8

.1   .2   1   5   10

Figure 15.7   Forest plot showing the effects of *antiplatelet therapy vs control* in patients with NRAF and a history of stroke or TIA on *major extracranial bleeding* complications at the end of follow-up. Reproduced from Koudstaal (1996), with permission from the authors and John Wiley & Sons Limited. Copyright Cochrane Library, reproduced with permission.

Review: Antiplatelet therapy for preventing stroke in patients with nonrheumatic atrial fibrillation and a history of stroke or transient ischemic attacks
Comparison: 01 Antiplatelets vs control
Outcome: 03 Any intracranial bleed

Study	Treatment n/N	Control n/N	Peto Odds Ratio 95% CI	Weight (%)	Peto Odds Ratio 95% CI
EAFT 1993	2 / 404	1 / 378		100.0	1.83 [0.19, 17.63]
Total (95% CI)	2 / 404	1 / 378		100.0	1.83 [0.19, 17.63]

Test for heterogeneity chi-square=0.00 df=0
Test for overall effect=0.52 p=0.6

.1   .2   1   5   10

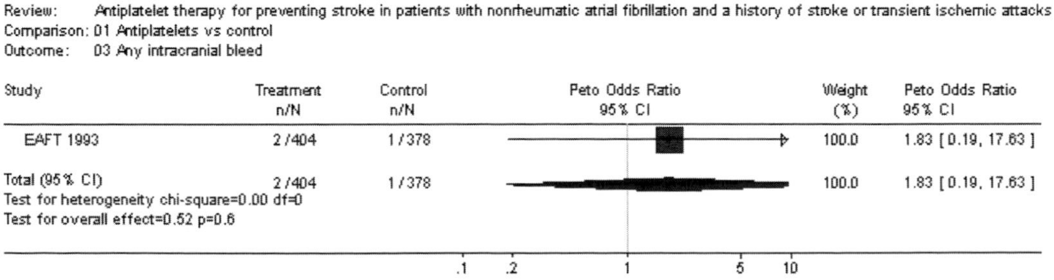

Figure 15.8   Forest plot showing the effects of *antiplatelet therapy vs control* in patients with NRAF and a history of stroke or TIA on *intracranial bleeding complications* at the end of follow-up. Reproduced from Koudstaal (1996), with permission from the authors and John Wiley & Sons Limited. Copyright Cochrane Library, reproduced with permission.

The EAFT randomised 455 patients within 3 months of TIA or minor stroke to receive either anticoagulants (INR: 2.5–4.0), or aspirin (300 mg/day) for a mean follow-up period of 2.3 years.

The Studio Italiano Fibrillazione Atriale (SIFA) trial randomised 916 patients with NRAF and a TIA or minor stroke within the previous 15 days to open-label anticoagulants (INR: 2.0–3.5) or indobufen (a reversible platelet cyclo-oxygenase inhibitor, 100 or 200 mg bid) for a follow-up period of 1 year.

Stroke   The combined results show that anticoagulants were significantly more effective than antiplatelet therapy in reducing the odds of recurrent stroke by about half (OR: 0.49, 95% CI: 0.33–0.72) (Fig. 15.9).

Serious vascular events   Anticoagulants were also significantly more effective than antiplatelet therapy in reducing the odds of all vascular events by about one-third (OR: 0.67, 95% CI: 0.50–0.91) (Fig. 15.10).

Bleeding   Anticoagulants increased the odds of major extracranial bleeding complications by about 5-fold compared with antiplatelet therapy (OR: 5.16, 95% CI: 2.08–12.83), but the absolute difference was small (2.8% per year (oral anticoagulants) vs 0.9% per year (antiplatelet therapy) in EAFT and 0.9% per year (oral anticoagulants) vs 0% (antiplatelet therapy) in SIFA) (Fig. 15.11).

Warfarin did not cause a significant increase of intracranial bleeds (Fig. 15.12).

Comment

Interpretation of the evidence   The evidence from two trials suggests that anticoagulant therapy is more effective than antiplatelet therapy for the prevention of

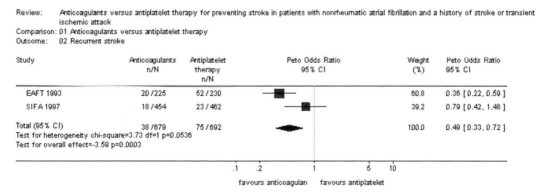

Figure 15.9   Forest plot showing the effects of *oral anticoagulants vs antiplatelet therapy* in patients with NRAF and a history of stroke or TIA on *recurrent stroke* at the end of follow-up. Reproduced from Saxena and Koudstaal (2003), with permission from the authors and John Wiley & Sons Limited. Copyright Cochrane Library, reproduced with permission.

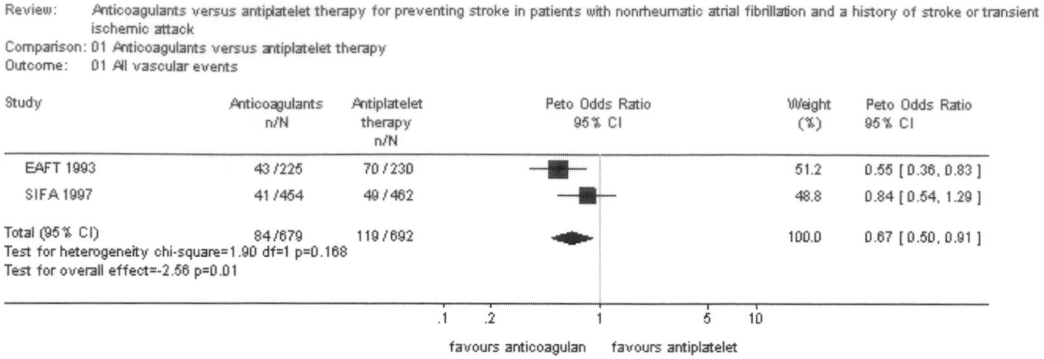

Review: Anticoagulants versus antiplatelet therapy for preventing stroke in patients with nonrheumatic atrial fibrillation and a history of stroke or transient
            ischemic attack
Comparison: 01 Anticoagulants versus antiplatelet therapy
Outcome: 01 All vascular events

Study	Anticoagulants n/N	Antiplatelet therapy n/N	Peto Odds Ratio 95% CI	Weight (%)	Peto Odds Ratio 95% CI
EAFT 1993	43 /225	70 /230		51.2	0.55 [0.36, 0.83]
SIFA 1997	41 /454	49 / 462		48.8	0.84 [0.54, 1.29]
Total (95% CI)	84/679	119/692		100.0	0.67 [0.50, 0.91]

Test for heterogeneity chi-square=1.90 df=1 p=0.168
Test for overall effect=-2.56 p=0.01

.1   .2   1   5   10

favours anticoagulan   favours antiplatelet

Figure 15.10 Forest plot showing the effects of *oral anticoagulants vs antiplatelet therapy* in patients
with NRAF and a history of stroke or TIA on *serious vascular events* at the end of
follow-up. Reproduced from Saxena and Koudstaal (2003), with permission from the
authors and John Wiley & Sons Limited. Copyright Cochrane Library, reproduced with
permission.

Review: Anticoagulants versus antiplatelet therapy for preventing stroke in patients with nonrheumatic atrial fibrillation and a history of stroke or transient
            ischemic attack
Comparison: 01 Anticoagulants versus antiplatelet therapy
Outcome: 04 Major extracranial bleed

Study	Antocoagulants n/N	Antiplatelet therapy n/N	Peto Odds Ratio 95% CI	Weight (%)	Peto Odds Ratio 95% CI
EAFT 1993	13 /225	2 /230		78.5	4.65 [1.66, 12.99]
SIFA 1997	4 /454	0 / 462		21.5	7.57 [1.06, 53.92]
Total (95% CI)	17/679	2/692		100.0	5.16 [2.08, 12.83]

Test for heterogeneity chi-square=0.19 df=1 p=0.666
Test for overall effect=3.53 p=0.0004

.1   .2   1   5   10

favours anticoagulan   favours antiplatelet

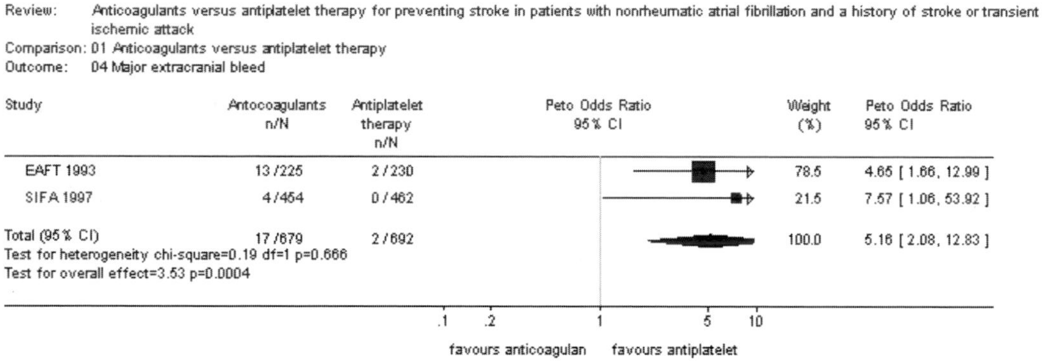

Figure 15.11 Forest plot showing the effects of *oral anticoagulants vs antiplatelet therapy* in patients with
NRAF and a history of stroke or TIA on *major extracranial bleeds* at the end of follow-up.
Reproduced from Saxena and Koudstaal (2003), with permission from the authors and
John Wiley & Sons Limited. Copyright Cochrane Library, reproduced with permission.

stroke in people with NRAF and recent non-disabling stroke or TIA despite a higher
risk of extracranial bleeding with anticoagulant therapy than with antiplatelet
therapy.

These results are consistent with a recently published individual patient meta-
analysis of 4052 patients with NRAF with (24%) or without (76%) a previous
stroke or TIA from six published randomised trials, in which oral anticoagulants were
compared with aspirin (Van Walraven *et al.*, 2002). Compared with aspirin, oral
anticoagulant significantly decreased the risk of all strokes, ischaemic strokes and
cardiovascular events but modestly increased the absolute risk of major bleeding.

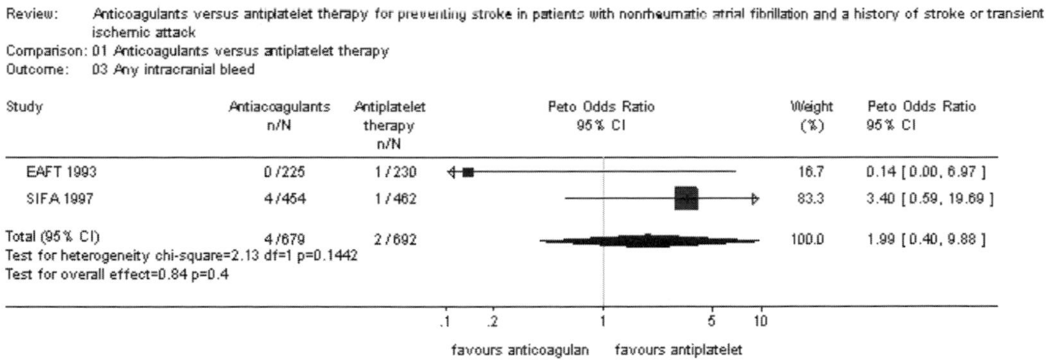

Review: Anticoagulants versus antiplatelet therapy for preventing stroke in patients with nonrheumatic atrial fibrillation and a history of stroke or transient ischemic attack
Comparison: 01 Anticoagulants versus antiplatelet therapy
Outcome: 03 Any intracranial bleed

Study	Antiacoagulants n/N	Antiplatelet therapy n/N	Peto Odds Ratio 95% CI	Weight (%)	Peto Odds Ratio 95% CI
EAFT 1993	0 /225	1 /230		16.7	0.14 [0.00, 6.97]
SIFA 1997	4 /454	1 /462		83.3	3.40 [0.59, 19.69]
Total (95% CI)	4 /679	2 /692		100.0	1.99 [0.40, 9.88]

Test for heterogeneity chi-square=2.13 df=1 p=0.1442
Test for overall effect=0.84 p=0.4

.1   .2   1   5   10

favours anticoagulan   favours antiplatelet

Figure 15.12 Forest plot showing the effects of *oral anticoagulants vs antiplatelet therapy* in patients with NRAF and a history of stroke or TIA on *intracranial bleeds* at the end of follow-up. Reproduced from Saxena and Koudstaal (2003), with permission from the authors and John Wiley & Sons Limited. Copyright Cochrane Library, reproduced with permission.

The relative risk reduction was similar to patients with a history of previous stroke or TIA, but was smaller in absolute terms because of the higher risk of recurrent stroke those with a history of stroke or TIA. For patients treated with aspirin, the risk of stroke was 10% per year in those with a previous stroke compared with only 2.7% per year in those without, and oral anticoagulation reduced these risks from 10% to 4%, and from 2.7% to 1.5%, per year, respectively (Van Walraven *et al.*, 2002).

Implications for practice   These results imply that anticoagulants should be prescribed to patients with NRAF and a recent TIA or minor ischaemic stroke if at all possible.

For patients with a contraindication for anticoagulant treatment, aspirin is a safe, but significantly less effective alternative.

Implications for research   Future research should aim to further refine the estimates of the relative effectiveness and safety of anticoagulation compared with antiplatelet therapy in acute ischaemic stroke due to embolism from the heart associated with AF; to improve stratification of the risks of recurrent cardioembolic stroke and intra- and extracranial haemorrhagic complications; and to determine whether combination therapy of aspirin plus anticoagulants is more effective and acceptably safe compared with either drug alone.

The Atrial fibrillation Clopidogrel Trial with Irbesartan for prevention of Vascular Events (ACTIVE) trial aims to determine whether the combination of clopidogrel 75 mg/day plus aspirin 75–100 mg/day is *superior* to aspirin among patients who are not suitable for anticoagulation (ACTIVE A).

Other antithrombotic regimens vs warfarin

Limitations of warfarin

The main limitation of oral vitamin K antagonists such as warfarin is that they cause twice as many intra- and extracranial haemorrhages as aspirin (see above), particularly in patients with a history of bleeding, the elderly, and those with common polymorphisms for genes encoding the hepatic microsomal enzyme CYP2C9 (Furuya *et al.*, 1995) and the factor IX propeptide (Oldenburg *et al.*, 1997). The excess bleeding associated with warfarin can be attributed in part to its narrow therapeutic window and numerous interactions with other drugs and foods (Hirsh *et al.*, 2001). Other practical limitations to long-term warfarin therapy are its need for regular coagulation monitoring and dose adjustment, its slow onset and offset of action, and the risk of foetal malformations. As a result, only one-third to one half of patients with AF who are appropriate candidates for warfarin therapy actually receive it (Peterson *et al.*, 2002; Bo *et al.*, 2003).

Possible alternatives to warfarin

Other regimens have been, or are being, compared with adjusted dose warfarin in patients with AF.

Ximelagatran   The Stroke Prevention using the ORal direct Thrombin Inhibitor ximelagatran in patients with non-valvular atrial Fibrillation (SPORTIF) III and V trials randomised a total of 7320 patients with non-valvular AF (persistent or paroxysmal) who had at least one additional risk factor for stroke into an open-label (SPORTIF III) and double-blind (SPORTIF V) RCTs of fixed dose ximelagatran 36 mg bid or adjusted-dose warfarin (INR: 2.0–3.0) (Executive Steering Committee on behalf of the SPORTIF III Investigators, 2003; SPORTIF executive steering committee for the SPORTIF V Investigators, 2005). The pooled results of the SPORTIF III and V trials demonstrated no significant difference in the risk of stroke or systemic embolism between ximelagatran (2.5%) and warfarin (2.5%) during a mean of 17 or 20 months of follow up, respectively (Eikelboom and Hankey, 2004; Hankey *et al.*, 2004). Both trials fulfilled the criterion for non-inferiority. However, ximelagatran significantly *reduced the risk of major bleeding* compared with warfarin (2.5% ximelagatran, 3.4% warfarin during a mean or 17 or 20 months of treatment in the SPORTIF III and V trials, respectively; estimated annualised ARR: 0.6%, number needed to treat (NNT) for 1 year to avoid one major bleed: 167) and *increased the risk of transiently elevated liver alanine-aminotransferase (ALT) enzymes* (6.1% ximelagatran, 0.8% warfarin; absolute risk increase (ARI) 5.3%, NNT with ximelagatran to harm (NNH) with increased ALT: 19). Raised ALT typically occurred 2–6 months after initiation of ximelagatran but was asymptomatic, transient (returning to baseline spontaneously or after cessation of treatment) and without sequelae in all cases reported in the SPORTIF trials (Lee *et al.*, 2005).

The advantages of ximelagatran are that it reduces the risk of major bleeding compared with warfarin and can be administered orally with a rapid onset of action. It has a predictable pharmacokinetic profile (uninfluenced by the patients age, sex, weight, ethnicity or food intake), and therefore it is not necessary to adjust the dose (except for patients with renal dysfunction in whom a decrease in dose or longer dosing interval is likely to be required) or monitor anticoagulation activity. Furthermore, ximelagatran has a wider therapeutic margin than warfarin, and a low potential for food and drug interactions.

The disadvantages of ximelagatran are the need for twice daily administration, excess occurrence of adverse hepatic effects in 6% of patients (thus potentially requiring monitoring of liver function for up to 6 months after treatment initiation), and the need to estimate creatinine clearance (because ximelagatran is primarily eliminated by the kidneys and data in patients with renal dysfunction are limited). In addition, the cost of ximelagatran for the patient and community is likely to be higher than warfarin.

There are two ongoing trials which are evaluating the relative safety and effectiveness of other antithrombotic strategies for preventing stroke and systemic embolism in patients with AF.

Idraparinux   The AF trial of Monitored, Adjusted Dose vitamin K antagonist, comparing Efficacy and safety with Unadjusted SanOrg 34006/idraparinux (AMADEUS) study is a multicentre, randomised, open-label, assessor-blind, trial which aims to determine whether once-weekly subcutaneous idraparinux (SanOrg34006, an inhibitor of activated factor X (Xa)) is *not inferior* to adjusted-dose oral vitamin K antagonists.

Clopidogrel plus aspirin   The ACTIVE trial aims to determine whether the combination of clopidogrel 75 mg/day plus aspirin 75–100 mg/day is *not inferior* to adjusted-dose oral vitamin K antagonist among patients who are suitable for anticoagulation (ACTIVE W).

Warfarin plus aspirin   Among all patients with TIA and ischaemic stroke, about 15% have AF, and up to one-third of these have atherothromboembolism as the cause of the stroke, and another substantial proportion also have ischaemic heart disease. These patients are therefore at risk of serious vascular events due to cardiogenic embolism and atherothromboembolism.

Antiplatelet therapy has been shown to effectively reduce the risk of recurrent serious vascular events due to presumed atherothromboembolism (see Chapter 10) and anticoagulation to effectively reduce the risk of stroke and systemic embolism due to AF. In theory, these patients would probably benefit from combination anticoagulation and antiplatelet therapy. However, it remains to be tested in large RCTs whether the theoretical benefits of combination therapy are real, and that they are not overshadowed by an excess risk of major bleeding. A small RCT compared the combination of triflusal (an antiplatelet drug which inhibits cyclo-oxygenase) and moderate intensity acenocumarol (an anticoagulant) in 235 patients in AF, with triflusal alone in 242 patients, and acenocumarol in 237 patients (Perez–Gomez, et al., 2004). After a median follow-up of 2.76 years, the primary outcome of stroke, systemic embolism or vascular death was lower among patients assigned combination therapy (0.92%) than triflusal (3.8%) or anticoagulation (2.7%) (HR: 0.33, 95% CI: 0.12–0.91, $P = 0.02$). There was no excess of severe bleeding with combination therapy (0.92% vs 1.80% anticoagulation, vs 0.35% antiplatelet therapy) (Perez–Gómez, et al., 2004).

Trials are to be encouraged comparing the 'gold standard' of warfarin with the combination of warfarin plus aspirin, or even perhaps better still, with the combination of warfarin plus clopidogrel, because of the lower rates of gastrointestinal (GI) haemorrhage with clopidogrel compared with aspirin (Chapter 10) in AF patients who have an ischaemic stroke or TIA due to presumed atherothromboembolism or who have concurrent ischaemic heart disease.

Patent foramen ovale

A patent foramen ovale (PFO) is a remnant of embryological development. It is common; echocardiographic and autopsy studies indicate that it fails to close completely after birth in about 25% (19–36%) of the general population, and is usually an incidental finding. The size of the defect varies from 1 to 19 mm (mean 4.9 mm), and is much like a flap valve, sealed closed by the higher pressure in the left atrium. However, at times of elevated right atrial pressure, blood may pass from the right atrium into the left atrium and, therefore, into the systemic arterial circulation.

This paradoxical route for venous embolic material to reach the systemic arterial circulation has been recognised by rare autopsy findings of thrombus straddling a PFO in the setting of a fatal stroke. Paradoxical embolism in the context of PFO has also been documented with stroke during pulmonary embolus, cerebral lesions from gas embolism in divers, and cerebral infarction from fat embolism post-orthopaedic trauma. However, these clinical settings are often associated with increased pressure in the right heart and therefore predispose to paradoxical embolism. Nevertheless, right-to-left shunting may occur with normal right heart pressures during normal respiration or the Valsalva manoeuvre.

The proposed mechanisms by which a PFO may cause a stroke include not only paradoxical embolisation, but also *in situ* thrombosis within the canal of the PFO, associated atrial dysrhythmias and concomitant hypercoagulable states (Horton and Bunch, 2004).

The possible predictors of an increased risk of stroke associated with a PFO are: larger size, greater shunting, association with an interseptal aneurysm (Mas *et al.*,

2001), evidence of a venous embolic source and clinical features supporting paradoxical embolism.

However, these parameters are yet to be confirmed, and indeed a clear relationship between PFO and stroke has yet to be proven (Tong and Becker, 2004). It is difficult, if not impossible, to reliably determine whether the presence of a PFO in a patient with an embolic ischaemic stroke is causal or coincidental. Furthermore, if it is thought to be causal, there is similar uncertainty as to how it should be treated, if at all.

Evidence

Several small uncontrolled studies suggest a relationship between PFO and stroke, but these studies may overestimate the association. A recent community-based case–control, study found a PFO in 20.8% of 519 randomly selected asymptomatic community-based controls and only 16.5% of 158 patients referred for evaluation of cryptogenic stroke, suggesting that there is no increase in the prevalence of PFO among patients with stroke compared with a random non-hospitalised reference population (Petty et al., 2003).

A systematic review identified six observational studies of medical therapy in a total of 895 patients with PFO (Khairy et al., 2003). The 1 year rate of recurrent neurological thromboembolism varied from 3.8% to 12.0%.

Most of these data came from two prospective multicentre observational studies of the risk of recurrent stroke in patients with PFO (Mas et al., 2001; Homma et al., 2002).

The French PFO-ASA Study Group registered 216 young patients (aged 18–55 years, mean 40 year) with PFO and cryptogenic stroke and 304 patients with cryptogenic stroke who did not have a PFO. All patients were treated with aspirin 300 mg/day. Over the next 4 years of follow-up, the rate of recurrent stroke was *lower* (2.3%) in patients with PFO than in those without a PFO (4.2%). Only patients with both a PFO and an atrial septal aneurysm (ASA) had an increased risk of recurrent stroke (15.2% at 4 years, OR: 4.17, 95% CI: 1.5–11.8) (Mas et al., 2001).

The second important study was the PFO in Cryptogenic Stroke Study (PICSS), which was a substudy of the Warfarin–Aspirin Recurrent Stroke Study (WARSS). The WARSS randomised 2206 patients with ischaemic stroke to either aspirin (325 mg/day) or adjusted-dose warfarin (target INR: 1.4–2.8), of whom 578 patients had cryptogenic stroke. There was no difference in recurrent ischaemic stroke among patients assigned aspirin or warfarin (Mohr et al., 2001). The PICSS evaluated 630 older stroke patients (aged 30–85 years, mean 59 years) in the WARSS trial by means of transoesophageal echocardiography (TOE) in a blinded fashion. They were randomised to either aspirin or adjusted-dose warfarin. Most of these 630 patients had cryptogenic (42%, $n = 265$) or lacunar (39%) stroke. Among the patients with TOE images adequate for analysis of PFO, a PFO was found in 39.2%

(98 of 250) of patients with cryptogenic stroke compared with 29.9% (105 of 351) of patients with a known cause of stroke ($P < 0.02$). Large PFOs were found in 20.0% (50 of 250) of patients with cryptogenic stroke compared with 9.7% (34 of 351) of those with a known stroke origin ($P < 0.001$). However, during the 2-year study the presence or absence of a PFO did not significantly affect the rate of recurrent stroke or death, regardless of aspirin or warfarin therapy (hazard ratio: 0.96, 95% CI: 0.62–1.48, $P > 0.2$) (Homma et al., 2002; Mohr, 2003). A similar lack of effect was found for the subset of patients with cryptogenic stroke (hazard ratio: 1.17, 95% CI: 0.60–2.37, $P > 0.2$).

Antithrombotic therapy

The role of antithrombotic therapy for the prevention of stroke associated with PFO is uncertain because of the absence of reliable evidence from RCTs.

The PICSS is the only RCT, albeit a substudy of a larger trial (WARSS), and it reported no significant different in the incidence of recurrent stroke or death among patients with PFO (aspirin 13.2%, warfarin 18.5%, $P = 0.49$) and patients without PFO (aspirin 17.4%, warfarin 13.4%, $P = 0.40$) assigned aspirin or warfarin. Among the 265 patients with cryptogenic stroke, the incidence of recurrent stroke or death among patients with PFO (aspirin 17.9%, warfarin 9.5%, $P = 0.28$) and patients without PFO (aspirin 16.3%, warfarin 8.3%, $P = 0.40$) was about 50% lower in patients assigned warfarin, but this difference did not reach statistical significance. The lower rate of stroke recurrence in patients taking warfarin was not influence by the presence of a PFO (9.5% with a PFO, 8.3% without a PFO). The size of the PFO and the presence of ASA also did not influence these findings (Homma et al., 2002). Indeed, larger PFOs were associated with a lower, not a higher, overall rate of recurrent stroke or death (18.5% small PFOs, 9.5% larger PFOs), in contrast to common reasoning that larger septal defects should be associated with higher risks of stroke.

Surgical closure of PFO

Open surgical closure of a PFO has not been evaluated by RCTs. Prospective observational studies suggest that some patients continue to experience recurrent stroke after surgical closure (indicating that the PFO may not have been the cause of the index stroke) (Homma et al., 1997) whereas others do not (Devuyst et al., 1996).

Transcatheter closure of PFO

In view of the morbidity of open-heart surgery, catheter-based approaches to PFO are an attractive alternative. Successful percutaneous implantation of PFO closure devices such as PFO-star device (Braun et al., 2002), the clamshell septal occluder (Hung et al., 2000) and other devices (Windecker et al., 2000; Martin et al., 2002) have been described.

A systematic review identified 10 observational studies of transcatheter closure for PFO in a total of 1355 patients (Khairy *et al.*, 2003).

The incidence of major complications was 1.5% and minor complications 7.9%. Peri-procedural complications included early device migration (requiring surgical intervention) and cardiac tamponade (requiring peri-cardiocentesis) (Martin *et al.*, 2002). Long-term complications included device malalignment and significant shunt (Martin *et al.*, 2002).

Overall, the 1-year rate of recurrent neurological thromboembolism with trans-catheter intervention was 0–4.9% (Hung *et al.*, 2000; Windecker *et al.*, 2000; Braun *et al.*, 2002; Martin *et al.*, 2002). As this rate may be no less than with best medical therapy alone (see results for literature controls above) after adjusting for differences in case mix, definitions, and vigilance of follow-up, it emphasises the need for RCTs to evaluate the relative risks and benefits of percutaneous trans-catheter closure of PFO.

A post-procedural shunt has been reported in one study to be a predictor of recurrent paradoxical embolism (relative risk: 4.2, 95% CI: 1.1–17.8) (Windecker *et al.*, 2000).

Comment

Interpretation of the evidence

Observational case series show that some stroke patients with PFO continue to have recurrent strokes, irrespective of whether they have been treated with aspirin (Homma *et al.*, 2002; Mas *et al.*, 2001), warfarin (Homma *et al.*, 2002), or surgical or percutaneous transcatheter closure (Hung *et al.*, 2000; Windecker *et al.*, 2000; Braun *et al.*, 2002; Martin *et al.*, 2002), presumably because the treatments are ineffective or there are other causes of stroke and the PFO may have been an innocent bystander.

However, the *relative* risks and benefits of these interventions (anatomical closure vs oral anticoagulation vs antiplatelet therapy vs no active treatment) for PFO remain uncertain due to the lack of reliable evidence from large RCTs.

Implications for clinicians

Given that secondary preventive measures (e.g. anatomical closure, warfarin, aspirin) are not without risk, the challenge is to identify patients in whom the PFO is causative and, therefore, who may gain benefit from anatomical closure or antithrombotic therapy. Those in whom the PFO is 'innocent' are unlikely to benefit from interventions targeted to the PFO, and closure of a PFO will not prevent embolism from the legs to the lungs in a patient with a treatable cause of deep venous thrombosis (e.g. thrombophilias).

While a patient preference of a 'once off' mechanical solution is intuitively appealing, it cannot yet be recommended until results of randomised trials are available.

In the absence of reliable evidence, the optimal approach is to be able to accurately identify high-risk patients and randomise them in a large RCT to device closure of the PFO by an experienced interventionalist or to long-term anticoagulant or antiplatelet therapy (see below) (Saver *et al.*, 2005). However, if such a trial is not available and accessible, one approach is to use standard antiplatelet therapy in patients with a PFO alone, without spontaneous shunting and a first event, and device closure by an experienced interventionalist for patients with a spontaneous right-to-left shunt and an associated ASA (Donnan and Davis, 2004). After percutaneous PFO closure, patients are usually treated empirically with aspirin indefinitely and with clopidogrel for 6 months.

In the USA, percutaneous PFO closure is permitted under a Food and Drug Administration (FDA) Humanitarian Device Exemption which states: The Cardio-SEAL Septal Occlusion System is indicated for the closure of a PFO in patients with recurrent crytogenic stroke due to presumed paradoxical embolism through a PFO and who have failed conventional drug therapy. Cryptogenic stroke is defined as a stroke occurring in the absence of potential phanerogenic cardiac, pulmonary, vascular or neurological sources. Conventional drug therapy is defined as a therapeutic INR on oral anticoagulants (US Food and Drug Administration, 2000).

Implications for researchers

Studies are required to better characterise which patients with PFO may be at sufficiently high risk of stroke to warrant costly and risk therapeutic interventions such as closure of the PFO or anticoagulation (e.g. is ASA really an adverse prognostic factor, is increasing age a protective factor? (Jones *et al.*, 1994)), and these patients then need to be randomised in large controlled trials to these interventions and followed-up over several years for the occurrence of important outcome events such as recurrent stroke and death which are reported and evaluated by observers blinded to the treatment allocation.

The REcurrent Stroke comparing PFO closure to Established Current standard of care Treatment (RESPECT) trial is a randomised, active control, blinded adjudicated outcome trial which aims to determine whether percutaneous PFO closure is superior to current standard medical treatment in the prevention of recurrent embolic stroke (Saver *et al.*, 2004). A total of 500 patients with PFO who have had a cryptogenic stroke due to presumed paradoxical embolism within the previous 90 days will be randomised to best medical therapy ($n = 250$) or best medical therapy plus PFO closure with the AMPLATZER PFO occluder ($n = 250$) and followed for the occurrence of recurrent non-fatal stroke, peri-procedural death and fatal stroke. Enrollment began in August 2003.

The patient-controlled (PC) trial is a randomised clinical trial comparing the efficacy of percutaneous closure of PFO using the amplatzer PFO occluder with best medical treatment (life-long anticoagulation or aspirin) in patients with cryptogenic embolism to the brain or peripheries (Mattle et al., 2005) (protocol see: http://www.drabo.de/dl/pctrial_ch.pdf). Warfarin for 6 months followed by aspirin is recommended as medical treatment. The primary outcome events are subsequent death, non-fatal stroke and peripheral embolism in the long term. Recruitment commenced in February 2000, and 211 patients had been randomised by November, 2004. The target sample size is 410 patients.

Infective endocarditis

Infective endocarditis causes ischaemic stroke or TIA in about one fifth of patients. The cause is embolism of valvular vegetations. Although TIA and stroke may be the initial manifestation, it more commonly manifests in patients who are unwell with uncontrolled infection (Jones and Siekert, 1989; Hart et al., 1990; Salgado, 1991; Moreillon and Que, 2004).

Infective endocarditis may also be complicated by haemorrhagic transformation of an infarct, sometimes as a consequence of unwise anticoagulation, and intracerebral or subarachnoid haemorrhage, due to a pyogenic vasculitis and vessel wall necrosis, or mycotic aneurysm(s) of the distal branches of the middle cerebral artery (Masuda et al., 1992; Krapf et al., 1999). Other non-stroke, neurological complications of infective endocarditis include meningitis; a diffuse encephalopathy, perhaps as a result of showers of small emboli; acute mononeuropathy; rarely, cerebral abscess; discitis and headache (Jones and Siekert, 1989; Kanter and Hart, 1991).

Patients with active endocarditis should not be treated with oral anticoagulants because of their high risk of intracerebral haemorrhage (Hart et al., 1995); bactericidal antibiotics with or without surgery (radical valve replacement, or vegetectomy and valve repair) are the cornerstone of therapy (Moreillon and Que, 2004).

The main indications for surgery comprise refractory cardiac failure caused by valvular insufficiency, persistent sepsis caused by a surgically removable focus or a valvular ring or myocardial abscess, and persistent life-threatening embolisation. Surgery for active endocarditis is associated with mortality rate of 8–16%, and actuarial survival rates of 75–76% at 5 years and 61% at 10 years (Moreillon and Que, 2004).

Mycotic aneurysms do not always rupture and tend to resolve with time so that, on balance, cerebral angiography to detect unruptured aneurysms with a view to surgery, and surgical repair of any asymptomatic aneurysm, are unnecessary (van der Meulen et al., 1992).

SUMMARY

Long-term anticoagulation with a vitamin K antagonist such as warfarin (target INR: 2.5, range 2.0–3.0) is the most effective treatment for patients with NRAF and recent ischaemic stroke or TIA to reduce recurrent stroke and systemic embolism. Compared with control, it reduces the odds of recurrent stroke by about two-thirds (OR: 0.36, 95% CI: 0.22–0.58) and the odds of all vascular events by almost half (OR: 0.55, 95% CI: 0.37–0.82) but increases the odds of major extracranial haemo-rrhage 4-fold (OR: 4.32, 95% CI: 1.55–12.10). The overall benefit to harm ratio is about 4.5 to 1 as oral anticoagulation saves 90 vascular events (80 recurrent strokes) and causes 21 major extracranial haemorrhages per 1000 patients treated per year.

Compared with aspirin, warfarin reduces the risk of serious vascular events by about one-third. Hence, for ischaemic stroke patients in AF who cannot, for what-ever reason, cope with anticoagulation, aspirin still offers some advantage.

Patients with TIA or very mild ischaemic strokes in AF can start oral anticoagu-lants within a day or so, but in patients with larger infarcts and high blood pressure anticoagulation should probably be delayed a week or two because of the risks of haemorrhagic transformation of the brain infarct.

A large PFO may be more common in cryptogenic stroke than stroke of known cause, but its presence may not increase the risk of recurrent stroke.
There is no reliable evidence to support or refute anticoagulation or closure of a PFO as a more effective strategy of stroke prevention than aspirin alone in patients with a PFO. Ongoing clinical trials are addressing this issue.

Infective endocarditis may be complicated by ischaemic stroke, haemorrhagic transformation of a brain infarct, and intracerebral or subarachnoid haemorrhage. The cause is septic embolism leading to focal cerebral ischaemia, pyogenic cere-bral vasculitis or mycotic aneurysm.

Patients with active endocarditis should not be treated with oral anticoagulants because of their high risk of intracerebral haemorrhage; bactericidal antibiotics (with or without valve surgery) are the mainstay of therapy.

Arterial dissection and arteritis

Arterial dissection

Extracranial arterial dissection can occur anywhere in the internal carotid artery (ICA) in the neck, but is unusual at the carotid bifurcation (the most common site for atheroma). In the vertebral artery it tends to affect the distal third. Sometimes carotid and vertebral dissection is a distal extension of aortic dissection.

Intracranial dissection is much rarer than extracranial dissection and more often appears to affect the vertebral and basilar arteries than the ICA and its branches.

Arterial dissection may be caused by trauma and even apparently trivial neck movement (Rothwell *et al.*, 2001). However, it may be spontaneous in patients with hereditary connective tissue disorders, in particular the vascular Ehler–Danlos syndrome (EDS) in which most patients carry mutations in the gene that encodes the pro-α1(III) collagen (Pepin *et al.*, 2000). Other causes include other subtypes of EDS (collagen defects due mostly to mutations in the pro-α1(V) and pro-α2(V) encoding genes), cystic medial necrosis, fibromuscular dysplasia, Marfan's syndrome, and α1 antitrypsin deficiency (Schievink *et al.*, 1998, 2001; Brandt and Grond-Ginsbach, 2002). Hyperhomocystinaemia and recent infection have also been suggested as possible causes (Grau *et al.*, 1999; Gallai *et al.*, 2001; Pezzini *et al.*, 2002).

Following a tear in the intima, blood penetrates the arterial wall to form an intra-mural haematoma of variable length, and this may expand with time. There may be one or more intimal tears so that the false and true lumens are in communication. Aneurysms sometimes form but seldom become symptomatic (Guillon *et al.*, 1999).

Dissection is the underlying stroke mechanism in about 2.5% of all strokes, and is the second leading cause of stroke in patients younger than 45 years of age. Ischaemic stroke and transient ischaemic attack (TIA) may be caused by occlusion of the true arterial lumen by the expanded vessel wall; occlusive and propagating thrombosis within the true lumen; and by embolism from thrombosis within the true lumen (O'Connell *et al.*, 1985). Usually only one artery is affected, but sometimes two or more appear to be affected simultaneously, perhaps because whatever caused the problem in one artery affected others at the same time (e.g. neck trauma, aortic arch dissection or even infection).

Intracranial dissection may not only present with ischaemic stroke but also subarachnoid haemorrhage, due to rupture of the aneurysmal bulging of the arterial adventitia, given the lack of external elastic lamina in the intradural section of the arteries, or dissection in the adventitial rather than medial layer of the arterial wall.

After the acute phase, remodelling and healing may, within a few months, lead to an arterial lumen which appears virtually normal (Mokri *et al.*, 1986; Sturzenegger *et al.*, 1995). In other cases, the artery remains occluded, but because the thrombus has probably been covered with endothelium, there is little risk of further thromboembolism.

Recurrence of symptomatic dissection, in the same or a different artery, is unusual; about 1% per annum, except in familial cases where it is more common (Leys *et al.*, 1995; Bassetti *et al.*, 1996; Schievink *et al.*, 1996). This argues against an underlying but as yet unrecognised abnormality of the arterial wall in most patients, and rather favours a 'one off' event such as trauma, although a combination of both is possible (Peters *et al.*, 1995).

The aim of treatment of patients with dissection of the extracranial carotid or vertebral arteries is to minimise adverse sequelae of any ischaemic stroke and prevent recurrent stroke by minimising arterial occlusion at the site of the dissection, and distal artery-to-artery embolisation of thrombus formed at the site of dissection.

Evidence

A systematic review for the Cochrane Library did not identify any randomised trials of antithrombotic drugs (Lyrer and Engelter, 2003, 2004).

A systematic review of the 26 non-randomised studies involving 327 patients who received with antiplatelet drugs or anticoagulants revealed there was no significant difference in the odds of death among patients who received antiplatelet drugs compared with anticoagulants (odds ratio (OR): 1.59, 95% confidence interval (CI): 0.22–11.59) (Lyrer and Engelter, 2003, 2004). There was also no significant difference in the odds of being dead or disabled comparing antiplatelet drugs with anticoagulants (OR: 1.94, 95% CI: 0.76–4.91) (Lyrer and Engelter, 2003, 2004). There were no intracranial haemorrhages reported for patients taking antiplatelet drugs and few (0.5%) among patients taking anticoagulants.

Comment

Interpretation of the evidence

There is no reliable evidence to support or refute the routine use of antithrombotic agents in patients with internal carotid or vertebral artery dissection. The available evidence does not reliably establish whether anticoagulants are more or less effective than antiplatelet drugs, or placebo, in these patients.

Implications for clinicians

Despite the lack of evidence of benefit from the trials of anticoagulants in ischaemic stroke in general (see Chapter 9), and the lack of any randomised evidence at all in patients with ischaemic stroke due to arterial dissection, many clinicians are still inclined to use anticoagulants. However, anticoagulants could increase bleeding into the dissected arterial wall, and therefore worsen the situation.

In a patient with a confirmed dissection, the factors which might justify the use of anticoagulants are sudden neurological deterioration presumed due to further embolism (after excluding other causes for deterioration such as cerebral herniation and pneumonia) and the presence of a coincidental prothrombotic state (e.g. acquired thrombophilia). Anticoagulants are probably to be avoided in patients who are clinically stable (or improving) and in whom the cerebral infarct is large and the blood pressure is high (and hence there is a high risk of haemorrhagic transformation).

In those patients with dissection who are anticoagulated, some clinicians find it helpful to re-image vessels non-invasively with ultrasound or magnetic resonance (MR) angiography a few months after the dissection and, if the vessel has returned to normal, they then stop any antithrombotic therapy. However, most clinicians do not routinely re-image the vessel before stopping treatment after a few months.

Implications for research

A randomised-controlled trial (RCT) including at least 1400 patients with internal carotid and vertebral artery dissection and comparing both aspirin and anticoagulants with control is needed.

Giant cell arteritis

Giant cell arteritis (GCA) (temporal arteritis) is probably the most common 'vasculitic' cause of ischaemic stroke but it still accounts for a very small minority ($<0.1\%$) of all ischaemic strokes.

Any medium or large artery may be affected (carotid, vertebral, coronary, femoral, aorta, etc.). The most commonly involved are the superficial temporal, occipital, and facial branches of the external carotid artery (which cause headache and facial pain, scalp tenderness and sometimes jaw claudication), the ophthalmic, posterior ciliary and central retinal arteries (which cause infarction of the optic nerve and retina), and the extradural vertebral and internal carotid arteries (which cause ischaemic stroke or TIAs) (Caselli et al., 1988; Hayreh, 2000). The intradural anterior, middle and posterior cerebral and basilar arteries and their branches are seldom affected.

Evidence

There have been no RCTs evaluating treatments for GCA.

Case series, when compared with literature, historical and concurrent controls, suggest that prompt treatment with corticosteroids is necessary to relieve symptoms and prevent blindness in patients with GCA (Swannell, 1997; Salvarani et al., 2002; Calvo-Romero, 2003). In the absence of reliable evidence, the use of non-steroidal anti-inflammatory drugs has been advocated in some cases, but most clinicians believe steroids to be necessary to achieve complete control of symptoms.

Initial therapy (empirical)

- Prednisolone 40–60 mg daily, as a single or divided dose (or pulsed intravenous (i.v.) methylprednisolone 1000 mg every day for 3 days may be considered for patients with recent or impending focal neurological dysfunction, such as visual loss).
- Maintain for 2–4 weeks.
- Then gradually reduce the dose every 1–2 weeks by 10% of the total daily dose (about 2.5–5 mg/day) until dose is 10 mg/day.
- Careful, frequent monitoring of clinical symptoms remains the best guide to management; the erythrocyte sedimentation rate (ESR) and C-reactive protein are not always reliable markers of disease activity although they correlate closely with symptoms in most patients.

Maintenance therapy (empirical)

- Prednisolone 5–7.5 mg/day for about 1–2 years.
- Then, if asymptomatic and ESR is normal, reduce dose gradually (e.g. by 1 mg/day every 2–3 months).

Comment

The response to steroids is usually rapid with resolution of many symptoms after a few days of therapy. A lack of improvement should alert clinicians to question the diagnosis.

There is a fine line between too rapidly reducing the dose of steroids, which leads to relapse, and too slowly reducing the dose, which leads to adverse effects such as hypertension, osteoporosis, skin fragility and diabetes mellitus.

Adverse effects of steroids are common and related to increasing age at diagnosis, female sex, the initial dose of prednisone of more than 40 mg/day, the total cumulative dose of at least 2 g of prednisone, and maintenance doses above 5 mg of prednisone a day. Calcium and vitamin D supplementation should be given with corticosteroid therapy in all patients. In patients with reduced bone mineral density, bisphosphonates are indicated (Salvarani et al., 2002).

There are no consistently reliable predictors to guide the duration of cortico-steroid therapy but most patients are still taking glucocorticoids after 2 years and up to half of them at 4 years. Judicious use of simple analgesia and non-steroidal anti-inflammatory drugs may help facilitate the withdrawal of steroids after about 2 years of stability on maintenance low-dose steroids.

For patients in whom reduction in corticosteroid dose is difficult (i.e. they need high doses of steroids to control active disease) or those who experience serious adverse effects of steroids, cytotoxic drugs such as methotrexate (7.5–20 mg/week) and azathioprine may allow a reduction in steroid dose. Intermittent cyclical etidronate may prevent some of the corticosteroid induced bone loss, if given when steroid treatment is begun. Alternate-day oral corticosteroid therapy is generally less effective in suppressing symptoms of GCA than daily administration (Salvarani *et al.*, 2002).

Primary angiitis of the central nervous system

Primary, or isolated, angiitis of the central nervous system (CNS) is rare. It affects the small leptomeningeal, cortical and spinal cord blood vessels. It may manifest clinically as a subacute multifocal or global encephalopathy or dementia, with or without stroke-like episodes due to focal or multifocal ischaemia, and sometimes haemorrhage, involving the brain, spinal cord or nerve roots (Hankey, 1991; Woolfenden *et al.*, 1998; Scolding *et al.*, 2002).

Evidence

There have been no RCTs of treatments for primary angiitis of the CNS.

Case series, compared with literature, historical and concurrent controls, suggest that prompt treatment with immunosuppressive therapy (e.g. corticosteroids with or without cyclophosphamide) may be effective (Hankey, 1991; Moore, 1998; Moore *et al.*, 1998). However, because the natural history of this condition is variable, it is difficult to distinguish any possible effects of treatment from the natural history.

Comment

As any evidence of effectiveness of treatments for CNS angiitis is anecdotal or inferred from clinical experience with systemic angiitis, the decision to treat and how to treat depend on the clinical condition of the patient, the course of the disease and the philosophies and experience of the attending clinician.

If the patient is stable, then time is available to allow a period of observation of the natural history of the disease. If the patient is unstable, and experiencing progressive or recurrent neurological deterioration, the attending clinician may feel compelled to initiate empirical immunosuppressive therapy whilst awaiting confirmation of the diagnosis of vasculitis by tissue biopsy.

Otherwise, a long-term course of anti-inflammatory and immunosuppressive therapy (with corticosteroids and/or cyclophosphamide), with its attendant risks, should ideally be withheld until the histological diagnosis of vasculitis is confirmed.

Induction therapy (empirical)

- Start with oral prednisolone 1 mg/kg/day (maximum dose 80 mg/day) or i.v. methylprednisolone 10 mg/kg/day. Rapidly reduce the dose of prednisolone by 50% over the first 2 weeks to 0.5 mg/kg/day, and by another 50% over the next 6 weeks so the patient is taking a dose of 0.25 mg/kg/day at week 8.

With/without

- Cyclophosphamide, 2 mg/kg/day orally, maximum dose 200 mg (reduce dose if age >60 years (reduce dose by 25%), age >70 years (reduce dose by 50%), infection or neutropenia).

Or

- Pulse cyclophosphamide can also be given as 10 pulses over 25 weeks (e.g. 0, 2, 4, 7, 10, 13 ….. 25 weeks) in a dose of 15 mg/kg i.v. Dose reductions must be made for increasing age and creatinine. White blood cell count (WBC) must be checked between day 10 and day 14 following pulse cyclophosphamide because the WBC count may decrease; if $<3 \times 10^9$/l, a suitable dose reduction must be made for the next pulse. If in remission after the first 6 pulses, methotrexate or azathioprine can be substituted for cyclophosphamide.
- Induction therapy is continued for 3 months following remission.

Maintenance therapy (empirical)

- Prednisolone, 5–10 mg/day.
- Azathioprine, 1.5 mg/kg/day, maximum dose 200 g.
- Alternatives to azathioprine include methotrexate, 0.15 mg/kg, maximum dose 15 mg once weekly (contraindicated in patients with creatinine >170 μmol/l), and mycophenolate mofetil.

Relapse therapy (empirical)

- *Major relapse*: return to initial induction therapy.
- *Minor relapse*: increase corticosteroid dose.

Strategies to minimise adverse effects of corticosteroids

- Calcium (1000 mg daily).
- Vitamin D 50,000 U one to three times weekly if 24-h urinary calcium excretion <120 mg (moniter for hypercalcaemia).
- Oestrogen replacement therapy if post-menopausal (despite small excess risk of thrombotic vascular events, see Chapter 14, pp 310–13).
- Calcitonin and bisphosphonates in patients with reduced bone mineral density.

- Hyperglycaemia, hypertension, oedema and hypokalaemia should be treated.
- Infections should be identified and treated early.
- Immunisations with influenza and pneumococcal vaccines are safe and should be given if disease is stable.

Toxicity of cyclophosphamide

- Nausea
- Alopecia
- Neutropenia
- Haemorrhagic cystitis
- Bladder cancer
- Infertility

Strategies to minimise adverse effects of cyclophosphamide

- Use lowest minimum effective doses of cyclophosphamide.
- Maintain fluid intake >3 l/day.
- Monitor the leucocyte count closely, keeping it above 3000/μl and the neutrophil count above 1500/μl.
- If severe neutropenia or bladder toxicity occurs despite low doses of cyclophosphamide and a fluid intake of >3 l/day, azathioprine 1–2 mg/kg/day or methotrexate can be used successfully with prednisone. A pulsed regimen of cyclophosphamide 10–15 mg/kg i.v. once every 4 weeks has less bladder toxicity than daily oral doses (1.5–2.5 mg/kg/day) but bone marrow suppression can be severe.

The role of antiplatelet agents and anticoagulants is uncertain.

SUMMARY

There is no reliable evidence to support or refute the routine use of antithrombotic agents in patients with internal carotid or vertebral artery dissection. The available evidence does not reliably establish whether anticoagulants are more or less effective than antiplatelet drugs, or placebo in these patients.

Long-term corticosteroids (with or without other immunomodulating therapies such as cyclophosphamide) are the mainstay of treatment for arteritis but their relative risks and benefits have not been evaluated in RCTs.

Treatment of intracerebral haemorrhage

Rupture of a blood vessel in the brain, resulting in intracerebral haemorrhage, causes immediate damage to neurones in the deep nuclei or cortex, and disruption of white matter tracts.

Direct mechanical compression of the brain tissue surrounding the haematoma and, to some extent, vasoconstrictor substances in extravasated blood, may compromise the local blood supply (Mendelow, 1993), and lead to cellular ischaemia which, in turn, leads to further swelling from cytotoxic, and later vasogenic, oedema. The zone of ischaemia around the haematoma may extend and swell through systemic factors such as hypoxia, hypotension and a loss of cerebral autoregulation in the vasculature supplying the region of the haematoma.

Haematomas adjacent to the ventricular system, such as cerebellar and large basal ganglia haematomas, may also directly compress the cerebrospinal fluid (CSF) pathway or rupture into the CSF pathway, and prevent outflow of the CSF from the brain, causing hydrocephalus (Ropper, 1986).

Due to the protective rigid encasement of the skull, the sudden increase in volume within the intracranial cavity due to the haemorrhage increases the intracranial pressure and threatens other parts of the brain, especially when the intracranial pressure reaches levels of the same order of magnitude as the arterial pressure, reducing the cerebral perfusion pressure close to zero.

About 25% of patients with intracerebral haematoma (ICH) die during the first day, and 40% within the first month, usually as a consequence of supratentorial haemorrhage large enough to cause transtentorial herniation, or haemorrhage in the posterior fossa causing direct brainstem compression and herniation upwards and downwards (Broderick *et al.*, 1999).

Survival and functional outcome depends on the following factors (Portenoy *et al.*, 1987; Daverat *et al.*, 1991; Tuhrim *et al.*, 1991; Lisk *et al.*, 1994):

- *Location of the haematoma*: worse outcome with posterior fossa, thalamic and putaminal haematoma, and intraventricular extension of blood.

- *Volume of the haematoma*: >50 ml, or volume of intraventricular haemorrhage >20 ml (Young *et al.*, 1990; Fogelholm *et al.*, 1997; Franke *et al.*, 1992; Hemphill *et al.*, 2001).
- *Level of consciousness on admission (e.g. Glasgow Coma Scale (GCS))*: stupor or coma is a grim prognostic sign except in thalamic haemorrhage.
- *Age of the patient*: worse prognosis in the elderly.
- *Pulse pressure.*
- *Extravasation of contrast material* during computerised tomography (CT) scanning is another relatively bad prognostic sign, probably reflecting ongoing haemorrhage (Becker *et al.*, 1999). A substantial (>33%) increase in ICH volume occurs in about 26% of patients within 1 h of onset and an additional 12% between 1 and 20 h (Brott *et al.*, 1997).
- *Later progression* of neurological signs and development of raised intracranial pressure.

Treatment

Decompressive surgical evacuation of supratentorial intracerebral haemorrhage

The four recognised surgical procedures to evacuate an ICH are simple aspiration, craniotomy with open surgery, endoscopic evacuation and stereotactic aspiration. Their use in clinical practice is inconsistent (Fernandes and Mendalow, 1999). In some countries (e.g. The Netherlands) they are rarely performed, in others (e.g. the USA) they are undertaken in about 20% of patients with ICH, and in others (e.g. some centres in Germany and Japan) they are offered to 50% or more of patients (Broderick *et al.*, 1994). Such wide variation in practice reflects uncertainty about the effectiveness and risks of surgery, due to a lack of appropriate evidence. The required evidence is evaluation by large randomised-controlled trials (RCTs).

Evidence

Simple aspiration
Simple aspiration was abandoned before it was properly evaluated because only small amounts of clot could be removed, and it could precipitate 'blind' re-bleeding.

Craniotomy with open surgery
A systematic review of five RCTs in a total of 305 patients indicated that craniotomy and open surgery combined with best medical therapy is associated with a non-significant increase in odds of death or dependency by 1.46 (95% confidence interval (CI): 0.87–2.45) compared with best medical therapy alone; surgery: $n = 114/147$ (77.6%); control: $n = 111/158$ (70.2%) (Figs 17.1 and 17.2) (McKissock *et al.*, 1961;

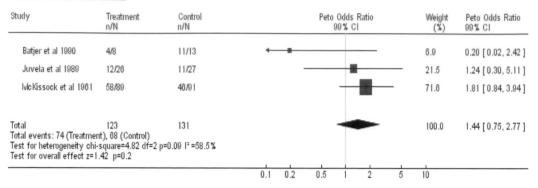

Review: Surgery for primary supratentorial intracerebral haemorrhage
Comparison: 01 Craniotomy plus medical vs medical: All trials
Outcome: 01 Death at six months

Figure 17.1   Forest plot showing the effects of *craniotomy vs no surgery* in acute primary supratentorial intracerebral haemorrhage on *death* at 6-month follow-up. Reproduced from Prasad and Shrivastava (1999), with permission from the authors and John Wiley & Sons Limited. Copyright Cochrane Library, reproduced with permission.

Review: Surgery for primary supratentorial intracerebral haemorrhage
Comparison: 01 Craniotomy plus medical vs medical: All trials
Outcome: 02 Death or dependence at six months

Study	Treatment n/N	Control n/N	Peto Odds Ratio 99% CI	Weight (%)	Peto Odds Ratio 99% CI
Batjer et al 1990	6/8	11/13		7.2	0.55 [0.03, 9.80]
Juvela et al 1989	25/26	22/27		12.2	4.20 [0.46, 38.34]
McKissock et al 1961	71/89	80/91		80.6	2.00 [0.85, 4.74]
Total	123	131		100.0	2.00 [0.92, 4.32]

Total events: 102 (Treatment), 93 (Control)
Test for heterogeneity chi-square=2.07 df=2 p=0.35 I²=3.5%
Test for overall effect z=2.31 p=0.02

0.1   0.2   0.5   1   2   5   10

Figure 17.2   Forest plot showing the effects of *craniotomy vs no surgery* in acute primary supratentorial intracerebral haemorrhage on *death or dependency* at 6-month follow-up. Reproduced from Prasad and Shrivastava (1999), with permission from the authors and John Wiley & Sons Limited. Copyright Cochrane Library, reproduced with permission.

Juvela *et al.*, 1989; Batjer *et al.*, 1990; Morgenstern *et al.*, 1998; Prasad and Shrivastava, 1999; Zuccarello *et al.*, 1999; Fernandes *et al.*, 2000).

After excluding the largest trial (McKissock *et al.*, 1961), because it was undertaken before CT brain scan, the four trials showed a modest non-significant

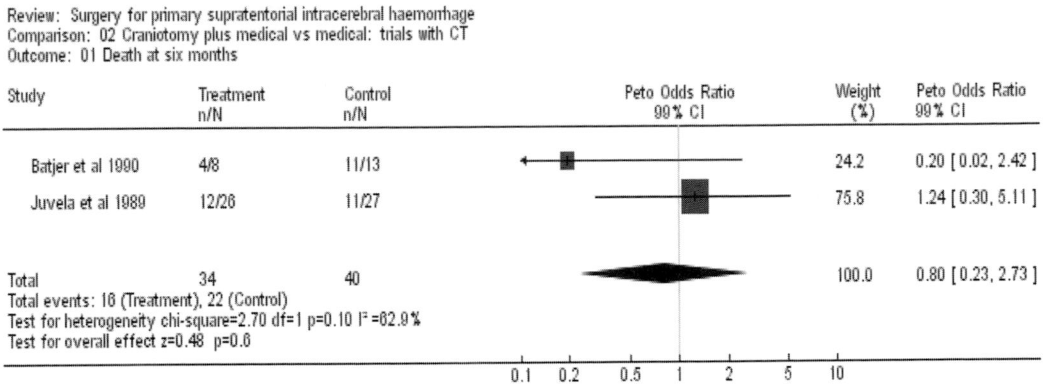

Review: Surgery for primary supratentorial intracerebral haemorrhage
Comparison: 02 Craniotomy plus medical vs medical: trials with CT
Outcome: 01 Death at six months

Study	Treatment n/N	Control n/N	Peto Odds Ratio 99% CI	Weight (%)	Peto Odds Ratio 99% CI
Batjer et al 1990	4/8	11/13		24.2	0.20 [0.02, 2.42]
Juvela et al 1989	12/26	11/27		75.8	1.24 [0.30, 5.11]
Total	34	40		100.0	0.80 [0.23, 2.73]

Total events: 16 (Treatment), 22 (Control)
Test for heterogeneity chi-square=2.70 df=1 p=0.10 I²=62.9%
Test for overall effect z=0.48 p=0.6

0.1   0.2   0.5   1   2   5   10

Figure 17.3   Forest plot showing the effects of *craniotomy vs no surgery* in acute primary supratentorial intracerebral haemorrhage on *death* at 6-month follow-up. Reproduced from Prasad and Shrivastava (1999), with permission from the authors and John Wiley & Sons Limited. Copyright Cochrane Library, reproduced with permission.

Review: Surgery for primary supratentorial intracerebral haemorrhage
Comparison: 02 Craniotomy plus medical vs medical: trials with CT
Outcome: 02 Death or dependence at six months

Study	Treatment n/N	Control n/N	Peto Odds Ratio 99% CI	Weight (%)	Peto Odds Ratio 99% CI
Batjer et al 1990	6/8	11/13		37.2	0.55 [0.03, 9.80]
Juvela et al 1989	25/26	22/27		62.8	4.20 [0.46, 38.34]
Total	34	40		100.0	1.97 [0.34, 11.40]

Total events: 31 (Treatment), 33 (Control)
Test for heterogeneity chi-square=2.07 df=1 p=0.15 I²=51.7%
Test for overall effect z=1.00 p=0.3

0.1   0.2   0.5   1   2   5   10

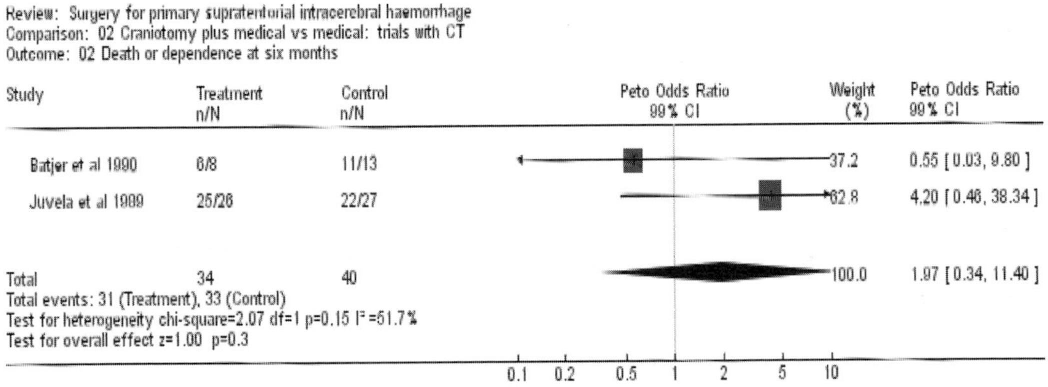

Figure 17.4   Forest plot showing the effects of *craniotomy vs no surgery* in acute primary supratentorial intracerebral haemorrhage on *death or dependency* at 6-month follow-up. Reproduced from Prasad and Shrivastava (1999), with permission from the authors and John Wiley & Sons Limited. Copyright Cochrane Library, reproduced with permission.

decrease in death or dependency (odds ratio (OR): 0.90, 95% CI: 0.40–2.03); surgery: 43/58 (74.1%); control: 51/67 (76.1%) (Figs 17.3 and 17.4) (Juvela *et al.*, 1989; Batjer *et al.*, 1990; Morgenstern *et al.*, 1998; Prasad and Shrivastava, 1999; Zuccarello *et al.*, 1999; Fernandes *et al.*, 2000).

International Surgical Trial in Intracerebral Haemorrhage   Subsequent to this review, the International Surgical Trial in Intracerebral Haemorrhage (International STICH) reported the results of an international multicentre randomised parallel group trial comparing a policy of 'early surgery' vs a policy of 'initial conservative treatment' in patients with spontaneous supratentorial ICHs (Mendelow *et al.*, 2005).

Among a total of 1033 patients from 83 centres in 27 countries, 503 patients were randomly allocated 'early surgery' and 530 'initial conservative treatment'. Patients were divided into a good and a poor prognosis group, based on their clinical status at randomisation.

At 6-month follow-up, 468 (93.0%) patients assigned 'early surgery' and 496 (93.8%) patients assigned 'initial conservative treatment' responded to a postal questionnaire sent directly to the patients.

The primary outcome measure was a favourable or unfavourable outcome as measured by the 8-point Glasgow Outcome Score (GOS) obtained by postal questionnaire. For the good prognosis group 'favourable outcome' was defined as 'good recovery' and 'moderate disability' on the GOS. For the poor prognosis group, 'favourable outcome' also included the upper level of severe disability (independence within the home). The same prognosis-based outcome methodology was used for the secondary outcome measures (Rankin and Barthel) and for the pre-specified subgroup analyses. All analyses were by 'intention to treat'.

The primary measure of efficacy, a favourable outcome at 6 months, was reported by 122 (26.1%) of the 468 patients assigned early surgery compared with 118 (23.8%) of the 496 patients assigned 'initial conservative treatment' group; OR: 0.89, 95% CI: 0.66–1.19, $P = 0.414$; absolute benefit 2.3% (95% CI: −3.2% to +7.7%); and relative benefit 10% (95% CI: −13% to +33%).

For the secondary outcomes, the absolute benefits were 1.2% (95% CI: −4.9 to +7.2%) for survival, 4.7% (95% CI: −1.2% to +10.5%) for a favourable prognosis based on the Rankin score (32.8% early surgery vs 28.1% initial conservative treatment); and 4.1% (95% CI: −1.4% to +9.5%) for a favourable prognosis based on the Barthel index (26.7% early surgery vs 22.6% initial conservative treatment).

The only significant interaction between treatment and any of the pre-specified subgroups was for depth of haematoma ($P = 0.020$). Patients in whom the haematoma was 1 cm or less from the cortical surface (one of the three minimisation criteria used at the time of randomisation through the Clinical Trials Service Unit in Oxford) were less likely to have an unfavourable outcome from early surgery (OR: 0.69, 95% CI: 0.47–1.01) than patients in whom the haematoma was more than 1 cm from the cortical surface (OR: 1.39, 95% CI: 0.86–2.25).

Endoscopic evacuation

One RCT indicated that endoscopic evacuation by stereotactic methods is associated with a statistically non-significant, but substantial, 54% (95% CI: −34% to 84%) reduction in odds of death or dependency; surgery: 28/50 (56%); control: 37/50

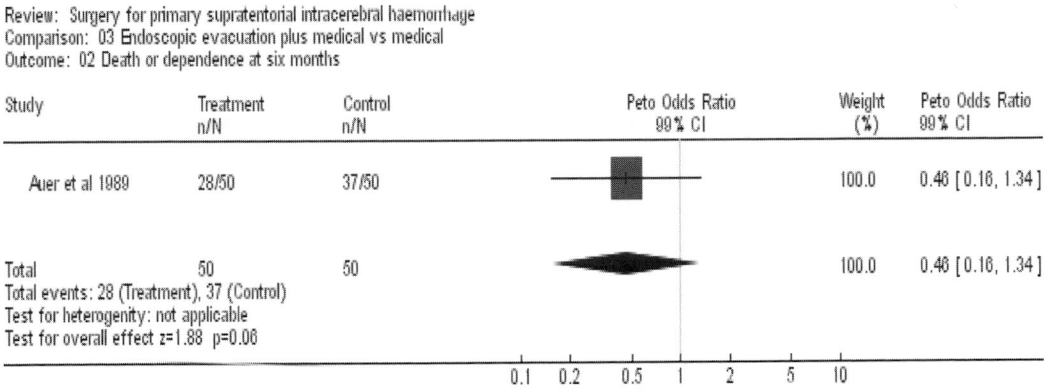

Review: Surgery for primary supratentorial intracerebral haemorrhage
Comparison: 03 Endoscopic evacuation plus medical vs medical
Outcome: 02 Death or dependence at six months

Study	Treatment n/N	Control n/N	Peto Odds Ratio 99% CI	Weight (%)	Peto Odds Ratio 99% CI
Auer et al 1989	28/50	37/50		100.0	0.46 [0.16, 1.34]
Total	50	50		100.0	0.46 [0.16, 1.34]

Total events: 28 (Treatment), 37 (Control)
Test for heterogenity: not applicable
Test for overall effect z=1.88 p=0.06

```
0.1   0.2    0.5    1    2    5   10
```

Figure 17.5   Forest plot showing the effects of *endoscopic evacuation vs no surgery* in acute primary supratentorial intracerebral haemorrhage on *death or dependency* at 6-month follow-up. Reproduced from Prasad and Shrivastava (2004), with permission from the authors and John Wiley & Sons Limited. Copyright Cochrane Library, reproduced with permission.

(74%) (Fig. 17.5) (Auer *et al.*, 1989). The absolute risk reduction was 18% (95% CI: −3% to 36%).

Stereotactic aspiration

The only RCT of CT-guided mechanical aspiration suggested a benefit but the number of patients was very small (Hosseini *et al.*, 2003). Among 37 patients with deep ICH of less than 24-h duration, 17 were randomised to medical treatment and 20 to stereotactic aspiration under general anaesthesia and CT control using a 2.5-mm diameter trocal (modified nucleosome). The mortality at 1 year was 52.9% among patients assigned medical treatment and 15% among patients assigned surgery (*P* = 0.017). Patients allocated surgery also had shorter length of intensive care stay (46.8 vs 24.3 days; *P* = 0.02), more rapid improvement in level of consciousness (*P* = 0.003 on day 24) and improved Karnofsky's score (*P* = 0.015). No complications related to the procedure were observed (Hosseini *et al.*, 2003).

A recent trial of stereotactic liquefaction of the blood clot by intracavity thrombolysis using plasminogen activator did not suggest a benefit from surgery (Teernstra *et al.*, 2003). A total of 71 patients with spontaneous supratentorial haematoma of >10 cm^3 volume were randomised within 72 h of onset to no surgery (*n* = 35) or surgery (*n* = 36). Surgery comprised insertion of a stereotactically placed catheter to instill urokinase to liquefy and drain the ICH in 6-h intervals over 48 h. Although stereotactic aspiration was associated with a reduction of haematoma volume by 18 ml over 7 days compared with control (relative reduction 34%), there was no difference in longer-term death or severe disability (modified Rankin scale score >5) at 180 days. After 180 days, the mortality rate was 56%

(20/36) among patients assigned surgery and 59% (20/34) among patients assigned no surgery (Teernstra *et al.*, 2003).

Comment

Interpretation of the evidence

It is sobering that surgical evacuation of ICH has been undertaken for nearly half a century on the basis of plausibility and general acceptance by the surgical community, without formal evaluation by the same regulatory standards that are applied to medical therapies. Although 'surgical studies with controls have tended to lack enthusiasm and surgical studies with enthusiasm have tended to lack controls' (David Sackett, 1985, personal communication), such double standards are no longer acceptable and the STICH trial investigators, and other trialists, are to be congratulated for their recent undertakings.

What can be deduced from the available evidence is that for patients with spontaneous supratentorial ICH in neurosurgical units, there is no evidence of an overall benefit with a policy of 'early surgery' when compared with 'initial conservative treatment'.

Implications for clinicians

There is insufficient evidence to justify a general policy of early operative intervention in patients with spontaneous supratentorial ICH, as opposed to one of initial conservative treatment.

Implications for research

Surgery, and particularly endoscopic stereotactic evacuation, *may* be effective and relatively safe, for some patients with supratentorial ICH who have specific prognostic factors, and for certain haematomas in particular sites of the brain.

The subgroup analyses from the International STICH and other trials justify further trials of early craniotomy in patients with superficial haematomas and stereotaxically-assisted ICH evacuation in patients with deep basal ganglia haematomas.

Decompressive surgical evacuation of infratentorial haematoma

Cerebellar haematomas

As observational studies consistently suggest that surgical evacuation of a cerebellar haematoma by suboccipital craniotomy has more than a modest favourable effect in saving the lives of patients with clinical features of progressive brainstem compression, and with surprisingly few adverse neurological sequelae, a RCT is unlikely to be ethically approved and undertaken (Fisher *et al.*, 1965, Lui *et al.*, 1985; Kobayashi *et al.*, 1994). The relative merits of conventional suboccipital craniotomy and stereotactic aspiration, with or without installation of fibrinolytic drugs, in this group of patients is uncertain.

Not all cerebellar haematomas require evacuation. The selection criteria for surgery ignite controversy, but probably include impaired consciousness with preserved brainstem reflexes, and perhaps large haematomas (>3–4 cm in diameter) and vermis haematomas distorting the quadrigeminal cistern, even in alert patients, because delayed decline in consciousness and death can be extremely rapid (Dunne *et al.*, 1987; Taneda *et al.*, 1987; Mathew *et al.*, 1995; St Louis *et al.*, 1998).

Pontine haematoma

Despite a case-fatality of up to about 60%, most patients with pontine haematoma are managed conservatively (Kushner and Bressman, 1985; Masiyama *et al.*, 1985). Apparently successful stereotactic aspiration has been reported in uncontrolled case series, but the effect on the prognosis remains uncertain (Beatty and Zervas, 1973; Bosch and Beute, 1985; Niizuma and Suzuki, 1987).

Fibrinolytic therapy for intraventricular haemorrhage

Spontaneous or secondary intraventricular haemorrhage can cause hydrocephalus, permanent neurological deficits and death. Ventricular shunt placement is commonly employed. Fibrinolytic agents injected into the ventricular system could dissolve blood clots, increase the clearance of blood from the ventricles and hence improve outcome.

Evidence

A systematic review of RCTs comparing intraventricular fibrinolytic therapy to placebo or open control for the management of intraventricular haemorrhage in adults identified no randomised trials of sufficient size and quality to evaluate the safety and efficacy of intraventricular fibrinolytic treatment (Lapointe and Haines, 2002).

Prevention of haematoma growth and re-bleeding by ultra-early haemostatic therapy

After ICH, the haematoma enlarges in up to 38% of patients scanned by CT within 3 h of onset, and in 16% of those scanned between 3 and 6 h (Kazui *et al.*, 1996; Brott *et al.*, 1997). Intervention with ultra-early haemostatic therapy in the emergency setting could potentially improve outcome after ICH by arresting ongoing bleeding and minimising haematoma growth.

Recombinant factor VIIa (rFVIIa) is currently approved to treat bleeding in hemophilia patients with inhibitors to factors VIII or IX, and is approved in Europe for the treatment of factor VII deficiency and Glanzmann thrombasthenia. After vascular damage and local initiation of the coagulation cascade, rFVIIa enhances thrombin generation on the surface of activated platelets, leading to the formation of a stable, lysis-resistant plug at the site of vessel injury (Monroe *et al.*, 1997). rFVIIa has been successfully used to control intracranial haemorrhage in patients with hemophilia or other coagulation disorders, and can arrest intra-operative bleeding and reverse coagulopathies in patients undergoing neurosurgical procedures (Arkin *et al.*, 1998; Park *et al.*, 2003; Fewel *et al.*, 2004). Although thromboembolic complications related to rFVIIa administration have occurred, with >400,000 doses administered for a growing number of clinical uses, the frequency of serious adverse events (SAEs) remains <1% (Roberts *et al.*, 2004).

Evidence

The European/Australasian NovoSeven ICH trial was a randomised, double-blind, placebo-controlled, dose-escalation trial involving 48 subjects with ICH diagnosed within 3 h of onset who were treated with placebo ($n = 12$) or rFVIIa (10, 20, 40, 80, 120 or 160 µg/kg; $n = 6$ per group). The primary endpoint was the frequency of adverse events (AEs). Safety assessments included serial electrocardiography (ECG), troponin I and coagulation testing, lower extremity Doppler ultrasonography and calculation of oedema:ICH volume ratios (Mayer *et al.*, 2005a).

The mean age of the patients was 61 years (range: 30–93) and 57% were male. At admission, the mean National Institutes of Health Stroke Scale (NIHSS) score was 14 (range: 1–26), the median GCS score was 14 (range: 6–15) and the mean ICH volume was 21 ml (range: 1–151). The mean time from onset to treatment was 181 min (range: 120–265). Twelve SAEs occurred, including five deaths (mortality 11%). Six AEs were considered possibly treatment-related, including rash, vomiting, fever, ECG T-wave inversion and two cases of deep vein thrombosis (DVT) (placebo and 20-µg/kg groups). No myocardial ischaemia, consumption coagulopathy or dose-related increase in oedema:ICH volume occurred.

A parallel study of 40 ICH patients that tested a lower range of doses demonstrated a similar safety profile (Mayer *et al.*, 2004).

A larger ($n = 399$), phase 26, dose-ranging, proof-of-concept trial of similar design comparing 40, 80 and 160 µg/kg rFVIIa with placebo has reported that among 399 patients with ICH diagnosed within 3 h of onset and treated within 4 h with placebo or rFVIIa (40, 80 or 160 µg/kg), there was a significant reduction in percentage change in mean volume (growth) of the ICH at 24 hours with increasing doses of rFVIIa (placebo: 29%; rFVIIa 40 µg/kg: 16%; rFVIIa 80 µg/kg: 14% and rFVIIa 160 µg/kg: 11%; $P = 0.01$ for the comparison of the three rFVIIa groups with placebo); and a significant increase in good outcome MRS ≥ 3 at 90 days (placebo: 31%; rFVIIa 40 µg/kg: 45%; rFVIIa 80 µg/kg: 51% and rFVIIa 160 µg/kg: 46%; $P = 0.004$ for the comparison of the three rFVIIIa groups with placebo); and a significant a reduction in mortality at 90 days (placebo: 29%; rFVIIa 40 µg/kg: 18%; rFVIIa 80 µg/kg: 18% and rFVIIa 160 µg/kg: 19%, $P = 0.02$). There was a non-significant increase in severe thrombotic events, mainly ischaemic stroke and myocardial infarction (placebo 2%, rFVIIa 7%, $P = 0.12$)(Mayer *et al.*, 2005b).

Comment

Two small phase II trials evaluated a wide range of rFVIIa doses in acute ICH and raised no major safety concerns.

A larger trial suggests that rFVIIa within four hours after onset of ICH can safely and effectively limit early ICH growth and improve outcome at 90 days, despite causing an excess of adverse thromboembolic events. However these results are preliminary and require confirmation in ongoing studies (Brown and Morgenstern, 2005; NINDS ICH workshop participants, 2005).

Iatrogenic intracerebral haemorrhage

Anticoagulant-associated intracerebral haemorrhage

Although never tested in a RCT, anticoagulant-associated intracerebral haemorrhage should probably be treated by reversing the deficiency of clotting factors as quickly as possible, because the patients frequently deteriorate neurologically (Kase *et al.*, 1985). The first step is intravenous (i.v.) injection of 10–20 mg of vitamin K, at not more than 5 mg/min, followed by infusion of a concentrate of the coagulation factors II, VII, IX and X, or of fresh frozen plasma. Infusion of the factors alone restores the coagulation system more rapidly than whole plasma, and is less likely to transmit virus particles (Fredriksson *et al.*, 1992). Alternatively, prothrombin complex concentrates can be used (Butler and Tait, 1998).

The appropriate time to resume anticoagulants in patients with a strong indication for anticoagulation (e.g. artificial heart valves) is uncertain; the only 'evidence' is anecdotal experience. The important determinants are the risk of thromboembolism without (and with) treatment and the risk of re-bleeding with treatment, which is more dependent on when the ruptured vessel is likely to have healed sufficiently, and not when blood has disappeared from the CT scan (which may take weeks or months). The ruptured vessel has probably healed sufficiently within 1 or 2 weeks if the underlying cause (e.g. hypertension, aneurysm, arteritis) is treated (Leker and Abramsky, 1998; Wijdicks *et al.*, 1998).

Thrombolytic therapy – associated intracerebral haemorrhage

Thrombolytic therapy after MI is complicated by intracerebral haemorrhage in only a small proportion of patients. However, because the case fatality is high, attempts at intervention are probably warranted, even without evidence of benefit from RCTs (Eleff *et al.*, 1990; Mahaffey *et al.*, 1999). Interventions include control of any hypertension and infusion of coagulation factors.

For patients who develop major intracerebral haemorrhage after thrombolytic treatment for ischaemic stroke there is no evidence about what to do (see Chapter 5) but in view of the lack of evidence of effectiveness of operative treatment for primary intracerebral haemorrhage in general, decompressive surgery is probably not indicated. The use of fresh frozen plasma and other measures to reverse the anticoagulant/thrombolytic state may also only result in further complications.

Aspirin-associated intracerebral haemorrhage

As aspirin treatment is associated with a small risk of intracerebral haemorrhage (see Chapter 10), it seems reasonable to stop aspirin in the presence of acute ICH. However, the antiplatelet effect of aspirin will continue to last for several days after discontinuing the drug (Patrono *et al.*, 1985), and there is no evidence that continuing aspirin is harmful. In the International Stroke Trial, there were more than 700 such patients (with acute haemorrhagic stroke who were randomised to aspirin), in 65% of whom the treatment was discontinued after the CT scan result became available, and there were no obviously untoward effects among patients with ICH who were treated with aspirin, but the confidence interval of the estimate was wide (Sandercock *et al.*, 1997; Keir *et al.*, 2000).

If aspirin is ceased, it is also not known when it is safe to restart aspirin. If there is a strong indication for aspirin, such as a high risk of thromboembolism, then perhaps aspirin should be started a week or so after the ICH, on the assumption that any ruptured blood vessel will be sufficiently healed by then (if the underlying cause of the haemorrhage is treated; e.g. hypertension).

Reduction of intracranial pressure

CSF drainage

CSF drainage can reduce intracranial pressure but there have been no RCTs which establish the true value (balance of risk and benefit) of any of the strategies.

Among 22 patients with supratentorial intracerebral haemorrhage and hydrocephalus who were treated with ventriculostomy, only one patient had any improvement in hydrocephalus and level of consciousness despite intracranial pressure being successfully controlled at <20 mmHg in 20 patients (Adams and Diringer, 1998). Furthermore, only three patients survived to 3 months, and they all had small haematoma volumes. The benefits of CSF diversion are therefore uncertain in patients with supratentorial haemorrhage and hydrocephalus.

For patients with extensive intraventricular haemorrhage secondary to deep intraparenchymal or aneurysmal rupture, a review of 22 observational studies suggested that CSF drainage may be helpful when it is combined with instillation of fibrinolytic drugs (Nieuwkamp *et al.*, 2000).

For patients with cerebellar haemorrhage and no signs of direct compression of the brainstem, insertion of a ventricular catheter may be a definitive measure (see above).

Hyperventilation

Hyperventilation sufficient to cause hypocapnia (down to about 4 kPa) causes cerebral vasoconstriction and thereby decreases intracranial pressure.

However, although this may relieve ischaemia caused by a compressive mass, it may exacerbate ischaemia by vasoconstriction. Furthermore, the effect of hypocapnia on the vessel diameter is short lived, about 6 h, and it is mainly in normal brain vasculature, so blood flow in the injured vessels may increase paradoxically and lead to increased oedema (Darby *et al.*, 1988).

Evidence

A RCT of prolonged hyperventilation in head-injured patients showed a worse outcome in the treatment group, although the numbers were small and the difference was statistically significant only after 3 and 6 months, but not at 1 year (Muizelaar *et al.*, 1991). For patients with ICHs, no RCTs of hyperventilation have been undertaken to determine whether the potential benefit exceeds the potential harm.

Comment

Provisionally, it seems best to reserve this treatment for bridging a few hours in patients for whom surgical evacuation is planned.

Osmotic agents

Osmotic agents such as mannitol, urea and glycerol, in doses between 0.5 and 2 g/kg, draw water from the extracellular into the intravascular compartment of the brain, provided the blood–brain barrier between these two compartments is still intact (refer to Chapter 8). The magnitude of the reduction in intracranial pressure parallels the amount of brain with preserved autoregulation (Muizelaar *et al.*, 1984; Bell *et al.*, 1987).

Evidence

Small controlled trials of i.v. glycerol have claimed benefit for patients with acute ischaemic stroke (see Chapter 8). However, a trial in patients with intracerebral haemorrhage showed no benefit (Yu *et al.*, 1992).

Comment

Despite the lack of evidence from controlled studies, mannitol (20–25% solution) has become the mainstay of osmotic therapy in many centres.

The correct dose cannot be predicted, but a safe regimen is 0.75–1 g/kg initially, then 0.25–0.5 kg every 3–5 h, depending on clinical findings and osmolality (the aim being 295–305 mOsm/l initially; if needed, 310–320 mOsm/l) (Ropper, 1993). With such regimens, the central venous pressure should ideally be monitored, and kept between 5 and 12 mmHg, to prevent hypovolaemia.

The interval between beginning the infusion and realising a decrease of intracranial pressure is usually less than 1 h, but the effect of a single dose lasts no more than 4–6 h, because the concentration of the solute becomes equilibrated between the intravascular and extracellular compartments.

Potential dangers include hypotension, hypokalaemia, renal failure from hyperosmolality, haemolysis and congestive heart failure (Yu *et al.*, 1992).

Corticosteroids

Corticosteroids reduce peritumoral oedema but probably not oedema around an ICH.

Evidence

There have been two small RCTs, the first undertaken in the early 1970s, before the advent of CT (Tellez and Bauer, 1973), and a subsequent study in Thailand (Poungvarin *et al.*, 1987).

Neither trial showed any difference in case fatality within the first 2–3 weeks between the treated and control groups (pooled OR: 1.0, 95% CI: 0.5–2.1).

Corticosteroid therapy was also not associated with any significant improvement in the proportion of patients making a complete recovery by the twenty-first day, despite a non-significant trend in favour of steroids (OR: 0.7; 95% CI: 0.2–2.4) (Poungvarin *et al.*, 1987).

Any modest benefits in terms of functional improvement were, in this trial at least, outweighed by the complications of steroid treatment (Poungvarin *et al.*, 1987); almost 50% of the steroid-treated group developed some complication (such as infection, diabetes or bleeding) compared with 13% amongst controls; this difference was highly significant.

The trial included patients with all levels of consciousness, in a stratified design. On the basis of a subgroup analysis it could be argued that corticosteroids might, after all, do some good in patients with a GCS score of eight or more, but apart from the pitfalls of data-dependent subgroup analyses an advantage emerged only for case fatality on day 7, and was lost on subsequent days. Thus, any benefit in terms of neurological function is moderate at best, whereas the adverse effects of corticosteroids in these patients are clearly substantial.

General supportive care

Blood pressure

The blood pressure (BP) is usually increased in patients with ICH, because of pre-existing hypertension, a response to a sudden increase in intracranial pressure or both.

As stated in Chapter 4, there are theoretical arguments in favour of decreasing the BP (in the hope of stopping ongoing bleeding from ruptured small arteries), and arguments in favour of increasing it further (in the hope of salvaging marginally perfused areas of brain that are compressed around the haematoma).

In the absence of any evidence from RCTs supporting one or other point of view, the only rational course is to leave the BP alone in the acute phase, unless it is elevated to such a degree that end-organ damage develops (especially in the retina, heart, brain and kidney). This is essentially the same advice as for patients with ischaemic stroke (see Chapter 4).

However, patients should not be discharged home with an elevated BP; adequate BP control in the long-term will substantially reduce the risk of recurrent stroke (including recurrent haemorrhage) and other cardiovascular events (refer to Chapter 12).

Prevention of DVT and pulmonary embolism

Patients with intracerebral haemorrhage have a substantial risk of DVT between 30% and 70%, depending on the severity of the stroke, the degree of immobilization and the rigour of the diagnostic process. The risk of pulmonary embolism (PE) is at least 1–5% (see Chapter 4) (Dickmann *et al.*, 1988).

The rationale for trialing antithrombotic drugs in patients with ICH is that although they may exacerbate any active intracerebral re-bleeding, they should not necessarily increase the risk of a small artery in the brain rupturing for a second time, and they may prevent a fatal pulmonary embolus as a consequence of venous stasis.

Subcutaneous heparin

Evidence   After general, orthopaedic and urologic surgery, subcutaneous heparin, usually given as 5000 U two or three times a day, reduces the relative risk (RR) of DVT by about 68% (Collins *et al.*, 1988).

After ICH, a single trial of this regimen, applied 4 days after the haemorrhage in the active treatment group and 10 days after the haemorrhage in the control group, to a total of 46 patients found that PE was detected by isotope perfusion lung scanning in 40% ($n = 9$) of 23 patients in the control group compared with 22% ($n = 5$) of 23 patients in the treated group (Dickmann *et al.*, 1988).

Comment   These results suggest that routine heparin prophylaxis for such patients could substantially reduce the risk of PE, but number of deaths was far too small to exclude the possibility that it could also increase the risk of fatal intracerebral re-bleeding.

Aspirin

Aspirin is effective in preventing DVT (approximately 39% RR reduction) and PE in the peri-operative period and in high risk medical patients but its safety in patients with intracerebral haemorrhage has not been studied. Nevertheless, it is unlikely that the risk of re-bleeding with aspirin is greater than with subcutaneous heparin.

Compression stockings

These are the safest method of prophylaxis in patients with ICH, although occasionally pressure sores may be induced.

Evidence   A systematic review of 12 RCTs of graduated compression stockings in patients at moderate risk of DVT, after abdominal, gynaecological and intracranial operations, indicates that compression stocking reduce the RR of DVT by about 70% (Wells *et al.*, 1994). Although the occurrence of PE was not included in this systematic review, a positive effect of compression stockings in preventing PE emerged from a large trial in patients who underwent cardiothoracic operations (Ramas *et al.*, 1996).

A systematic review identified two RCTs which compared physical methods for preventing DVT in stroke patients (Grandi *et al.*, 2005). In one trial of 97 patients, compression stockings were associated with a non significant trend toward a reduction in DVT detected by doppler ultrasound. In the other RCT of 26 patients, an intermittent compression device was not associated with a significant reduction in DVT detected by 125-I-Fibrinogen scanning. Overall, physical methods were not associated with a significant reduction in DVT during the treatment period in survivors (OR: 0.54; 95% CI: 0.18–1.57), death (OR: 1.54; 95% CI: 0.5–4.8), or death or DVT (OR: 0.88; 95% CI: 0.4–2.0) (Grandi *et al.*, 2005).

There have been no RCTs of graduated compression stockings in patients with PICH specifically.

Comment   Graduated compression stockings may effectively reduce the risk of DVT in patients with PICH, but evidence is lacking. They are not associated with an increased risk of bleeding (like heparin and aspirin) but their application is fairly labour intensive, the stockings can be uncomfortable after a time, and occasionally pressure sores may be induced.

Clinical trials of therapies to prevent venous thromboembolism in patients with PICH are needed. One such trial is the CLOTS trial (Clots in Legs Or Teds after Stroke), which aims to determine whether graded compression stockings are effective, and for patients with a clear indication for graded compression stockings, whether below-knee or full-length stockings is best (www.dcn.ed.ac.uk/clots/).

SUMMARY

There is insufficient evidence to justify a general policy of early operative intervention in patients with spontaneous supratentorial ICH, as opposed to one of initial conservative treatment. However, further research should explore the potential benefits and risks in certain subgroups of patients, and of stereotactic aspiration of deep ICHs under computed tomographic control.

Surgical evacuation of cerebellar haematomas can be life saving, and with surprisingly few neurological sequelae. Sound (but not evidence-based) indications for evacuation are the combination of a depressed level of consciousness with signs of progressive brainstem compression (unless all brainstem reflexes have been lost for more than a few hours, in which case a fatal outcome is unavoidable), or haematoma greater than 3–4 cm in diameter. If the patient has a depressed level of consciousness and hydrocephalus, without signs of brainstem compression and with a haematoma less than 3 cm, ventriculostomy can be carried out as an initial (and perhaps only) procedure.

Preliminary evidence suggests that early haemostatic treatment with rFVIIa can safely and effectively limit ICH growth and improve outcome.

Mannitol is widely used in patients with primary intracerebral haemorrhage and a depressed level of consciousness, to decrease intracranial pressure and to alleviate the space-occupying effect of the haematoma in a deteriorating patient, although this custom is not backed up by RCTs that have measured clinical effect rather than pressure as the outcome. With corticosteroids, it has not been shown that the benefits outweigh the disadvantages.

Subcutaneous heparin and graduated compression stockings both decrease the risk of DVT in bedridden patients by approximately 70% and aspirin by approximately 39%, as judged from clinical trials in a variety of post-operative conditions. As the safety of heparin and aspirin is largely unknown in patients with primary intracerebral haemorrhage, compression stockings are the preferred method of prophylaxis, despite being labour-intensive and despite the lack of any direct randomised trial evidence in patients with primary intracerebral haemorrhage.

Treatment of subarachnoid haemorrhage

The fundamentals of managing patients with aneurysmal subarachnoid haemorrhage (SAH) is to make the diagnosis, locate the aneurysm and occlude it. And yet, as simple as that sounds, about half of the patients in the general population still die, half of the survivors remain severely disabled and many functionally independent patients have impaired quality of life (Hijdra *et al.*, 1987a; Hop *et al.*, 1997; Olafsson *et al.*, 1997; Hop *et al.*, 1998).

The opportunities to improve the outcome of patients with SAH are to minimise the early and late deaths, and the many complications of the disease such as re-bleeding, delayed cerebral ischaemia, hydrocephalus and a variety of systemic disorders.

About 15% of patients die outside hospital within hours of the onset and, of those patients who reach hospital alive, a further 10–12% die within 24 h of the first bleed (Crawford and Sarner, 1965; Ljunggren *et al.*, 1985; Inagawa *et al.*, 1995; Schievink *et al.*, 1995). Re-bleeding is the cause of death in 50% of patients who die within the first day of admission to hospital (Locksley, 1966; Hijdra and van Gijn, 1982; Broderick *et al.*, 1994). The other common cause of early death is primary dysfunction of the brainstem from massive intraventricular haemorrhage, including distension of the fourth ventricle with blood (Shimoda *et al.*, 1999).

The 25% of patients who die within 24 h of the onset of SAH, outside or just inside hospital, are unlikely to be prevented by medical and surgical interventions in the near future. A more realistic target for intervention is the 35% of patients who survive the first day but die within the subsequent 3 months, due to poor condition from the initial haemorrhage (e.g. raised intracranial pressure), re-bleeding and delayed cerebral ischaemia (in roughly equal proportions) (Hijdra *et al.*, 1987a; Hop *et al.*, 1997).

The three major prognostic factors associated with a poor outcome are reduced level of consciousness, increasing age and increasing amounts of subarachnoid blood on the computed tomographical (CT) scan (Kassell *et al.*, 1990).

Treatment of raised intracranial pressure by immediate operation

Intracranial haematomas

Intraparenchymal haematomas occur in up to 30% of patients with ruptured aneurysms (van Gijn and van Dongen, 1982), and the average outcome is worse than in patients with purely subarachnoid blood (Hauerberg *et al.*, 1994).

Evidence

There has been only one small randomised-controlled trial (RCT) of immediate surgical evacuation of an intraparenchymal haematoma in 30 patients with SAH. Among the 15 patients assigned operation, 11 survived compared with three of 15 assigned conservative treatment (relative risk (RR): 0.27, 95% confidence interval (CI): 0.09–0.74) (Heiskanen *et al.*, 1988).

Comment

These data suggest that if a large haematoma is the most likely cause of gradual deterioration in the level of consciousness within the first few hours after SAH (usually temporal haematomas causing impending transtentorial herniation), patients should undergo magnetic resonance (MR) angiography or CT angiography to search for an aneurysm, and then immediate evacuation should be seriously considered (with simultaneous clipping of the aneurysm, if it can be identified).

Similarly, an acute subdural haematoma associated with recurrent aneurysmal rupture should be evacuated if it is life threatening (O'Sullivan *et al.*, 1994).

Symptomatic hydrocephalus

Patients with intraventricular blood or with extensive haemorrhage in the peri-mesencephalic cisterns are predisposed to developing acute hydrocephalus. Acute hydrocephalus usually causes a gradual obtundation within 24 h of haemorrhage, sometimes accompanied by slow pupillary responses to light and downward deviation of the eyes (van Gijn *et al.*, 1985; Rinkel *et al.*, 1990). Repeat CT scanning is required to diagnose or exclude hydrocephalus in such patients with SAH who deteriorate within hours or days of the initial event, with or without eye signs of hydrocephalus (small, unreactive pupils and downward deviation of gaze). As some patients improve spontaneously in the first 24 h, there are three main therapeutic options, none of which have been evaluated properly by RCTs.

Wait-and-see

For patients who are alert with dilated ventricles but not massive intraventricular haemorrhage, it is reasonable to adopt a conservative approach and 'wait-and-see' because only about one-third will become symptomatic in the next few days

(Hasan *et al.*, 1989c). However, another third of patients may temporarily improve to some extent, but then reach a plateau phase or again deteriorate warranting active intervention (Hasan *et al.*, 1989c).

Lumbar puncture

Until data from RCTs become available, it seems from a prospective uncontrolled study that lumbar puncture is a safe and reasonably effective way of treating acute hydrocephalus which is not caused by intraventricular obstruction (i.e. neither a haematoma nor gross intraventricular haemorrhage, i.e. less than complete filling of the third or fourth ventricle) (Hasan *et al.*, 1991). In this study, between one and seven spinal taps per patient were performed in the first 10 days, the number depending on the rate of improvement; each time, a maximum of 20 ml of cerebrospinal fluid was removed, the aim being to achieve a closing pressure of 15 cmH$_2$O. Five of the 17 patients had a decreased level of consciousness on admission, and in these patients the lumbar punctures were started immediately; in 11 of the remaining 12 patients, deterioration occurred a few days after admission, and the last patient had a fluctuating level of consciousness. Of the 17 patients, 12 showed initial improvement, and of these six fully recovered, two showed incomplete improvement but fully recovered after insertion of an internal shunt and the four others died of other complications several days after the lumbar punctures had been started. Of the five remaining patients in whom lumbar puncture had no effect, two recovered after an internal shunt and three died of other complications. The rate of re-bleeding (two of the 17 patients) was similar to what might have been expected, but of course the numbers were small (Hasan *et al.*, 1991).

External ventricular drainage

External drainage of the cerebral ventricles by a catheter inserted through a burr hole is the most commonly employed method of treating acute hydrocephalus. Internal drainage, to the right atrium or the peritoneal cavity, is rarely considered in the first few days, because the blood in the cerebrospinal fluid will almost inevitably block the shunt. After insertion of an external catheter, the improvement is usually rapid and sometimes dramatic (van Gijn *et al.*, 1985; Hasan *et al.*, 1989c). Unfortunately other problems tend to intervene soon, particularly re-bleeding and ventriculitis (Hasan *et al.*, 1989c; Paré *et al.*, 1992; Kawai *et al.*, 1997).

Prevention of re-bleeding

The two most common complications of SAH are re-bleeding and cerebral ischaemia.

In the first few hours after hospital admission for the initial SAH, up to 15% of patients experience sudden deterioration that suggests re-bleeding (Kassell and

Torner, 1983; Inagawa *et al.*, 1987; Hijdra *et al.*, 1987b; Fujii *et al.*, 1996). In patients who survive the first day, the risk of re-bleeding without medical or surgical intervention in the 4 weeks after the first day is about 35–40%, and is more or less evenly distributed over the next 4 weeks (Hijdra *et al.*, 1987b). Between 4 weeks and 6 months after the haemorrhage, the risk of re-bleeding gradually decreases, from the initial level of 1–2% per day to a constant level of about 3% per year, if they do not have their ruptured aneurysm occluded. Re-bleeding of a ruptured aneurysm cannot be predicted reliably.

The case fatality of re-bleeding is high, around 50%, compared with the 35% overall case fatality within 3 months for patients who survive the first day (Hijdra *et al.*, 1987b). Consequently, re-bleeding is still the main cause of a poor outcome, even in centres aiming at early occlusion of the aneurysm (Roos *et al.*, 1997; Vermeij *et al.*, 1998).

Operative aneurysmal occlusion by clipping, and its timing

Evidence

The first RCT of operative occlusion of the symptomatic aneurysm reported that operation (at that time mainly carotid ligation) was more effective than conservative management for patients who had recovered from the immediate effects of rupture of an aneurysm of the posterior communicating artery (McKissock *et al.*, 1960).

A subsequent similar RCT, but of aneurysms of the anterior communicating artery complex, showed no difference between surgical and conservative treatment (McKissock *et al.*, 1965).

A systematic review of the timing of surgery for aneurysmal SAH identified only one RCT which randomised 216 patients with aneurysmal SAH to surgery within 3 days of SAH, between days 3 and 7 of SAH and more than 7 days after SAH (Öhman and Heiskanen, 1989; Whitfield and Kirkpatrick, 2001). Patients undergoing early surgery tended to fare better than those undergoing late surgery but the difference was not statistically significant for the composite outcome of death or dependency at 3 months (odds ratio (OR): 0.37, 95% CI: 0.13–1.02) (Fig. 18.1) or the singular outcome of death at 3 months (OR: 0.40, 95% CI: 0.12–1.38) (Fig. 18.2) (Whitfield and Kirkpatrick, 2001). Patients undergoing early surgery appeared to have a lower odds of death or dependency than those undergoing surgery in the intermediate time period (OR: 0.34, 95% CI: 0.12–0.93), but the estimate of the magnitude of the effect was imprecise due to the wide 95% CI of the estimate of the OR.

The same result – no statistically significant difference in outcome after early or late operation – emerged from observational studies: a multicentre study from North America (Kassell *et al.*, 1990), and a single-institution review in Cambridge, England (Whitfield *et al.*, 1996). The US study found the worst outcome in patients

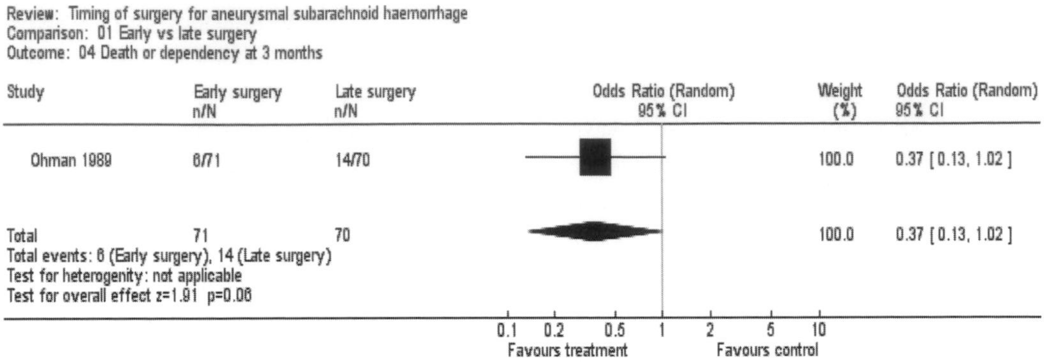

Review: Timing of surgery for aneurysmal subarachnoid haemorrhage
Comparison: 01 Early vs late surgery
Outcome: 04 Death or dependency at 3 months

Study	Early surgery n/N	Late surgery n/N	Odds Ratio (Random) 95% CI	Weight (%)	Odds Ratio (Random) 95% CI
Ohman 1989	8/71	14/70		100.0	0.37 [0.13, 1.02]
Total	71	70		100.0	0.37 [0.13, 1.02]

Total events: 8 (Early surgery), 14 (Late surgery)
Test for heterogenity: not applicable
Test for overall effect z=1.91 p=0.06

0.1   0.2   0.5   1   2   5   10
Favours treatment   Favours control

Figure 18.1 Forest plot showing the effects of *early surgery vs late surgery* in acute SAH on *death or dependency* at 3-month follow-up. Reproduced from Whitfield and Kirkpatrick (2001), with permission from the authors and John Wiley & Sons Limited. Copyright Cochrane Library, reproduced with permission.

Review: Timing of surgery for aneurysmal subarachnoid haemorrhage
Comparison: 01 Early vs late surgery
Outcome: 01 Death by 3 months

Study	Early surgery n/N	Late surgery n/N	Odds Ratio (Random) 95% CI	Weight (%)	Odds Ratio (Random) 95% CI
Ohman 1989	4/71	9/70		100.0	0.40 [0.12, 1.38]
Total	71	70		100.0	0.40 [0.12, 1.38]

Total events: 4 (Early surgery), 9 (Late surgery)
Test for heterogenity: not applicable
Test for overall effect z=1.44 p=0.1

0.1   0.2   0.5   1   2   5   10
Favours treatment   Favours control

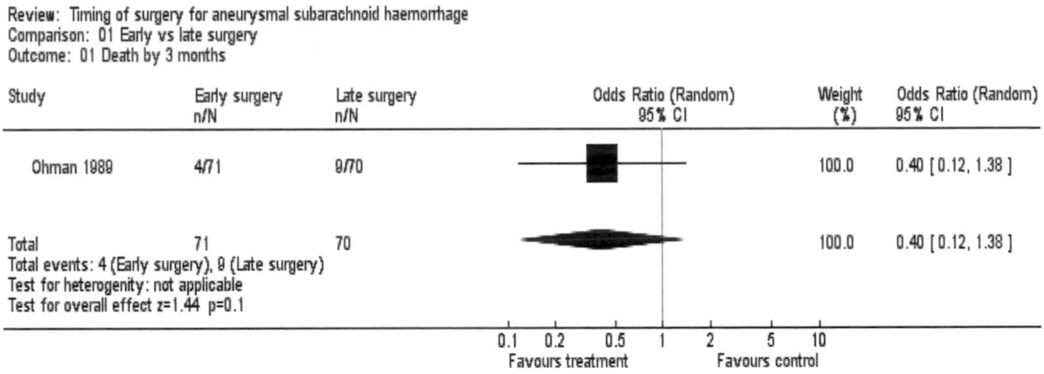

Figure 18.2 Forest plot showing the effects of *early surgery vs late surgery* in acute SAH on *death* at 3-month follow-up. Reproduced from Whitfield and Kirkpatrick (2001), with permission from the authors and John Wiley & Sons Limited. Copyright Cochrane Library, reproduced with permission.

who underwent surgery between days 7 and 10 after the initial haemorrhage. This disadvantageous period for performing the operation, in the second week after SAH, coincided with the peak time of cerebral ischaemia (Hijdra *et al.*, 1986) and of cerebral vasospasm (Weir *et al.*, 1978), which were both most common between days 4 to 12.

Comment

In the absence of further evaluation by RCTs, surgical treatment of intracranial aneurysms became the standard treatment for aneurysmal SAH. Initially, the aneurysm was usually clipped after at least 12 days had elapsed because the second week was notorious for its ischaemic complications, and attempts at very early intervention were disappointing.

Improvements in anaesthetic technique, and the introduction of the operating microscope, subsequently prompted earlier surgery (i.e. within 3 days of the initial bleed) to mainly prevent re-bleeding, and perhaps cerebral ischaemia in the second week (Mizukami *et al.*, 1982). Another theoretical advantage of early aneurysm clipping was that if cerebral ischaemia does develop, there is an opportunity for hypertensive and hypervolaemic treatment without the danger of re-bleeding.

However, the theoretical advantages of early surgery remain to be proven in any RCTs. Since the publication of the only RCT in 1989, techniques for the treatment of SAH have progressed, questioning the validity of the conclusions in the modern era. Currently, most neurovascular surgeons elect to operate within 3 or 4 days of the bleed in good-grade patients to minimise the chances of a devastating re-bleed. However, the treatment of patients in poorer grades certainly warrants further scrutiny in RCTs.

Endovascular occlusion of the aneurysm by coiling

Until the 1990s, endovascular treatment of aneurysms was restricted to patients in whom the aneurysm was unsuitable for clipping because of its size or location (especially in the posterior circulation), or in whom operation was contraindicated. The technique consisted initially of balloon occlusion, but a more novel development was to pack the aneurysm with coils, first of a pushable kind and subsequently with a system for controlled detachment (Guglielmi *et al.*, 1992). Ideally, after coiling, the remaining aneurysmal lumen becomes occluded by a process of reactive thrombosis; post-mortem studies have shown, however, that endothelialisation of the aneurysm orifice after placement of coils is the exception rather than the rule (Stiver *et al.*, 1998; Bavinzski *et al.*, 1999a). In large aneurysms, the process of intra-aneurysm clot organisation seems to be delayed and incomplete; tiny open spaces between the coils and an incomplete membranous covering in the region of the neck are frequently encountered (Molyneux *et al.*, 1995; Bavinzski *et al.*, 1999a).

The appeal of endovascular occlusion is that it is much less invasive than surgical treatment. However, it is not without its hazards. Firstly, the aneurysm may rupture during the procedure, a complication much more difficult to control than during surgical exploration (McDougall *et al.*, 1998). Secondly, if the process of reactive thrombosis extends to the parent vessel, infarction of brain tissue may occur. Of course, in patients with ruptured aneurysms, ischaemic complications may occur even without any intervention at all, but the rate may be as high as 38% in patients treated within 3 days of coil deployment, against 22% in patients treated surgically (Gruber *et al.*, 1998a). For that reason, most interventional radiologists institute heparin after the procedure, at least for a few days. Finally, one or more coils may become dislodged and herniate or embolise into the parent vessel, which again may lead to ischaemic brain damage (Spetzger *et al.*, 1997). The risk of this complication is greater with wide-necked aneurysms; special coils that can expand in three dimensions have been devised to minimise this danger (Malek *et al.*, 1999). With detachable coils, the overall rate of ischaemic complications is of the order of 8–9% and that of re-bleeding 2–3% (Brilstra *et al.*, 1999).

Evidence

The first RCT of surgical clipping vs endovascular coiling involved 109 patients and reported no difference in outcome at 3 months between the surgical group and the endovascular group (Vanninen *et al.*, 1999; Koivisto *et al.*, 2000).

The subsequent International Subarachnoid Aneurysm Trial (ISAT) was a randomised, multicentre trial which aimed to compare the safety and efficacy of endovascular coiling with standard neurosurgical clipping for aneurysms judged to be suitable for both treatments (International Subarachnoid Aneurysm Trial (ISAT) Collaborative Group, 2002). A total of 9559 patients with SAH within the previous 28 days were assessed for eligibility. Of these patients, 7416 were excluded (77.6%); 671 patients refused the study, 2737 patients were considered to be better candidates for endovascular coiling, 3615 patients for neurosurgical clipping and 1064 were treated in some other unknown manner. This left 2143 patients (22.4% of total) with ruptured intracranial aneurysms in the previous 28 days who were randomly assigned to neurosurgical clipping ($n = 1070$) or endovascular treatment by detachable platinum coils ($n = 1073$). The majority of patients' randomised were in good clinical condition prior to treatment. Eighty-eight per cent of the endovascular group and 88% of the surgical group were World Federation of Neurological Surgery (WFNS) grade 1 or 2. The majority of patients entered in the study had anterior circulation aneurysms (97.3%), and the target aneurysms were 10 mm or smaller in diameter in 93% of patients.

Clinical outcomes were assessed at 2 months and at 1 year with interim ascertainment of re-bleeds and death. The primary outcome was the proportion of patients with a modified Rankin scale score of 3–6 (dependency or death) at 1 year.

Trial recruitment was stopped by the steering committee after a planned interim analysis.

Among the 801 patients allocated endovascular treatment, 190 (23.7%) were dependent or dead (modified Rankin outcome scale score of 3–6, pooled results) at 1 year compared with 243 of the 793 (30.6%) allocated neurosurgical treatment ($P = 0.0019$). This was a RR reduction of 22.6% (95% CI: 8.9–34.2%) and absolute risk reduction 6.9% (95% CI: 2.5–11.3%) over 1 year.

The risk of re-bleeding from the ruptured aneurysm after 1 year was 2/1276 and 0/1081 patient-years for patients allocated endovascular and neurosurgical treatment, respectively.

Comment

Interpretation of the evidence

In patients with a ruptured intracranial aneurysm, for which endovascular coiling and neurosurgical clipping are therapeutic options, the outcome in terms of survival free of disability at 1 year is significantly better with endovascular coiling.

The risks of further bleeding from the treated aneurysm within the first year are low with either therapy, and they are somewhat more frequent with endovascular coiling. In the ISAT trial, 23 patients assigned neurosurgical clipping re-bled before the first procedure, compared with 14 in the endovascular group. This result may be secondary to the small but statistically significant difference in the time between randomisation and the first procedure (1.7 days for neurosurgery *vs* 1.1 days for endovascular), and underscores the importance of early treatment of ruptured cerebral aneurysms.

Implications for clinicians

These data suggest that the small subgroup of good-grade, anterior circulation, small ruptured saccular aneurysms, of such morphology that they would be considered a reasonable candidate for neurosurgical or endovascular therapy, should be considered for coiling if such expertise is available on an emergency basis. However, these data cannot be extrapolated to all other ruptured aneurysms, or to the entire population of unruptured aneurysms.

The results can also not be generalised beyond 1 year of follow-up. During the first year of follow-up, six patients in the endovascular group and five in the neurosurgical group re-bled after the aneurysm was deemed to be completely coiled or clipped.

Implications for researchers

Long-term follow-up of patients randomised in the ISAT and other trials is needed to answer questions about the long-term durability of each procedure in terms of re-bleeding rates, risks of recanalisation of the aneurysm and need for repeat procedures.

Antifibrinolytic drug therapy

Re-bleeding after SAH is thought to originate from dissolution of the clot at the site of the ruptured aneurysm by natural fibrinolytic activity in the cerebrospinal fluid after the SAH. Antifibrinolytic drugs cross the blood–brain barrier rapidly after SAH and reduce fibrinolytic activity (Fodstad *et al.*, 1981). The two most commonly used drugs are tranexamic acid (TEA; usual dose 1 g intravenously or 1.5 g orally, four to six times daily) and ε-aminocaproic acid (EACA; 3–4.5 g/3 h intravenously or orally). Both agents are structurally similar to lysine and so block the lysine sites by which the plasminogen molecules bind to complementary sites on fibrin. In this way, these drugs prevent fibrinolysis in general and lysis of the clot around the recently ruptured aneurysm in particular. It is assumed that it takes 36 h to achieve complete inhibition of fibrinolysis in the cerebrospinal fluid.

Evidence

A systematic review for the Cochrane Library identified nine RCTs which evaluated the effect of antifibrinolytic treatment in a total of 1399 patients with aneurysmal SAH (Roos *et al.*, 2003).

Death

Among all 1399 patients enrolled in the nine RCTs trials, random assignment to antifibrinolytic treatment was not associated with any reduction in the odds of death from all causes (OR: 0.99, 95% CI: 0.79–1.24) (Fig. 18.3).

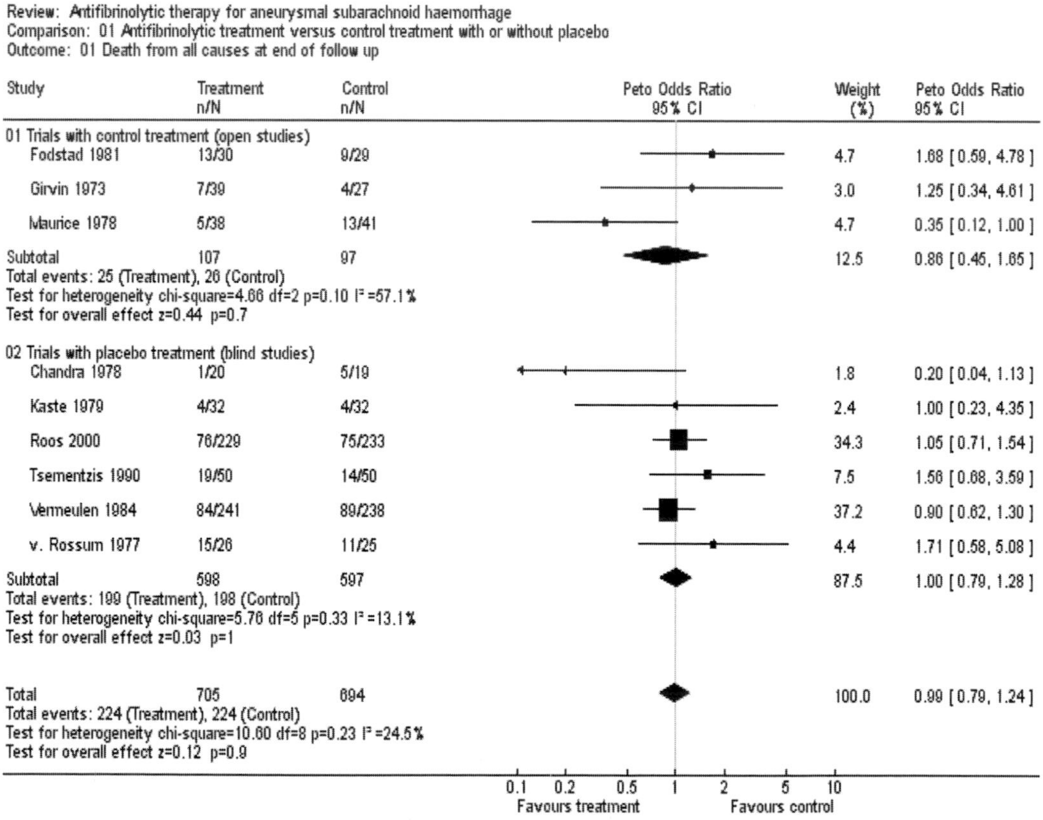

Review: Antifibrinolytic therapy for aneurysmal subarachnoid haemorrhage
Comparison: 01 Antifibrinolytic treatment versus control treatment with or without placebo
Outcome: 01 Death from all causes at end of follow up

Study	Treatment n/N	Control n/N	Peto Odds Ratio 95% CI	Weight (%)	Peto Odds Ratio 95% CI
01 Trials with control treatment (open studies)					
Fodstad 1981	13/30	9/29		4.7	1.68 [0.59, 4.78]
Girvin 1973	7/39	4/27		3.0	1.25 [0.34, 4.61]
Maurice 1978	5/38	13/41		4.7	0.35 [0.12, 1.00]
Subtotal	107	97		12.5	0.86 [0.45, 1.65]
Total events: 25 (Treatment), 26 (Control)					
Test for heterogeneity chi-square=4.66 df=2 p=0.10 I²=57.1%					
Test for overall effect z=0.44 p=0.7					
02 Trials with placebo treatment (blind studies)					
Chandra 1978	1/20	5/19		1.8	0.20 [0.04, 1.13]
Kaste 1979	4/32	4/32		2.4	1.00 [0.23, 4.35]
Roos 2000	76/229	75/233		34.3	1.05 [0.71, 1.54]
Tsementzis 1990	19/50	14/50		7.5	1.56 [0.68, 3.59]
Vermeulen 1984	84/241	89/238		37.2	0.90 [0.62, 1.30]
v. Rossum 1977	15/26	11/25		4.4	1.71 [0.58, 5.08]
Subtotal	598	597		87.5	1.00 [0.79, 1.28]
Total events: 199 (Treatment), 198 (Control)					
Test for heterogeneity chi-square=5.76 df=5 p=0.33 I²=13.1%					
Test for overall effect z=0.03 p=1					
Total	705	694		100.0	0.99 [0.79, 1.24]
Total events: 224 (Treatment), 224 (Control)					
Test for heterogeneity chi-square=10.60 df=8 p=0.23 I²=24.5%					
Test for overall effect z=0.12 p=0.9					

0.1   0.2   0.5   1   2   5   10
Favours treatment   Favours control

Figure 18.3   Forest plot showing the effects of *antifibrinolytic therapy vs control* in acute SAH on *death* at end of follow-up. Reproduced from Roos *et al.* (2003), with permission from the authors and John Wiley & Sons Limited. Copyright Cochrane Library, reproduced with permission.

Poor outcome

Among 1041 patients enrolled in three trials, for which data on functional outcome were available, random assignment to antifibrinolytic treatment was not associated with any reduction in the odds of a poor outcome, as defined by death, vegetative state or severe disability (OR: 1.12, 95% CI: 0.88–1.43) (Fig. 18.4).

Re-bleeding

Antifibrinolytic treatment reduced the odds of re-bleeding reported at the end of follow-up, (OR: 0.55, 95% CI: 0.42–0.71) with some heterogeneity between the trials ($p = 0.01$) (Fig. 18.5).

Cerebral ischaemia

Antifibrinolytic treatment increased the odds of cerebral ischaemia in five trials (OR: 1.39, 95% CI: 1.07–1.82) but there was considerable heterogeneity between the most recent study (Roos, 2000), in which specific treatments to prevent cerebral ischaemia were used, and the four earlier studies (Fig. 18.6).

Hydrocephalus

Antifibrinolytic treatment showed no effect on the reported rate of hydrocephalus in five trials (OR: 1.14, 95% CI: 0.86–1.51).

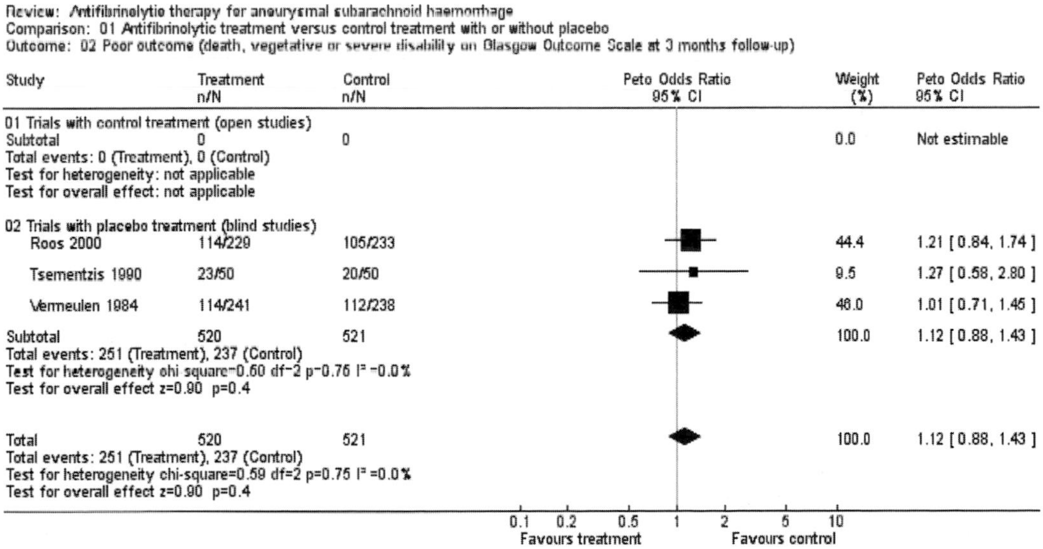

Figure 18.4 Forest plot showing the effects of *antifibrinolytic therapy vs control* in acute SAH on *poor outcome* at 3-month follow-up. Reproduced from Roos *et al.* (2003), with permission from the authors and John Wiley & Sons Limited. Copyright Cochrane Library, reproduced with permission.

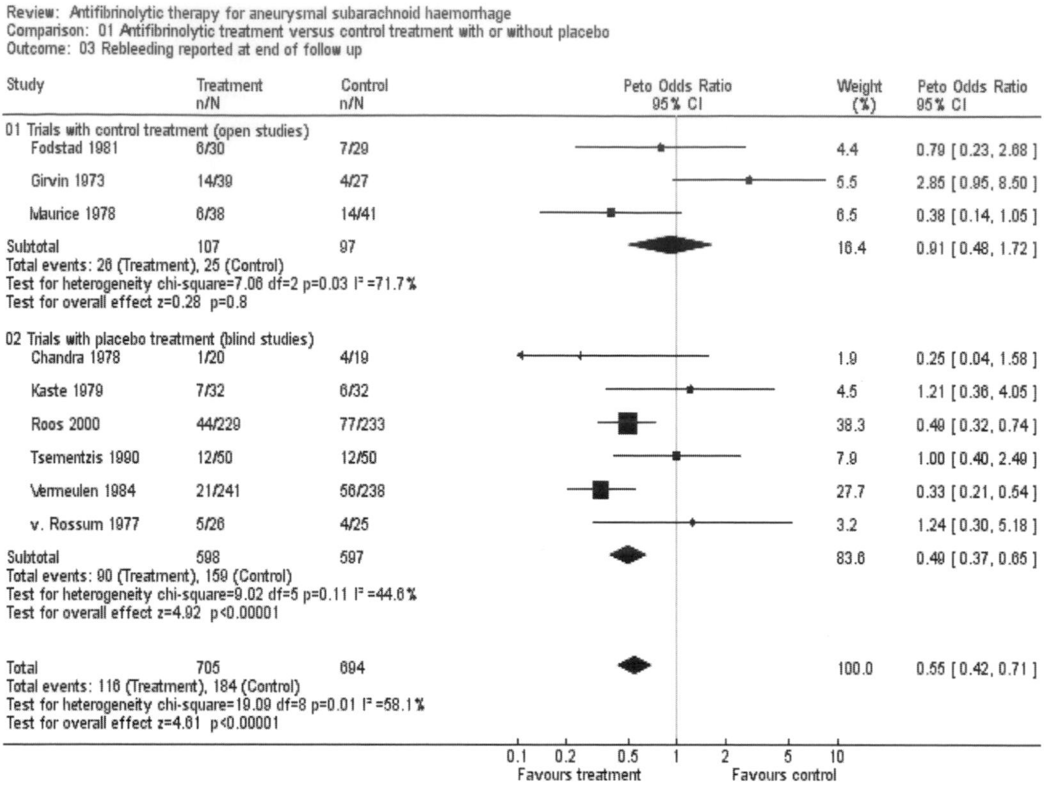

Review: Antifibrinolytic therapy for aneurysmal subarachnoid haemorrhage
Comparison: 01 Antifibrinolytic treatment versus control treatment with or without placebo
Outcome: 03 Rebleeding reported at end of follow up

Study	Treatment n/N	Control n/N	Peto Odds Ratio 95% CI	Weight (%)	Peto Odds Ratio 95% CI
01 Trials with control treatment (open studies)					
Fodstad 1981	8/30	7/29		4.4	0.79 [0.23, 2.68]
Girvin 1973	14/39	4/27		5.5	2.85 [0.95, 8.50]
Maurice 1978	6/38	14/41		8.5	0.38 [0.14, 1.05]
Subtotal	107	97		18.4	0.91 [0.48, 1.72]

Total events: 28 (Treatment), 25 (Control)
Test for heterogeneity chi-square=7.08 df=2 p=0.03 I²=71.7%
Test for overall effect z=0.28 p=0.8

02 Trials with placebo treatment (blind studies)					
Chandra 1978	1/20	4/19		1.9	0.25 [0.04, 1.58]
Kaste 1979	7/32	6/32		4.5	1.21 [0.36, 4.05]
Roos 2000	44/229	77/233		38.3	0.49 [0.32, 0.74]
Tsementzis 1990	12/50	12/50		7.9	1.00 [0.40, 2.49]
Vermeulen 1984	21/241	56/238		27.7	0.33 [0.21, 0.54]
v. Rossum 1977	5/26	4/25		3.2	1.24 [0.30, 5.18]
Subtotal	598	597		83.6	0.49 [0.37, 0.65]

Total events: 90 (Treatment), 159 (Control)
Test for heterogeneity chi-square=9.02 df=5 p=0.11 I²=44.6%
Test for overall effect z=4.92 p<0.00001

Total	705	694		100.0	0.55 [0.42, 0.71]

Total events: 118 (Treatment), 184 (Control)
Test for heterogeneity chi-square=19.09 df=8 p=0.01 I²=58.1%
Test for overall effect z=4.61 p<0.00001

0.1   0.2   0.5   1   2   5   10
Favours treatment   Favours control

Figure 18.5 Forest plot showing the effects of *antifibrinolytic therapy vs control* in acute SAH on *re-bleeding* at the end of follow-up. Reproduced from Roos *et al.* (2003), with permission from the authors and John Wiley & Sons Limited. Copyright Cochrane Library, reproduced with permission.

Comment

Interpretation of the evidence

Antifibrinolytic treatment does not improve clinical outcome after SAH because the benefit in preventing re-bleeding is offset by an increase in cerebral ischaemia.

Implications for clinicians

These data do not support the routine use of antifibrinolytic drugs in the treatment of patients with aneurysmal SAH.

Implications for researchers

Although antifibrinolytic drugs 'work' in preventing re-bleeding, they do not improve patient outcome. However, they could improve outcome if the attendant cerebral ischaemia could be concurrently prevented. Further research should aim to improve

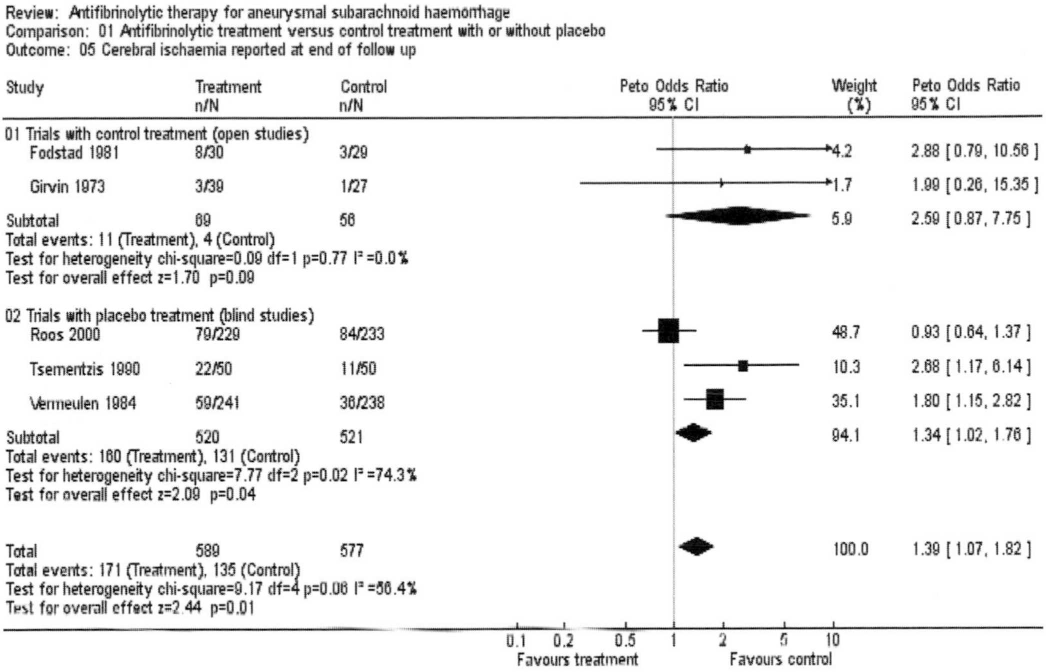

Review: Antifibrinolytic therapy for aneurysmal subarachnoid haemorrhage
Comparison: 01 Antifibrinolytic treatment versus control treatment with or without placebo
Outcome: 05 Cerebral ischaemia reported at end of follow up

Study	Treatment n/N	Control n/N	Peto Odds Ratio 95% CI	Weight (%)	Peto Odds Ratio 95% CI
01 Trials with control treatment (open studies)					
Fodstad 1981	8/30	3/29		4.2	2.88 [0.79, 10.56]
Girvin 1973	3/39	1/27		1.7	1.99 [0.26, 15.35]
Subtotal	69	56		5.9	2.59 [0.87, 7.75]
Total events: 11 (Treatment), 4 (Control)					
Test for heterogeneity chi-square=0.09 df=1 p=0.77 I²=0.0%					
Test for overall effect z=1.70 p=0.09					
02 Trials with placebo treatment (blind studies)					
Roos 2000	79/229	84/233		48.7	0.93 [0.64, 1.37]
Tsementzis 1990	22/50	11/50		10.3	2.68 [1.17, 6.14]
Vermeulen 1984	59/241	36/238		35.1	1.80 [1.15, 2.82]
Subtotal	520	521		94.1	1.34 [1.02, 1.76]
Total events: 160 (Treatment), 131 (Control)					
Test for heterogeneity chi-square=7.77 df=2 p=0.02 I²=74.3%					
Test for overall effect z=2.09 p=0.04					
Total	589	577		100.0	1.39 [1.07, 1.82]
Total events: 171 (Treatment), 135 (Control)					
Test for heterogeneity chi-square=9.17 df=4 p=0.06 I²=56.4%					
Test for overall effect z=2.44 p=0.01					

0.1   0.2   0.5   1   2   5   10
Favours treatment   Favours control

Figure 18.6   Forest plot showing the effects of *antifibrinolytic therapy vs control* in acute SAH on *cerebral ischaemia*. Reproduced from Roos *et al.* (2003), with permission from the authors and John Wiley & Sons Limited. Copyright Cochrane Library, reproduced with permission.

our understanding of how antifibrinolytic treatment precipitates cerebral ischaemia, in order to develop strategies to minimise it. Possible explanations for the increase in cerebral ischaemia include increased blood viscosity, the development of microthrombi, delayed clearance of blood clots around the arteries at the base of the brain and the development of hydrocephalus through delayed resorption of blood.

Prevention of delayed cerebral ischaemia

Cerebral ischaemia or infarction is a complication of SAH that tends to peak around days 4–12 after SAH. Its cause remains uncertain. It is not confined to the territory of a single cerebral artery or one of its branches (Hijdra *et al.*, 1986), and it occurs only if the source is a ruptured aneurysm. It is strongly related to the total amount of subarachnoid blood. However, any causal relationship between the amount of extravasated blood and the development of delayed cerebral ischaemia is not sufficiently explained by the production of putative toxic substances released from clots around the large arteries at the base of the brain. As loss of consciousness at the time of the haemorrhage is an important and independent predictive factor for delayed cerebral ischaemia (Brouwers *et al.*, 1992; Hop *et al.*, 1999) it is conceivable that global ischaemia during this brief period, along with a massive increase in intracranial pressure, may sensitise neurones to marginal perfusion associated with later complications, such as diffuse vasospasm or hypovolaemia.

The prophylactic treatments for cerebral ischaemia which have been evaluated by means of RCTs are the administration of calcium antagonists, magnesium sulphate and volume expansion therapy.

Calcium antagonists

Calcium entry blocking drugs have been used to prevent cerebral ischaemia because they inhibit the contractile properties of smooth-muscle cells, particularly those in cerebral arteries, and because they may protect neurones against the deleterious effect of calcium influx after ischaemic damage (Greenberg, 1987).

Evidence

A systematic review for the Cochrane Library identified 12 RCTs which aimed to determine whether calcium antagonists improved the outcome of patients with aneurysmal SAH (Rinkel *et al.*, 2005).

A total of 2844 patients with SAH were randomised to active treatment with a calcium antagonist ($n = 1396$) or to control ($n = 1448$). The drugs analysed were: nimodipine (eight trials, 1574 patients), nicardipine (two trials, 954 patients),

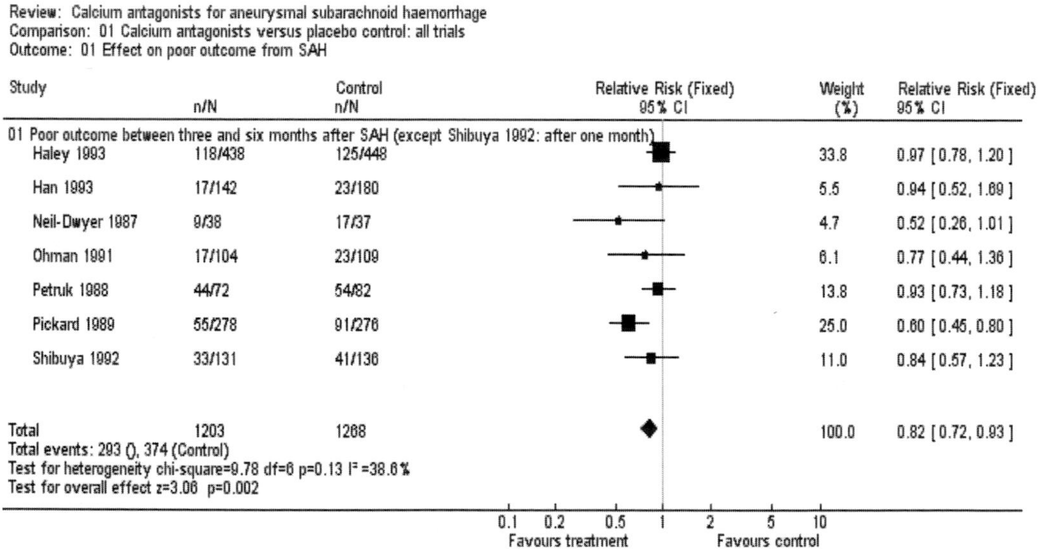

Review: Calcium antagonists for aneurysmal subarachnoid haemorrhage
Comparison: 01 Calcium antagonists versus placebo control: all trials
Outcome: 01 Effect on poor outcome from SAH

Study	Treatment n/N	Control n/N	Relative Risk (Fixed) 95% CI	Weight (%)	Relative Risk (Fixed) 95% CI
01 Poor outcome between three and six months after SAH (except Shibuya 1992: after one month)					
Haley 1993	118/438	125/448		33.8	0.97 [0.78, 1.20]
Han 1993	17/142	23/180		5.5	0.94 [0.52, 1.69]
Neil-Dwyer 1987	9/38	17/37		4.7	0.52 [0.26, 1.01]
Ohman 1991	17/104	23/109		6.1	0.77 [0.44, 1.36]
Petruk 1988	44/72	54/82		13.8	0.93 [0.73, 1.18]
Pickard 1989	55/278	91/276		25.0	0.60 [0.45, 0.80]
Shibuya 1992	33/131	41/136		11.0	0.84 [0.57, 1.23]
Total	1203	1268		100.0	0.82 [0.72, 0.93]

Total events: 293 (), 374 (Control)
Test for heterogeneity chi-square=9.78 df=6 p=0.13 I²=38.6%
Test for overall effect z=3.06 p=0.002

```
            0.1  0.2   0.5   1   2    5   10
           Favours treatment      Favours control
```

Figure 18.7   Forest plot showing the effects of a *calcium antagonist vs control* in acute SAH on *poor outcome* at final follow-up. Reproduced from Rinkel *et al.* (2005), with permission from the authors and John Wiley & Sons Limited. Copyright Cochrane Library, reproduced with permission.

AT877 (one trial, 276 patients) and magnesium (one trial, 40 patients). In 92% of the patients aneurysms were confirmed by angiography or autopsy.

Poor outcome

Overall, random allocation to treatment with a calcium antagonist was associated with a statistically significantly reduction in the RR of a poor outcome compared with control (RR: 0.82, 95% CI: 0.72–0.93) (Fig. 18.7).

The absolute risk reduction was 5.1%, and so the corresponding number of patients needed to treat to prevent a single poor outcome event was 20.

Treatment with oral nimodipine alone was associated with a reduction in the RR of a poor outcome compared with control (RR: 0.69, 95% CI: 0.58–0.84) (Fig. 18.8).

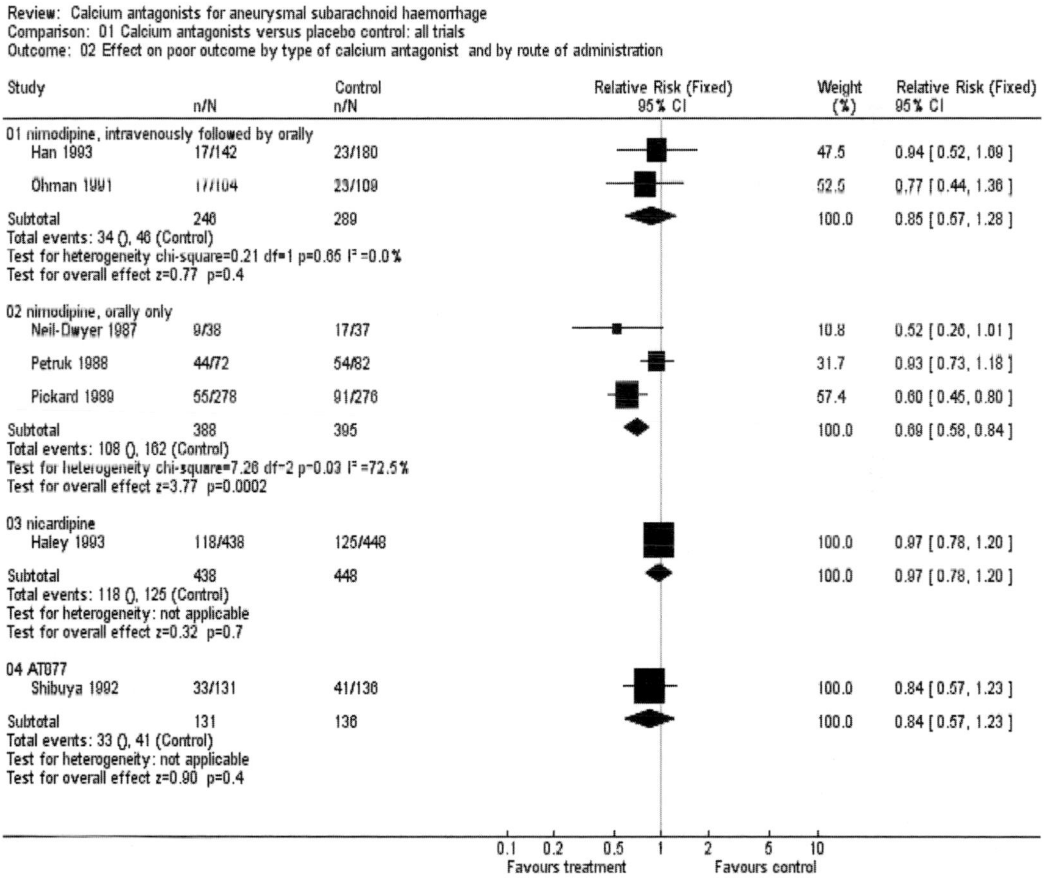

Review: Calcium antagonists for aneurysmal subarachnoid haemorrhage
Comparison: 01 Calcium antagonists versus placebo control: all trials
Outcome: 02 Effect on poor outcome by type of calcium antagonist and by route of administration

Study	n/N	Control n/N	Relative Risk (Fixed) 95% CI	Weight (%)	Relative Risk (Fixed) 95% CI
01 nimodipine, intravenously followed by orally					
Han 1993	17/142	23/180		47.5	0.94 [0.52, 1.69]
Ohman 1991	17/104	23/109		52.5	0.77 [0.44, 1.36]
Subtotal	246	289		100.0	0.85 [0.57, 1.28]
Total events: 34 (), 46 (Control)					
Test for heterogeneity chi-square=0.21 df=1 p=0.65 I²=0.0%					
Test for overall effect z=0.77 p=0.4					
02 nimodipine, orally only					
Neil-Dwyer 1987	9/38	17/37		10.8	0.52 [0.26, 1.01]
Petruk 1988	44/72	54/82		31.7	0.93 [0.73, 1.18]
Pickard 1989	55/278	91/276		57.4	0.60 [0.45, 0.80]
Subtotal	388	395		100.0	0.69 [0.58, 0.84]
Total events: 108 (), 162 (Control)					
Test for heterogeneity chi-square=7.26 df=2 p=0.03 I²=72.5%					
Test for overall effect z=3.77 p=0.0002					
03 nicardipine					
Haley 1993	118/438	125/448		100.0	0.97 [0.78, 1.20]
Subtotal	438	448		100.0	0.97 [0.78, 1.20]
Total events: 118 (), 125 (Control)					
Test for heterogeneity: not applicable					
Test for overall effect z=0.32 p=0.7					
04 AT877					
Shibuya 1992	33/131	41/138		100.0	0.84 [0.57, 1.23]
Subtotal	131	138		100.0	0.84 [0.57, 1.23]
Total events: 33 (), 41 (Control)					
Test for heterogeneity: not applicable					
Test for overall effect z=0.90 p=0.4					

```
         0.1   0.2   0.5    1     2    5   10
              Favours treatment      Favours control
```

Figure 18.8   Forest plot showing the effects of a *calcium antagonist vs control* in acute SAH on *poor outcome* at final follow-up *by drug administration and its route of administration*. Reproduced from Rinkel *et al.* (2005), with permission from the authors and John Wiley & Sons Limited. Copyright Cochrane Library, reproduced with permission.

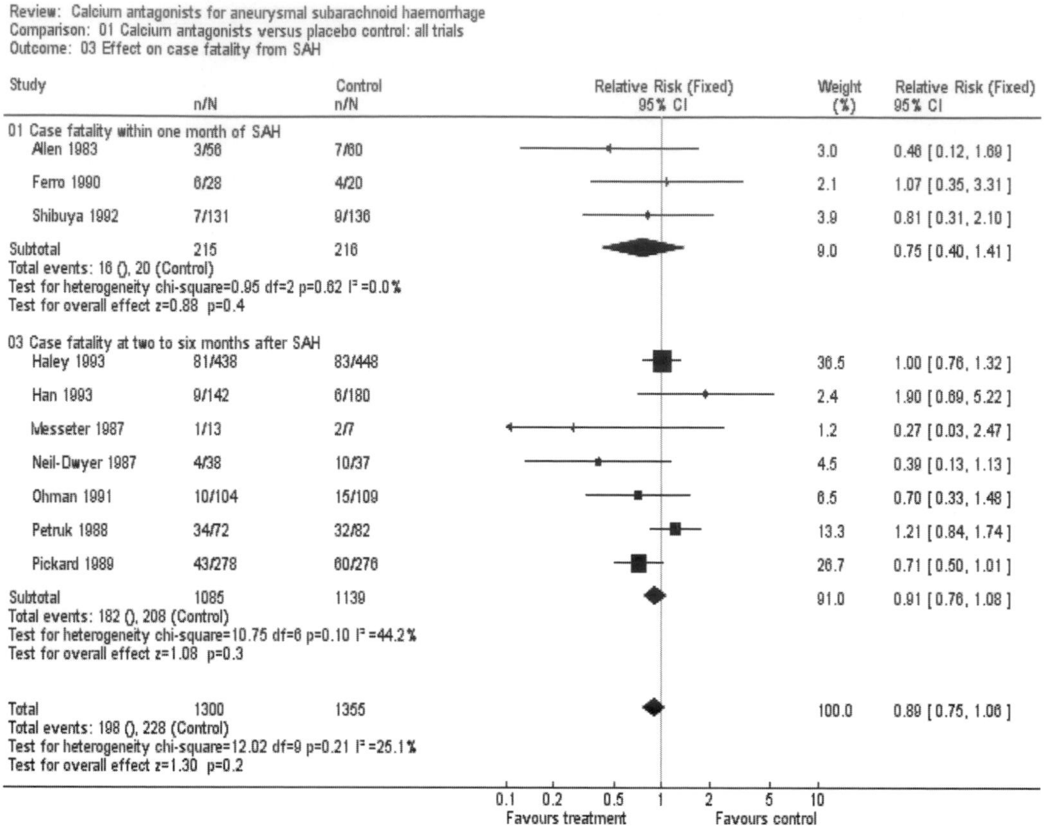

Review: Calcium antagonists for aneurysmal subarachnoid haemorrhage
Comparison: 01 Calcium antagonists versus placebo control: all trials
Outcome: 03 Effect on case fatality from SAH

Study		Control	Relative Risk (Fixed)	Weight	Relative Risk (Fixed)
	n/N	n/N	95% CI	(%)	95% CI
01 Case fatality within one month of SAH					
Allen 1983	3/58	7/60		3.0	0.48 [0.12, 1.89]
Ferro 1990	6/28	4/20		2.1	1.07 [0.35, 3.31]
Shibuya 1992	7/131	9/136		3.9	0.81 [0.31, 2.10]
Subtotal	215	216		9.0	0.75 [0.40, 1.41]
Total events: 16 (), 20 (Control)					
Test for heterogeneity chi-square=0.95 df=2 p=0.62 I²=0.0%					
Test for overall effect z=0.88 p=0.4					
03 Case fatality at two to six months after SAH					
Haley 1993	81/438	83/448		36.5	1.00 [0.76, 1.32]
Han 1993	9/142	6/180		2.4	1.90 [0.69, 5.22]
Messeter 1987	1/13	2/7		1.2	0.27 [0.03, 2.47]
Neil-Dwyer 1987	4/38	10/37		4.5	0.39 [0.13, 1.13]
Ohman 1991	10/104	15/109		8.5	0.70 [0.33, 1.48]
Petruk 1988	34/72	32/82		13.3	1.21 [0.84, 1.74]
Pickard 1989	43/278	60/276		26.7	0.71 [0.50, 1.01]
Subtotal	1085	1139		91.0	0.91 [0.76, 1.08]
Total events: 182 (), 208 (Control)					
Test for heterogeneity chi-square=10.75 df=6 p=0.10 I²=44.2%					
Test for overall effect z=1.08 p=0.3					
Total	1300	1355		100.0	0.89 [0.75, 1.06]
Total events: 198 (), 228 (Control)					
Test for heterogeneity chi-square=12.02 df=9 p=0.21 I²=25.1%					
Test for overall effect z=1.30 p=0.2					

0.1   0.2   0.5   1   2   5   10
Favours treatment   Favours control

Figure 18.9 Forest plot showing the effects of a *calcium antagonist vs control* in acute SAH on *case fatality* at final follow-up. Reproduced from Rinkel *et al.* (2005), with permission from the authors and John Wiley & Sons Limited. Copyright Cochrane Library, reproduced with permission.

Death

Treatment with a calcium antagonist was not associated with a statistically significant reduction in the RR of death compared with control (RR: 0.89, 95% CI: 0.75–1.06) (Fig. 18.9).

Cerebral ischaemia

Calcium antagonists were associated with a significant reduction in clinical signs of ischaemic neurological deficits (RR: 0.67, 95% CI: 0.59–0.76) and CT-scan documented cerebral infarction (RR: 0.80, 95% CI: 0.71–0.89) (Fig. 18.10).

Re-bleeding

Calcium antagonists were not associated with any significant excess of re-bleeding (RR: 0.77, 95% CI: 0.58–1.02) (Fig. 18.11).

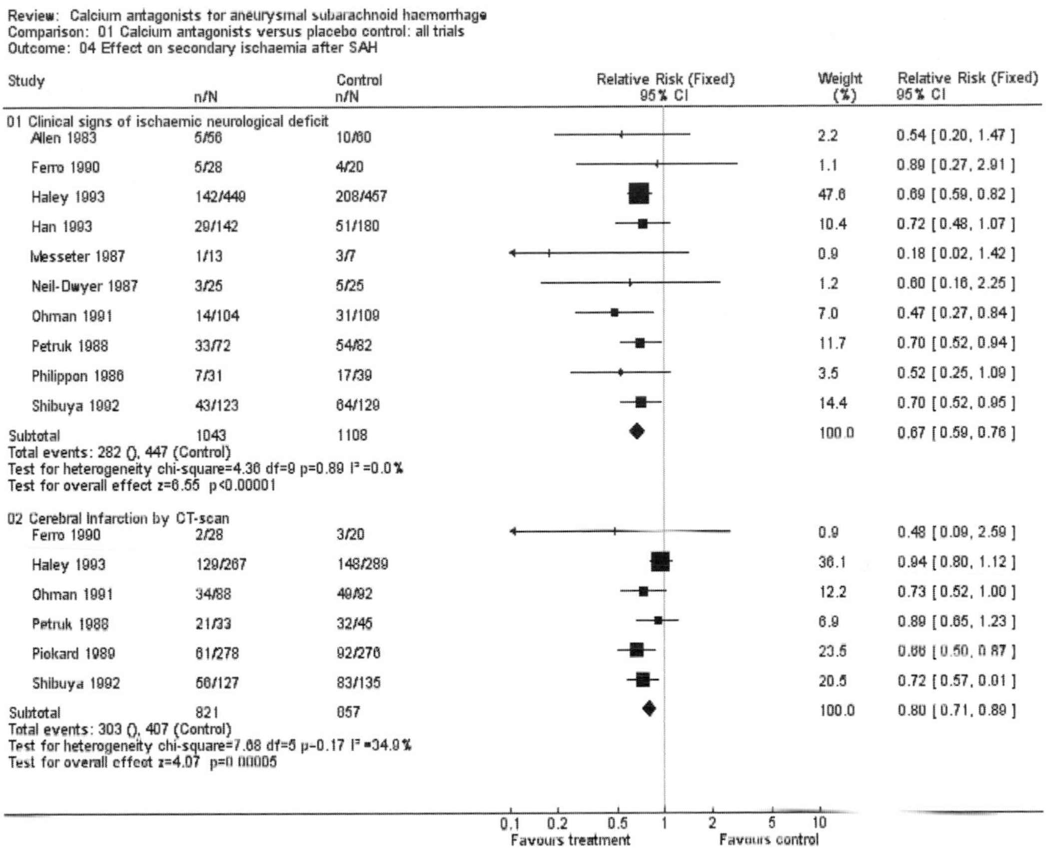

Review: Calcium antagonists for aneurysmal subarachnoid haemorrhage
Comparison: 01 Calcium antagonists versus placebo control: all trials
Outcome: 04 Effect on secondary ischaemia after SAH

Study	n/N	Control n/N	Relative Risk (Fixed) 95% CI	Weight (%)	Relative Risk (Fixed) 95% CI
01 Clinical signs of ischaemic neurological deficit					
Allen 1983	5/58	10/60		2.2	0.54 [0.20, 1.47]
Ferro 1990	5/28	4/20		1.1	0.89 [0.27, 2.91]
Haley 1993	142/449	208/457		47.6	0.69 [0.59, 0.82]
Han 1993	29/142	51/180		10.4	0.72 [0.48, 1.07]
Messeter 1987	1/13	3/7		0.9	0.18 [0.02, 1.42]
Neil-Dwyer 1987	3/25	5/25		1.2	0.60 [0.16, 2.25]
Ohman 1991	14/104	31/109		7.0	0.47 [0.27, 0.84]
Petruk 1988	33/72	54/82		11.7	0.70 [0.52, 0.94]
Philippon 1986	7/31	17/39		3.5	0.52 [0.25, 1.09]
Shibuya 1992	43/123	64/129		14.4	0.70 [0.52, 0.95]
Subtotal	1043	1108		100.0	0.67 [0.59, 0.76]

Total events: 282 (), 447 (Control)
Test for heterogeneity chi-square=4.36 df=9 p=0.89 I²=0.0%
Test for overall effect z=6.55 p<0.00001

02 Cerebral Infarction by CT-scan					
Ferro 1990	2/28	3/20		0.9	0.48 [0.09, 2.59]
Haley 1993	129/267	148/289		36.1	0.94 [0.80, 1.12]
Ohman 1991	34/88	49/92		12.2	0.73 [0.52, 1.00]
Petruk 1988	21/33	32/45		6.9	0.89 [0.65, 1.23]
Pickard 1989	61/278	92/276		23.5	0.66 [0.50, 0.87]
Shibuya 1992	56/127	83/135		20.5	0.72 [0.57, 0.91]
Subtotal	821	857		100.0	0.80 [0.71, 0.89]

Total events: 303 (), 407 (Control)
Test for heterogeneity chi-square=7.68 df=5 p=0.17 I²=34.9%
Test for overall effect z=4.07 p=0.00005

0.1 0.2 0.5 1 2 5 10
Favours treatment   Favours control

Figure 18.10 Forest plot showing the effects of *a calcium antagonist vs control* in acute SAH on *cerebral ischaemia* at final follow-up. Reproduced from Rinkel *et al.* (2005), with permission from the authors and John Wiley & Sons Limited. Copyright Cochrane Library, reproduced with permission.

Comment

Interpretation of the evidence

Calcium antagonists reduce the proportion of patients with poor outcome after aneurysmal SAH, mainly by reducing the risk of ischaemic neurological deficits.

The results are statistically robust, but depend largely on one large trial with oral nimodipine (Pickard *et al.*, 1989); the evidence for nicardipine and AT877 is inconclusive.

Therefore, the evidence for calcium antagonists, and even nimodipine, is not beyond every doubt. However, given the potential benefits and modest risks associated with this treatment, against the background of a devastating natural history, oral nimodipine (60 mg every 4 h) is indicated in patients with aneurysal SAH.

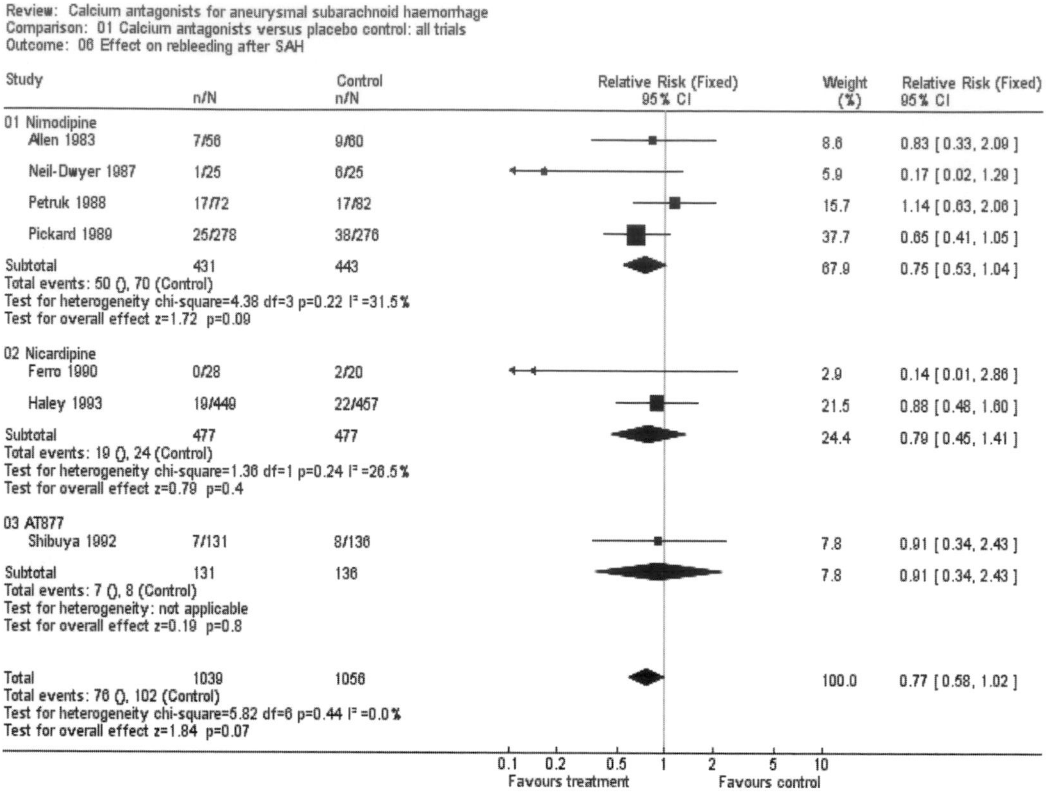

Review: Calcium antagonists for aneurysmal subarachnoid haemorrhage
Comparison: 01 Calcium antagonists versus placebo control: all trials
Outcome: 06 Effect on rebleeding after SAH

Study	n/N	Control n/N	Relative Risk (Fixed) 95% CI	Weight (%)	Relative Risk (Fixed) 95% CI
01 Nimodipine					
Allen 1983	7/56	9/60		8.6	0.83 [0.33, 2.09]
Neil-Dwyer 1987	1/25	6/25		5.9	0.17 [0.02, 1.29]
Petruk 1988	17/72	17/82		15.7	1.14 [0.63, 2.06]
Pickard 1989	25/278	38/276		37.7	0.65 [0.41, 1.05]
Subtotal	431	443		67.9	0.75 [0.53, 1.04]
Total events: 50 (), 70 (Control)					
Test for heterogeneity chi-square=4.38 df=3 p=0.22 I²=31.5%					
Test for overall effect z=1.72 p=0.09					
02 Nicardipine					
Ferro 1990	0/28	2/20		2.9	0.14 [0.01, 2.86]
Haley 1993	19/449	22/457		21.5	0.88 [0.48, 1.60]
Subtotal	477	477		24.4	0.79 [0.45, 1.41]
Total events: 19 (), 24 (Control)					
Test for heterogeneity chi-square=1.36 df=1 p=0.24 I²=26.5%					
Test for overall effect z=0.79 p=0.4					
03 AT877					
Shibuya 1992	7/131	8/136		7.8	0.91 [0.34, 2.43]
Subtotal	131	136		7.8	0.91 [0.34, 2.43]
Total events: 7 (), 8 (Control)					
Test for heterogeneity: not applicable					
Test for overall effect z=0.19 p=0.8					
Total	1039	1056		100.0	0.77 [0.58, 1.02]
Total events: 76 (), 102 (Control)					
Test for heterogeneity chi-square=5.82 df=6 p=0.44 I²=0.0%					
Test for overall effect z=1.84 p=0.07					

```
        0.1   0.2   0.5    1    2    5    10
          Favours treatment    Favours control
```

Figure 18.11   Forest plot showing the effects of *a calcium antagonist vs control* in acute SAH on *re-bleeding* at final follow-up. Reproduced from Rinkel *et al.* (2001), with permission from the authors and John Wiley & Sons Limited. Copyright Cochrane Library, reproduced with permission.

Implications for clinicians

Nimodipine trial (60 mg orally every 4 h, continued for 3 weeks) is the standard treatment in patients with aneurysmal SAH. If the patient is unable to swallow, the tablets should be crushed and washed down a nasogastric tube with normal saline. Intravenous administration of calcium antagonists cannot be recommended on the basis of the present evidence.

Low blood pressure may complicate administration of nimodipine, not only with the intravenous route but also when the drug is given orally (Rinkel *et al.*, 2001). In the presence of hypotension, if no blood loss has occurred or any other cause for hypotension is found, the dose of nimodipine should be halved (to 60 mg tds), and subsequently discontinued if the blood pressure does not come back to initial levels.

Implications for researchers

Almost all the evidence about efficacy and dosage of nimodipine hinges on this single, large clinical trial (Pickard *et al.*, 1989). Given the uncertain effect on overall case fatality, and the possibility that the results of the meta-analysis might be affected by unpublished negative trials, the benefits of nimodipine cannot be regarded as being beyond all reasonable doubt.

For oral nimodipine uncertainty also remains regarding the (dis)advantages in patients in poor clinical condition on admission or in patients with established cerebral ischaemia, the optimal dose and time window, the question whether other types of calcium antagonists offer better protection and the intermediate factors through which nimodipine exerts its beneficial effect after aneurysmal SAH.

Magnesium sulphate

A randomised, double-blind, placebo-controlled trial showed that a continuous intravenous dose of 64 mmol/day, started within 4 days after SAH and continued until 14 days after occlusion of the aneurysm, reduced the risk of delayed cerebral ischaemia by 34% (hazard ratio, 0.66; 95% CI: 0.38 to 1.14). After 3 months, the risk reduction for poor outcome was 23% (risk ratio 0.77; 95% CI: 0.54 to 1.09). [van den Bergh, on behalf of the MASH study group, 2005]. Phase III trials are warranted.

Circulatory volume expansion therapy

A systematic review for the Cochrane Library of circulatory volume expansion therapy (hypervolaemia) in patients with SAH to prevent or treat secondary ischaemia identified one truly randomised trial and one quasi-randomised trial with comparable baseline characteristics for both groups (Rinkel *et al.*, 2004, 2005).

Evidence

Poor outcome
Among a total of 114 patients with SAH randomly assigned volume expansion therapy after occlusion of the aneurysm or no volume expansion therapy, there was no difference in the rate of subsequent poor outcome (RR: 1.0, 95% CI: 0.5–2.2) (Fig. 18.12).

Case fatality
Random assignment to volume expansion therapy after occlusion of the aneurysm was also not associated with any significant reduction in case fatality (RR: 0.75, 95% CI: 0.18–3.20) (Fig. 18.13).

Secondary cerebral ischaemia
Volume expansion therapy was not associated with any reduction in clinical signs of secondary cerebral ischaemia (RR: 1.08, 95% CI: 0.54–2.16) (Fig. 18.14).

Review: Circulatory volume expansion therapy for aneurysmal subarachnoid haemorrhage
Comparison: 01 poor outcome
Outcome: 02 treatment started after occlusion of the aneurysm

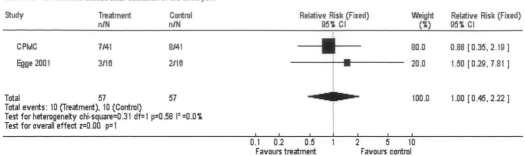

Figure 18.12   Forest plot showing the effects of *circulatory volume expansion therapy vs control* started after occlusion of the aneurysm in patients with acute SAH on *poor outcome* at final follow-up. Reproduced from Rinkel *et al.* (2004), with permission from the authors and John Wiley & Sons Limited. Copyright Cochrane Library, reproduced with permission.

Review: Circulatory volume expansion therapy for aneurysmal subarachnoid haemorrhage
Comparison: 02 case fatality
Outcome: 02 treatment started after occlusion of the aneurysm

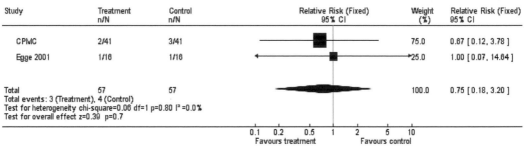

Figure 18.13   Forest plot showing the effects of *circulatory volume expansion therapy vs control* started after occlusion of the aneurysm in patients with acute SAH on *case fatality* at final follow-up. Reproduced from Rinkel *et al.* (2004), with permission from the authors and John Wiley & Sons Limited. Copyright Cochrane Library, reproduced with permission.

Complications

There was a non-significant trend towards hypervolaemia increasing the rate of complications (RR: 1.8, 95% CI: 0.9–3.7).

Comment

The effects of volume expansion therapy have been studied properly in only two trials of patients with aneurysmal SAH, with very small numbers. At present, there is no sound evidence for the use of volume expansion therapy in patients with aneurysmal SAH. However, there was a trend to more complications with the

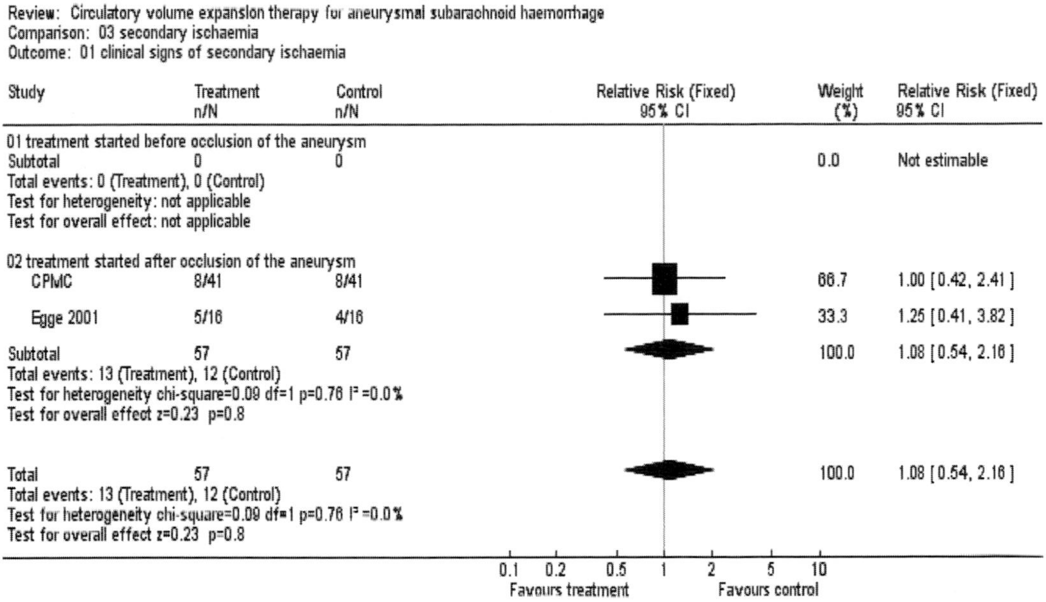

Review: Circulatory volume expansion therapy for aneurysmal subarachnoid haemorrhage
Comparison: 03 secondary ischaemia
Outcome: 01 clinical signs of secondary ischaemia

Study	Treatment n/N	Control n/N	Relative Risk (Fixed) 95% CI	Weight (%)	Relative Risk (Fixed) 95% CI
01 treatment started before occlusion of the aneurysm					
Subtotal	0	0		0.0	Not estimable
Total events: 0 (Treatment), 0 (Control)					
Test for heterogeneity: not applicable					
Test for overall effect: not applicable					
02 treatment started after occlusion of the aneurysm					
CPMC	8/41	8/41		66.7	1.00 [0.42, 2.41]
Egge 2001	5/16	4/16		33.3	1.25 [0.41, 3.82]
Subtotal	57	57		100.0	1.08 [0.54, 2.18]
Total events: 13 (Treatment), 12 (Control)					
Test for heterogeneity chi-square=0.09 df=1 p=0.76 I²=0.0%					
Test for overall effect z=0.23 p=0.8					
Total	57	57		100.0	1.08 [0.54, 2.18]
Total events: 13 (Treatment), 12 (Control)					
Test for heterogeneity chi-square=0.09 df=1 p=0.76 I²=0.0%					
Test for overall effect z=0.23 p=0.8					

```
0.1   0.2   0.5    1    2    5   10
   Favours treatment      Favours control
```

Figure 18.14   Forest plot showing the effects of *circulatory volume expansion therapy vs control* started after occlusion of the aneurysm in patients with acute SAH on *clinical signs of secondary cerebral ischaemia* at final follow-up. Reproduced from Rinkel *et al.* (2004), with permission from the authors and John Wiley & Sons Limited. Copyright Cochrane Library, reproduced with permission.

intervention strategy. Because volume expansion is often used to treat patients with aneurysmal SAH, further evaluation, by means of RCTs, is urgently needed.

Fludrocortisone

Fludrocortisone possesses mineralocorticoid activity (reabsorption of sodium (and water) in the distal tubules of the kidney) which, in theory, may prevent a negative sodium balance, hypovolaemia and so ischaemic complications (Wijdicks *et al.*, 1988a).

Evidence

A randomised trial of 91 patients with SAH who were randomised soon after admission showed that fludrocortisone acetate significantly reduced natriuresis in the first 6 days after the haemorrhage, but there was no significant reduction in plasma volume depletion and ischaemic complications compared with control (Hasan *et al.*, 1989b). This may have been because patients in the control group were often treated with plasma expanders after they had developed clinical signs of ischaemia.

A smaller RCT in 30 patients supported the above results (Mori *et al.*, 1999).

Comment

The available evidence is insufficient to support routine administration of fludrocortisone to all patients with SAH.

5% Albumin

Evidence

A small RCT of 5% albumin (2 h, until central venous pressures of 5–8 mmHg
were reached) compared with control (in which central venous pressure was kept
below 5 mmHg) in 43 patients with SAH showed that the 19 patients assigned
albumin maintained an even sodium balance compared with the 24 controls who
experienced an average sodium loss. There was no difference in blood volume
however between the two groups and the number of patients was too small to
allow conclusions about prevention of ischaemia (Mayer *et al.*, 1998).

Other strategies to maintain plasma volume to prevent delayed cerebral ischaemia

Practical measures that may help to prevent ischaemia are an adequate intake of
fluid and sodium, and avoidance of antihypertensive drugs. However, the benefit
of such regimens is supported by indirect evidence only (Rosenwasser *et al.*, 1983;
Hasan *et al.*, 1989a; Vermeij *et al.*, 1998).

Early intra-operative thrombolysis

A controlled clinical trial of intra-operative thrombolysis with recombinant tissue
plasminogen activator (rt-PA) failed to show any convincing benefit (Findlay *et al.*,
1995). An uncontrolled and small study also reported no difference in outcome
according to the dose of rt-PA that was used (Öhman *et al.*, 1991).

Free radical scavengers

Tirilazad mesylate, a 21-aminosteroid free radical scavenger, has so far failed to
show consistent improvement of outcome in four RCTs, involving a total of more
than 3500 patients (Kassell *et al.*, 1996; Haley *et al.*, 1997; Lanzino and Kassell,
1999; Lanzino *et al.*, 1999b).

N'-propylenedinicotinamide (nicaraven), another hydroxyl radical scavenger, was
shown in a single trial involving 162 patients to be associated with a decreased rate
of delayed cerebral ischaemia, but no reduction in the rate of poor outcomes at
3 months after SAH (Asano *et al.*, 1996).

Ebselen, a seleno-organic compound with antioxidant activity through a gluta-
thione peroxidase-like action, was shown in a trial of 286 patients to be associated
with improved outcome at 3 months after SAH, but without any reduction in the
frequency of delayed ischaemia (Saito *et al.*, 1998).

Antiplatelet therapy

A systematic overview of six RCTs of antiplatelet therapy identified no significant difference in outcome between patients treated with antiplatelet agents and controls (Mendelow *et al.*, 1982; Saito *et al.*, 1983; Shaw *et al.*, 1985; Suzuki *et al.*, 1989; Tokiyoshi *et al.*, 1991; Raupp *et al.*, unpublished review).

General care

Blood pressure

Following intracranial haemorrhage, the range between the upper and lower limits of the autoregulation of cerebral blood flow becomes narrower, which makes the perfusion of brain more dependent on arterial blood pressure (Kaneko *et al.*, 1983). Consequently, aggressive treatment of surges of blood pressure entails a definite risk of ischaemia in brain areas with no autoregulation.

Evidence

In the American Cooperative Study, conducted between 1963 and 1970, 1005 patients with ruptured aneurysms were randomised between four treatment modalities; one arm consisted of drug-induced lowering of the blood pressure, another of bed rest alone, and the other two arms were surgical: carotid ligation and intracranial surgery. In the intention-to-treat analysis, antihypertensive drugs failed to reduce either case fatality or the rate of re-bleeding within the first 6 months after the initial event; on-treatment analysis suggested that induced hypotension did decrease the rate of re-bleeding in comparison with bed rest, but not the case fatality (Torner *et al.*, 1981b). However, the diagnosis of re-bleeding was made in the pre-CT era and was therefore probably inaccurate. The same caveat applies to the finding from the same study that the rate of re-bleeding was not dependent on the degree of blood pressure reduction (Nibbelink *et al.*, 1981).

An observational study, in which all events had been documented by serial CT scanning, compared patients in whom hypertension had been newly treated with normotensive controls. The rate of re-bleeding was lower, but the rate of cerebral infarction was higher, than in untreated controls, despite the blood pressures still being, on average, higher than in the controls (Wijdicks *et al.*, 1990). This suggests that hypertension after SAH is a compensatory phenomenon, at least to some extent, and one that should not be interfered with. In keeping with this, a further observational study from the same centre (Rotterdam) suggested that the combined strategy of avoiding antihypertensive medication and increasing fluid intake may decrease the risk of cerebral infarction (Hasan *et al.*, 1989a).

Comment

These data support the avoidance of treating hypertension with antihypertensive drugs following aneurysmal rupture. In many patients, surges of high blood pressure can be attenuated by adequate pain management or sedation; for example, when the patient is resisting the ventilator.

Antihypertensive therapy should only be started (in addition to other drugs the patient is already taking) in patients with extreme elevations of blood pressure and rapidly progressive end-organ deterioration (e.g. new retinopathy, left-ventricular failure, proteinuria or oliguria with a rapid rise of plasma creatinine levels).

Effective antihypertensive treatments are:

- diazoxide (50–150 mg by intravenous bolus, repeated after 5–10 min, or 15–30 mg/min by intravenous infusion, up to 600 mg);
- labetalol hydrochloride (20–80 mg by intravenous bolus every 10 min, or 2 mg/min by intravenous infusion, up to 300 mg) (Calhoun and Oparil 1990; Gifford et al., 1991). Labetalol, however, may be ineffective in patients previously treated with β-blockers and is contraindicated in heart failure and asthma;
- nitroprusside (intravenously) has also been advocated in hypertensive crises, but is probably not a first-line drug in this situation because animal studies have shown that it increases intracranial pressure (Candia et al., 1978).

It is probably reasonable to aim for a 25% decrease in mean arterial pressure below the initial baseline. Intra-arterial monitoring of the blood pressure is recommended in these situations.

Fluids and electrolytes

In about one-third of patients with SAH, the plasma volume decreases by more than 10% between the second and tenth day after the haemorrhage due to a loss of sodium and water (cerebral salt wasting), which causes negative sodium balance (Wijdicks et al., 1985a; Hasan et al., 1990).

The rationale for fluid replacement is to prevent a reduction in plasma volume, which may contribute to the development of cerebral ischaemia (Wijdicks et al., 1985b).

Evidence

Two RCTs of fluid supplementation (a daily intake of at least 3 l of saline) have been undertaken in patients with SAH.

The first trial included only 30 patients (Rosenwasser et al., 1983). Treatment allocation was not blinded and outcome was not assessed beyond the time of operation (days 7–10). At days 7–10, the rate of delayed ischaemia was reduced by two-thirds (67%; 95% CI: 1–89%) among patients assigned hypervolaemic therapy.

The second trial randomised 82 patients between normovolaemia and hypervolaemia (monitored by means of cardiac filling pressures). There was no difference in outcome: 20% in each group had an episode of secondary deterioration interpreted as delayed cerebral ischaemia, and blood volume and cerebral blood flow measurements were also similar in the two groups (Lennihan *et al.*, 2000).

Comment

Despite the incomplete evidence, it seems reasonable to prevent hypovolaemia by giving 2.5–3.5 l/day of normal saline, unless contraindicated by signs of impending cardiac failure. The amount of intravenous saline should be reduced if the patient is also receiving nutritional solution via the enteral route; most commercially prepared enteral solutions deliver 1–2 cal/ml (4–8 J/ml).

Otherwise, a daily fluid intake of 4–6 l (sometimes as much as 10 l) may be needed to balance the loss of sodium and water in the urine plus estimated insensible losses via perspiration and expired air (which are greater in patients with fever).

Fluid requirements should be guided by frequent calculation of fluid balance (four times per day until approximately day 10), with or without recording the central venous pressure (the directly measured value should be above 8 mmHg) or pulmonary wedge pressure (to be kept above 7 mmHg). Central venous pressure should be measured, via a catheter in the subclavian or internal jugular vein, in patients who develop hyponatraemia or a negative fluid balance; pulmonary artery balloon catheters are used in patients with a history of cardiopulmonary disease.

Analgesics and general nursing care

Bed rest

Until the aneurysm has been occluded, the patient should be confined to complete bed rest, laying flat in dimmed light, because it is assumed that any form of excitement may increase blood pressure and increase the risk of re-bleeding. If a good angiographical study has not shown an aneurysm, the patient can be allowed to sit up as soon as their headache subsides. However, if there is an aneurysmal pattern of haemorrhage on the CT scan it is wise to keep the patient under the close supervision of the nursing staff until the angiogram has been done.

Headache

Headache can sometimes be managed with mild analgesics such as paracetamol, with or without dextropropoxyphene; salicylates should be avoided until the aneurysm has been occluded, because of their inhibitory effect on haemostasis. However, usually the pain is so severe that tramadol or codeine needs to be added, and this will not mask neurological signs. Sometimes, pain can be alleviated with anxiolytic drugs such as midazolam. Even a synthetic opiate such as piritramide may be needed to obtain relief. As a last resort, severe headache can be treated with morphine given intravenously in small increments of 1–2 mg; many patients benefit from the euphoriant effect. A potential adverse effect of morphine is hypotension, because it is a potent vasodilator. The blood pressure should be checked frequently until the pain has subsided. Constipation is a common disadvantage of morphine, as well as of codeine.

Fever

The body temperature should be frequently measured, up to four times per day, depending on the interval after SAH and the level of consciousness. In the first few days, mild fever (up to 38.5°C) often results from the inflammatory reaction in the subarachnoid space; in that case, the pulse rate is characteristically normal (Rousseaux *et al.*, 1980). Infection should be suspected if the temperature exceeds 38.5°C, if the pulse rate is elevated as well or if the patient has vomited.

Coughing and straining

Coughing and straining must be prevented because of the attendant overshoots in arterial blood pressure. Stool softeners should be prescribed routinely. Enemas are contraindicated because they markedly increase intra-abdominal pressure and secondarily intracranial pressure. A urinary catheter is almost always needed, except in men who are alert and have perfect bladder control. Proper control of fluid balance requires the volume of urine to be precisely measured; condom devices leak or slip off too often to be of any use in these critically ill patients. Intermittent catheterisation may substantially decrease the risk of urinary infections and promote bladder 're-training', but the procedure is commonly very stressful for patients with SAH.

Gastric bleeding prophylaxis

Oral administration of antacids is said to be sufficient to protect against stress-induced gastric bleeding; H2-receptor antagonists or proton-pump inhibitors are expensive and should be considered only in mechanically ventilated patients, or in patients with a previous history of peptic ulcers.

Venous thromboembolism prophylaxis

Deep venous thrombosis (DVT) is not as common after SAH as ischaemic stroke, presumably because the patients are restless, mostly younger and have no paralysed leg. In a large and prospective series, DVT was diagnosed clinically in only 4% of patients. (Vermeulen *et al.*, 1984a).

In general, DVT can be prevented by subcutaneous low-dose heparin or heparinoids (Chapter 9), but the concern is that the risk of aneurysmal re-bleeding will be increased.

In patients undergoing general surgical, neurosurgical or orthopaedic procedures, graduated compression stockings significantly reduced the risk of DVT by
about two-thirds (Wells *et al.*, 1994; Nurmohamed *et al.*, 1996; Agnelli *et al.*, 1998).
In patients with SAH, a study with non-randomised controls also suggested DVT
could be successfully prevented in this way (Black *et al.*, 1986).

There have been no RCTs of stockings (or antithrombotic agents) for the prevention of venous thromboembolism (VTE) in patients with SAH.

Epileptic seizure prophylaxis

The prophylactic use of antiepileptic medication is controversial. Seizures in the
first few weeks after aneurysmal rupture occur in about 10% of patients, and most
occur soon after the initial haemorrhage (Rose and Sarner, 1965; Hart *et al.*, 1981;
Hasan *et al.*, 1993; Pinto *et al.*, 1996). Intracranial haematoma and intracranial
surgery probably increase the risk.

Evidence

A randomised trial of anticonvulsants after supratentorial craniotomy for benign
lesions (not only aneurysms) failed to show benefit in terms of seizure rate or case
fatality, although the CI was wide (Foy *et al.*, 1992).

Comment

As the possible disadvantage of a serious drug reaction may well outweigh the benefits, antiepileptic drugs should probably not be administered routinely, unless
there is a history of seizures. If phenytoin is given, absorption by the oral route is
severely impaired when patients receive continuous nasogastric tube feeding
(Bauer, 1982). Absorption will improve if the continuous feeding is stopped 2 h
before the dose is given, the suspension or crushed tablets are flushed down the
nasogastric tube with 60 ml of water, and two additional hours are allowed to
elapse before feeding is resumed; but larger than usual doses may still be required.

Management of re-bleeding

Sudden apnoea in a patient with SAH usually signifies re-bleeding.

Resuscitation

With full resuscitative measures, spontaneous respiration will rapidly return in
approximately 50% of the cases, followed within hours by return of consciousness
and of brainstem reflexes if these were lost at the same time. If spontaneous
respiration does not return, then organ donation should be considered (Hijdra
et al., 1984).

Emergency clipping or coiling of the aneurysm

Emergency clipping or coiling of the aneurysm should be considered in patients who regain consciousness after re-bleeding, despite the increased risk of the operation after a re-bleed, because 50–75% of survivors have a further re-bleed if the aneurysm is not occluded (Hijdra *et al.*, 1987b; Inagawa *et al.*, 1987).

For the 10% of cases with re-bleeding in whom there is a large haematoma that causes brain shift without gross intraventricular haemorrhage, evacuation of the haematoma may be indicated.

Management of cerebral ischaemia

The clinical manifestations of delayed cerebral ischaemia evolve gradually, over several hours, and usually between days 4 and 12 after the haemorrhage. In a quarter of the patients, ischaemia causes hemispheric focal deficits; in another quarter, a decrease in the level of consciousness; and in the remaining half of the patients, these two features develop at the same time (Hijdra *et al.*, 1986). The CT brain scan identifies ischaemic changes in about 80% of patients within a few days (Hijdra *et al.*, 1986). MR imaging is more sensitive but the acquisition time needed to obtain good images is often too long for ill and restless patients. Transcranial Doppler sonography may suggest impending cerebral ischaemia by means of the increased blood flow velocity from arterial narrowing in the middle cerebral artery or in the posterior circulation (Vora *et al.*, 1999).

Induced hypertension and volume expansion

Volume expansion and induced hypertension have been used to combat ischaemic deficits in patients with SAH for several decades (Farhat and Schneider, 1967; Kosnik and Hunt, 1976).

Evidence

Although not evaluated by RCTs, cases have served as their own controls in a larger series of 58 patients with progressive neurological deterioration and angiographically confirmed 'vasospasm' (Kassell *et al.*, 1982). Volume expansion and induced hypertension reversed the deficits in 47 of the 58 cases, and permanently in 43. In 16 patients who responded to this treatment, the neurological deficits recurred when the blood pressure transiently dropped, but again resolved when the pressure increased. Similar results have been obtained in two other series (Awad *et al.*, 1987; Miller *et al.*, 1995).

Comment

The most plausible explanation for the apparent effectiveness of volume expansion and induced hypertension in the treatment of delayed cerebral ischaemia is a defect of cerebral autoregulation that makes the perfusion of the brain passively dependent on the systemic blood pressure.

The risks of deliberately increasing the arterial pressure and plasma volume include re-bleeding of an untreated aneurysm, increased cerebral oedema or haemorrhagic transformation in areas of infarction (Amin-Hanjani et al., 1999), myocardial infarction and congestive heart failure. Consequently, the circulatory system should be closely monitored with an arterial line and either a central venous or pulmonary artery catheter, despite the risks of infection, pneumothorax, haemothorax, ventricular dysrhythmias and pulmonary infarction (Rosenwasser et al., 1995).

A recommended regimen, although not supported by RCTs, is to start with plasma volume expansion with hetastarch or another colloid solution. The aim is to raise the central venous filling pressure to approximately 8–12 mmHg or the pulmonary capillary wedge pressure to about 14–18 mmHg. If no clinical improvement is obtained with these measures, other strategies are to raise the blood pressure to 20–40 mmHg above pretreatment values by using dopamine or dobutamine (Biller et al., 1988).

Transluminal angioplasty

Evidence

Reports of case series of an endovascular approach to the treatment of 'symptomatic vasospasm' document sustained improvement in more than half the cases, but the series were uncontrolled and are likely to be prone to publication bias (Higashida et al., 1989; Newell et al., 1989; Bejjani et al., 1998; Eskridge et al., 1998).

Complications included hyperperfusion injury (Schoser et al., 1997) and re-bleeding, even after the aneurysm has been clipped (Newell et al., 1989; Linskey et al., 1991; Honma et al., 1995). Hyperperfusion injury has also been reported (Schoser et al., 1997).

Comment

In view of the lack of evidence of effectiveness from RCTs and the documented risks, and known high costs, transluminal angioplasty should presently be regarded as an experimental procedure.

Calcitonin gene-related peptide

Calcitonin gene-related peptide (CGRP) is a potent vasodilator in the carotid vascular bed, but a randomised, multicentre, single-blind clinical trial in 62 patients failed to show any benefit in terms of overall outcome: the RR of a poor outcome in CGRP-treated patients was 0.88 (95% CI: 0.60–1.28) (Anon., 1992).

Management of systemic complications

Hyponatraemia

Hyponatraemia, with or without intravascular volume change, is the most common electrolyte disturbance following aneurysmal rupture. It develops most commonly between the second and tenth day (Wijdicks *et al.*, 1985a).

Plasma sodium concentrations below 125 mmol/l cause irritability, restlessness, confusion, an impaired consciousness, asterixis, hemiparesis and seizures. Sodium levels below 100 mmol/l almost always give rise to seizures, and rarely ventricular tachycardia or fibrillation. However, the most feared complication of hyponatraemia is the precipitation of delayed cerebral ischaemia, through associated hypovolaemia.

Hyponatraemia after SAH results from excessive natriuresis, or *cerebral salt wasting*, and not inappropriate secretion of antidiuretic hormone (sodium dilution) (Harrigan, 1996). The negative sodium balance leads to a decrease in plasma volume (Wijdicks *et al.*, 1985a).

The treatment of hyponatraemia after SAH is to correct the volume depletion. A mild degree of hyponatraemia (125–134 mmol/l) is usually well tolerated and self-limiting, and need not be treated. Moderate hyponatraemia in patients with evidence of a negative fluid balance, or excessive natriuresis, is corrected with saline (0.9%; sodium concentration: 150 mmol/l) or with a mixture of glucose and saline. Acute symptomatic hyponatraemia is rare, and requires urgent treatment with hypertonic saline (1.8% or even 3%). However, over-rapid infusion of sodium may precipitate myelinolysis in the pons and the white matter of the cerebral hemispheres. A retrospective survey suggests that the maximal rate of correction should be by 12 mmol/l/day (Sterns *et al.*, 1986), but others maintain that more rapid correction is safe as long as the plasma sodium level does not exceed 126 mmol/l during the first 24 h (Ayus *et al.*, 1987).

Disorders of heart rhythm

Cardiac dysrhythmias and electrocardiographical (ECG) abnormalities are common after SAH. The most common ECG abnormalities are ST segment and T segment changes, prominent U waves, QT prolongation and sinus dysrhythmias. Life-threatening dysrhythmias such as ventricular fibrillation or *torsade de pointes* may be seen on 24-h monitoring, but are extremely rare (Brouwers *et al.*, 1989).

The prognostic value of ECG changes after SAH is unclear, but they are more important as indicators of severe intracranial disease than as predictors of potentially serious cardiac complications (Brouwers *et al.*, 1989; Manninen *et al.*, 1995).

In patients with SAH, routine administration of antidysrhythmic drugs is not warranted until there is evidence of improved overall outcome; the net benefits may be disappointing because some, such as β-blockers, also lower blood pressure.

Neurogenic pulmonary oedema

Neurogenic pulmonary oedema is a dramatic and dangerous complication of SAH, seen in less than 10% of patients (Wijdicks *et al.*, 1998). It usually evolves rapidly within hours of SAH. The cause it uncertain but it is related to the severity of aneurysmal haemorrhage. One explanation is that the elevated intracranial pressure provokes a massive sympathetic discharge mediated by the anterior hypothalamus which leads to vasoconstriction of the pulmonary (and other) vasculature. If severe, there may be severe vasoconstriction of the vasa vasorum, causing ischaemic damage to endothelial cells, resulting in increased permeability (Theodore and Robin, 1976).

Diuretics are often used as standard therapy, and labetalol or chlorpromazine may be also beneficial (Wohns *et al.*, 1985; Harrier, 1988).

SUMMARY

The fundamentals of treating aneurysmal SAH are to prevent re-bleeding by occluding the aneurysm, and prevent and treat the complications of intracranial blood such as raised intracranial pressure, delayed cerebral ischaemia and hypovolaemia.

Immediate neurosurgery is indicated in patients with large intraparenchymal or subdural haematomas caused by a ruptured aneurysm, who become increasingly drowsy in the first few hours after SAH, to evacuate the haematoma. The operation is preferably preceded by CT angiography to display the relevant aneurysm, so it can also be clipped at the time of decompressive surgery.

In patients deteriorating from acute hydrocephalus after SAH, it is worth trying serial lumbar punctures if spontaneous improvement does not occur within 24 h, and if the probable site of obstruction is in the subarachnoid space, not in the ventricular system.

The risk of re-bleeding after rupture of an intracranial aneurysm, without medical or surgical intervention is about 20% on the first day; and in survivors of the first day, about 40% in the first month. Therefore, the cumulative risk for all patients in the first month is about 50%.

Early neurosurgical clipping of the aneurysm is now the usual practice for patients in good clinical condition but this policy is vulnerable to challenge and reversal because it has not been supported by any RCT.

Endovascular coiling of the aneurysm is more effective than neurosurgical clipping in reducing death or dependency at 1 year among the small subgroup (one-fifth to one-quarter) of patients with good-grade, anterior circulation, small ruptured saccular aneurysms, providing expert neuroradiological intervention is available.

Antifibrinolytic drugs prevent re-bleeding after aneurysmal rupture, but because they increase the risk of cerebral ischaemia there is no useful effect on overall outcome.

Effective strategies for preventing ischaemic complications include calcium antagonists, maintenance of an adequate intake of water and sodium and, if necessary, plasma volume expansion and avoidance of antihypertensive treatment.

Oral nimodipine probably reduces the risk of a poor outcome after SAH by about one-third.

A high fluid intake is essential in patients with aneurysmal SAH to compensate for 'cerebral salt wasting' and to prevent hypovolaemia, because this predisposes to cerebral ischaemia. The daily minimum is 2.5–3.5 l of normal saline, by the oral or intravenous route; more may be needed to balance the volume of urine, or with fever.

Other theoretically attractive pharmacological interventions to prevent cerebral ischaemia, such as maintaining plasma volume by means of fludrocortisone acetate or albumin, neuroprotection via hydroxyl radical scavengers, and – after aneurysm occlusion – prophylaxis with antithrombotic drugs such as aspirin, are unproven.

Hypertension in the acute phase of SAH can be left untreated unless there are signs of end-organ damage by high blood pressure. Existing antihypertensive drugs can be continued.

Headache is a typical and distressing problem in patients with SAH. In those with a decreased level of consciousness, it may manifest as restlessness. The 'analgesic staircase' consists of frequent doses (every 3–4 h) of paracetamol 500 mg orally; add codeine 20 mg orally; piritramide 20 mg subcutaneously; morphine 2 mg intravenously, with 1–2 mg increments.

Hyponatraemia after SAH usually reflects cerebral salt wasting (sodium depletion) and not secretion of antidiuretic hormone (sodium dilution). As hyponatraemia may lead to hypovolaemia, it should be vigorously treated to prevent cerebral ischaemia.

Abnormalities of heart rhythm after SAH represent 'smoke' rather than 'fire', and rarely need to be treated.

References

Preface

Alderson P. Absence of evidence is not evidence of absence. *British Medical Journal* 2004; 328: 476–477.

Warlow C, Sudlow C, Dennis M, Wardlaw J, Sandercock P. Stroke. *Lancet* 2003; 362: 1211–1224.

Chapter 1. The size of the problem of stroke

Bonita R, Stewart A, Beaglehole R. International trends in stroke mortality 1970–1985. *Stroke* 1990; 21: 989–992.

Bonita R, Solomon N, Broad JB. Prevalence of stroke and stroke-related disability: estimates from the Auckland Stroke Studies. *Stroke* 1997; 28: 1898–1902.

Bonita R, Mendis S, Truelsen T, Bogousslavsky J, Toole J, Yatsu F. The global stroke initiative. *Lancet Neurology* 2004; 3: 391–393.

Bots ML, Looman SJ, Koudstaal PJ, Hofman A, Hoes AW, Grobbee DE. Prevalence of stroke in the general population. The Rotterdam study. *Stroke* 1996; 27: 1499–1501.

Coull AJ, Lovett JK, Rothwell PM, for the Oxford Vascular Study. Population based study of early risk of stroke after transient ischemic attack or minor stroke: implications for public education and organisation of services. *British Medical Journal* 2004; 328: 326–328.

Counsell C, Dennis M, McDowall M, Warlow C. Predicting outcome after acute and subacute stroke: development and validation of new prognostic models. *Stroke* 2002; 33: 1041–1047.

Dennis MS, Burn JP, Sandercock PAG et al. Long-term survival after first-ever stroke: the Oxfordshire community stroke project. *Stroke* 1993; 24: 796–800.

Dewey HM, Thrift AG, Mihalopoulos C, Macdonell RAL, McNeil JJ, Donnan GA. Cost of stroke in Australia from a societal perspective. Results from the North East Melbourne Stroke Incidence Study (NEMESIS). *Stroke* 2001; 32: 2409–2416.

Dippel DW, Wijnhoud AD, Koudstaal PJ. Prediction of major vascular events after TIA or minor stroke. A comparison of 6 models. *Cerebrovascular Diseases* 2004; 17 (Suppl 5): 35.

Evers SMAA, Engel GL, Ament AJHA. Cost of stroke in the Netherlands from a societal perspective. *Stroke* 1997; 28: 1375–1381.

Evers SM, Struijs JN, Ament AJ et al. International comparison of stroke cost studies. *Stroke* 2004; 35: 1209–1215.

Feigin VL, Lawes CMM, Bennett DA, Anderson CA. Stroke epidemiology: a review of population-based studies of incidence, prevalence, and case-fatality in the late 20th century. *Lancet Neurology* 2003; 2: 43–53.

Feigin VL. Stroke epidemiology in the developing world. Lancet 2005; 365: 2160–1.

Geddes JML, Fear J, Tennant A, Pickering A, Hillman M, Chamberlain MA. Prevalence of self reported stroke in a population in northern England. *Journal of Epidemiology and Community Health* 1996; 50, 140–143.

Gross CP, Anderson GF, Powe NR. The relation between funding by the National Institutes of Health and the burden of disease. *New England Journal of Medicine* 1999; 340: 1881–1887.

Hankey GJ. Preventing stroke – what is the real progress? *Medical Journal of Australia* 1999; 171: 285–286.

Hankey GJ. Redefining risks after TIA and minor ischaemic stroke. *Lancet* 2005; 365: 2065–6.

Hankey GJ, Jamrozik K, Broadhurst RJ, Forbes S, Burvill PW, Anderson CS, Stewart-Wynne EG. Long-term risk of recurrent stroke in the Perth Community Stroke Study. *Stroke* 1998; 29: 2491–2500.

Hankey GJ, Jamrozik K, Broadhurst RJ, Forbes S, Burvill PW, Anderson CS, Stewart-Wynne EG. Five year survival after first-ever stroke and related prognostic factors in the Perth Community Stroke Study. *Stroke* 2000; 31: 2080–2086.

Hankey GJ, Jamrozik K, Broadhurst RJ, Forbes S, Anderson CS. Long-term disability after first-ever stroke and related prognostic factors in the Perth Community Stroke Study, 1989–1990. *Stroke* 2002; 33: 1034–1040.

Hardie K, Hankey GJ, Jamrozik K, Broadhurst R, Anderson C. Ten-year survival after first-ever stroke in the Perth Community Stroke Study. *Stroke* 2003; 34: 1842–1846.

Hardie K, Hankey GJ, Jamrozik K, Broadhurst RJ, Anderson CS. Ten-year risk of first recurrent stroke and disability after first-ever stroke in the Perth Community Stroke Study. *Stroke* 2004; 35: 731–735.

Hill MD, Yiannakoulias N, Jeerakathil T, Tu JV, Svenson LW, Schopflocher DP. The high risk of stroke immediately after transient ischemic attack. A population-based study. *Neurology* 2004; 62: 2015–2020.

Isaard PA, Forbes JF. The cost of stroke to the National Health Service in Scotland. *Cerebrovascular Diseases* 1992; 2: 47–50.

Jamrozik K, Broadhurst R, Lai N, Hankey GJ, Burvill PW, Anderson CS. Trends in the incidence, severity and short-term outcome of stroke in Perth, Western Australia. *Stroke* 1999; 30: 2105–2111.

Lavados PM, Sacks C, Prina L, et al. Incidence, 30-day case-fatality rate, and prognosis of stroke in iquique, chile: a 2-year community-based prospective study (PISCIS project). Lancet 2005; 365: 2206–15.

Levy E, Gabriel S, Dinet J. The comparative medical costs of atherothrombotic disease in European countries. *Pharmacoeconomics* 2003; 21: 651–659.

Lopez AD, Murray CC. The global burden of disease, 1990–2020. *Nature Medicine* 1998; 4: 1241–1243.

Lovett JK, Coull A, Rothwell PM, on behalf of the Oxford Vascular Study. Early risk of recurrence by subtype of ischemic stroke in population-based incidence studies. *Neurology* 2004; 62: 569–574.

Malmgren R, Bamford J, Warlow C, Sandercock P, Slattery J. Projecting the number of patients with first-ever strokes and patients newly handicapped by stroke in England and Wales. *British Medical Journal* 1989; 298: 656–660.

Martinez-Vila E, Irimia P. The cost of stroke. *Cerebrovascular Diseases* 2004; 17 (Suppl 1): 124–129.

Murray CJL, Lopez AD. *The Global Burden of Disease: A Comprehensive Assessment of Mortality and Disability from Diseases, Injuries and Risk Factors in 1990 and Projected to 2020.* Boston: Harvard University Press, 1996.

Murray CJL, Lopez AD. Mortality by cause for eight regions of the world: global burden of disease study. *Lancet* 1997; 349: 1269–1276.

Payne K, Huybrechts K, Caro J *et al.* Long term cost-of-illness in stroke: an international review. *Pharmacoeconomics* 2002; 20: 813–825.

Pendlebury ST, Rothwell PM, Algra A *et al.* Underfunding of stroke research: a Europe-wide problem. *Stroke* 2004; 35: 2368–2371.

Rose G. *The Strategy of Preventive Medicine.* Oxford: Oxford University Press, Oxford Medical Publications, 1992.

Rothwell PM. The high cost of not funding stroke research: a comparison with heart disease and cancer. *Lancet* 2001; 357: 1612–1616.

Rothwell P, Coull AJ, Giles MF *et al.*, for the Oxford Vascular Study. Change in stroke incidence, mortality, case-fatality, severity and risk factors in Oxfordshire, United Kingdom, from 1981 to 2004 (Oxford Vascular Study). *Lancet* 2004; 363: 1925–1933.

Rothwell PM, Giles MF, Flossmann E, Lovelock CE, Redgrave JNE, Warlow CP, Mehta Z. A simple score (ABCD) to identify individuals at high early risk of stroke after transient ischaemic attack. Lancet 2005; 366: 29–36.

Sarti C, Rastenyte D, Cepaitis Z, Tuomilehto J. International trends in mortality from stroke, 1968 to 1994. *Stroke* 2000; 31: 1588–1601.

Sudlow CLM, Warlow CP, for the International Stroke Incidence Collaboration. Comparable studies of the incidence of stroke and its pathological subtypes. Results from an International Collaboration. *Stroke* 1997; 28: 491–499.

Taylor T, Davis P, Torner J *et al.* Lifetime cost of stroke in the United States. *Stroke* 1996; 27: 1459–1466.

van Wijk I, Kappelle LJ, van Gijn J, Koudstaal PJ, Franke CL, Vermeulen M, Gorter JW, Algra A, for the LILAC Study Group. Long-term survival and vascular event risk after transient ischaemic attack or minor ischaemic stroke. *Lancet* 2005; 365: 2098–104.

Warlow C, Sudlow C, Dennis M, Wardlaw J, Sandercock P. Stroke. *Lancet* 2003; 362: 1211–1224.

Wyller TB, Bautz-Holter E, Holmen J. Prevalence of stroke and stroke-related disability in North Trondelag County, Norway. *Cerebrovascular Diseases* 1994; 4: 421–427.

Chapter 2. Understanding evidence

Alderson P. Absence of evidence is not evidence of absence. *British Medical Journal* 2004; 328: 476–477.

Alderson P, Chalmers I. Survey of claims of no effect in abstracts of Cochrane Reviews. *British Medical Journal* 2003; 326: 475.

Altman DG, Bland JM. Absence of evidence is no evidence of absence. *British Medical Journal* 1995; 311: 485.

Altman DG, Schulz KF, Moher D, *et al.*, for the CONSORT group. The revised CONSORT statement for reporting randomised trials: explanation and elaboration. *Annals of Internal Medicine* 2001; 134: 663–694.

Antithrombotic Trialists' Collaboration. Collaborative meta-analysis of randomised trials of antiplatelet therapy for prevention of death, myocardial infarction, and stroke in high risk patients. *British Medical Journal* 2002; 324: 71–86.

Ashcroft R. Giving medicine a fair trial. *British Medical Journal* 2000; 320: 1686.

Bekelman JE, Yi Y, Gross CP. Scope and impact of financial conflicts of interest in biomedical research – a systematic review. *Journal of the American Medical Association* 2003; 289: 454–465.

De Bruijn SFTN, Stam J. Randomized placebo-controlled trial of anticoagulant treatment with low-molecular-weight heparin for cerebral sinus thrombosis. *Stroke* 1999; 30: 484–488.

The Canadian Cooperative Study Group. A randomized trial of aspirin and sulfinpyrazone in threatened stroke. *New England Journal of Medicine* 1978; 299: 53–59.

Chalmers I. Well informed uncertainties about the effects of treatments. *British Medical Journal* 2004; 328: 475–476.

Cochran WG. The combination of estimates from different experiments. *Biometrics* 1954; 10: 101–129.

Collins R, Gray R, Goodwin J, Peto R. Avoidance of large biases and large random errors in the assessment of moderate treatment effects. The need for systematic overviews. *Statistics in Medicine* 1987; 6: 245–250.

Collins R, MacMahon S. Reliable assessment of the effects of treatment on mortality and major morbidity. I: Clinical trials. *Lancet* 2001; 357: 373–380.

Cook DI, Gebski VJ, Keech AC. Subgroup analysis in clinical trials. *Medical Journal of Australia* 2004; 180: 289–291.

Donnan GA, Davis SM, Kaste M, for the International Trial Subcommittee of the International Stroke Liaison Committee, American Stroke Association. Recommendations for the relationship between sponsors and investigators in the design and conduct of clinical stroke trials. *Stroke* 2003; 34: 1041–1045.

Der Simonian R, Laird N. Meta-analysis in clinical trials. *Controlled Clinical Trials* 1986; 7: 177–188.

Diener HC, Cunha L, Forbes C *et al.* European Stroke Prevention Study 2. Dipyridamole and acetylsalicylic acid in the secondary prevention of stroke. *Journal of the Neurological Sciences* 1996; 143: 1–13.

Doust J, Del Mar C. Why do doctors use treatments that do not work? *British Medical Journal* 2004; 328: 474–475.

Easterbrook PJ, Berlin JA, Gopalan R, Matthews DR. Publication bias in clinical research. *Lancet* 1991; 337: 865–872.

EC-IC Bypass Study Group. Failure of extracranial–intracranial arterial bypass to reduce the risk of ischaemic stroke: results of an international randomised trial. *New England Journal of Medicine* 1985; 313: 1191–1200.

Gardner MJ, Altman DG. Confidence intervals rather than *p* values: estimation rather than hypothesis testing. *British Medical Journal* 1986; 292: 746–750.

Gardner MJ, Altman DG. Calculating confidence intervals for odds ratios. In: Gardner MJ, Altman DG (eds), *Statistics with Confidence. Confidence Intervals and Statistical Guidelines.* Belfast: Universities Press. *British Medical Journal* 1989; 53–59.

Gelmers, HJ, Gorter K, de Weerdt CJ *et al.* A controlled trial of nimodipine in acute ischaemic stroke. *New England Journal of Medicine* 1998; 318: 203–237.

Glasziou P, Vandenbroucke J, Chalmers I. Assessing the quality of research. *British Medical Journal* 2004; 328: 39–41.

Harbour R, Miller J, for the Scottish Intercollegiate Guidelines Network Grading Review Group. A new system for drafting recommendations in evidence-based guidelines. *British Medical Journal* 2001; 323: 334–336.

Higgins JPT, Thompson SG, Deeks JJ, Altman DG. Measuring inconsistency in meta-analyses. *British Medical Journal* 2003; 327: 557–560.

Horn J, Limburg M. Calcium antagonists for acute ischemic stroke. *The Cochrane Database of Systematic Reviews* 2000, Issue 1. Art. No.: CD001928. DOI: 10.1002/14651858.CD001928.

International Subarachnoid Aneurysm Trial (ISAT) Collaborative Group. International Subarachnoid Aneurysm Trial (ISAT) trial of neurosurgical clipping versus endovascular coiling in 2143 patients with ruptured intracranial aneurysms: a randomised trial. *Lancet* 2002; 360: 1267–1274.

Lader EW, Cannon CP, Ohman EM *et al.*, The clinician as investigator. Participating in clinical trials in the practice setting. *Circulation* 2004, 109: 2672–2679, e302–e304, e305–e307.

Lees KR, Hankey GJ, Hacke W. Design of future acute-stroke treatment trials. *Lancet Neurology* 2003; 2: 54–61.

Lexchin J, Bero LA, Djulbegovic B *et al.* Pharmaceutical industry sponsorship and research outcome and quality: systematic review. *British Medical Journal* 2003; 326: 1167–1170.

Lewis SC, Warlow CP. How to spot bias and other potential problems in randomised controlled trials. *Journal of Neurology Neurosurgery and Psychiatry* 2004; 75: 181–187.

MacMahon S, Collins R. Reliable assessment of the effects of treatment on mortality and major morbidity. I: Observational studies. *Lancet* 2001; 357: 455–462.

Moher D, Schulz KF, Altman D. The CONSORT statement: revised recommendations for improving the quality of parallel-group randomised trials. *Journal of the American Medical Association* 2001; 285: 1987–1991.

National Health and Medical Research Council. A guide to the development, implementation and evaluation of clinical practice guidelines. Canberra: NHMRC, AusInfo, 1999.

O'Connell RL, Gebski VJ, Keech AC. Making sense of trial results: outcomes and estimation. *Medical Journal of Australia* 2004; 180: 128–130.

Peto R. Why do we need systematic reviews of randomised trials? *Statistics in Medicine* 1987; 6: 233–240.

Peto R, Baigent C. Trials: the next 50 years. *British Medical Journal* 1998; 317: 1170–1171.

Rothwell PM. External validity of randomised controlled trials: "To whom do the results of this trial apply?" *Lancet* 2005a; 365: 82–93.

Rothwell PM. Subgroup analysis in randomised controlled trials: importance, indications, and interpretation. *Lancet* 2005b; 365: 176–186.

Rothwell PM, Metha Z, Howard SC, Gutnikov SA, Warlow CP. From subgroups to individuals: general principles and the example of carotid endarterectomy. *Lancet* 2005; 365: 256–265.

Sackett DL, Straus SE, Richardson WS, Rosenberg W, Haynes RB. *Evidence-Based Medicine. How to Practice and Teach EBM*. Edinburgh: Churchill Livingstone, 2000.

Sandercock P. The odds ratio: a useful tool in neurosciences. *Journal of Neurology Neurosurgery and Psychiatry* 1989; 52: 817–820.

Shaw GB (ed.). *The Doctor's Dilemma*. London: Penguin Books, 1908.

Shultz KF, Chalmers I, Grimes DA *et al*. Assessing the quality of randomisation from reports of controlled trials published in obstetrics and gynaecology reports. *Journal of the American Medical Association* 1994; 272: 125–128.

Toole JF, Malinow R, Chambless L, Spence JD, Pettigrew LC, Howard VJ, Sides EG, Wang C-H, Stampfer M. Lowering homocysteine in patients with ischemic stroke to prevent recurrent stroke, myocardial infarction and death. The Vitamin Intervention for Stroke Prevention (VISP) randomised controlled trial. *Journal of the American Medical Association* 2004; 291: 565–575.

van Gijn J. Evidence-based stroke medicine. Plenary lecture at *The European Stroke Conference*, Mannheim, Germany, May, 2004.

van Gijn J. From randomised trials to rational practice. *Cerebrovascular Diseases* 2005; 19: 69–76.

Warlow C. The Willis Lecture 2003. Evaluating treatments for stroke patients too slowly. Time to get of out second gear. *Stroke* 2004; 35: 2211–2219.

Chapter 3. Organised acute stroke care

Caplan L. Neurologist, internist, strokologist? *Stroke* 2003; 34: 2765.

Donnan GA, Davis SM. Stroke is best managed by a neurologist: battle of the titans. *Stroke* 2003; 34: 2764–2765.

Early Supported Discharge Trialists. Services for reducing duration of hospital care for acute stroke patients. *The Cochrane Database of Systematic Reviews* 2001, Issue 3. Art. No.: CD000443. DOI: 10.1002/14651858.CD000443.

Evans A, Perez I, Harraf F, Melbourn A, Steadman J, Donaldson N, Kalra L. Can differences in management processes explain different outcomes between stroke unit and stroke-team care? *Lancet* 2001; 358: 1586–1592.

Evans A, Harraf F, Donaldson N, Kalra L. Randomised controlled study of stroke unit care versus stroke team care in different stroke subtypes. *Stroke* 2002; 33: 449–455.

Fjaertoft H, Indredavik B, Lydersen S. Stroke unit care combined with early supported discharge. Long-term follow-up of a randomised controlled trial. *Stroke* 2003; 34: 2687–2692.

Fuentes B, Diez TE, Lara M, Frank A, Barriero P. Stroke units: which stroke subtypes benefit the most (abstract). *Cerebrovascular Diseases* 2001; 11 (Suppl 4): 121.

Glader E-L, Stegmayr B, Johannson L *et al*. Differences in long-term outcome between patients treated in stroke units and in general wards: a 2 year fellow up of stroke patients in Sweden. *Stroke* 2001; 32: 2124–2130.

Hacke W. A late step in the right direction of stroke care. *Lancet* 2000; 356: 869–870.

Hydo B. Designing an effective clinical pathway for stroke. *American Journal of Nursing* 1995; 95: 44–50.

Indredavik B, Bakke F, Slørdahl SA, Rokseth R, Haheim LL. Treatment in a combined acute and rehabilitation stroke unit: which aspects are most important? *Stroke* 1999; 30: 917–923.

Indredavik B, Fjkaertoft H, Ekeberg G, Løge AD, Mørch B. Benefit of an extended stroke unit service with early supported discharge: a randomised controlled trial. *Stroke* 2000; 31: 2989–2994.

Intercollegiate Stroke Working Party. National Sentinel Stroke Audit 2001/2. Trust Report: Clinical Effectiveness and Evaluation Unit, Royal College of Physicians, 2002.

Jorgensen HS, Kammersgard LP, Houth J *et al.* Who benefits from treatment and rehabilitation in a stroke unit? A community based study. *Stroke* 2000; 31: 434–439.

Kalra L, Evans A, Perez I, Knapp M, Donaldson N, Swift C. Alternative strategies for stroke: a prospective randomised controlled trial. *Lancet* 2000; 356: 894–899.

Kwakkel G, van Peppen R, Wagenaar RC *et al.* Effects of augmented exercise therapy time after stroke. A meta-analysis. *Stroke* 2004; 35: 2529–2536.

Kwan J, Sandercock P. In-hospital care pathways for stroke. An updated systematic review. *Stroke* 2005; 36: 1348–9.

Kwan J, Sandercock P. In-hospital care pathways for stroke. *The Cochrane Database of Systematic Reviews* 2004, Issue 4. Art. No.: CD002924. DOI: 10.1002/14651858.CD002924.pub2.

Langhorne P. How should stroke services be organised? *Lancet Neurology* 2002; 1: 62–63.

Langhorne P. Early supported discharge: an idea whose time has come? *Stroke* 2003; 34: 2691–2692.

Langhorne P, Dennis M. *Stroke Units: An Evidence-Based Approach*. London: BMJ Books, 1998.

Langhorne P, Dennis MS, Kalra L, Shepperd S, Wade DT, Wolfe CDA. Services for helping acute stroke patients avoid hospital admission. *The Cochrane Database of Systematic Reviews* 1999, Issue 3. Art. No.: CD000444. DOI: 10.1002/14651858.CD000444.

Langhorne P, Pollock A, in conjunction with The Stroke Unit Trialists' Collaboration. What are the components of effective stroke unit care? *Age and Ageing* 2002; 31: 365–371.

Langhorne P, Dennis M. Stroke units: the next 10 years. *Lancet* 2004; 363: 834–835.

Langhorne P, Taylor G, Murray G *et al.* Early supported discharge services for stroke patients. *Lancet* 2005; 365: 501–506.

Lanska DJ. The role of clinical pathways in reducing the economic burden of stroke. *Pharmacoeconomics* 1998; 14: 151–158.

Legg L, Langhorne P. Therapy-based rehabilitation for stroke patients living at home. *Stroke* 2004; 35: 1022.

Lees KR. Stroke is best managed by a neurologist: battle of the titans. *Stroke* 2003; 34: 2764–2765.

Major K, Walker A. Economics of stroke unit care. In: Langhorne P, Dennis M (eds), *Stroke Units: An Evidence-Based Approach*. London: BMJ Books, 1998; 56–65.

Meijer R, van Limbeek J. early supported discharge: A valuable alternative for some stroke patients. *Lancet* 2005; 365: 455–456.

Patel A, Knapp M, Perez I, Evans A, Kalra L. Alternative strategies for stroke care. Cost-effectiveness and cost-utility analyses from a prospective randomised controlled trial. *Stroke* 2004; 35: 196–204.

Rudd AG, Hoffman A, Irwin P, Lowe D, Pearson MG. Stroke unit care and outcome. Results from the 2001 National Sentinel Audit of Stroke (England, Wales, and Northern Ireland). *Stroke* 2005; 36: 103–106.

Shepperd S, Iliffe S. Hospital at home versus in-patient hospital care. *The Cochrane Database of Systematic Reviews* 2001, Issue 2. Art. No.: CD000356. DOI: 10.1002/14651858.CD000356.

Stegmayr B, Asplund K, Hutter-Åsperg *et al.* Stroke units in the natural habitat-can results of randomised trials be reproduced in clinical practice? *Stroke* 1999; 30: 709–714.

Stroke Unit Trialists' Collaboration. Organised inpatient (stroke unit) care for stroke. *The Cochrane Database of Systematic Reviews* 2001, Issue 3. Art. No.: CD000197. DOI: 10.1002/14651858.CD000197.

Stone S. Every patient with a stroke should be treated in a stroke unit. *British Medical Journal* 2002; 325: 291–292.

Sulter G, Elting JW, Langedijk M, Maurits NM, Keyser J. Admitting acute ischaemic stroke patients to a stroke care monitoring unit versus a conventional stroke unit: a randomised pilot study. *Stroke* 2003; 34: 101–104.

References to trials included in the Cochrane Review by the Stroke Unit Trialists' Collaboration, Organised inpatient (stroke unit) care for stroke (Cochrane Review). *The Cochrane Database of Systematic Reviews* 2001, Issue 3. Art. No.: CD000197. DOI: 10.1002/14651858.CD000197

Akershus {published and unpublished data}
*Ronning OM, Guldvog B. Stroke units versus general medical wards. II: Neurological deficits and activities of daily living: a quasi-randomised controlled trial. *Stroke* 1998; 29: 586–590.

Birmingham {published data only}
*Peacock PB, Riley CHP, Lampton TD, Raffel SS, Walker JS. The Birmingham stroke, epidemiology and rehabilitation study. In: Stewart GT (ed.), *Trends in Epidemiology*. Springfield, IL: Thomas, 1972: 231–345.

Dover {published and unpublished data}
*Stevens RS, Ambler NR, Warren MD. A randomised controlled trial of a stroke rehabilitation ward. *Age and Ageing* 1984; 13: 65–75.

Edinburgh {published and unpublished data}
*Garraway, WM, Akhtar AJ, Hockey L, Prescott RJ. Management of acute stroke in elderly: follow up of a controlled trial. *British Medical Journal* 1980; 281: 827–829.

Goteborg-Ostra {unpublished data only}
Svensson, Harmsen P, Wilhelmsen L. {Unpublished trial}
Goteborg-Sahlgren {unpublished data only}
Claeesson L, Gosman-Hedstrom G, Johannnesson M, Fagerberg B, Blomstrand C. Resource utilization and costs of stroke unit care integrated in a care continuum: a 1-year controlled, prospective, randomized study in elderly patients. The Goteborg 70+ stroke study. *Stroke* 2000; 31: 2569–2577.

Classson L, Gosman-Hedstrom G, Johannesson M, Fagerberg B, Blomstrand C. Stroke unit care – effects on ADL, health-related quality of life and health economy (abstract). *Cerebrovascular Diseases* 1999; 9 (Suppl 1): 115.

Fagerberg B, Blomstrand C. Do stroke units save lives? (letter) *Lancet* 1993; 342: 992.

*Fagerberg B, Claesson L, Gosman-Hedstrom G, Blomstrand C. Effect of acute stroke unit care integrated with care continuum versus conventional treatment: a randomized 1-year study of elderly patients. The Goteborg 70+ stroke study. *Stroke* 2000; 31: 2578–2584.

Helsinki {published and unpublished data}
Kaste M, Palomaki H. By whom should elderly stroke patients be treated? (abstract). *Stroke* 1992; 23: 163.

Kaste M, Palomaki H. Who should treat elderly stroke patients? (abstract). *Journal of Stroke and Cerebrovascular Diseases* 1992; 2 (Suppl 1): S27.

*Kaste M, Palomaki H, Sarna S. Where and how should elderly stroke patients be treated? A randomised trial. *Stroke* 1995; 26: 249–253.

Illinois {published data only}

*Gordon EE, Kohn KH. Evaluation of rehabilitation methods in the hemiplegic patient. *Journal of Chronic Diseases* 1966; 19: 3–16.

Kuopio {published and unpublished data}

*Sivenius J, Pyorala K, Heinonen OP, Salonen JT, Reikkinen P. The significance of intensity of rehabilitation after stroke – a controlled trial. *Stroke* 1985; 16: 928–931.

Montreal {published and unpublished data}

*Wood-Dauphinee S, Shapiro S, Bass E, Fletcher C, Georges P, Hensby V *et al.* A randomised trial of team care following stroke. *Stroke* 1984; 5: 864–872.

Montreal-Home {published data only}

Montreal-Transfer {published data only}

New York {published data only}

*Feldman DJ, Lee PR, Unterecker J, Lloyd K, Rusk HA, Toole A. A comparison of functionally orientated medical care and formal rehabilitation in the management of patients with hemiplegia due to cerebrovascular disease. *Journal of Chronic Diseases* 1962; 15: 297–310.

Newcastle {published and unpublished data}

*Aitken PD, Rodgers H, French JM, Bates D, James OFW. General medical or geriatric unit care for acute stroke? A controlled trial. *Age and Ageing* 1993; 22 (Suppl 2): 4–5.

Nottingham {published and unpublished data}

Husbands SL, Lincoln NB, Drummond AER, Gladman J, Trescoli C. Five-year results of a randomized controlled trial of a stroke rehabilitation unit (abstract). *Clinical Rehabilitation* 1999; 13: 530–531.

*Juby LC, Loncoln NB, Berman P. The effect of a stroke rehabilitation unit on functional and psychological outcome. A randomised controlled trial. *Cerebrovascular Diseases* 1996; 6: 106–110.

Lincoln NB, Husbands S, Trescoli C, Drummond AER, Gladman JRF, Berman P. Five year follow up of a randomised controlled trial of a stroke rehabilitation unit. *British Medical Journal* 2000; 320: 549.

Orpington-1993 {published and unpublished data}

*Kalra L, Dale P, Crome P. Improving stroke rehabilitation: a controlled study. *Stroke* 1993; 24: 1462–1467.

Orpington-1995 {published and unpublished data}

*Kalra L, Eade J. Role of stroke rehabilitation units in managing severe disability after stroke. *Stroke* 1995; 26: 2031–2034.

Orpington-2000 {published and unpublished data}

Evans A, Perez I, Melbourn A, Steadman J, Kalra L. Alternative strategies in stroke: a randomised controlled trial of three strategies of stroke management and rehabilitation (abstract). *Cerebrovascular Diseases* 2000; 10 (Suppl 2): 60.

*Kalra LL, Evaans A, Perez I, Knapp M, Donaldson N, Swift C. Alternative strategies for stroke: a prospective randomised controlled trial. *Lancet* 2000; 356: 894–899.

Orpington-Mild {published data only}

Orpington-Moderate {published data only}

Orpington-Severe {published data only}

Perth {published and unpublished data}

*Hankey GJ, Deleo D, Stewart-Wynne EG. Stroke units: an Australian perspective. *Australian and New Zealand Journal of Medicine* 1997; 27: 437–438.

Stockholm {published data only}

*von Arbin M, Britton M, de Faire U, Helmers C, Miah K, Murray V. A study of stroke patients treated in a non-intensive stroke unit or in general medical wards. *Acta Medica Scandinavica* 1980; 208: 81–85.

Svendborg {published data only}

Henriksen IO, Laursen SO. Acute stroke – treatment in a non-intensive stroke unit (abstract). *Scandinavian Journal of Rehabilitation Medicine* 1992; Suppl 26: 153.

*Laursen SO, Henriksen IO, Dons U, Jacobsen B, Gundertofte L. Intensive rehabilitation following stroke: controlled pilot study. *Ugeskrift for Laeger* 1995; 157: 1996–1999.

Tampere {unpublished data only}

*Ilmavirta M, Frey H, Erila T, Fogelholm R. Stroke outcome and outcome of brain infarction. A prospective randomised study comparing the outcome of patients with acute brain infarction treated in a stroke unit and in an ordinary neurological ward (academic dissertation), Vol. 410, Series A. Tampere, Finland: University of Tampere Faculty of Medicine, 1994.

Trondheim {published and unpublished data}

Indredavik B, Bakke F, Slordahl SA, Rokseth R, Haheim LL. Stroke unit treatment improves long-term quality of life: a randomized controlled trial. *Stroke* 1998; 29: 895–899.

Indredavik B, Bakke F, Slordahl SA, Rokseth R, Haheim LL. Stroke unit treatment: 10 year follow-up. *Stroke* 1999; 30: 1524–1527.

Indredavik B, Bakke F, Slordahl SA, Rokseth R, Haheim LL. Treatment in a combined acute and rehabilitation stroke unit. Which aspects are important? *Stroke* 1999; 30: 917–923.

*Indredavik B, Bakke F, Solberg R Rokseth R, Haahein LL, Home I. Benefit of stroke unit: a randomised controlled trial. *Stroke* 1991; 22: 1026–1031.

Indredavik B, Slordahl SA, Bakke F. Stroke unit treatment – 10 years follow-up (abstract). *Cerebrovascular Diseases* 1999; 9 (Suppl 1): 122.

Indredavik B, Slordahl SA, Bakke F, Rokseth R, Haheim LL. Stroke unit treatment: long-term effects. *Stroke* 1997; 28: 1861–1866.

Umea {published and unpublished data}

*Strand T, Asplund K, Eriksson S, Hagg E, Lithner F, Wester PO. A non-intensive stroke unit reduced functional disability and the need for long-term hospitalisation. *Stroke* 1985; 16: 29–34.

Uppsala {published and unpublished data}

*Hamrin E. Early activation after stroke: does it make a difference? *Scandinavian Journal of Rehabilitation Medicine* 1982; 14: 101–109.

Chapter 4. General supportive acute stroke care

Adams Jr HP. Effective prophylaxis for deep vein thrombosis after stroke. Low-dose anticoagulation rather than stockings alone: For. *Stroke* 2004; 35: 2911–2912.

Adams Jr HP, Brott TG, Crowell RM, Furlan AJ, Gomez CR, Grotta J, Helgason CM, Marler JR, Woolson RF, Zivin JA *et al.* Guidelines for the management of patients with acute ischemic stroke. A statement for healthcare professionals from a special writing group of the Stroke Council, American Heart Association. *Stroke* 1994; 25: 1901–1914.

Adams Jr HP, Adams RJ, Brott T *et al.* Guidelines for the early management of patients with ischaemic stroke. A scientific statement from the Stroke Council of the American Stroke Association. *Stroke* 2003; 34: 1056–1083.

Adams H, Adams R, Del Zoppo G, Goldstein L. Guidelines for the early management of patients with ischaemic stroke. 2005 guidelines update. A scientific statement from the stroke council of the American Heart Association/American Stroke Association. *Stroke* 2005; 36: 916–921.

Ahmed N, Nasman P, Wahlgren NG. Effect of intravenous nimodipine on blood pressure and outcome after acute stroke. *Stroke* 2000; 31: 1250–1255.

[AU2]Ahmed N, Wahlgren G. High initial blood pressure after acute stroke is associated with poor functional outcome. *Journal of Internal Medicine* 2001; 249: 467–473.

Antiplatelet Trialists' Collaboration. Collaborative overview of randomised trials of antiplatelet therapy. III: Reduction in venous thrombosis and pulmonary embolism by antiplatelet prophylaxis among surgical and medical patients. *British Medical Journal* 1994; 308: 235–246.

Aslanyan S, Fazekas F, Weir CJ, Horner S, Lees KR, for the GAIN International Steering Committee and Investigators. Effect of blood pressure during the acute period of ischaemic stroke on stroke outcome. A tertiary analysis of the GAIN international trial. *Stroke* 2003; 34: 2420–2425.

Bath FJ, Bath PMW. What is the correct management of blood pressure in acute stroke? The Blood Pressure in Acute Stroke Collaboration. *Cerebrovascular Diseases* 1997; 7: 205–213.

Bath PMW, Bath FJ, Smithard DG. Interventions for dysphagia in acute stroke. *The Cochrane Database of Systematic Reviews* 1999, Issue 3. Art. No.: CD000323. DOI: 10.1002/14651858. CD000323.

Bath P. Efficacy of Nitric Oxide in Stroke (ENOS) trial – a prospective randomised controlled trial in acute stroke. Ongoing Clinical Trial Abstracts, *29th International Stroke Conference*, 2004, American Stroke Association, CTP39.

Bhalla A, Sankaralingam S, Dundas R, Swaminathan R, Wolfe CD, Rudd AG. Influence of raised plasma osmolality on clinical outcome after acute stroke. *Stroke* 2000; 31: 2043–2048.

Blood Pressure in Acute Stroke Collaboration (BASC). Interventions for deliberately altering blood pressure in acute stroke (Cochrane Review). In: *The Cochrane Library*, Issue 1, 2001. Oxford: Update Software.

The Blood Pressure in Acute Stroke Collaboration (BASC). Vasoactive drugs for acute stroke (Cochrane Review). In: *The Cochrane Library*, Issue 2, 2004. Chichester, UK: John Wiley & Sons, Ltd.

Boysen G. Editorial comment – persisting dilemma: to treat or not to treat blood pressure in acute ischaemic stroke. *Stroke* 2004; 35: 526–527.

Britton M, Carlsson A, de Faire U. Blood pressure course in patients with acute stroke and matched controls. *Stroke* 1986; 17: 861–864.

Broderick JP, Phillips SJ, O'Fallon WM, Frye RL, Whisnant JP. Relationship of cardiac disease to stroke occurrence, recurrence, and mortality. *Stroke* 1992; 23: 1250–1256.

Capes SE, Hunt D, Malmberg K, Pathak P, Gerstein HC. Stress hyperglycemia and prognosis of stroke in nondiabetic and diabetic patients: a systematic overview. *Stroke* 2001; 32: 2426–3223.

Carlsson A, Britton M. Blood pressure after stroke. A 1 year follow up study. *Stroke* 1993; 24: 195–199.

Carlberg B, Asplund K, Hagg E. Factors influencing admission blood pressure levels in patients with acute stroke. *Stroke* 1991; 22: 527–530.

Castillo J, Leira R, Garcia MM, Serena J, Blanco M, Dávalos A. Blood pressure decrease during the acute phase of ischaemic stroke is associated with brain injury and poor stroke outcome. *Stroke* 2004; 35: 520–527.

Choi-Kwon S, Yang YH, Kim EK, Leon MY, Kim JS. Nutritional status in acute stroke: undernutrition versus overnutrition in different stroke subtypes. *Acta Neurologica Scandinavica* 1998; 98: 187–192.

Corbett D, Thornhill J. Temperature modulation (hypothermic and hyperthermic conditions) and its influence on histological and behavioral outcomes following cerebral ischemia. *Brain Pathology* 2000; 10: 145–152.

Counsell C, Sandercock P. Low-molecular-weight heparins or heparinoids versus standard unfractionated heparin for acute ischaemic stroke stroke (Cochrane Corner). *Stroke* 2002; 33: 1925–1926.

Davenport RJ, Dennis MS, Wellwood I, Warlow CP. Complications after acute stroke. *Stroke* 1996; 27: 415–420.

Davis M, Hollymann C, McGiven M, Chambers I, Egbuji J, Barer D. Physiological monitoring in acute stroke. *Age and Ageing* 1999; 28 (Suppl 1): P45.

Davis SM, Donnan GA. Effective prophylaxis for deep vein thrombosis after stroke. Both low-dose anticoagulation and stockings for most cases. *Stroke* 2004; 35: 2910.

Dennis MS. Effective prophylaxis for deep vein thrombosis after stroke. Low-dose anticoagulation rather than stockings alone: Against. *Stroke* 2004; 35: 2912–2913.

Dippel DWJ, van Breda EJ, van Gemert HMA, van der Worp HB, Kappelle LJ, Koudstaal PJ. The effect of paracetamol (acetaminophen) on body temperature in acute ischaemic stroke. A double blind, randomised phase-II clinical trial. *Cerebrovascular Diseases* 2001; 11 (Suppl 4): 79.

Diringer MN. Management of sodium abnormalities in patients with CNS disease. *Clinical Neuropharmacology* 1992; 15: 427–447.

Eames PJ, Blake MJ, Dawson SL, Panerai RB, Potter JF. Dynamic cerebral autoregulation and beat to beat blood pressure control are impaired in acute ischaemic stroke. *Journal of Neurology Neurosurgery and Psychiatry* 2002; 72: 467–472.

The European Stroke Initiative Executive Committee and the EUSI Writing Committee. European Stroke Initiative Recommendations for stroke management – Update 2003. *Cerebrovascular Diseases* 2003; 16: 311–337.

European Stroke Initiative. Recommendations for stroke management: Update 2003. *Cerebrovascular Diseases* 2004; 17 (Suppl 2): 1–46.

Evans A, Perez I, Harraf F, Melbourn A, Steadman J, Donaldson N, Kalra. Can differences in management processes explain different outcomes between stroke unit and stroke-team care? *Lancet* 2001; 358: 1586–1592.

Finestone HM. Safe feeding methods in stroke patients. *Lancet* 2000; 355: 1662–1663.

The FOOD Trial Collaboration. Poor nutritional status on admission predicts poor outcomes after stroke: observational data from the FOOD trial. *Stroke* 2003; 34: 140–156.

The FOOD Trial Collaboration. Routine oral nutritional supplementation for stroke patients in hospital (FOOD): a multicentre randomised controlled trial. *Lancet* 2005a; 365: 755–763.

The FOOD Trial Collaboration. Effect of timing and method of enteral tube feeding for dysphagic stroke patients (FOOD): a multicentre, randomised controlled trial. *Lancet* 2005b; 365: 764–772.

Fukuda H, Kitani M, Takahashi K. Body temperature correlates with functional outcome and the lesion size of cerebral infarction. *Acta Neurologica Scandinavica* 1999; 100: 385–390.

Gariballa SE, Parker SG, Taub N, Castleden CM. A randomised controlled single-blind trial of nutritional supplementation after acute stroke. *Journal of Parenteral Enteral Nutrition* 1998; 22: 315–319.

Gilbertson L, Langhorne P, Walker A, Allen A, Murray GD. Domiciliary occupational therapy for patients with *stroke* discharged from hospital: a randomised controlled trial. *British Medical Journal* 2000; 320: 603–606.

GIST-UK Protocol, 2004. http://www.gist-uk.org. Accessed January 3, 2005.

Grandi FC, Sandrock P, Miccio M, Salvi RM. Physical methods for preventing deep vein thrombosis in stroke. *Stroke* 2005; 36: 1102–1103.

Grau AJ, Buggle F, Schnitzler P, Spiel M, Lichy C, Hacke W. Fever and infection early after ischemic stroke. *Journal of Neurological Science* 1999; 171: 115–120.

Grau AJ, Boddy AW, Dukovic DA *et al*. Leucocyte count as an independent predictor of recurrent ischaemic events. *Stroke* 2004; 35: 1147–1152.

Gray CS, Hildreth AJ, Alberti GKMM, O'Connell JE, on behalf of the GIST Collaboration. Poststroke hyperglycaemia. Natural history and immediate management. *Stroke* 2004; 35: 122–126.

Grossman E, Messerli FH, Grodzicki T, Kowey P. Should a moratorium be placed on sublingual nifedipine capsules given for hypertensive emergencies and pseudoemergencies? *Journal of the American Medical Association* 1996; 276: 1328–1331.

Gubitz G, Sandercock P, Counsell C. Anticoagulants for acute ischaemic stroke. *The Cochrane Database of Systematic Reviews* 2004, Issue 2. Art. No.: CD000024. DOI: 10.1002/14651858. CD000024.pub2.

Hajat C, Hajat S, Sharma P. Effects of post-stroke pyrexia on stroke outcome: a meta-analysis of studies in patients. *Stroke* 2000; 31: 410–414.

Harper G, Castleden CM, Potter JF. Factors affecting changes in blood pressure after acute stroke. *Stroke* 1994; 25: 1726–1729.

Hillbom M, Erila T, Sotaniemi K, Tatlisumak T, Sarna S, Kaste M. Enoxaparin vs heparin for prevention of deep-vein thrombosis in acute ischaemic stroke: a randomised, double-blind study. *Acta Neurologica Scandinavica* 2002; 106: 84–92.

Huff JS. Stroke mimics and chameleon. *Emergency Medicine Clinics of North America* 2002; 20: 583–595.

Indredavik B, Bakke F, Slordahl SA *et al.* Treatment in a combined acute and rehabilitation stroke unit: which aspects are most important? *Stroke* 1999; 30: 917–923.

International Society of Hypertension Writing Group. International Society of Hypertension (ISH): Statement on the management of blood pressure in acute stroke. *Journal of Hypertension* 2003; 21: 665–672.

Kalra L, Yu G, Wilson K *et al.* Medical complications during stroke rehabilitation. *Stroke* 1995; 26: 990–994.

Kasner SE, Wein T, Piriyawat P, Villar-Cordova CE, Chalela JA, Krieger DW, Morgenstern LB, Kimmel SE, Grotta JC. Acetaminophen for altering body temperature in acute stroke: a randomized clinical trial. *Stroke* 2002; 33: 130–134.

Kelly J, Rudd A, Lewis R, Hunt BJ. Venous thromboembolism after acute stroke. *Stroke* 2001; 32: 262–267.

Langhorne P, Stott DJ, Robertson L, MacDonald J, Jones L, McAlpine C, Dick F, Taylor GS, Murray G. Medical complications after stroke. A multicenter study. *Stroke* 2000; 31: 1223–1229.

Langhorne P, Tong BLP, Stott DJ. Association between physiological homeostasis and early recovery after stroke. *Stroke* 2000; 31: 2526–2527.

Leonardi-Be J, Bath PMW, Phillips SJ, Sandercock PAG, for the IST Collaborative Group. Blood pressure and clinical outcomes in the International Stroke Trial. *Stroke* 2002; 33: 1315–1320.

Lindsberg PJ, Roine RO. Hyperglycaemia in acute stroke. *Stroke* 2004; 35: 363–364.

Lindsberg PJ, Grau AJ. Inflammation and infections as risk factors for ischaemic stroke. *Stroke* 2003; 34: 2518–2532.

Mann G, Hankey GJ, Cameron D. Swallowing disorders after acute stroke. Prevalence and diagnostic accuracy. *Cerebrovascular Diseases* 2000; 10: 380–386.

Mann G, Hankey GJ, Cameron D. Swallowing dysfunction after acute stroke. Prognosis and prognostic factors at 6 months. *Stroke* 1999; 30: 744–748.

Mazzone C, Chiodo Grandi F, Sandercock P, Miccio M, Salvi R. Physical methods for preventing deep vein thrombosis in stroke (Cochrane Methodological Review). In: *The Cochrane Library*, Chichester, UK: John Wiley & Sons, Ltd, Issue 4, 2004.

McClatchie G. Survey of the rehabilitation outcomes of stroke. *Medical Journal of Australia* 1980; 1: 649–651.

Meyer JS, Shimazu K, Fukuhuchi, Ohuchi T, Okamoto S, Koto A. Impaired neurogenic cerebrovascular control and dysautoregulation after stroke. *Stroke* 1973; 4: 169.

Muir KW, Watt A, Baxter G, Grosset DG, Lees KR. Randomised trial of graded compression stockings for prevention of deep-vein thrombosis after acute stroke. *Quarterly Journal of Medicine* 2000; 93: 359–364.

Myers M, Norris J, Hachinski V *et al.* Cardiac sequelae of acute stroke. *Stroke* 1982; 13: 838–842.

Nachtmann A, Siebler M, Rose G *et al.* Cheyne-Strokes respiration in ischemic stroke. *Neurology* 1995; 45: 820–821.

Nakayama H, Jorgensen HS, Pedersen PM *et al.* Prevalence and risk factors for incontinence after stroke. The Copenhagen stroke study. *Stroke* 1997; 28: 58–62.

Nuffield Institute of Health. Effective health care. The prevention and treatment of pressure sores. *Effective Health Care* 1995; 2: 1–16.

Oppenheimer SM, Keden G, Martin WM. Left-insular cortex lesions perturb cardiac autonomic tone in humans. *Clinical Autonomic Research* 1996; 6: 131–140.

Parsons MW, Barber PA, Desmond PM *et al.* Acute hyperglycaemia adversely affects stroke outcome: a magnetic resonance imaging and spectroscopy study. *Annals of Neurology* 2002; 52: 20–28.

Reith J, Jorgensen HS, Pedersen PM *et al.* Body temperature in acute stroke: relation to stroke severity, infarct size, mortality, and outcome. *Lancet* 1996; 347: 422–425.

Ronning OM, Guldvog B. Should stroke victims routinely receive supplemental oxygen? A quasi-randomised controlled trial. *Stroke* 1999; 30: 2033–2037.

Rusymiak DE, Kirk MA, May JD *et al.* Hyperbaric oxygen therapy in acute ischaemic stroke. Results of the hyperbaric oxygen in acute ischaemic stroke trial pilot study. *Stroke* 2003; 34: 571–574.

Sandercock P, Gubitz G, Foley P, Counsell C. Antiplatelet therapy for acute ischaemic stroke. *The Cochrane Database of Systematic Reviews* 2003, Issue 2. Art. No.: CD000029. DOI: 10.1002/14651858.CD00002.

Sandercock P, Counsell C, Stobbs SL. Low-molecular-weight heparins or heparinoids versus standard unfractionated heparin for acute ischaemic stroke stroke. *The Cochrane Database of Systematic Reviews* 2005, Issue 2. Art. No.: CD000119. DOI: 10.1002/14651858.CD000119.pub2.

Schrader J, Luders S, Kulschewski A, Berger J, Zidek W, Treib J, Einhaupl K, Diener HC, Dominiak P, for the Acute Candesartan Cilexetil Therapy in Stroke Survivors Study Group. The ACCESS study: evaluation of Acute Candesartan Cilexetil Therapy in Stroke Survivors. *Stroke* 2003; 34: 1699–1703.

Schwab S, Schwarz S, Spranger M *et al.* Moderate hypothermia in the treatment of patients with severe middle cerebral artery infarction. *Stroke* 1998; 29: 2461–2466.

Scott JF, Gray CS, O'Connell JE *et al.* Glucose and insulin therapy in acute stroke; why delay further? *Quarterly Journal of Medicine* 1998; 91: 511–515.

Scott JF, Robinson GM, O'Connell JE *et al.* Glucose potassium insulin (GKI) infusions in the treatment of acute stroke patients with mild to moderate hyperglycaemia: the Glucose Insulin in Stroke Study (GIST). *Stroke* 1999; 30: 793–799.

Singhal AB, Benner T, Roccatagliata L *et al.* A pilot study of normobaric oxygen therapy in acute ischaemic stroke. *Stroke* 2005; 36: 797–802.

Smithard DG, O'Neill PA, Park C *et al.* Complications and outcome after stroke. Does dysphagia matter? *Stroke* 1996; 27: 1200–1204.

Sulter G, Elting JW, Langedijk M, Maurits NM, De Keyser J. Admitting acute ischemic stroke patients to a stroke care monitoring unit versus a conventional stroke unit. A randomised pilot study. *Stroke* 2003; 34: 101–104.

Sulter G, Elting JW, Maurits N, Luyckx GJ, De Keyser J. Acetylsalicyclic acid and acetaminophen to combat elevated body temperature in acute ischaemic stroke. *Cerebrovascular Diseases* 2004; 17: 118–122.

Unosson M, Ek AC, Bjurulf P, von Schenck H, Larsson J. Feeding dependence and nutritional status after acute stroke. *Stroke* 1994; 25: 366–371.

Vemmos KN, Tsivgoulis G, Spengos K *et al.* Association between 24-h blood pressure monitoring variables and brain oedema in patients with hyperacute stroke. *Journal of Hypertension* 2003; 21: 2167–2173.

Vemmos KN, Tsivgoulis G, Spengos K *et al.* U-shaped relationship between mortality and admission blood pressure in patients with acute stoke. *Journal of Internal Medicine* 2004a; 255: 257–265.

Vemmos KN, Spengos K, Tsivgoulis G *et al.* Factors influencing acute blood pressure values in stroke subtypes. *Journal of Human Hypertension* 2004b; 18: 253–259.

Vingerhoets F, Bogousslavsky J, Regli F, Van Melle G. Atrial fibrillation after acute stroke. *Stroke* 1993; 24: 26–30.

Wahlgren NG, MacMahon DG, DeKeyser J, Indredavik B, Ryman T. Intravenous Nimodipine West European Stroke Trial (INWEST) of nimodipine in the treatment of acute ischaemic stroke. *Cerebrovascular Diseases* 1994; 4: 204–210.

Wallace JD, Levy LL. Blood pressure after stroke. *Journal of the American Medical Association* 1981; 246: 2177–2180.

Warlow C, Ogston D, Douglas AS. Venous thrombosis following strokes. *Lancet* 1972; I: 1305–1306.

Warlow C. Venous thromboembolism after stroke. *American Heart Journal* 1978; 96: 283–285.

Wells PA, Lensing AWA, Hirsch J. Graduated pressure stockings in the prevention of postoperative venous thromboembolism: a meta analysis. *Archives of Internal Medicine* 1994; 154: 67–72.

Willmot M, Leonardi-Bee J, Bath PM. High blood pressure in acute stroke and subsequent outcome: a systematic review. *Hypertension* 2004; 43: 18–24.

Chapter 5. Reperfusion of ischaemic brain by thrombolysis and other strategies

Adams H, Adams R, Del Zoppo G, Goldstein L. Guidelines for the early management of patients with ischaemic stroke. 2005 Guidelines Update. A scientific statement from the stroke council of the American Heart Association/American Stroke Association. *Stroke* 2005; 36: 916–921.

Alexandrov AV, Molina CA, Grotta JC *et al.*, for the CLOTBUST investigators. Ultrasound-enhanced systemic thrombolysis for acute ischaemic stroke. *New England Journal of Medicine* 2004; 351: 2170–2178.

Alvarez-Sabín J, Molina CA, Ribó M *et al.* Impact of admission hyperglycaemia on stroke outcome after thrombolysis. Risk stratification in relations to time to reperfusion. *Stroke* 2004; 35: 2493–2499.

The ATLANTIS, ECASS, and NINDS rt-PA Study Group Investigators. Association of outcome with early stroke treatment: pooled analysis of ATLANTIS, ECASS, and NINDS rt-PA stroke trials. *Lancet* 2004; 363: 768–774.

Auderbert HJ, Kukla C, Clarmann von Claranau S *et al.* for the TEMPiS group. Telemedicine for safe and extended use of thrombolysis in stroke. The TeleMedic Pilot project for integrative Stroke care (TEMPiS) in Bavaria. *Stroke* 2005; 36: 287–291.

Barber PA, Demchuk AM, Zhang J, Buchan AM. Validity and reliability of a quantitative computed tomography score in predicting outcome of hyperacute stroke before thrombolytic therapy. *Lancet* 2000; 355: 1670–1674.

Buchan AM, Barber PA, Newcommon N, Karbalai HG, Demchuk AM, Hoyte KM, Klein GM, Feasby TE. Effectiveness of t-PA in acute ischaemic stroke. Outcome relates to appropriateness. *Neurology* 2000; 54: 679–684.

Caplan LR. Treatment of patients with stroke. *Archives of Neurology* 2002; 59: 703–707.

Chalela JA, Kang D-W, Luby M *et al.* Early MRI findings in patients receiving tissue plasminogen activator predict outcome: insights into the pathophysiology of acute stroke in the thrombolysis era. *Annals of Neurology* 2004; 55: 105–112.

Ciccone A, Boccardi E, Cantisani TA *et al.* A randomised comparison of intra arterial with intravenous thrombolysis for acute ischaemic stroke: The SYNTHESIS trial. Ongoing Clinical Trial Abstracts, *29th International Stroke Conference*, 2004, American Stroke Association, CTP42.

Coutts SB, Demchuk AM, Barber PA *et al.*, for the VISION Study Group. Interobserver variation of ASPECTS in real time. *Stroke* 2004; 35: e103–e105.

Daffertshofer M, Hennerici M. Ultrasound in the treatment of ischaemic stroke. *Lancet Neurology* 2003; 2: 283–290.

Davis SM, Donnan GA, Butcher KS, Parsons M. Selection of thrombolytic therapy beyond 3H using magnetic resonance imaging. *Curr Opin Neurology* 2005; 18: 47–52.

Donnan GA, Davis SM. Neuroimaging, the ischaemic penumbra, and selection of patients for acute stroke therapy. *Lancet Neurology* 2002; 1: 417–423.

Dunn B, Warach S. ReoPro Retavase Reperfusion of Stroke Safety Study: Imaging Evaluation. Ongoing Clinical Trial Abstracts, *International Stroke Conference* 2005, New Orleans, Louisiana, CTP58.

Foerch C, du Mesnil de Rochemont R, Singer O *et al.* S100B as a surrogate marker for successful clot lysis in hyperacute middle cerebral artery infarction. *Journal of Neurology Neurosurgery and Psychiatry* 2003; 74: 322–325.

Frey JL, Jahnke HK, Goslar PW, Partovi S, Flaster MS. tPA by telephone: extending the benefits of a comprehensive stroke centre. *Neurology* 2005; 64: 154–156.

Furlan A, Higashida R, Weschler L, Gent M, Rowley H, Kase C, Pessin M, Ahuja A, Callahan F, Clark WM, Silver F, Rivera F, for the PROACT Investigators. Intraarterial Pro-Urokinase for acute ischaemic stroke. The PROACT II Study: A randomised controlledd trial. *Journal of the American Medical Association* 1999; 282: 2003–2011.

Gilligan AK, Markus R, Read SJ *et al.* Baseline blood pressure but not early computed tomography changes predicts major haemorrhage in acute ischaemic stroke. *Stroke* 2002; 33: 2236–2242.

Hacke W, Albers G, Al-Rawi Y *et al.*, for the DIAS study Group. The Desmoteplase in Acute Ischaemic Stroke Trial (DIAS). A phase II MRI-based 9-hour window acute stroke thrombolysis trial with intravenous desmoteplase. *Stroke* 2005; 36: 66–73.

Heuschmann PU, Kolominsky-Rabas PL, Roether J *et al.*, for the German Stroke Registers Study Group. Predictors of in-hospital mortality in patients with acute ischaemic stroke treated with thrombolytic therapy. *Journal of the American Medical Association* 2004; 292: 1831–1838.

Hill MD, Lye T, Moss H *et al.* Hemi-orolingual angioedema and ACE inhibition after alteplase treatment of stroke. *Neurology* 2003; 60: 1525–1527.

Hill MD, Rowley HA, Adler F *et al.* Selection of acute ischaemic stroke patients for intra-arterial thrombolysis with pro-urokinase by using ASPECTS. *Stroke* 2003; 34: 1925–1931.

Hill MD, Buchan AM, for the Canadian Alteplase for Stroke Effectiveness Study (CASES) investigators. Thrombolysis for acute ischaemic stroke. Results of the Canadian Alteplase for Stroke Effectiveness Study. *Canadian Medical Association Journal* 2005; 172: 1307–1312.

Hjort N, Butcher K, Davis SM *et al.* Magnetic resonance imaging criteria for thrombolysis in acute cerebral infarct. *Stroke* 2005; 36: 388–397.

Ingall TJ, O'Fallon WM, Asplund K *et al.* Findings from the reanalysis of the NINDS tissue plasminogen activator for acute ischemic stroke treatment trial. *Stroke* 2004; 35: 2418–2424.

Kalafut MA, Schriger DL, Saver JL, Starkman S. Detection of early CT signs of >1/3 middle cerebral artery infarctions. Interrater reliability and sensitivity of CT interpretation by physicians involved in acute stroke care. *Stroke* 2000; 31: 1667–1671.

Kane I, Sandercock P. Third International Stroke Trial. Ongoing Clinical Trial Abstracts, *29th International Stroke Conference*, 2004, American Stroke Association, CTP26.

Kidwell CS, Saver JL, Starkman S *et al.* Late secondary ischaemic injury in patients receiving intraarterial thrombolysis. *Annals of Neurology* 2002; 52: 698–703.

Kidwell CS, Alger JR, Saver JL. Beyond mismatch. Evolving paradigms in imaging the ischaemic penumbra with multimodal magnetic resonance imaging. *Stroke* 2003; 34: 2729–2735.

Kidwell CS, Jahan R, Starkman S, Saver JL. MR and recanalisation of stroke clots using embolectomy (MR rescue). Ongoing Clinical Trials Abstracts, *International Stroke Conference*, New Orleans, Louisiana, 2005, CTP59.

Kwan J, Hand P, Sandercock P. A systematic review of barriers to delivery of thrombolysis for acute stroke. *Age and Ageing* 2004; 33: 116–121.

Kwiatkowski T, Libman R, Tilley BC *et al.* The impact of imbalances in baseline stroke severity on outcome in the national institute of neurological disorders and stroke recombinant tissue plasminogen activator stroke study. *Annals of Emergency Medicine* 2005; 45: 377–384.

Labiche LA, Shaltoni H, Choi J *et al.* Combined cytoprotection tPA trial. Ongoing Clinical Trial Abstracts, *29th International Stroke Conference*, 2004, American Stroke Association, CTP25.

Lewandowski CA, Frankel M, Tomsick TA *et al.* Combined intravenous and intra-arterial rt-PA versus intra-arterial therapy of acute ischaemic stroke; Emergency Management of Stroke (EMS) Briding Trial. *Stroke* 1999; 30: 2598–2605.

Liberatore GT, Samson A, Bladin C, Schleuning WD, Medcalf RL. Vampire bat salivary plasminogen activator (desmoteplase): a unique fibrinolytic enzyme that does not promote neurodegeneration. *Stroke* 2003; 34: 537–543.

Lyden P, Jacoby M, Schim J *et al.* The Clomethiazole Acute Stroke Study in tissue-type plasminogen activator-treated stroke (CLASS-T). Final results. *Neurology* 2001; 57: 1199–1205.

Magid D, Naviaux N, Wears RL. Stroking the data: re-analysis of the NINDS trial. *Annals of Emergency Medicine* 2005; 45: 385–387.

Mielke O, Wardlaw J, Liu M. Thrombolysis (different doses, routes of administration and agents) for acute ischaemic stroke. *The Cochrane Database of Systematic Reviews* 2004, Issue 1, Art. No.: CD000514. DOI: 10.1002/14651858.CD000514.pub2.

Noser EA, Shaltoni HM, Hall CE *et al*. Aggressive mechanical clot disruption. A safe adjunct to thrombolytic therapy in acute stroke? *Stroke* 2005; 36: 292–296.

Nighoghossian N, Hermier M, Adeleine P *et al*. Old microbleeds are a potential risk factor for cerebral bleeding after ischaemic stroke. A gradient-echo T2*-weighted brain MRI study. *Stroke* 2002; 33: 735–742.

Oh S-H, Lee J-G, Na S-J *et al*. Prediction of early clinical severity and extent of neuronal damage in anterior circulation infarction using the initial serum neuron-specific enolase. *Archives of Neurology* 2003; 60: 37–41.

Pancioli AM, Broderick JP. The Combined approach to Lysis utilising Eptifibatide And rt-PA in acute ischaemic stroke (the CLEAR Stroke trial). Ongoing Clinical Trial Abstracts, *29th International Stroke Conference*, 2004, American Stroke Association, CTP16.

Patel SC, Levine S, Tilley BC *et al*. Lack of clinical significance of early ischaemic changes on computed tomography in acute stroke. *Journal of the American Medical Association* 2001; 286: 2830–2838.

The National Institute of Neurological Disorders and Stroke (NINDS) rt-PA Stroke Study Group. A systems approach to immediate evaluation and management of hyperacute stroke: experience at eight centers and implications for community practice and patient care. *Stroke* 1997; 28: 1530–1540.

Reddrop C, Moldrich RX, Beart PM, Farso M, Liberatore GT, Howells DW, Petersen K-U, Schleuning WD, Medcalf RL. Vampire bat salivary plasminogen activator (desmoteplase) inhibits tissue-type plasminogen activator-induced potentitation of excitotoxic injury. *Stroke* 2005; 36: 1241–6.

Sandercock P, Berge E, Dennis M *et al*. A systematic review of the effectiveness, cost-effectiveness and barriers to implementation of thrombolytic and neuroprotective therapy for acute ischaemic stroke in the NHS. *Health Technological Assessment* 2002; 6: 35–57.

Sandercock P, Berge E, Dennis M *et al*. Cost-effectiveness of thrombolysis with recombinant tissue plasminogen activator for acute ischaemic stroke assessed by a model based on UK NHS costs. *Stroke* 2004; 35: 1490–1498.

Saposnik G, Young B, Silber B *et al*. Lack of improvement in patients with acute stroke after treatment with thrombolytic therapy. Predictors and association with outcome. *Journal of the American Medical Association* 2004; 292: 1839–1844.

Schellinger PD, Feiback JB, Hacke W. Imaging-based decision making in thrombolytic therapy for ischaemic stroke. Present status. *Stroke* 2003; 34: 575–583.

Seitz RJ, Meisel S, Moll M *et al*. The effect of combined thrombolysis with rtPA and tirofiban on ischaemic brain lesions. *Neurology* 2004; 62: 2110–2112.

Shih LC, Saver JL, Alger JR *et al*. Perfusion-weighted magnetic resonance imaging thresholds identifying core, irreversibly infarcted tissue. *Stroke* 2003; 34: 1425–1430.

Teal P. Thrombolysis in the real world. The Canadian experience: the CASES study. Presented at the *5th World Stroke Congress*, Vancouver, Canada, June 23–26, 2004.

Toni D. Update on SITS-MOST. Presented at *New Insights-Stroke Management Meeting*, Germany: Mainz; September 9–11, 2004.

Warach S. Thrombolysis in stroke beyond three hours: targeting patients with diffusion and perfusion MRI. *Annals of Neurology* 2002; 51: 11–13.

Warach S. Stroke neuroimaging. *Stroke* 2003; 34: 345–347.

Warach S, Davis L, for the ROSIE Study Group. ReoPro Retavase Reperfusion of Stroke Safety Study: Imaging Evaluation (ROSIE). In: The American Stroke Association, *28th International Stroke Conference*, Phoenix, Arizona, USA, 2003 (Conference Proceedings).

Wardlaw JM, Sandercock PAG, Warlow CP, Lindley RI. Trials of thrombolysis in acute ischaemic stroke. Does the choice of primary outcome measure really matter? *Stroke* 2000; 31: 1133–1135.

Wardlaw JM, Sandercock PAG, Berge E. Thrombolysis therapy with recombinant tissue plasminogen activator for acute ischaemic stroke. Where do we go from here? A cumulative meta-analysis. *Stroke* 2003; 34: 1437–1442.

Wardlaw JM, Farrell AJ. Diagnosis of stroke on neuroimaging. *British Medical Journal* 2004; 328: 655–656.

Wardlaw JM, del Zoppo G, Yamaguchi T, Berge E. Thrombolysis for acute ischaemic stroke. *The Cochrane Database of Systematic Reviews* 2003, Issue 3. Art. No.: CD000213. DOI: 10.1002/14651858.CD000213.

Wardlaw J, Berge E, del Zoppo G, Yamaguchi T. Thrombolysis for acute ischemic stroke (Cochrane Corner). *Stroke* 2004; 35: 2914–2915.

Warlow CP, Dennis MS, van Gijn J, Hankey GJ, Sandercock PAG, Bamford J, Wardlaw J. *Stroke: A Practical Guide to Management*, 2nd edition. Blackwell Scientific Publications, Oxford, UK, 2000.

Warlow C, Wardlaw J. Therapeutic thrombolysis for acute ischaemic stroke. What is good for heart attacks is still not good enough for brain attacks. *British Medical Journal* 2003; 326: 233–234.

References to studies included in the Cochrane Review by Wardlaw *et al*. Thrombolysis for acute ischaemic stroke. In: The Cochrane Library, Issue 4, 2004

Abe 1981 {published and unpublished data}

*Abe T, Kazama M, Naito I *et al*. Clinical evaluation for efficacy of tissue cultured urokinase (TCUK) on cerebral thrombosis by means of multi-centre double blind study (translated from Japanese). *Blood-Vessel* 1981; 12: 321–341.

Abe T. Thrombolytic therapy for cerebral infarction. *International Angiology* 1984; 3: 359–365.

ASK 1996 {published data only}

*Donnan G, Davis SM, Chambers BR, Gates PC, Hankey GJ, McNeill JJ, Rosen D, Stewart-Wynne EG, Tuck RR, for the Australian Streptokinase Trial Investigators. Streptokinase in acute ischaemic stroke: Does time of therapy administration affect outcome? *Journal of the American Medical Association* 1996; 271: 961–966.

Davis S, Donnan G, Mitchell P, Fitt G, Chambers B, Gates PC, Hankey GJ, McNeill JJ, Rosen D, Stewart-Wynne EG, Tuck RR, for the ASK Study Group. Australian Streptokinase trial: clinical and CT outcome predictors (abstract). *Cerebrovascular Diseases* 1996; 6 (Suppl 2): 128.

Donnan G, Davis S. ASK Trial: risk factors for poor outcome (abstract). *Cerebrovascular Diseases* 1996; 6: 182.

Donnan G, Davis S. ASK Trial – predictors of good outcome. *Cerebrovascular Diseases* 1996; 6: 183.

Donnan GA, Davis SM, Chambers BR, Gates PC, Hankey GJ, McNeil JJ, Rosen D, Stewart-Wynne EG, Tuck RR. Trials of streptokinase in severe acute ischaemic stroke. *Lancet* 1995; 345: 578–579.

Gilligan AK, Markus R, Read SJ, Srikanth V, Fitt G, Chambers BR, Donnan GA. Early CT changes do not predict parenchymal haemorrhage following streptokinase therapy in acute stroke. *Stroke* 2001; 32 (1): 370.

Yasaka M, O'Keefe GJ, Chambers BR, Davis SM, Infield B, O'Malley H, Baird AE, Hirano T, Donnan GA. Streptokinase in acute stroke: effect on reperfusion and recanalisation. *Neurology* 1998; 50: 626–632.

Atarashi 1985 {published and unpublished data}

Atarashi J, Ohtomo E, Araki G, Itoh E, Togi H, Matsuda T. Clinical utility of urokinase in the treatment of acute stage cerebral thrombosis: multi-center double blind study in comparison with placebo (translated from Japanese). *Clinical Evaluation* 1985; 13: 659–709.

ATLANTIS A 2000 {published and unpublished data}

Clark WM, Albers GW, for the ATLANTIS Stroke Study Investigators. The ATLANTIS rt-PA (Alteplase) Acute Stroke Trial – Final Results. *Stroke* 1999 1999; 30: 234.

Clark WM, Albers GW, Madden KP, Hamilton S, for the Thrombolytic Therapy in Acute Ischaemic Stroke Study Investigators. The rt-PA (Alteplase) 0- to 6-hour Acute Stroke Trial, Part A (A027g). Results of a double-blind, placebo-controlled, multicentre study. *Stroke* 2000; 31: 811–816.

Marks M, Holmgren EB, Fox AJ, Patel S, von Kummer R, Froehlich J. Evaluation of early computed tomographic findings in acute ischaemic stroke. *Stroke* 1999; 30: 389–392.

ATLANTIS B 1999 {unpublished data only}

Albers GW, Clark WM, for the ATLANTIS Study Investigators. The ATLANTIS rt-TP (Alteplase) acute stroke trial: final results. *Cerebrovascular Diseases* 1999; 9 (Suppl 1): 126.

Albers GW, Clark WM, Madden KP, Hamilton SA. The ATLANTIS trial: results for patients treated within three hours of stroke onset. *Stroke* 2002; 33: 493–496.

Clark WM, Albers GW, for the ATLANTIS Stroke Study Investigators. The ATLANTIS rt-PA (Alteplase) Acute Stroke Trial – Final Results. *Stroke* 1999; 30: 234.

Clark WM, Wissman S, Albers GW, Jhamandas JH, MAdden KP, Hamilton S, for the ATLANTIS Study Investigators. Recombinant tissue-type plasminogen activator (Alteplase) for ischaemic stroke 3 to 5 hours after symptom onset. The ATLANTIS Study: a randomised controlled trial. *Journal of the American Medical Association* 1999; 282: 2019–2026.

Kent D, Ruthazer R, Selker HP. Do some patients benefit from rt-PA treatment for acute ischaemic stroke even when treated more than 3 hours after the onset of symptoms? Abstracts of the *7th International Symposium on Thrombolysis and Acute Ischaemic. Stroke*, 27–28 May 2002, Lyon, 2002: 79.

Chinese UK 2003 {published and unpublished data}

The study group of a 5 year National Project of the People's Republic of China, conducted by Qingtang Chen and Maolin He. Intravenous thrombolysis with Urokinase for acute cerebral infarctions. *Chinese Journal of Neurology* (full reference awaited) 2002.

ECASS 1995 {published and unpublished data}

Ciccone A, Motta C, Aritzu E, Candelise L. Letter to the editor. *Journal of the American Medical Association* 1996; 275: 983–984.

Davalos A, Toni D, Iweins F, Lesaffre E, Bastianello S, Castillo J, for the ECASS Group. Neurological deterioration in acute ischaemic stroke. Potential predictors and associated factors in the European Cooperative Acute Stroke Study (ECASS) I. *Stroke* 1999; 30: 2631–2636.

ECASS Study Group. Very early identification of lacunar infarcts in the ECASS Study. *Cerebrovascular Diseases* 1997; 7 (Suppl 4): 29.

European Cooperative Acute Stroke Study (ECASS). Intravenous thrombolysis with recombinant tissue plasminogen activator for acute hemispheric stroke. *The Journal of the American Medical Association* 1995; 274: 1017–1025.

Fieschi C, Argentino C, Fiorelli M, Mau J, Roine RO, Willig V, for the ECASS 1 Study Group. Frequency and consequences of medical complications of ischaemic stroke. *The Challenge of Stroke Lancet Conference Book of Abstracts*, Montreal 15–16 October 1999, 1999: 35.

Fiorelli M, Argentino C, Falcou A, Meier D, Kaste M, Hacke W, Mau J, Fieschi C. Natural history of ischaemic stroke in ECASS 1 and ECASS II placebo cohorts. *Cerebrovascular Diseases* 1999; 9 (Suppl 1): 14.

Fiorelli M, Bastianello S, von Kummer R, del Zoppo GJ, Larrue V, Lesaffre E, Ringleb AP, Lorenzano S, Manelfe C, Bozzao L, for the ECASS Study I Group. Hemorrhagic transformation within 36 hours of a cerebral infarct. Relationships with early clinical deterioration and three month outcome in the European Cooperative Acute Stroke Study I (ECASS I) Cohort. *Stroke* 1999; 30: 2280–2284.

Fiorelli M, Busse O, Mau J, Bozzao L, Bastianello S, Fieschi C, Hacke W, Kaste M, Von Kummer R, for the ECASS 1 Study Group. Cortical extension of the infarction at 24 hours in patients with isolated hypodensity of the lentiform nucleus on 1–6 hour CT: Incidence, predictors and outcome in the ECASS 1 Cohort (abstract). *Cerebrovascular Diseases* 1998; 8 (Suppl 4): 19.

Fisher M, Pessin M, Furlan A. ECASS: lessons for future thrombolytic stroke trials. *Journal of the American Medical Association* 1996; 274: 1058–1059.

Hacke W, Bluhmki E, Steiner T, Tatlisumak T, Mahagne M-H, Sacchetti M-L, Meier D, for the ECASS Study Group. Dichotomized efficacy end points and global end-point analysis applied to the ECASS intention-to-treat data set. *Post hoc* analysis of ECASS 1. *Stroke* 1998; 29: 2073–2075.

Hacke W, Kaste M, Fieschi C. Reply to letter to the editor. *Journal of the American Medical Association* 1996; 275: 984–985.

Hacke W, Steiner T, Bluhmki E, Tatlisumak T, Mahagne MH, Meier D, for the ECASS Study Group. Dichotomised endpoints and combined global endpoint statistics applied to the ECASS intention-to-treat data set (abstract). *Stroke* 1998; 29: 303.

Hacke W, Toni D, Steiner T, Kaste M, von Kummer R, Fieschi C, Bluhmki E, for the ECASS Study Group. rt-PA in acute ischaemic stroke – results from the ECASS three hour cohort. *Stroke* 1997; 28: 272.

Kaste M, for the ECASS Study Group. Potential contributors to bad functional outcome or death in European Cooperative Acute Stroke Study (ECASS). *Cerebrovascular Diseases* 1996; 6: 181.

Kaste M, Fieschi C, Hacke W, Lesaffre E, Verstraete M, Frohlich J. The European Cooperative Acute Stroke Study (ECASS). In: Del Zoppo G, Mori E, Hacke W (eds), *Thrombolytic Therapy in Acute Ischaemic Stroke*. Berlin: Springer Verlag, 1993: 66–71.

Kaste M, Mau J, Bluhmki E, Del Zoppo GJ, Orgogozo J-M, Overgaard K, Von Kummer R, Wahlgren N-G, for the ECASS Study Group. Risk/benefit assessment for mortality and handicap in ECASS randomised and treated patients: A *post-hoc* analysis (abstract). *Stroke* 1998; 29: 288.

Kaste M, Mau J, Bluhmki E, Del Zoppo GJ, Orgogozo J-M, Overgaard K, Von Kummer R, Wahlgren N-G, for the ECASS Study Group. A *post-hoc* risk/benefit assessment for mortality and handicap in 615 ECASS patients randomised and treated. *Upsala Journal of Medical Sciences* 1997; Suppl 53.

Kaste M, Mau J, Bluhmki E, Del Zoppo GJ, Orgogozo J-M, Overgaard K, Von Kummer R, Wahlgren N-G, for the ECASS Study Group. Risk/benefit assessment for mortality and handicap among 615 patients randomised and treated in ECASS. *European Journal of Neurology* 1998; 5 (Suppl 1): S20.

Kaste M, Overgaard K, Del Zoppo GJ, Von Kummer R, Orgogozo J-M, Wahlgren N-G, Bluhmki E, Mau J, for the ECASS Study Group. Potential contributors for good vs bad functional outcome or death in European Cooperative Acute Stroke Study (ECASS). *Cerebrovascular Diseases* 1996; 6 (Suppl 2): 129.

Larrue V, Von Kummer R, Hoxter G, Bluhmki E, Manelfe G, Regesta G, Bes A, for the ECASS Study Group. Predictors of hemorrhagic transformation in the ECASS trial. *Cerebrovascular Diseases* 1996; 6: 181.

Larrue V, Von Kummer R, del Zoppo GJ, Bluhmki E. Hemorrhagic transformation in acute ischaemic stroke. Potential contributing factors in the European Cooperative Acute Stroke Study. *Stroke* 1997; 28: 957–960.

Manelfe C, Larrue V, Von Kummer R, Bozzao L, Ringleb P, Bastianello S, Iweins F, Lessaffre E. Association of hyperdense middle cerebral artery sign with clinical outcome in patients treated with tissue plasminogen activator. *Stroke* 1999; 30: 769–772.

Mau J, Kaste M, Bluhmki E, del Zoppo G, Orgogozo JM, Overgaard K, von Kummer R, Wahlgren NG, for the ECASS Group. A risk/benefit assessment of 1.1 mg/kg i.v. rt-PA in 615 acute stroke patients of ECASS. *Cerebrovascular Diseases* 1997; 7 (Suppl 4): 1.

Mau J, Kaste M, Del Zoppo GJ, Von Kummer R, Orgogozo JM, Overgaard K, Wahlgren N, for the ECASS Study Group. Risk profile comparison in 615 patients randomised to either 1.1 mg/kg intravenous rt-PA or placebo of ECASS 1. *Stroke* 1999; 30: 247.

Pantano P, Caramina F, Bozzao L, Dieler C, Von Kummer R. Delayed increase in infarct volume after cerebral ischaemia. Correlations with thrombolytic treatment and clinical outcome. *Stroke* 1999; 30: 502–507.

Steiner T, Bluhmki E, Kaste M, Toni D, Trouillas P, Von Kummer R, Hacke W, for the ECASS Study Group. The ECASS 3-hour cohort. Secondary analysis of ECASS data by time stratification. *Cerebrovascular Diseases* 1998; 8: 198–203.

The ECASS Study Group. European Cooperative Acute Stroke Study (ECASS): (rt-PA – Thrombolysis in acute stroke) study design and progress report. *European Journal of Neurology* 1995; 1: 213–219.

The ECASS Trial. Predictors of good outcome – ECASS Trial. *Cerebrovascular Diseases* 1996; 6: 182.

von Kummer R, Allen KL, Holle R, Bozzao L, Bastianello S, Manelfe C, Bluhmki E, Ringleb P, Meier DH, Hacke W. Acute stroke – usefulness of early CT findings before thrombolytic therapy. *Radiology* 1997; 205: 327–333.

Willig V, Hoxter G, Steiner T, Fiorelli M, von Kummer R, Hacke W, for the ECASS Study Group. Causes of death in ECASS. *Cerebrovascular Diseases* 1996; 6 (Suppl 2): 129.

Willig V, Pawelec D, Mau J, Hoxter G, Hacke W. Heparin effects in the European Cooperative Acute Stroke Study. *Stroke* 1997; 28: 272.

Wood L. Letter to the editor. *Journal of the American Medical Association* 1996; 275: 983.

von Kummer R, Bozzao L. Letter to the editor. *Journal of the American Medical Association* 1996; 275: 13.

ECASS II 1998 {published and unpublished data}

Barer D. Letter to the editor. *Lancet* 1999; 353: 66–67.

Berrouschot J, Barthel H, Hesse S, Knapp WH, Schneider D, von Kummer R. Reperfusion and metabolic recovery of brain tissue and clinical outcome after ischaemic stroke and thrombolytic therapy. *Stroke* 2000; 31: 1545–1551.

Berrouschot J, Barthel H, von Kummer R, Hesse S, Schneider D. Reperfusion after focal cerebral ischaemia does not increase the rate and severity of secondary haemorrhage (abstract). *Cerebrovascular Diseases* 1999; 9 (Suppl 1): 95.

Berrouschot J, Barthel H, von Kummer R, Koester J, Knapp W, Schneider D. Thrombolysis with rt-PA: A SPECT study. *Stroke* 1999; 30: 267.

Davalos A, Mostacero E, Castillo J, Larracoechea J, Ruiz-Peris M, on behalf of the ECASS II Spanish Group. Type of acute stroke care, stroke outcome and safety parameters in the ECASS II trial: the Spanish experience. *Cerebrovascular Diseases* 1999; 9 (Suppl 1): 33.

Davalos A, on behalf of the ECASS II Spanish Group. Fibrinolytic therapy for acute stroke: the Spanish experience. *Cerebrovascular Diseases* 1999; 9 (Suppl 3): 9–15.

Fieschi C, Hacke W, Kaste M, for the ECASS II Study Group. Final results of the second European–Australasian Acute Stroke Study of intravenous alteplase in acute ischaemic stroke (ECASS II). *Cerebrovascular Diseases* 1999; 9 (Suppl 1): 128.

Fiorelli M, Argentino C, Falcou A, Meier D, Kaste M, Hacke W, Mau J, Fieschi C. Natural history of ischaemic stroke in ECASS I and ECASS II placebo cohorts. *Cerebrovascular Diseases* 1999; 9 (Suppl 1): 14.

Ford G, Freemantle N, Lees KR, Raha S, Barer D, Jenkinson D, Hacke W, Davalos A, Von Kummer R, Kaste M, Larrue V, for the Steering Committee and authors of the ECASS II Study Group. ECASS II: Intravenous alteplase in acute ischaemic stroke. *Lancet* 1999; 353: 65–68.

Hacke W. The results of the European Co-operative Stroke Study II (ECASS II), a placebo-controlled, randomized study of thrombolytic therapy. *European Journal of Neurology* 1998; 5 (Suppl 3): S9.

Hacke W, Davalos A, Von Kummer R, Kaste M, Larrue V, for the steering committee and authors of the ECASS II Study Group. Authors' reply. *Lancet* 1999; 353: 67–68.

Hacke W, Kaste M, Fieschi C, Von Kummer R, Davalos A, Meier D, Larrue V, Bluhmki E, Davis S, Donnan G, Schneider D, Diez-Tejedor E, Trouillas P, for the Second European–Australasian Acute Stroke Study Investigators. Randomised double-blind placebo-controlled trial of thrombolytic therapy with intravenous alteplase in acute ischaemic stroke (ECASS II). *Lancet* 1998; 352: 1245–1251.

Hacke W, for the ECASS II Study Group. Thrombolysis in acute ischaemic stroke: ECASS II. *The Challenge of Stroke Lancet Conference Montreal*, 15–16 October 1999, Book of Abstracts, 1999.

Jenkinson D. Letter to the editor. *Lancet* 1999; 353: 67.

Larrue V, Bluhmki E, Muller A, Von Kummer R. Risk factors for haemorrhagic transformation in ECASS II. *Stroke* 2000; 31: 278.

Larrue V, von Kummer R, Muller A, Bluhmki E. Risk factors for severe hemorrhagic transformation in ischemic stroke patients treated with recombinanat tissue plasminogen activator. *Stroke* 2001; 32: 438–441.

Lees KR. Letter to the editor. *Lancet* 1999; 353: 65–66.

Raha S. Letter to the editor. *Lancet* 1999; 353: 66.

Schaefer E, Hacke W, Davalos A, Donnan GA, Fieschi C, Kaste M, Von Kummer R, Larrue V, Bluhmki E, Meier D, for the ECASS II Investigators. European–Australian cooperative acute stroke study II (ECASS II) – interim demographics and baseline characteristics (abstract). *Cerebrovascular Diseases* 1998; 8 (Suppl 4): 82.

Stingele R, Bluhmki E, Hacke W. Bootstrap statistics of ECASS II data: Just another *post hoc* analysis of a negative stroke trial? *Cerebrovascular Diseases* 2001; 11: 30–33.

von Kummer R, Berrouschot J, Henrik B, Swen H, Deiler C, Schneider D. The effect of early and late brain tissue reperfusion on infarct volume. *Stroke* 2000; 31: 275.

Haley 1993 {published data only}

Haley EC, Brott TG, Sheppard GL *et al*. Pilot randomized trial of tissue Plasminogen Activator in acute Ischemic Stroke. *Stroke* 1993; 24: 1000–1004.

JTSG 1993 {published and unpublished data}

Yamaguchi T, Japanese Thrombolysis Study Group. Intravenous tissue plasminogen activator in acute thromboembolic stroke: a placebo controlled, double blind trial. In: Del Zoppo GJ, Mori E, Hacke W (eds), *Thrombolytic Therapy in Acute Ischemic Stroke II*. New York: Springer Verlag, 1993; 59–65.

Yamaguchi T, Hayakawa T, Kiuchi H, for the Japanese Thrombolysis Study Group. Intravenous tissue plasminogen activator ameliorates the outcome of hyperacute embolic stroke. *Cerebrovascular Diseases* 1993; 3: 269–272.

MAST-E 1996 {published and unpublished data}

Hommel M, Besson G, Jaillard Serradj A, for the MAST-E Group. Multicentre Acute Stroke Trial-Europe: risk factors for the development of oedema, haemorrhage, bad neurological, bad functional outcome and death. *Cerebrovascular Diseases* 1996; 6: 182.

Hommel M, Besson G, Jaillard Serradj A, for the MAST-E Group. Multicentre Acute Stroke Trial-Europe: predictors of good outcome. *Cerebrovascular Diseases* 1996; 6: 183.

Hommel M, Boissel JP, Cornu C, Boutitie F, Lees KR, Besson G, Leys D, Amarenco P, Bogaert M, for the MAST Study Group. Termination of trial of streptokinase in severe acute ischaemic stroke. *Lancet* 1995; 345: 57.

Hommel M, Boissel JP, on behalf of the MAST Group. Authors' reply. *Lancet* 1995; 345: 578–579.

Jaillard A, Cornu C, Durieux A, Moulin T, Boutitie F, Lees KR, Hommel M, on behalf of the MAST-E Group. Haemorrhagic transformation in acute ischaemic stroke. The MAST-E Study. *Stroke* 1999; 30: 1326–1332.

Jaillard AS, Hommel M. Predictive factors related to outcome at one year after intravenous thrombolysis: the MAST-E Study. *Cerebrovascular Diseases* 2000; 10 (Suppl 2): 797.

Jaillard AS, Hommel M. Predictive factors related to outcome at one year after iv thrombolysis: the MAST-E Study. *Stroke* 2000; 31: 2887.

Moulin T, Besson G, Crepin-Leblond, Garnier P, Tau L, Chavot D, and the MAST-E Group. Haemorrhagic transformation in MAST-E trial: predictive factors. *Cerebrovascular Diseases* 1996; 6: 182.

The Multicentre Acute Stroke Trial-Europe Study Group (Hommel M, Cornu C, Boutitie F, Boissel JP). Thrombolytic therapy with streptokinase in acute ischaemic stroke. *New England Journal of Medicine* 1996; 335: 145–150.

MAST-I 1995 {published and unpublished data}

Aritzu E, Candelise L, Motto C, Ciccone A, Piana A. Long term effect of thrombolytic treatment in acute ischaemic stroke. *Cerebrovascular Diseases* 1996; 6 (Suppl 2): 129.

Aritzu E, Motto C, Ciccone A, Candelise L, and the MAST-I Study Group. Prognostic value of haemorrhagic transformation in acute ischaemic stroke. *Cerebrovascular Diseases* 1996; 6: 190.

Barer D. Letter to the editor. *Lancet* 1996; 347: 391–392.

Candelise L. The long term effects of acute treatment with streptokinase and/or aspirin. Book of Abstracts *Proceedings of the 6th International Conference on Thrombolysis in Acute Ischaemic Stroke*, Hamilton Island, November 2000, 2000: 3.

Candelise L, for the MAST-I Study Group. Risk factors in the MAST-Italy Trial. *Cerebrovascular Diseases* 1996; 6: 181.

Candelise L, Aritzu E, Ciccone A, Ricci S, Wardlaw J. Multicentre Acute Stroke Trial-Italy (Authors' Reply). *Lancet* 1996; 347: 393.

Candelise L, Aritzu E, Ciccone A, Ricci S, Wardlaw JM. Authors' reply. *Lancet* 1996; 347: 393.

Candelise L, Ciccone A, Motto C. Letter to the editor. *Stroke* 2000; 31 (7): 1785.

Candelise L, Motto C, Aritzu E, Ciccone A, Ricci S, and the MAST-I Study Group. Aspirin given within six hours reduces long term case fatality but not stroke related disability. *Cerebrovascular Diseases* 1996; 6 (Suppl 2): 23.

Candelise L, Roncaglione C, Aritzu E, Ciccone A, Maggioni AP, and the MAST-I Group. Thrombolytic therapy. From myocardial to cerebral infarction. *Italian Journal of Neurological Science* 1996; 17: 5–21.

Carolei A, Marini C, Motolese M. Letter to the editor. *Lancet* 1996; 347: 392.

Ciccone A, Motto C, Aritzu E, Piana A, Candelise L, on behalf of the MAST-I Collaborative Group. Risk of aspirin use plus thrombolysis after acute ischaemic stroke: a further MAST-I analysis. *Lancet* 1998; 352: 880.

Ciccone A, Motto C, Aritzu E, Piana A, Candelise L, on behalf of the MAST-I Collaborative Group. Negative interaction of aspirin and streptokinase in acute ischaemic stroke: Further analysis of the Multicentre Acute Stroke Trial-Italy. *Cerebrovascular Diseases* 2000; 10: 61–64.

Motto C, Candelise L, Aritzu E, Ciccone A, Piana A, on behalf of the MAST-I Group. Aspirin in combination with thrombolysis increases the risk of early death but not of intracranial bleeding in patients with acute ischaemic stroke. *Cerebrovascular Diseases* 1996; 6 (Suppl 2): 129.

Motto C, Ciccone A, Aritzu E, Boccardi E, De Grandi C, Piana A, Candelise L, and the MAST-I Collaborative Group. Haemorrhage after an acute ischaemic stroke. *Stroke* 1999; 30: 761–764.

Muir KW. Letter to the editor. *Lancet* 1996; 347: 391.

Multicentre Acute Stroke Trial-Italy (MAST-I) Group (Candelise L, Aritzu E, Ciccone A, Ricci S, Wardlaw J). Randomised controlled trial of streptokinase, aspirin, and combination of both in treatment of acute ischaemic stroke. *Lancet* 1995; 346: 1509–1514.

Rothwell P. Letter to the editor. *Lancet* 1996; 347: 393.

Sandercock PAG. Thrombolytic therapy for acute ischaemic stroke: promising, perilous or unproven? *Lancet* 1996; 346: 1504–1505.

The MAST-I Collaborative Group. Is thrombolysis useful for acute stroke patients? The experience of the MAST-I Study. In: Yamaguchi T, Mori E, Minematsu K, Del Zoppo GJ (eds), *Thrombolytic Therapy in Acute Ischaemic Stroke*. Tokyo: Springer Verlag, 1995; 198–205.

Tognoni G, Roncaglione MC. Dissent: an alternative interpretation of MAST-I. *Lancet* 1996; 346: 1515.

Wardlaw JM, for the MAST-I Group. Predictors of good outcome in the MAST-I trial. *Cerebrovascular Diseases* 1996; 6: 183.

Mori 1992 {published and unpublished data}

Mori E, Yoneda Y, Tabuchi M *et al*. Intravenous recombinant tissue plasminogen activator in acute carotid artery territory stroke. *Neurology* 1992; 42: 976–982.

Morris 1995 {published data only}

Morris AD, Ritchie C, Grosset DG, Adams FG, Lees KR. A pilot study of streptokinase for acute cerebral infarction. *Quarterly Journal of Medicine* 1995; 88: 727–731.

NINDS 1995 {published data only}

Food and Drug Administration. http://www.fda.gov/cber/products/altegen061896.htm see *Clinical Review* 2.

Anonymous. Heart treatment reduces damage from stroke. *Laboratory Medicine* 1996; 27 (5): 296.

Barch C, Spilker J, Bratina P, Rapp K, Daley S, Donnarumma R, Sailor S, Braimah J, Kongable G, and the NINDS rt-PA Stroke Study Group. Nursing management of acute complications following rt-PA in acute ischaemic stroke. *Journal of Neuroscience and Nursing* 1997; 29: 367–372.

Broderick J, Lu M, Jackson C, Pancioli A, Tilley BM, Fagan S, Kothari R, Levine S, Marler J, Lyden P, Haley E, Brott T, Grotta K, the NINDS t-PA Stroke Study Group. Apo E Phenotype and the efficacy of intravenous t-PA in acute ischemic stroke. *Stroke* 2000; 31 (11): 2828.

Broderick JP, Lu M, Kothari R, Levine SR, Lyden PD, Haley C, Brott TG, Grotta J, Tilley BC, Marler JR, Frankel M, and the NINDS rt-PA Stroke Study Group. Finding the most powerful measures of the effectiveness of tissue plasminogen activator in the NINDS t-PA Stroke Trial. *Stroke* 2000; 31: 2335–2341.

Brott T, Kothari R, Fagan S, Frankel M, Grotta JC, Broderick J, Kwiatkowski T, Lewandowski C, Haley EC, Marler JR, Tilley BC, for the NINDS rt-PA Stroke Study Group. Hypertension and its treatment in the NINDS rt-PA Stroke Trial. *Stroke* 1998; 29: 1504–1509.

Fagan SC, Morgenstern LB, Petitta A, Ward RE, Tilley BC, Marler JR, Levine SR, Broderick JP, Kwiatkowski TG, Frankel M, Brott TG, Walker MD, and the NINDS rt-PA Stroke Study Group. Cost-effectiveness of tissue plasminogen activator for acute ischaemic stroke. *Neurology* 1998; 50: 883–890.

Freidman HS. Tissue plasminogen activator for acute ischaemic stroke; letter to the editor. *New England Journal of Medicine* 1996; 334: 1405.

Grotta J, and the NINDS Investigators. The NINDS Stroke Study Group Response. British Medical Journal online 02.07.2002; electronic letter in response to paper by Lenzer *et al.* *British Medical Journal* 2002; 324: 723–729 (online).

Grotta JC, Chiu D, Lu M, Patel S, Levine SR, Tilley BC, Brott TG, Haley EC, Leyden PD, Kothari R, Frankel M, Lewandowski CA, Libman R, Kwiatkowski T, Broderick JP, Marler JR, COrrigan J, Huff S, Mitsias P, Talati S, Tanne D, and the NINDS Study Group. Agreement and variability in the interpretation of early CT changes in stroke patients qualifying for intravenous rtPA therapy. *Stroke* 1999; 30: 1528–1533.

Grotta JC, Welch K, Fagan SC, Lu Mei, Frankel MR, Brott T, Levine SR, Lyden PD, and the NINDS rt-PA Stroke Study Group. Clinical deterioration following improvement in the NINDS rt-PA stroke trial. *Stroke* 2001; 32: 661–668.

Haley EC, Lewandowski C, Tilley BC, and the NINDS rtPA Stroke Study Group. Myths regarding the NINDS rt-PA Stroke Trial: Setting the record straight. *Annals of Emergency Medicine* 1997; 30: 676–682.

Koroshetz WJ. Tissue plasminogen activator for acute ischaemic stroke; letter to the editor. *New England Journal of Medicine* 1999; 334: 1405–1406.

Kwiatkowski TG, Libman R, Frankel M, Tilley B, Morganstern L, Lu M, Broderick J, Marler J, Brott T, and the NINDS RT-PA Stroke Study Group. The NINDS RT-PA stroke study – sustained benefit at one year (abstract). *Stroke* 1998; 29: 288.

Kwiatkowski TG, Libman RB, Frankel M, Tilley BC, Morgenstern LB, Lu M, Broderick JP, Lewandowski CA, Marler JR, Levine SR, Brott T, for the National Institute of Neurological Disorders and Stroke Recombinant Tissue Plasminogen Activator Stroke Study Group. Effects of tissue plasminogen activator for acute ischaemic stroke at one year. *New England Journal of Medicine* 1999; 340 (23): 1781–1787.

Li J. Questioning thrombolytic use for cerebrovascular accidents. *Journal of Emergency Medicine* 1998; 16 (5): 757–758.

Lyden P, Lu M, Jackson C, Marler J, Kothari R, Brott T, Zivin J, and the NINDS rt-PA Stroke Study Investigators. Underlying structure of the National Institutes of Health Stroke Scale. Results of a factor analysis. *Stroke* 1999; 30: 2347–2354.

Lyden P, Lu M, Jackson CM, Marler J, Kothari R, Brott T, Zivin JA. Underlying structure of the NIH Stroke Scale. Results of a factor analysis. *Stroke* 2000; 31: 307.

Marler JR, for the NINDS rt-PA Stroke Study Group. Tissue plasminogen activator for acute ischaemic stroke; letter to the editor – authors' reply. *New England Journal of Medicine* 1999; 334: 1406.

Marler JR, Tilley B, Lu M, Brott T, Lyden P, Broderick JP, Grotta J, Levine S, Frankel M, Horowitz S, Kwaitkowski T, and for the NINDS rt-PA Stroke Study Group. Earlier treatment associated with better outcome in the NINDS t-PA Stroke Study. *Stroke* 1999; 30: 244.

Morgenstern L. Recent results from the NINDS-tPA trial. *Acta Neurologica Scandinavica – Proceedings of the 31st Scandinavian Congress of Neurology* 1996; 94 (167): 28–29.

Patel SC, Levine S, Tilley BC, Grotta JC, Lu M, Frankel M, Haley EC, Brott TG, Broderick JP, Horowitz S, Lyden PD, Lewandowski CA, Marler JR, Welch KMA, for the National Institute of Neurological Disorders and Stroke rt-PA Stroke Study Group. Lack of clinical significance of early ischaemic changes on computed tomography in acute stroke. *Journal of the American Medical Association* 2001; 286: 2830–2838.

Quereshi N. Tissue plasminogen activator for acute ischaemic stroke; letter to the editor. *New England Journal of Medicine* 1999; 334: 1406.

The NINDS rt-PA Stroke Study Group. Effect of rt-PA on ischaemic stroke lesion size by computed tomography: preliminary results from the NINDS rt-PA Stroke Trial. *Proceedings of the 23rd International Joint Conference on Stroke and Cerebral Circulation.*

The NINDS rt-PA Stroke Study Group. A systems approach to immediate evaluation and management of hyperacute stroke. Experience at eight centres and implications for community practice and patient care. *Stroke* 1997; 28: 1530–1540.

The NINDS rt-PA Stroke Study Group. Effect of rt-PA on CT lesion volume over time. *Stroke* 2000; 31 (11): 2828.

The NINDS rt-PA Stroke Trial. Predictors of an unfavourable outcome. *Cerebrovascular Diseases* 1996; 6: 181.

The NINDS rt-PA Trial. Predictors of favourable outcome. *Cerebrovascular Diseases* 1996; 6: 182.

The NINDS t-PA Stroke Study Group. Generalised efficacy of t-PA for Acute Stroke: Subgroup analysis of the NINDS t-PA Stroke Trial. *Stroke* 1997; 28: 2119–2125.

The NINDS t-PA Stroke Study Group. Intracerebral haemorrhage after intravenous t-PA therapy for ischaemic stroke. *Stroke* 1997; 28: 2109–2118.

The National Institute of Neurological Disorders and Stroke rt-PA Stroke Study Group. Tissue Plasminogen Activator for Acute Ischaemic Stroke. *New England Journal of Medicine* 1995; 333: 1581–1587.

Tilley BC, Lyden PD, Brott TG, Lu M, Levine SR, Welch KMA, for the National Institute of Neurological Disorders and Stroke rt-PA Stroke Study Group. Total quality improvement method for reduction of delays between emergency department admission and treatment of acute ischemic stroke. *Archives of Neurology* 1997; 54: 1466–1474.

Wein TH, Hickenbottom SL, Morgenstern LB, Demchuk AM, Grotta JC. Safety of tissue plasminogen activator for acute stroke in menstruating women. *Stroke* 2002; 33: 2506–2508.

del Zoppo GJ. Tissue plasminogen activator for acute ischaemic stroke; letter to the editor – authors' reply. *New England Journal of Medicine* 1996; 334: 1406.

von Kummer R, Hacke W. Letter to the editor. *Stroke* 2000; 31: 231–232.

Ohtomo 1985 {published data only}

Ohtomo E, Araki G, Itoh E, Toghi H, Matsuda T, Atarashi J. Clinical efficacy of urokinase in the treatment of cerebral thrombosis. Multi-center double-blind study in comparison with placebo (translated from Japanese). *Clinical Evaluation* 1985; 15 (3): 711–731.

Ohtomo E, Araki G, Itoh E, Toghi H, Matsuda T, Atarashi J. Clinical efficacy of urokinase in patients with cerebral thrombosis: multicentre double blind study (translation from Japanese awaited). *Kiso-to-Rinshyo (Basic and Clinical)* 1985; 19: 445–478.

PROACT 1998 {published and unpublished data}

Furlan AJ, Putney K, Barker W, del Zoppo GJ, Higashida R, Pessin M, and the PROACT Investigators. The clinical trials acceleration program: experience from the Prolyse in Acute Cerebral Thromboembolism Trial (PROACT). *Stroke* 1996; 27 (1): 171.

del Zoppo GJ, Higashida RT, Furlan AJ, Pessin MS, Rowley HA, Gent M, and the PROACT Investigators. PROACT: A phase II randomised trial of recombinant pro-urokinase by direct arterial delivery in acute middle cerebral artery stroke. *Stroke* 1998; 29: 4–11.

PROACT 2 1999 {published and unpublished data}

Furlan A, Higashida R, Wechsler L, Schulz G, on behalf of the PROACT II Investigators. PROACT II: Recombinant prourokinase (r-ProUK) in acute cerebral thromboembolism. *Proceedings of the 23rd Joint International Conference on Stroke and Cerebral Circulation*, Orlando, Florida, February 5–7, 1998.

Furlan A, Higashida R, Weschler L, Gent M, Rowley H, Kase C, Pessin M, Ahuja A, Callahan F, Clark WM, Silver F, Rivera F, for the PROACT Investigators. Intraarterial pro-urokinase for acute ischaemic stroke. The PROACT II Study: A randomised controlled trial. *Journal of the American Medical Association* 1999; 282: 2003–2011.

Furlan AJ, Higashida R, Wechsler L, Schulz G, for the PROACT 2 Investigators: PROACT II. Recombinant prourokinase (r-ProUK) in acute cerebral thromboembolism: initial trial results. *Stroke* 1999; 30: 234.

Kase CS, Furlan AJ, Wechsler LR, Higashida RT, Rowley HA, Hart RG, Molinari GF, Frederick S, Roberts HC, Gebel JM, Sila CA, Roberts RS, Gent M, Schulz GA, and the PROACT II Investigators. Symptomatic intracranial hemorrhage after intraarterial thrombolysis with recombinant prourokinase in acute ischaemic stroke: The PROACT II Study. *Neurology* 2000; 54 (Suppl 3): A260–A261.

Roberts HC, Dillon WP, Furlan AJ, Rowley HA, Fischbein NJ, Higashida RT, Wechsler LR, Kase C, Schulz GA. Angiographic collaterals in acute stroke – relationship to clinical presentation and outcome: The PROACT II Trial. *Stroke* 2001; 32: 336.

Roberts HC, Dillon WP, Furlan AJ, Wechsler LR, Rowley HA, Fischbein NJ, Higashida RT, Kase C, Schulz GA, Lu Y, Firszt CM. Computed tomographic findings in patients undergoing intra-arterial thrombolysis for acute ischaemic stroke due to middle cerebral artery occlusion: results from the PROACT II trial. *Stroke* 2002; 33: 1557–1565.

Roberts HC, Rowley HA, Dillon WP, Fischbein NJ, Furlan AJ, Higashida RT, Kase CS, Weschler LR, Gent M, Schulz GA. Effect of intraarterial prourokinase on CT infarct volume: results of PROACT II. *Stroke* 2000; 31: 278.

Wechsler LR, Roberts R, Furlan AJ, Higashida R, Dillon WP, Roberts HC, Pettigrew LC, Callahan A, Bruno A, Smith WS, Schula GA. Factors influencing outcome and treatment effect in PROACT II. *Stroke* 2001; 32: 319.

Chapter 6. Augmentation of cerebral blood flow: fibrinogen-depleting agents, haemodilution, and pentoxifylline

Asplund K. Haemodilution for acute ischaemic stroke. *The Cochrane Database of Systematic Reviews* 2002, Issue 4. Art. No.: CD000103. DOI: 10.1002/14651858.CD000103.

Bath PMW, Bath-Hextall FJ. Pentoxifylline, propentofylline and pentifylline for acute ischaemic stroke. *The Cochrane Database of Systematic Reviews* 2004, Issue 3. Art. No.: CD000162. DOI: 10.1002/14651858.CD000162.pub2.

Liu M, Counsell C, Zhao XL, Wardlaw J. Fibrinogen-depleting agents for acute ischaemic stroke (Cochrane Corner). *Stroke* 2004; 36: 173–174.

Liu M, Counsell C, Zhao XL, Wardlaw J. Fibrinogen-depleting agents for acute ischaemic stroke. *The Cochrane Database of Systematic Reviews* 2003, Issue 3, Art. No.: CD000091. DOI: 10.1002/14651858.CD000091.

Sherman DG, Atkinson RP, Chippendale T *et al*. Intravenous ancrod for treatment of acute ischaemic stroke: the STAT study: a randomised controlled trial. Stroke Treatment with Ancrod Trial. *Journal of the American Medical Association* 2000; 283: 2395–2403.

References to studies included in the Cochrane Review of fibrinogen-depleting agents by Liu *et al.* (2003)

AISS 1994 {published and unpublished data}

Glas-Greenwalt P, Levy DE. Ancrod causes rapid and efficient activation of fibrinolysis in patients with acute stroke. *Thrombosis and Haemostasis* 1995; 73 (6): 1151.

Jahnke H. Experimental ancrod (Arvin) for acute ischaemic stroke: nursing implications. *Journal of Neuroscience Nursing* 1991; 23: 386–389. 1992211153.

Ringelstein EB, Olinger CP. The Ancrod Ischaemic Stroke Study: study design and demographics with initial clinical data from the first 60 patients. A multicenter placebo-controlled double-blind trial (abstract). *International Conference on Stroke*, Geneva, Switzerland, 1991: 40.

*The Ancrod Stroke Study Investigators. Ancrod for the treatment of acute ischaemic brain infarction. *Stroke* 1994; 25: 1755–1759. 1994353427.

Hossmann 1983 {published and unpublished data}

Hossmann V, Heiss WD, Bewermeyer H. Controlled trial of ancrod induced hypofibrinogenemia. In: Meyer JS, Lechner H, Reivich M, Ott EO, Aranibar (eds), *Cerebral Vascular Disease 3. Proceedings of the 10th International Salzburg Conference*, Amsterdam: 1981: 36–39.

*Hossmann V, Heiss WD, Bewermeyer H, Wiedemann G. Controlled trial of ancrod in ischaemic stroke. *Archives of Neurology* 1983; 40: 803–808. 1984051898.

Olinger 1988 {published data only}

Olinger CP, Brott TG, Barsan WG, Hedges JR, Glas-Greenwalt P, Pollak VE. Double-blind, randomised placebo-controlled study of ancrod as therapy for acute cerebral infarction (abstract). *Stroke* 1988; 19: 133.

*Olinger CP, Brott TG, Barsan WG, Hedges JR, Glas-Greenwalt P, Pollak VE, Spilker J, Eberle R. Use of ancrod in acute or progressing ischaemic cerebral infarction. *Annals of Emergency Medicine* 1988; 17: 1208–1209. 1989048552.

Pollack VE, Glas-Greenwalt P, Olinger CP, Wadhwa NK. Ancrod, a safe thrombolytic agent, causes rapid thrombolysis in acute stroke (abstract). *Clinical Research* 1989; 37: A549.

Pollack VE, Glas-greenwalt P, Olinger CP, Wadhwa NK, Myre SA. Ancrod causes rapid thrombolysis in patients with acute stroke. *American Journal of the Medical Sciences* 1990; 299: 319–325. 1990247444.

RDTCI 2000 {published data only}

The Cooperative Group for Reassessment of Defibrase, China. Reassessment of defibrase in treatment of cerebral infarction. *Chinese Journal of Neurology* 2000; 33 (5): 263–267.

STAT 2000 {published data only}

Levy DE. Stroke Treatment with Ancrod Trial (STAT) (abstract). *Stroke* 1994; 25: 544.

Sherman D. STAT: Stroke treatment with ancrod trial (abstract). *Cerebrovascular Diseases* 1996; 6: 189.

*Sherman DG, Atkinson RP, Chippendale T, Levin KA, Ng K, Futrell N, Hsu CY, Levy DE. Intravenous ancrod for treatment of acute ischemic stroke: the STAT study: a randomized controlled trial. Stroke Treatment with Ancrod Trial. *Journal of the American Medical Association* 2000; 283 (18): 2395–2403.

References to studies included in the Cochrane Review of Haemodilution for acute ischaemic stroke by Asplund (2002)

Austrian multic 1998 {published data only}

Aichner FT, Fazekas F, Brainin M, Polz W, Mamoli B, Zeiler K. Hypervolemic hemodilution in acute ischemic stroke: the Multicenter Austrian Hemodilution Stroke Trial (MAHST). *Stroke* 1998; 29: 743–749.

Bornstein 1981 {published data only}

Bornstein N, Regev I, Flechater S, Streifler M, Vardi J. (Dextran-40 in nonhemorrhagic cerebrovascular accidents) (in Hebrew). *Harefuah* 1981; 100: 455–456.

Frei *et al.*, 1987 {published data only}

Frei A, Cottier C, Wunderlich P, Ladin E. Glycerol and dextran combined in the therapy of acute stroke. A placebo-controlled, double-blind trial with a planned interim analysis. *Stroke* 1987; 18: 373–379.

Gilroy *et al.*, 1969 {published data only}

Gilroy J, Barnhardt MI, Meyer JS. Treatment of acute stroke with Dextran 40. *Journal of the American Medical Association* 1969; 210: 293–298.

Goslinga *et al.*, 1992 {published data only}

Goslinga H, Eijzenbach V, Heuvelmans JHA, van de Nes JCM, Kurk RM, Bezemer PD. Haemodilution in acute cerebral infarction; administration of albumin solution and crystalline infusion fluid guided by the haematocrit (Hemodilutie op maat bij het acute herseninfarct met behulp van een 20%-albumine-oplossing en fysiologische zoutoplossing). Ned Tidschr Geneeskd 1992; 136: 2422–2428.

*Goslinga H, Eijzenbach V, Heuvelmans JHA, van der Laan de Vries E, Melis VMJ, Schmid-Schonbein H, Bezemer PD. Custum-tailored hemodilution with albumin and crystalloids in acute ischemic stroke. *Stroke* 1992; 23: 181–188.

Haass *et al.*, 1989 {published and unpublished data}

Haass A, Decker I, Hamann G, Stoll M, Schimrigk K, Kasser U. Hemodilution therapy of acute stroke. Paper presented at the *Satellite Symposium on Haemodilution at the First European Stroke Conference*, Dusseldorf, FRG, May 10–12, 1990.

Krack P, Haass A. Hemodynamic effect of hemodliution with hydroxyethyl starch (abstract). *Stroke* 1989; 20: 137.

Hartmann *et al.*, 1987 {published data only}

Hartmann A. Regional cerebral blood flow in acute cerebral infarction during hypervolemic hemodilution. In: Meyer JS, Lechner H, Reivich M, Ott EO (eds), *Cerebral Vascular Disease 5*. Amsterdam: Excerpta Medica, 1985; 206–214.

*Hartmann A, Tsuda Y, Lagreze H, Dettmers C. Effect of hemodilution on regional cerebral blood flow in patients with acute cerebral infarction. In: Hartmann A, Kuschinsky W (eds), *Cerebral Ischemia and Hemorheology*. Berlin: Springer-Verlag, 1987: 423–428.

Italian multic 1988 {published data only}

Italian Acute Stroke Study Group. Haemodilution in acute stroke: results from the Italian Haemodilution Trial. *Lancet* 1988; i: 318–320.

Kaste *et al.*, 1976 {published data only}

Kaste M, Fogelholm R, Waltimo O. Combined dexamethasone and low-molecular-weight dextran in acute brain infarction: double-blind study. *British Medical Journal* 1976; 2: 1409–1410.

Koller *et al.*, 1990 {published data only}

Koller M, Haenny P, Hess K, Weniger D, Zangger P. Adjusted hypervolemic hemodilution in acute ischemic stroke. *Stroke* 1990; 21: 1429–1434.

Mast *et al.*, 1991 {published data only}

Mast H, Marx P. Neurological deterioration under isovolemic hemodilution with hydroxyethyl starch in acute cerebral ischemia. *Stroke* 1991; 22: 680–683.

Mast H, Vogel H-P, Marx P. Hemodilution in ischemic stroke (letter). *Stroke* 1991; 22: 955.

Matthews *et al.*, 1976 {published data only}

Matthews WB, Oxbury JM, Grainger KMR, Greenhall RCD. A blind controlled trial of dextran 40 in the treatment of ischemic stroke. *Brain* 1976; 99: 193–206.

Popa *et al.*, 1989 {published data only}

Popa G, Popa C, Stanescu A, Ionescu G, Lugoji G, Radula D, Popescu A. Haemodilution therapy in acute ischaemic stroke. Rev Roum – *Neurology Psychiatry* 1989; 27: 79–90.

Rudolf *et al.*, 2002 {unpublished data only}

Heiss W-D, for the HES Study Group. Hypervolemic hemodilution by hydroxyethyl starch in acute ischemic stroke (abstract). *Stroke* 1999; 30: 270.

*Rudolf J. Hydroxyethyl starch for hypervolemic hemodilution in patients with acute ischemic stroke: a randomized, placebo-controlled phase II safety study. *Cerebrovascular Diseases* 2002; 14: 33–41.

Rudolf J. Evaluation of safety of hydroxyethyl starch (HES) in hypervolemic hemodilution in patients with acute ischemic stroke – an explanatory pilot study. *Cerebrovascular Diseases* 2001; 11 (Suppl 4): 121.

Scand multic 1987 {published data only}

Scandinavian Stroke Study Group. Hemodilution in acute ischemic stroke – a randomized multicenter trial (abstract). *Stroke* 1986; 17: 143.

Scandinavian Stroke Study Group (clinical coordinator K Asplund). Multicenter trial of hemodilution in acute ischemic stroke: background and study protocol. *Stroke* 1985; 16: 885–890.

Scandinavian Stroke Study Group (clinical coordinator K Asplund). Multicenter trial of hemodilution in acute ischemic stroke: I. Results in the total patient population. *Stroke* 1987; 18: 691–699.

Scandinavian Stroke Study Group (clinical coordinator K Asplund). Multicenter trial of hemodilution in acute ischemic stroke: results of subgroup analyses. *Stroke* 1988; 19: 464–471.

Spudis *et al.*, 1973 {published data only}

Spudis EV, de la Torre E, Pikula L. Management of completed stroke with dextran 40. A community hospital failure. *Stroke* 1973; 4: 895–897.

Strand *et al.*, 1984 {published data only}

Asplund K, Eriksson S, Hagg E, Lithner F, Strand T, Wester PO. Ischemic stroke treated by haemodilution: an interim report of a randomized trial. In: Meyer JS, Lechner H, Reivich M,

Ott EO (eds), Cerebral Vascular Disease 4. I.C.S. No. 616. Elsevier Science Publishing Co., 1982: 148–150.

Strand T, Asplund K, Eriksson S, Hagg E, Lithner F, Wester PO. A randomized controlled trial of hemodilution therapy in acute ischemic stroke. *Stroke* 1984; 15: 980–989.

Strand T, Asplund K, Eriksson S, Hagg E, Lithner F, Wester PO. Hemodilution treatment of ischemic stroke (abstract). *Stroke* 1983; 14: 122.

US multicentre 1989 {published data only}

The Hemodilution in Stroke Study Group. Hypervolemic hemodilution treatment of acute stroke. Results of a randomized multicenter trial using pentastarch. *Stroke* 1989; 20: 317–323.

Chapter 7. Neuroprotection

Albers GW, Bogousslavsky J, Bozik MA *et al.* Recommendations for clinical trial evaluation of acute stroke therapies: Stroke Therapy Academic Industry Roundtable II (STAIR II). *Stroke* 2001; 32: 1598–1606.

Baird AE, Benfield A, Schlaug G *et al.* Enlargement of human cerebral ischemic lesion volumes measured by diffusion-weighted magnetic resonance imaging. *Annals of Neurology* 1997; 41: 581–589.

Bernard SA, Gray TW, Buist MD *et al.* Treatment of comatose survivors of out-of-hospital cardiac arrest with induced hypothermia. *New England Journal of Medicine* 2002; 346: 557–563.

Bogousslavsky J, Victor SJ, Salinas EO, Pallay A, Donnan GA, Fieschi C, Kaste M, Orgogozo J-M, Chammorro A, Desmet A, for the European-Australian Fiblast (Trafermin) in Acute Stroke Group. Fiblast (Trafermin) in acute stroke: results of the European–Australian phase II/III safety and efficacy trial. *Cerebrovascular Diseases* 2002; 14: 239–251.

Candelise L, Ciccone A. Gangliosides for acute ischaemic stroke (Cochrane Corner). *Stroke* 2002; 33: 2336.

Candelise L, Ciccone A. Gangliosides for acute ischaemic stroke. *The Cochrane Database of Systematic Reviews* 2000, Issue 4. Art. No.: CD000094. DOI: 10.1002/14651858.CD000094.

Correia M, Silva M, Veloso M. Cooling therapy for acute stroke. *The Cochrane Database of Systematic Reviews* 1999, Issue 3. Art. No.: CD001247. DOI: 10.1002/14651858.CD001247.

Crowther CA, Hiller JE, Doyle LW, Haslam RR. Effect of magnesium sulfate given for neuroprotection before preterm birth: a randomised controlled trial. *Journal of the American Medical Association* 2003; 290: 2669–2676.

Dávalos A, Castillo J, Álavarez-Sabin J *et al.* Oral citicoline in acute ischemic stroke. An individual patient data pooling analysis of clinical trials. *Stroke* 2002; 33: 2850–2857.

Enlimomab Acute Stroke Trial Investigators. Use of anti-ICAM-1 therapy in ischemic stroke: results of the Enlimomab Acute Stroke Trial. *Neurology*, 2001; 57 (8): 1428–1434.

Falcao ALE, Reutens DC, Markus R *et al.* The resistance to ischaemia of white and gray matter after stroke. *Annals of Neurology* 2004; 56: 695–701.

Finkelstein SP, Fisher M, Furlan AJ *et al.* Recommendations for standards regarding preclinical neuroprotective and restorative drug development. Stroke Therapy Academic Industry Roundtable (STAIR). *Stroke* 1999; 30: 2752–2758.

Fisher M, Cyrus PA, Davis SM *et al.* Recommendations for advancing development of acute stroke therapies: Stroke Therapy Academic Industry Roundtable-3. *Stroke* 2003; 34: 1539–1546.

Gandolfo C, Sandercock P, Conti M. Lubeluzole for acute ischaemic stroke. *The Cochrane Database of Systematic Reviews* 2002, Issue 1. Art. No.: CD001924. DOI: 10.1002/14651858.CD001924.

Ginsberg MD. Injury mechanisms in the ischaemic penumbra – approaches to neuroprotection in acute ischaemic stroke. *Cerebrovascular Diseases* 1997; 7 (Suppl 2): 7–12.

Gladstone DJ, Black SE, Hakim AM, for the Heart and Stroke Foundation of Ontario Centre of Excellence in Stroke Recovery. Toward wisdon from failure. Lesson from neuroprotective stroke trials and new therapeutic directions. *Stroke* 2002; 33: 2123–2136.

Goldstein LB. Neuroprotective therapy for acute ischaemic stroke: down, but not out. *Lancet* 2004; 363: 414–415.

Hankey GJ. Clomethiazole: an unsuccessful bachelor, but perhaps a prosperous married man? *Stroke* 2002; 33: 128–129.

Horn J, Limburg M. Calcium antagonists for acute ischemic stroke. *The Cochrane Database of Systematic Reviews* 2000, Issue 1. Art. No.: CD001928. DOI: 10.1002/14651858.CD001928.

Horn J, Limburg M. Calcium antagonists for acute ischemic stroke. A systematic review. *Stroke* 2001; 32: 570–576.

Hypothermia after Cardiac Arrest Study Group. Mild therapeutic hypothermia to improve the neurologic outcome after cardiac arrest. *New England Journal of Medicine* 2002; 346: 549–556.

Internet Stroke Centre: http://www.strokecenter.org/trials/

Intravenous Magnesium Efficacy in Stroke (IMAGES) Investigators. Magnesium for acute stroke (Intravenous Magnesium Efficacy in Stroke trial): randomised controlled trial. *Lancet* 2004; 363: 439–445.

Kramss M, Lees KR, Hacke W *et al.* Acute stroke therapy by inhibition of neutrophils (ASTIN). An adaptive dose-response study of UK-279,276 in acute ischaemic stroke. *Stroke* 2003; 34: 2543–2548.

Lee JM, Zipfel GJ, Choi DW. The changing landscape of ischaemic brain injury mechanisms. *Nature* 1999; 399 (Suppl); A7–A14.

Lyden PD, Shuaib A, Ng K, Levin K, Atkinson RP, Rajput A, Wechsler LR, Ashwood T, Claesson L, Odergren T, Salazar-Grueso. Clomethiazole Acute Stroke Study in ischemic stroke (CLASS-I): final results. *Stroke.* 2002; 33: 122–128.

Marler JR, Tilley BC, Lu M *et al.* Early stroke treatment associated with better outcome: the NINDS rt-PA Stroke Study. *Neurology* 2000; 55: 1649–1655.

Muir KW, Lees KR. Excitatory amino acid antagonists for acute stroke. *The Cochrane Data-base of Systematic Reviews* 2003, Issue 2. Art. No.: CD001244. DOI: 10.1002/14651858. CD001244.

Ricci S, Celani MG, Cantisani AT, Righetti E. Piracetam for acute ischaemic stroke. *The Cochrane Database of Systematic Reviews* 2002, Issue 4. Art. No.: CD000419. DOI: 10.1002/14651858. CD000419.

Reith J, Jorgensen HS, Pedersen PM *et al.* Body temperature in acute stroke: relation to stroke severity, infarct size, mortality, and outcome. *Lancet* 1996; 347: 422–425.

Sandercock P, Berge E, Dennis M *et al.* A systematic review of the effectiveness, cost-effectiveness and barriers to implementation of thrombolytic and neuroprotective therapy for acute ischaemic stroke in the NHS. *Health Technology Assessment* 2002; 6: 35–57.

Saver JL, Kidwell CS, Eckstein M, Starkman S. FAST-MAG Pilot Trail investigators. Prehospital neuroprotective therapy for acute stroke: results of the Field Administration of Stroke Therapy-Magnesium (FAST-MAG) Pilot Trial. *Stroke* 2004; 35: e106–e108.

Schmid-Elsaesser R, Hungerhuber E, Zausinger S *et al.* Combination drug therapy and mild hypothermia: a promising treatment strategy for reversible, focal cerebral ischaemia. *Stroke* 1999; 30: 1891–1899.

The Tirilazad International Steering Committee. Tirilazad for acute ischaemic stroke. A systematic review. *Stroke* 2000; 31: 2257–2265.

The Tirilazad International Steering Committee. Tirilazad for acute ischaemic stroke. *The Cochrane Database of Systematic Reviews* 2001, Issue 4. Art. No.: CD002087. DOI: 10.1002/14651858. CD002087.

Wahlgren N-G, Ranasinha KW, Rosolacci T, Francke CL, van Erven PM, Ashwood T, Claesson L, for the CLASS Study Group. Clomethiazole Acute Stroke Study (CLASS): results of a randomized, controlled trial of clomethiazole versus placebo in 1360 acute stroke patients. *Stroke* 1999; 30: 21–28.

Zivin JA. SLOW-MAG. *Stroke* 2004; 35: 1776–1777.

Zweifler RM, Voorhees ME, Mahmood A, Parnell M. Magnesium sulphate increases the rate of hypothermia via surface cooling and improves comfort. *Stroke* 2004; 35: 2331–2334.

References to studies included in the Cochrane Review of excitatory amino acids by Muir and Lees (2003)

AR-R15896AR {published and unpublished data}

*Lees KR, Dyker AG, Sharma A, Ford GA, Ardron ME, Grosset DG. Tolerability of the low-affinity, use-dependent NMDA antagonist AR-R15896AR in stroke patients: a dose-ranging study. *Stroke* 2001; 32: 466–472.

Lees KR, Dyker AG, Sharma A, Ford GA, Ardron ME, Grosset DG, Dean A. AR-R15896AR in patients with acute stroke: a dose-finding study. *Cerebrovascular Diseases* 1999; 9 (Suppl 1): 102.

ASSIST Protocols 7&10 {published and unpublished data}

Davis SM, Albers GW, Diener HC, Lees KR, Norris J. Termination of Acute Stroke Studies Involving Selfotel Treatment. ASSIST Steering Committee. *Lancet* 1997; 349: 32.

CNS1102-003 {published data only}

*Block GA. Final results from a dose-escalating safety and tolerance study of the non-competitive NMDA antagonist CNS1102 in patients with acute cerebral ischemia. *Stroke* 1995; 26: 185.

Fisher M. Cerestat (CNS 1102), a non-competitive NMDA antagonist, in ischemic stroke patients: dose-escalating safety study. *Cerebrovascular Diseases* 1994; 4: 245.

McBurney RN. Development of the NMDA ion-channel blocker, aptiganel hydrochloride, as a neuroprotective agent for acute CNS injury. In: Green AR, Cross AJ (eds), *Neuroprotective Agents and Cerebral Ischaemia*, Vol. 40. San Diego: Academic Press, 1997: 173–195.

CNS1102-008 {unpublished data only}

*Edwards K. Cerestat (aptiganel hydrochloride) in the treatment of acute ischemic stroke: results of a phase II trial. *Neurology* 1996; 46 (Suppl 2): A424.

CNS1102-010 {unpublished data only}

*Dyker AG, Edwards KR, Fayad PB, Hormes JT, Lees KR. Safety and tolerability study of aptiganel hydrochloride in patients with an acute ischemic stroke. *Stroke* 1999; 30 (10): 2038–2042.

CNS1102-011 {published data only}

CNS 1102-011 Trial Synopsis 1997.

*Albers GW, Goldstein LB, Hall D, Lesko LM. Aptiganel hydrochloride in acute ischemic stroke: a randomized controlled trial. *Journal of the American Medical Association* 2001; 286 (21): 2673–2682.

CVD 715 {unpublished data only}

*Depierre C. Clinical evaluation of eliprodil in the acute phase of stroke. *Sanofi-Synthelabo Report* 2000.

Dextrorphan {published data only}

*Albers GW, Atkinson RP, Kelley RE, Rosenbaum DM. Safety, tolerability, and pharmacokinetics of the N-methyl-D-aspartate antagonist dextrorphan in patients with acute stroke. *Stroke* 1995; 26: 254–258.

Eliprodil {unpublished data only}

Depierre C. Clinical evaluation of eliprodil in the acute phase of stroke. *Sanofi-Synthelabo Report* 2000.

Fosphenytoin IIa {published data only}

*Tietjen GE, Dombi T, Pulsinelli W, Becske T, Kugler AR, Mann ME. A double-blind, safety, and tolerance study of single intravenous doses of fosphenytoin in patients with acute ischemic stroke. *Neurology* 1996; 46 (Suppl 2): A424–A425.

GAIN ICH {published data only}

*Davis S, Zafar K, Vohora S, Okubo S, Nagashima J, Ito T, Katayama Y. Efficacy and safety of GV150526 in primary intracerebral haemorrhage: data from the GAIN trials (Glycine Antagonist in Neuroprotection). *Stroke* 2000; 31 (11): 2865.

GAIN-A {published data only}

Sacco RL. GV150526 in the treatment of acute stroke: results of the GAIN Americas trial. *Cerebrovascular Diseases* 102001: 106.

*Sacco RL, DeRosa JT, Haley Jr EC, Levin B, Ordronneau P, Phillips SJ *et al.* Glycine antagonist in neuroprotection for patients with acute stroke: GAIN Americas: a randomized controlled trial. *Journal of the American Medical Association* 2001; 285 (13): 1719–1728.

GAIN-I {published data only}

*Lees KR, Asplund K, Carolei A, Davis SM, Diener HC, Orgogozo JM, Whitehead J. Glycine antagonist (gavestinel) in neuroprotection (GAIN International) in patients with acute stroke: a randomised controlled trial. *Lancet* 2000; 355: 1949–1954.

GLYA2001 {unpublished data only}

*Phase II studies of the glycine antagonist GV150526 in acute stroke: the North American experience. The North American Glycine Antagonist in Neuroprotection (GAIN) Investigators. *Stroke* 2000; 31 (2): 358–365.

GLYA2005 {unpublished data only}

*Phase II studies of the glycine antagonist GV150526 in acute stroke: the North American experience. The North American Glycine Antagonist in Neuroprotection (GAIN) Investigators. *Stroke* 2000; 31 (2): 358–365.

GLYB2001 {unpublished data only}

*Dyker AG, Lees KR. Safety and tolerability of GV150526 (a glycine site antagonist at the N-methyl-D-aspartate receptor) in patients with acute stroke. *Stroke* 1999; 30 (5): 986–992.

GLYB2002 {unpublished data only}

GAIN European Study Group. Safety and tolerability of GV150526 in acute stroke (GLYB 2002). *Cerebrovascular Diseases* 1998; 8 (Suppl 4): 20.

*Lees KR, Lavelle JF, Cunha L, Diener HC, Sanders EA, Tack P *et al.* Glycine antagonist (GV150526) in acute stroke: a multicentre, double-blind placebo-controlled phase II trial. *Cerebrovascular Diseases* 2001; 11 (1): 20–29.

GLYB2003 {unpublished data only}

*Dyker AG, Lees KR. Safety and tolerability of GV150526 (a glycine site antagonist at the N-methyl-D-aspartate receptor) in patients with acute stroke. *Stroke* 1999; 30 (5): 986–992.

IMAGES pilot {published data only}

*IMAGES Study Group, Bradford APJ, Muir KW, Lees KR. IMAGES pilot study of intravenous magnesium in acute stroke. *Cerebrovascular Diseases* 1998; 8 (Suppl 4): 86.

LES 01 {unpublished data only}

*Depierre C. Clinical evaluation of eliprodil in the acute phase of stroke. *Sanofi-Synthelabo Report* 2000.

LES 02 {unpublished data only}

*Depierre C. Clinical evaluation of eliprodil in the acute phase of stroke. *Sanofi-Synthelabo Report* 2000.

Licostinel {published data only}

*Albers GW, Clark WM, Atkinson RP, Madden K, Data JL, Whitehouse MJ. Dose escalation study of the NMDA glycine-site antagonist licostinel in acute ischemic stroke. *Stroke* 1999; 30 (3): 508–513.

Lifarizine {published and unpublished data}

*Squire IB, Lees KR, Pryse-Phillips W, Kertesz A, Bamford J. The effects of lifarizine in acute cerebral infarction: a pilot safety study. *Cerebrovascular Diseases* 1996; 6: 156–160.

Lub-Int 13 {published data only}

*Diener HC, Cortens M, Ford G, Grotta J, Hacke W, Kaste M *et al.* Lubeluzole in acute ischemic stroke treatment: A double-blind study with an 8-hour inclusion window comparing a 10-mg daily dose of lubeluzole with placebo. *Stroke* 2000; 31 (11): 2543–2551.

Lub-Int 4 {published data only}

Diener HC, Hacke W, Hennerici M, Radberg J, Hantson L, De Keyser J. Lubeluzole in acute ischemic stroke. A double-blind, placebo-controlled phase II trial. Lubeluzole International Study Group. *Stroke* 1996; 27: 76–81.

Lub-Int 5 {published and unpublished data}

Diener HC. Multinational randomised controlled trial of lubeluzole in acute ischaemic stroke. European and Australian Lubeluzole Ischaemic Stroke Study Group. *Cerebrovascular Diseases* 1998; 8: 172–181.

Lub-Int 7 {published data only}

*Hacke W, Lees KR, Timmerhuis T, Haan J, Hantson L, Hennerici M *et al.* Cardiovascular safety of lubeluzole (prosynap®) in patients with ischemic stroke. *Cerebrovascular Diseases* 1998; 8 (5): 247–254.

Lub-Int 9 {published data only}

Grotta J. Lubeluzole treatment of acute ischemic stroke. The US and Canadian Lubeluzole Ischemic Stroke Study Group. *Stroke* 1997; 28: 2338–2346.

Lub-USA 6 {published data only}

*Grotta J. Combination Therapy Stroke Trial: recombinant tissue-type plasminogen activator with/without lubeluzole. *Cerebrovascular Diseases* 2001; 12 (3): 258–263.

Grotta JC. Combination therapy stroke trial: rtPA +/− lubeluzole. *Stroke* 2000; 31 (1): 278.

Muir & Lees (1) {published data only}

Muir KW, Lees KR. A randomised, double-blind, placebo-controlled pilot trial of intravenous magnesium sulfate in acute stroke. *Stroke* 1995; 26: 183–188.

Muir & Lees (2) {published data only}

Muir KW, Lees KR. Dose optimization of intravenous magnesium sulfate after acute stroke. *Stroke* 1998; 29: 918–923.

Remacemide phase 2 {unpublished data only}

*Dyker AG, Lees KR. Remacemide hydrochloride: a double-blind, placebo-controlled, safety and tolerability study in patients with acute ischemic stroke. *Stroke* 1999; 30 (9): 1796–1801.

Selfotel IIa {published data only}

Grotta J, Clark W, Coull B *et al.* Safety and tolerability of the glutamate antagonist CGS 19755 (selfotel) in patients with acute ischemic stroke: results of a phase IIa randomized trial. *Stroke* 1995; 26: 602–605.

Selfotel IIb {published data only}

*Markabi S. Selfotel (CGS 19755): the preliminary clinical experience. In: Krieglstein J, Oberpichler-Schwenk H (eds), *Pharmacology of Cerebral Ischemia*. Stuttgart: Medpharm, 1994: 635–642.

Sipatrigine 137-101 {published data only}

Hussein Z, Fraser IJ, Lees KR *et al.* Pharmacokinetics of 619C89, a novel neuronal sodium channel inhibitor, in acute stroke patients after loading and discrete maintenance infusions. *British Journal of Clinical Pharmacology* 1996; 41: 505–511.

Muir KW, Hamilton SJC, Lunnon MW, Hobbiger S, Lees KR. Safety and tolerability of 619C89 after acute stroke. *Cerebrovascular Diseases* 1998; 8: 31–37.

Sipatrigine 137-102 {unpublished data only}

*Hainsworth AH, Stefani A, Calabresi P, Smith TW, Leach MJ. Sipatrigine (BW619C89) is a neuroprotective agent and a sodium and calcium channel inhibitor. *CNS Drug Reviews 2000*; 6 (2): 111–134.

Sipatrigine 137-104 {unpublished data only}

*Hainsworth AH, Stefani A, Calabresi P, Smith TW, Leach MJ. Sipatrigine (BW619C89) is a neuroprotective agent and a sodium and calcium channel inhibitor. *CNS Drug Reviews 2000*; 6 (2): 111–134.

Sipatrigine 137-121 {published data only}

Muir KW, Holzapfel L, Lees KR. Phase II clinical trial of sipatrigine (619C89) by continuous infusion in acute stroke. *Cerebrovascular Diseases* 2000; 10 (6): 431–436.

Wester {published data only}

*Wester PO, Asplund K, Eriksson S, Hagg E, Lithner F, Strand T. Infusion of magnesium in patients with acute brain infarction. *Acta Neurologica Scandinavica* 1984; 70 (2): 143.

References to studies included in the Cochrane Review of Lubeluzole for acute ischaemic stroke by Gandolfi *et al.* (2002)

LUB-INT-13 1996 {published data only}

Diener HC. Lubeluzole in acute ischaemic stroke treatment: lack of efficacy in a large phase III study with an 8-hour window (abstract). *Stroke* 1999; 30: 234.

Diener HC, Cortens M, Ford G, Grotta J, Hacke W, Kaste M, Koudstaal PJ, Wessel T. Lubeluzole in acute stroke treatment. A double-blind study with an 8-hour inclusion window comparing a 10-mg daily dose of Lubeluzole with placebo. *Stroke* 2000; 31: 2543–2551.

Hantson L, Wessel T. Therapeutic benefits of lubeluzole in ischaemic stroke (abstract). *Stroke* 1998; 29: 287.

Janssen Research Foundation. Lubeluzole in acute ischaemic stroke treatment: a double-blind study with an 8-hour inclusion window, comparing a 10 mg daily dose of lubeluzole with placebo. LUB-INT-13 Study Protocol 1996.

Wessel TC. Determinants of outcome in the lubeluzole clinical trial (abstract). Proceedings of the IBC's Seventh Annual Conference on Ischaemic Stroke. Advances in Novel Therapeutic Development. 1998, November 19–20. USA, Washington DC: IBC, 1998.

LUB-INT-4 1995 {published data only}

Anonymous. [LUB-INT-4].

Day L. New stroke treatment (abstract). *Journal of Neuroscience Nursing* 1995; 27: 260.

De Ryck, Janssen. Lubeluzole: a novel experimental neuroprotective agent in the acute treatment of ischemic stroke.

Diener HC. Clinical experience with lubeluzole in patients with acute ischaemic stroke. *Cerebrovascular Diseases* 1997; 7 (Suppl 2): 35–38.

Diener HC. Lubeluzole (abstract). *Cerebrovascular Diseases* 1996; 6: 189.

Diener HC, Hacke W, Hennerici M, De Keyser J, Hantson L. Lubeluzole in the acute treatment of ischemic stroke: results of a phase II trial (abstract). *Journal of Stroke Cerebrovascular Diseases* 1995; 5: 101.

Diener HC, Hacke W, Hennerici M, De Keyser J, Radberg J, Hantson L. Lubeluzole in the acute treatment of ischemic stroke: results of a phase 2 trial (abstract). *Journal of Cerebral Blood Flow and Metabolism* 1995; 15 (Suppl 1): S128.

Diener HC, Hacke W, Hennerici M, De Keyser J, Radberg J, Hantson L, for the LUB-INT-4 Study Group. The effects of lubeluzole in the acute treatment of ischemic stroke: results of a phase 2 trial (abstract). *Stroke* 1995; 26: 185.

Diener HC, Hacke W, Hennerici M, De Keyser J, Radberg J, Hantson L, for the LUB-INT-4 Study Group. Lubeluzole reduces mortality and improves functional outcome in the acute treatment of ischaemic stroke. Results of a phase-2 trial (abstract). *Proceeding of the 8th Scandinavian Meeting on Cerebrovascular Diseases*, 26–29 August 1995, Trondheim, Norway, 1995. Norway, Trondheim: 1995.

Diener HC, Hacke W, Hennerici M, Radberg J, Hantson L, De Keyser J. Lubeluzole in acute ischemic stroke. A double blind, placebo controlled phase II trial. *Stroke* 1996; 27: 76–81.

Hennerici M, Diener HC, Hacke W, De Keyser J, Radberg J, Hantson L. The effect of lubeluzole in the acute treatment of ischemic stroke: results of a late phase 2 trial (abstract). *Journal of Clinical Neuroscience* 1995; 2 (1): 91.

Hennerici M, Diener HC, Hacke W, De Keyser J, Radberg J, Hantson L, LUB-INT-4 Study Group. Lubeluzole in the acute treatment of ischaemic stroke: results of a late phase II trial (abstract). *Cerebrovascular Diseases* 1995; 5: 235.

Radberg J, Diener HC, Hacke M, Hennerici M, Eriksson B. Lubeluzole in the acute treatment of ischemic stroke (abstract). *Proceedings of the Paneuropean Consensus Meeting on Stroke Management*, November 1995, Sweden, Helsingborg: World Health Organisation & European Stroke Council, 1995.

Radberg J, Diener HC, Hacke W, Hennerici M, Eriksson B, for the Lubeluzole International Study Group. Lubeluzole in the acute treatment of ischaemic stroke (abstract). *Acta Neurologica Scandinavica* 1996; 94 (Suppl 167): 21.

LUB-INT-5 1997 {published data only}

Diener HC, Kaste M, Hacke W, Koudstaal P, Hennerici M, Wessel T, Hanson L. Lubeluzole in acute ischemic stroke (abstract). *Proceedings of the 22nd International Joint Conference on Stroke and Cerebral Circulation*, 1997, USA, Anaheim. CA: 1997.

Diener HC, Kaste M, Hacke W, Koudstaal P, Hennerici M, for the LUB-INT-5 Lubeluzole Study Group. Lubeluzole in acute ischemic stroke: international trial (abstract). *Journal of the Neurological Sciences* 1997; 150 (Suppl): S199.

Diener HC, for the European and Australian Lubeluzole Ischemic Stroke Study Group. Multinational randomised controlled trial of Lubeluzole in acute ischaemic stroke. *Cerebrovascular Diseases* 1998; 8: 172–181.

Hantson L, Wessel T. Therapeutic benefits of lubeluzole in ischemic stroke (abstract). *Stroke* 1998; 29: 287.

Jannsen. Lubeluzole in acute stroke treatment.

Jannsen Research Foundation. LUB-INT-5 study protocol: Lubeluzole in acute stroke treatment.

Jannsen Research Foundation. Lubeluzole in acute stroke treatment. Inclusion/exclusion criteria and European Stroke Scale. LUB-INT-5.

LUB-INT-7 1996 {published and unpublished data}

Diener HC, Hacke W, Lees K, Timmerhuis T, Haan J, Hantson L, Hennerici M. Cardiovascular safety of Lubeluzole in patients with acute ischemic stroke.

Diener HC. Clinical experience with Lubeluzole in patients with acute ischaemic stroke. *Cerebrovascular Diseases* 1997; 7 (Suppl 2):35–38.

Diener HC, Hacke W, Lees K, Timmerhuis T, Haan J, Hantson L, Hennerici M. Cardiovascular safety of Lubeluzole in patients with acute ischaemic stroke (abstract). *Cerebrovascular Diseases* 1996; 6 (Suppl 2): 77.

Hacke W, Hennerici H, Hantson L, Diener HC. Lubeluzole – A new neuroprotectant agent in the treatment of acute ischaemic stroke: results of a cardiovascular safety study in stroke patients (abstract). *Neurology* 1996; 46: A429.

Hacke W, Lees KR, Timmerhuis T, Haan J, Hantson L, Hennerici M, Diener HC. Cardiovascular safety of Lubeluzole (Prosynap) in patients with ischemic stroke. *Cerebrovascular Diseases* 1998; 8: 247–254.

Hantson L, De Keyser J, Tritsmans L, Gheuens J, Wessel T, Smith DB. The safety and tolerability of Lubeluzole in patients with acute ischaemic stroke (abstract). J Stroke *Cerebrovascular Diseases* 1997; 6 (3): 153.

LUB-INT-9 1997 {published data only}

Grotta J, Hantson L, Wessel T. The efficacy and safety of lubeluzole in patients with acute ischemic stroke (abstract). *Stroke* 1997; 28: 271.

Grotta J, for the LUB-INT-9 Lubeluzole Study Group. The efficacy and safety of lubeluzole in patients with acute ischemic stroke (abstract). *Journal of Neurological Science* 1997; 150 (Suppl): S199.

Grotta J, for the US and Canadian Lubeluzole Ischaemic Stroke Study Group. Lubeluzole treatment of acute ischemic stroke. *Stroke* 1997; 28: 2338–2346.

Krieger DW, Demchuk AM, Kasner SE, Jauss M, Hantson L. Early clinical and radiological predictors of fatal brain swelling in ischemic stroke. *Stroke* 1999; 30: 287–292.

Lodder J. Lubeluzole treatment in acute ischemic stroke (letter). *Stroke* 1998; 29: 1067.

References to studies included in the Cochrane Review of calcium channel antagonists by Horn and Limburg (2000)

ASCLEPIOS 1990 {unpublished data only}

Azcona A, Lataste X. Isradipine in patients with acute ischemic cerebral infarction. An overview of the ASCLEPIOS programme. *Drugs* 1990; 40 (Suppl 2): 52–57.

Bogousslavsky 1990 {published and unpublished data}

Bogousslavsky J, Regli F, Zumstein V, Kobberling W. Double-blind study of nimodipine in non-severe stroke. *European Journal of Neurology* 1990; 30: 23–26.

Bridgers 1991 {published and unpublished data}

Bridgers SL, Koch G, Munera C *et al.* Intravenous nimodipine in acute stroke: interim analysis of randomized trials. *Stroke* 1991; 22: 153.

Canwin 1993 {published and unpublished data}

Norris JW, LeBrun LH, Anderson BA. The Canwin Study Group. Intravenous Nimodipine in acute ischaemic stroke. *Cerebrovascular Diseases* 1994; 4: 194–196.

Capon 1983 {unpublished data only}

[AQ30a]Unpublished study

Chandra 1995 {published data only}

Chandra B. A New form of management of stroke. *Journal of Stroke and Cerebrovascular Diseases* 1995; 5: 241–243.

FIST 1990 {published and unpublished data}

Franke CL, Palm R, Dalby M *et al.* Flunarizine in stroke treatment (FIST). A double-blind, placebo-controlled trial in Scandinavia and the Netherlands. *Acta Neurologica Scandinavica* 1996; 93: 56–60.

Gelmers 1984 {published and unpublished data}

Gelmers HJ. The effects of nimodipine on the clinical course of patients with acute ischemic stroke. *Acta Neurologica Scandinavica* 1984; 69: 232–239.

Gelmers 1988 {published and unpublished data}

Gelmers HJ, Gorter K, De Weerdt CJ, Wiezer HJA. A controlled trial of nimodipine in acute ischemic stroke. *New England Journal of Medicine* 1988; 318: 203–207.

German-Austrian 1994 {published and unpublished data}

Kramer G, Tettenborn B, Schmutzhard E *et al.* Nimodipine in acute ischemic stroke. Results of the nimodipine German-Austrian stroke trial. *Cerebrovascular Diseases* 1994; 4: 182–188.

Heiss 1990 {published and unpublished data}

Heiss WD, Holthoff V, Pawlik G, Neveling M. Effect of nimodipine on regional cerebral glucose metabolism in patients with acute ischemic stroke as measured by positron emission tomography. *Journal of Cerebral Blood Flow and Metabolism* 1990; 10: 127–132.

INWEST 1990 {published and unpublished data}

Wahlgren NG, MacMahon DG, De Keyser J, Ryman T, INWEST Study Group. Intravenous nimodipine West European Stroke Trial (INWEST) of nimodipine in the treatment of acute ischaemic stroke. *Cerebrovascular Diseases* 1994; 4: 204–210.

Kaste 1994 {published and unpublished data}

Kaste M, Fogelholm R, Erila T *et al.* A randomized, double-blind, placebo-controlled trial of nimodipine in acute ischemic hemishperic stroke. *Stroke* 1994; 25: 1348–1353.

Kornhuber 1993 {published data only}

Kornhuber HH, Hartung J, Herrlinger JD *et al.* Flunarizine in ischemic stroke; a randomised, multicentre, placebo-controlled, double blind study. *Neurology Psychiatry and Brain Research* 1993; 1: 173–180.

Limburg 1990 {published and unpublished data}

Limburg M, Hijdra A. Flunarizine in acute ischemic stroke: A pilot study. *European Neurology* 1990; 30: 121–122.

Lisk 1993 {published data only}

Lisk DR, Grotta JC, Lamki LM *et al.* Should hypertension be treated after acute stroke? A randomized controlled trial using single photon emission computed tomography. *Archives of Neurology* 1993; 50: 855–862.

Lowe 1989 {unpublished data only}

Lowe G. Nimodipine in acute cerebral hemispheric infarction. Unpublished data, University of Glasgow.

Martinez-Vila 1990 {published and unpublished data}

Martinez-Vila E, Guillen F, Villanueva JA *et al.* Placebo-controlled trial of nimodipine in the treatment of acute ischemic cerebral infarction. *Stroke* 1990; 21: 1023–1028.

Mohr 1992 {published and unpublished data}

The American Nimodipine Study Group. Clinical trial of nimodipine in acute ischemic stroke. *Stroke* 1992; 23: 3–8.

NEST 1993 {published and unpublished data}

Hennerici M, Kramer G, North PM, Schmitz H, Tettenborn D, Nimodipine European Stroke Trial Group (NEST). Nimodipine in the treatment of acute MCA ischemic stroke. *Cerebrovascular Diseases* 1994; 4: 189–193.

NIMPAS 1999 {published and unpublished data}

Infeld B, Davis SM, Donnan GA *et al.* Nimodipine and perfusion changes after stroke. *Stroke* 1999; 30: 1417–1423.

Oczkowski 1989 {published data only}

Oczkowski WJ, Hachinski VC, Bogousslavsky JB *et al.* A double-blind, randomized trial of PY 108–068 in acute ischemic cerebral infarction. *Stroke* 1989; 20: 604–608.

Paci 1989 {published data only}

Paci A, Ottaviano P, Trenta A *et al.* Nimodipine in acute ischemic stroke: a double-blind controlled study. *Acta Neurologica Scandinavica* 1989; 80: 282–286.

Sherman 1986 {published data only}

Sherman DG, Easton JD, Hart RG, Sherman CP. Nimodipine in acute cerebral infarction. A double-blind study of safety and efficacy. In: Battistini N *et al.* (eds). *Acute Brain Ischaemia: Medical and Surgical Therapy.* New York: Raven Press, 1986: 257–262.

TRUST 1990 {published and unpublished data}

TRUST Study Group. Randomised, double-blind, placebo-controlled trial of nimodipine in acute stroke. *Lancet* 1990; 336: 1205–1209.

Uzunur 1995 {published and unpublished data}

Uzuner N, Ozdemir G, Gucuyener D. The interaction between nimodipine and systemic blood pressure and pulse rate. *Proceedings of the WHO Pan-European Consensus Meeting on Stroke Management,* Helsingborg, Sweden, November 1995.

VENUS 1999 {published and unpublished data}

VENUS: Very Early Nimodipine Use in Stroke. *Stroke* 1995; 26 (2): 353.

Wimalaratna 1994 {published and unpublished data}

Wimalaratna HSK, Capildeo R. Nimodipine in acute ischaemic cerebral hemisphere infarction. *Cerebrovascular Diseases* 1994; 4: 179–181.

Yordanov 1984 {unpublished data only}

Unpublished study

References to studies included in the Cochrane Review of Gangliosides for acute ischaemic stroke by Candelise and Ciccone (2000)

Angeleri 1992 {published data only}

Angeleri F, Scarpino O, Martinazzo C, Mauro A, Magi A, Pelliccioni G, Rapex G, Bruno R. GM1 ganglioside therapy in acute ischemic stroke. *Cerebrovascular Diseases* 1992; 2: 163–169.

Argentino 1989 {published data only}

*Argentino C, Sacchetti ML, Toni D, Savoini G, D'Arcangelo E, Erminio F, Federico F, Ferro Milone F, Gallai V, Gambi D, Mamoli A, Ottonello GA, Ponari O, Rebucci G, Senin U, Fieschi C. GM1 ganglioside therapy in acute ischemic stroke. *Stroke* 1989; 20: 1143–1149.

Argentino C, Toni D, Sacchetti ML, Savoini G, Fieschi C, for the Italian Acute Stroke Study Group. Ischemic stroke therapy with ganglioside GM1 within 12 hours from onset of symptoms (abstract). *Stroke* 211990: 1–96 (Abst OS-12–07).

Oppenheimer S, Argentino C, Sacchetti ML, Toni D. GM1 ganglioside therapy in acute ischemic stroke (letter). *Stroke* 1990; 21: 825.

Silvestrini M, Argentino C, Giubilei F, Sacchetti ML, Savoini G, Fieschi C. Italian acute stroke hemodilution + drug (Protocol presentation). *Minerva Medica* 1988; 79: 695–696.

Argentino plus haemo {published data only}

See Argentino 1989.

Bassi 1984 {published data only}

Apollonio I, Frattola L, Massarotti M. Trial of ganglioside GM1 in acute stroke (letter). *Journal of Neurology Neurosurgery and Psychiatry* 1989; 52: 685–686.

*Bassi S, Albizzati MG, Sbacchi M, Frattola L, Massarotti M. Double-blind evaluation of mono-sialoganglioside (GM1) therapy in stroke. *Journal of Neuroscience Research* 1984; 12: 493–498.

Bassi S, Albizzati MG, Sbacchi M, Frattola L, Massarotti M. Monosialoganglioside therapy in stroke (letter). *Stroke* 1985; 899–900.

Battistin 1985 {published data only}

Battistin L, Cesari A, Galligioni F, Marin G, Massarotti M, Paccagnella D, Pellegrini A, Testa G, Tonin P. Effects of GM1 gangliosides in *cerebrovascular disease*: a double blind trial in 40 cases. *European Neurology* 1985; 24: 343–351.

EST 1994 {published data only}

Carolei A. The Early Stroke Trial (EST): safety and efficacy of GM1 in acute ischaemic stroke (abstract). *Neurology* 1993; 43 (Suppl): A263.

Fieschi C, Carolei A, Argentino C, Bottacchi E, Brambilla GL, Gambi D, Inzitari D, Mamoli A, Senin U, Gerstenbrand F, Ott EO, Bes A, Bogousslavsky J, Portera-Sanchez A, Horowitz S, Einhaeupl K, Hopf HC, Lenzi GL, Bruno R. Early Stroke Trial (EST): a multicenter study on acute ischemic stroke (abstract). *International Conference on Stroke*, 1991: 67.

Fiorentini R, Friday G, Dorsey F. Clinical studies of monosialotetrahexosyl-ganglioside for the treatment of central nervous system injuries. *Journal of Neurochemistry* 1993; 61 (Suppl): S7.

*Lenzi GL, Grigoletto F, Gent M, Roberts RS, Walker MD, Easton D, Carolei A, Dorsey FC, Rocca WA, Bruno R, Patarnello F, Fieschi C, Early Stroke Trial Group. Early treatment of stroke with monosialoganglioside GM-1. Efficacy and safety results of the Early Stroke Trial. *Stroke* 1994; 25: 1552–1558.

Rocca WA, Dorsey FC, Grigoletto F, Gent M, Roberts RS, Walker MD, Easton JD, Bruno R, Carolei A, Sancesario G, Fieschi C. Design and baseline results of the monosialoganglioside Early Stroke Trial. *Stroke* 1992; 23: 519–526.

Giraldi 1990 {published data only}

Giraldi C, Masi MC, Manetti M, Carabelli E, Martini A. A pilot study with monosialoganglioside GM1 on acute cerebral ischemia. *Acta Neurologica* (Napoli) 1990; 12: 214–221.

Heiss 1989 {published and unpublished data}

Heiss WD, Pawlik G, Helbold I, Beil C, Herholz K, Szelies B, v Einsiedel R, Wienhard K. Can PET estimate functional recovery and indicate therapeutic strategy in stroke?. In: Krieglstein J (ed.), Pharmacology of cerebral ischemia. 1st edition. Stuttgart: Wissenschaftliche Verlagsgesellschaft mbH, 1989: 433–438.

Hoffbrand 1988 {published data only}

Hoffbrand BI, Bingley PJ, Oppenheimer SM, Sheldon CD. Trial of ganglioside GM1 in acute stroke. *Journal of Neurology Neurosurgery and Psychiatry* 1988; 51: 1213–1214.

Kirczynska 1994 {published data only}

Kirczynska-Zaderwialy A, Kruszewska J, Lechowicz W, Czlonkowska A. [Zastosowanie gangliozydu GM1 we wczesney fazie udaru mózgu]. Neur Neurochir Pol 1993; 28: 643–649.

Monaco 1991 {published data only}

Monaco P, Pastore L, Cottone S, Conti A, Bellinvia S. Early treatment of patients with ischemic stroke: a double blind study with monosialotetraesosiganglioside (GM1) (abstract). *Proceedings of the 1st International Conference on Stroke*, Geneva, Switzerland, 1991: 7.

SASS 1994 {published data only}

Alter M, SASS Study Group. The Sygen (GM1) Acute Stroke Study (SASS) (abstract). *Journal of Stroke Cerebrovascular Disease* 1992; 1 (Suppl 1): S12.

Fiorentini R, Friday G, Dorsey F. Clinical studies of monosialotetrahexosyl-ganglioside for the treatment of central nervous system injuries. *Journal of Neurochemistry* 1993; 61 (Suppl): S7.

*SASS investigators. Ganglioside GM1 in acute ischemic stroke. The SASS trial. *Stroke* 1994; 25: 1141–1148.

Wender 1993 {unpublished data only}

Wender M, Mularek J, Godlewski A, Losy J, Michatowska-Wender G, Sniata-Kamasa M, Wojcicka M. (Proby leczenia monosialogangliozydem (Sygenem) chorych z niedokrwiennym udarem mozgu). *Neur Neurochir Pol* 1993; 27: 31–38.

References to studies included in the Cochrane Review of Piracetam for acute ischaemic stroke by Ricci *et al.* (2002)

Ming 1990 {published data only}

Ming A, Fritz V, Winterton R, Esser J, Hinton S. Piracetam versus placebo in first, acute, non-haemorrhagic, carotid territory stroke: a double-blind pilot study. *Symposium Piracetam*, Athens, 29 April 1990: 139–151.

PASS 1997 {published and unpublished data}

De Deyn P, De Reuck J, Deberdt W, Vlietnick R, Orgogozo J, for members of the Piracetam in Acute Stroke Study (PASS) Group. Treatment of acute ischemic stroke with piracetam. *Stroke* 1997; 28: 2347–2352.

Platt 1993 {published data only}

Platt D, Horn J, Summa J, Shimitt-Ruth R, Kaunntz J, Kronert E. On the efficacy of piracetam in geriatric patients with acute cerebral ischemia: a clinical controlled double-blind study. *Archives of Gerontology and Geriatrics* 1993; 16: 149–164.

Chapter 8. Treatment of brain oedema

Bereczki D, Liu M, Fernandez do Prado G, Fekete I. Cochrane Report. A systematic review of mannitol therapy for acute ischaemic stroke and cerebral parenchymal haemorrhage. *Stroke* 2000; 31: 2719–2722.

Bereczki D, Liu M, do Prado GF, Fekete I. Mannitol for acute stroke. *The Cochrane Database of Systematic Reviews* 2001, Issue 1, Art. No.: CD001153. DOI: 10.1002/14651858.CD001153.

Brown MM. Surgical decompression of patients with large middle cerebral artery infarcts is effective: not proven. *Stroke* 2003; 34: 2305–2306.

Chen HJ, Lee TC, Wei CP. Treatment of cerebellar infarction by decompressive suboccipital craniectomy. *Stroke* 1992; 23: 957–961.

Cockroft KM. Hemicraniectomy after massive hemispheric cerebral infraction: are we ready for a prospective randomised controlled trial? *Journal of Neurology Neurosurgery and Psychiatry* 2004; 75: 179–80.

Donnan GA, Davis SM. Surgical decompression for malignant middle cerebral artery infarction: a challenge to conventional thinking. *Stroke* 2003; 34: 2307.

Davis SM, Donnan GA. Steroids for stroke: another potential therapy discarded prematurely? *Stroke* 2004; 35: 230–231.

Frank JI. A randomised multi-center trial of hemicraniectomy and durotomy for deterioration from infarction related swelling: HEADFIRST. www.strokecenter.org, Stroke trials directory, Internet stroke center, 2000.

Frank JI, Krieger D, Chyatte DM, Cancian S. HEADFIRST: Hemicraniectomy and durotomy upon deterioration from massive hemispheric infarctions. A proposed multicenter, prospective randomized study (abstract). *Stroke* 1999; 30: 243 (Abstract 67).

Gujjar AR, Deibert E, Manno EM, Duff S, Diringer MN. Mechanical ventilation for ischemic stroke and intracerebral haemorrhage: indications, timing, and outcome. *Neurology* 1998; 51: 447–451.

Gupta R, Connolly ES, Mayer S, Elkind MSV. Hemicraniectomy for massive middle cerebral artery territory infarction. A systematic review. *Stroke* 2004; 35: 539–543.

Hofmeijer J, van der Worp HB, Amelink GJ, Algra A. Kappelle LJ. Decompressive surgery in space-occupying hemispheric infarction: a randomised controlled trial. (abstract). *Cerebrovascular Diseases* 2001; 11 (Suppl 4): 34.

Jamora RD, Nigos J, Collantes E, Vahedi K, Vicaut E, Blanquet A *et al.* Hemicraniectomy for Malignant Middle cerebral artery Infarcts (HeMMI). Ongoing Clinical Trial Abstracts, *29th International Stroke Conference*, 2004, American Stroke Association, CTP50.

Kaufmann AM, Carduso ER. Aggravation of vasogenic cerebral oedema by multiple doses mannitol. *Journal of Neurosurgery* 1992; 77: 584–589.

Maramattom BV, Bahn MM, Wijdicks EFM. Which patient fares worse after early deterioration due to swelling from hemispheric stroke? *Neurology* 2004; 63: 2142–2145.

Morley NCD, Berge E, Cruz-Flores S, Whittle IR. Surgical decompression for cerebral oedema in acute ischaemic stroke. *The Cochrane Database of Systematic Reviews* 2002, Issue 3. Art. No.: CD003435. DOI: 10.1002/14651858.CD003435.

Morley NCD, Berge E, Cruz-Flores S, Whittle IR. Surgical decompression for cerebral oedema in acute ischaemic stroke (Cochrane Corner). *Stroke* 2003; 34: 1337.

Norris JW. Steroids may have a role in stroke therapy. *Stroke* 2004; 35: 228–229.

Poungvarin N, Bhoopat W, Viriyavejakul A *et al.* Effects of dexamethasone in primary supratentorial intracerebral haemorrhage. *New England Journal of Medicine* 1987; 316: 1229–1233.

Poungvarin N. Steroids have no role in stroke therapy. *Stroke* 2004; 35: 229–230.

Qizilbash N, Lewington SL, Lopez-Arrieta JM. Corticosteroids for acute ischaemic stroke. *The Cochrane Database of Systematic Reviews* 2001, Issue 4. Art. No.: CD000064. DOI: 10.1002/14651858.CD000064.

Righetti E, Celani MG, Cantisani T, Sterzi R, Boysen G, Ricci S. Glycerol for acute stroke. *The Cochrane Database of Systematic Reviews* 2003, Issue 4. Art. No.: CD000096. DOI: 10.1002/14651858.CD000096.pub2.

Righetti E, Celani MG, Cantisani T, Sterzi R, Boysen G, Ricci S. Glycerol for acute stroke (Cochrane Corner). *Stroke* 2004; 36: 171–172.

Ropper AH, Shafran B. Brain oedema after stroke: clinical syndrome and intracranial pressure. *Archives of Neurology* 1984; 41: 26–29.

Santambrogio S, Martinotti R, Sardella F *et al.* Is there a real treatment for stroke? Clinical and statistical comparison of different treatments in 300 patients. *Stroke* 1978; 9: 130–132.

Schlaug G, Siewert B, Benfield A, Edelman RR, Warach S. Time course of the apparent diffusion coefficient (ADC) abnormality in human stroke. *Neurology* 1997; 49: 113–119.

Schwab S, Aschoff A, Spranger M, Albert F, Hacke W. The value of intracranial pressure monitoring in acute hemispheric stroke. *Neurology* 1996; 51: 447–451.

Schwab S, Spranger M, Schwarz S, Hacke W. Barbiturate coma in severe hemispheric stroke: useful or obsolete? *Neurology* 1997; 48: 1608–1613.

Schwab S, Spranger M, Aschoff A, Steiner T, Hacke W. Brain temperature monitoring and modulation in patients with severe MCA infarction. *Neurology* 1997; 48: 762–767.

Schwab S, Hacke W. Surgical decompression of patients with large middle cerebral artery infarcts is effective. *Stroke* 2003; 34: 2304–2305.

Uhl E, Kreth FW, Elias B *et al.* Outcome and prognostic factors of hemicraniectomy for space occupying cerebral infarction. *Journal of Neurology Neurosurgery and Psychiatry* 2004; 75: 270–274.

Vahedi K, Vicaut E, Blanquet A *et al.* DECIMAL trial: DEcompressive Craniectomy In MALignant middle cerebral artery infarcts: a sequential design, multicentre, randomised controlled trial. Ongoing Clinical Trial Abstracts, *29th International Stroke Conference*, 2004, American Stroke Association, CTP27.

Videen TO, Zazulia AR, Manno EM *et al.* Mannitol bolus preferentially shrinks non-infarcted brain in patients with ischaemic stroke. *Neurology* 2001; 57: 2120–2122.

Winkler ST, Munoz-Ruiz L. Mechanism of action of mannitol. *Surgical Neurology* 1995; 43: 59.

van der Worp HB, Hofmeijer J, Amelink J, Algra A, van Gijn J, Kappelle LJ. HAMLET. Hemicraniectomy After Middle cerebral artery infarction with Life-threatening Edema Trial. Ongoing Clinical Trial Abstracts, *29th International Stroke Conference*, 2004, American Stroke Association, CTP24.

References to studies included in the Cochrane Review of Corticosteroids in acute ischaemic stroke by Qizilbash *et al.* (2001)

Bauer 1973 {published data only}

Bauer RB, Tellez H. Dexamethasone as treatment in cerebrovascular disease. 2. A controlled study in acute cerebral infarction. *Stroke* 1973; 4: 547–555.

Gupta 1978 {published data only}

Gupta RC, Bhatnagar HN, Gambhir MS, Shah DR. Betamethasone therapy in acute cerebrovascular accidents. *Journal of Association of Physicians of India* 1978; 26: 589–594.

McQueen 1978 {published and unpublished data}

McQueen EG. Betamethasone in stroke (letter). *New Zealand Medical Journal* 1978; 87: 103–104.

Mulley 1978 {published and unpublished data}

Mulley G, Wilcox RG, Mitchell JR. Dexamethasone in acute stroke. *British Medical Journal* 1978; 2: 994–996.

Norris 1976 {published and unpublished data}

Norris JW. Steroid therapy in acute cerebral infarction. *Archives of Neurology* 1976; 33: 69–71.

Norris 1986 {published and unpublished data}

Norris JW, Hachinski VC. High dose steroid treatment in cerebral infarction. *British Medical Journal* 1986; 292: 21–23.

Patten 1972 {published and unpublished data}

Patten BM, Mendell J, Bruun B, Curtin W, Carter S. Double-blind study of the effects of dexamethasone on acute stroke. *Neurology* 1972; 22: 377–383.

References to studies included in the Cochrane Review of Mannitol for acute stroke by Bereczki *et al.* (2001)

Santambrogio 1978 {published data only}

*Santambrogio S, Martinotti R, Sardella F, Porro F, Randazzo A. Is there a real treatment for stroke? Clinical and statistical comparison of different treatments in 300 patients. *Stroke* 1978; 9: 130–132.

References to studies included in the Cochrane Review of Glycerol for acute stroke by Righetti *et al.* (2003)

Albizzati 1979 {published data only}

Albizzati MG, Candelise L, Capitani E, Colombo A, Spinnler H. Association of glycerol to dexamethasone in treatment of stroke patients. *Acta Neurologica Scandinavica* 1979; 60: 77–84.

Azzimondi {unpublished data only}

*Azzimondi G, Casmiro M, D'Alessandro R, Fiorani L, Nonino F, Rinaldi R, Bassein L. Intravenous glycerol in acute ischemic stroke. A multicentre randomised placebo-controlled trial. Unpublished data.

Bayer 1987 {published data only}

Bayer AJ, Pathy MS, Newcombe R. Double-blind randomised trial of intravenous glycerol in acute stroke (plus letters). *Lancet* 1987; 1: 405–408.

Fawer 1978 {published data only}

Fawer R, Justafre JC, Berger JP, Schelling JL. Intravenous glycerol in cerebral infarction: a controlled 4-month trial. *Stroke* 1978; 9: 484–486.

Frei 1987 {published data only}

Frei A, Cottier C, Wunderlich P, Ludin E. Glycerol and dextran combined in the therapy of acute stroke. A placebo-controlled, double-blind trial with a planned interim analysis. *Stroke* 1987; 18: 373–379.

Friedli 1979 {published data only}

Friedli W, Imbach P, Ghisleni-Steinegger S, Schwarz C, Maire P. Treatment with 10% glycerin in acute ischemic cerebral infarct. Double blind study. *Schweizeriche Medizinische Wochenschrift* 1979; 109: 737–742.

Frithz 1975 {published data only}

Frithz G, Werner I. The effect of glycerol infusion in acute cerebral infarction. *Acta Medica Scandinavica* 1975; 198: 287–289.

Larsson 1976 {published data only}

Larsson O, Marinovich N, Barber K. Double-blind trial of glycerol therapy in early stroke. *Lancet* 1976; 1: 832–834.

Mathew 1972 {published data only}

Mathew NT, Rivera VM, Meyer JS, Charney JZ, Hartmann A. Double-blind evaluation of glycerol therapy in acute cerebral infarction. *Lancet* 1972; 2: 1327–1329.

Yu 1992 {published data only}

Yu YL, Kumana CR, Lauder IJ, Cheung YK, Chan FL, Kou M, Chang CM, Cheung RTF, Fong KY. Treatment of acute cerebral haemorrhage with intravenous glycerol. A double-blind, placebo-controlled randomised trial. *Stroke* 1992; 23: 967–971.

Yu 1993 {published data only}

Kumana CR, Chan GT, Yu YL, Lauder IJ, Chan TK, Kou M. Investigation of intravascular haemolysis during treatment of acute stroke with intravenous glycerol. *British Journal of Clinical Pharmacology* 1990; 29: 347–353.

Yu YL, Kumana CR, Lauder IJ, Cheung YK, Chan FL, Kou M, Fong KY, Cheung RTF, Chang CM. Treatment of acute cortical infarct with intravenous glycerol. A double-blind randomised controlled trial. *Stroke* 1993; 24: 1119–1124.

Chapter 9. Anticoagulation

Acute ischaemic stroke

Al-Sadat A, Sunbulli M, Chaturvedi S. Use of heparin by North American Neurologists: do the data matter? *Stroke* 2002; 33: 1574–1577.

Bath PMW, Iddenden R, Bath FJ. Low-molecular-weight heparins and heparinoidss in acute ischaemic stroke. A meta-analysis of randomised controlled trials. *Stroke* 2000; 31: 1770–1778.

Berge E, Abdelnoor M, Nakstad PH, Sandset PM. Low molecular-weight heparin versus aspirin in patients with acute ischaemic stroke and atrial fibrillation: a double-blind randomised study. HAEST Study Group. Heparin in Acute Embolic Stroke Trial. *Lancet* 2000; 355: 1205–1210.

Burak CR, Bowen MD, Barron TF. The use of enoxaparin in children with acute nonhemorrhagic ischemic stroke. *Paediatric Neurology* 2003; 29: 295–298.

Cerebral Embolism Study Group. Immediate anticoagulation of embolic stroke – a randomised trial. *Stroke* 1983; 14: 668–676.

Coull AJ, Lovett JK, Rothwell PM, for the Oxford Vascular Study. Population based study of early risk of stroke after transient ischemic attack or minor stroke: implications for public education and organisation of services. *British Medical Journal* 2004; 328: 326–328.

Counsell C, Sandercock P. Low-molecular-weight heparins or heparinoids versus standard unfractionated heparin for acute ischaemic stroke stroke (Cochrane Corner). *Stroke* 2002; 33: 1925–1926.

Dippel DW, Wijnhoud AD, Koudstaal PJ. Prediction of major vascular events after TIA or minor stroke. A comparison of 6 models (abstract). *Cerebrovascular Diseases* 2004; 17 (Suppl 5): 35.

Gubitz G, Sandercock P, Counsell C. Anticoagulants for acute ischaemic stroke. *The Cochrane Database of Systematic Reviews* 2004, Issue 2. Art. No.: CD000024. DOI: 10.1002/14651858. CD000024.pub2.

Hankey GJ, Slattery JM, Warlow CP. Transient ischaemic attacks: Which patients are at high (and low) risk of serious vascular events? *Journal of Neurology Neurosurgery and Psychiatry* 1992; 55: 640–652.

Hankey GJ. Redefining risks after TIA and minor ischaemic stroke. *Lancet* 2005; 365: 2065–6.

Hart RG, Palacio S, Pearce LA. Atrial fibrillation, stroke and acute antithrombotic therapy. Analysis of randomised clinical trials. *Stroke* 2002; 33: 2722–2727.

Kernan WN, Viscoli CM, Brass LM, Makuch RW, Sarrel PM, Roberts RS, Gent M, Rothwell PM, Sacco R, Liu RC, Boden-Albala B, Horowitz RI: The Stroke Prognosis Instrument II (SPI II): A clinical prediction instrument for patients with transient ischaemia and non-disabling ischaemic stroke. *Stroke* 2000; 31: 456–462.

LaMonte MP, Nash ML, Wang DZ *et al*. Argatroban anticoagulation in patients with acute ischaemic stroke (ARGIS-I): a randomised, placebo-controlled safety study. *Stroke* 2004; 35: 1677–1682.

Langhorne P, Stott DJ, Robertson L, MacDonald J, Jones L, McAlpine C, Dick F, Taylor GS, Murray G. Medical complications after stroke. A multicenter study. *Stroke* 2000; 31: 1223–1229.

Lovett J, Dennis M, Sandercock PAG, Bamford J, Warlow CP, Rothwell PM. The very early risk of stroke following a TIA. *Stroke* 2003; 34: e138–e140.

Lovett JK, Coull A, Rothwell PM, on behalf of the Oxford Vascular Study. Early risk of recurrence by subtype of ischaemic stroke in population-based incidence studies. *Neurology* 2004; 62: 569–574.

Sandercock P, Gubitz G, Counsell C. Anticoagulants for acute ischaemic stroke (Cochrane Corner). *Stroke* 2004; 35: 2916–2917.

Sandercock P, Counsell C, Stobbs SL. Low-molecular-weight heparins or heparinoids versus standard unfractionated heparin for acute ischaemic stroke. *The Cochrane Database of Systematic Reviews* 2005, Issue 2. Art. No.: CD000119. DOI: 10.1002/14651858.CD000119.pub2.

Saxena R, Lewis S, Berge E, Sandercock PAG, Koudstaal PJ, for the International Stroke Trial Collaborative Group. Risk of Early Death and Recurrent Stroke and Effect of Heparin in 3169 Patients With Acute Ischemic Stroke and Atrial Fibrillation in the International Stroke Trial. *Stroke* 2001; 32: 2333.

Schmulling S, Rudolf J, Strotmann-Tack T *et al*. Acetylsalicylic acid pretreatment, concomitant heparin therapy and the risk of early intracranial haemorrhage following systemic thrombolysis for acute ischaemic stroke. *Cerebrovascular Diseases* 2003; 16: 183–190.

Warlow C, Ogston D, Douglas AS. Venous thrombosis following strokes. *Lancet* 1972; I: 1305–1306.

Warlow C. Venous thromboembolism after stroke. *American Heart Journal* 1978; 96: 283–285.

Warlow CP, Dennis MS, van Gijn J, Hankey GJ, Sandercock PAG, Bamford J, Wardlaw J. What caused this transient or persisting ischaemic event? In: *Stroke: A Practical Guide to Management*, 2nd edition. Blackwell Science, Oxford, UK, 2000: 223–300.

Wijdicks EF, Scott JP. Pulmonary embolism associated with acute stroke. *Mayo Clinic Proceedings* 1997; 72: 297–300.

References to studies included in the Cochrane Review by Gubitz *et al.* (2004) of anticoagulants vs control in acute ischaemic stroke

Cazzato 1989 {published and unpublished data}

**Cazzato G, Zorzon M, Mase G, Antonutto L, Iona LG. Mesoglycan in the treatment of acute cerebral infarction (Il mesoglicano nelle ischemie cerebrali acute a focolaio). *Rivista di Neurologia* 1989; 59: 121–126.

CESG 1983 {published and unpublished data}

**Hakim AM, Furlan AJ, Hart RG. Immediate anticoagulation of embolic stroke: a randomized trial. The Cerebral Embolism Study Group. *Stroke* 1983; 14: 668–676.

Hakim AM, Ryder-Cooke A, Melanson D. Sequential computerized tomographic appearances of strokes. *Stroke* 1983; 14: 893–897.

Duke 1983 {published and unpublished data}

**Duke RJ, Turpie AGG, Bloch RF, Trebilcock RG. Clinical trial of low-dose subcutaneous heparin for the prevention of stroke progression: natural history of acute partial stroke and stroke-in-evolution. In: Reivich M, Hurtig HI (eds), *Cerebrovascular Disease*. New York: Raven Press, 1983: 399–405.

Duke RJ, Turpie AGG, Bloch RF, Derby IR, Kronby MH, Bayer NH. Clinical trial of low-dose heparin for the prevention of stroke progression (abstract). *Circulation* 1980; (Suppl III): 21.

Duke 1986 {published and unpublished data}

**Duke RJ, Bloch RF, Turpie AGG, Trebilcock RG, Bayer N. Intravenous heparin for the prevention of stroke progression in acute partial stable stroke. *Annals of Internal Medicine* 1986; 105: 825–828.

Duke RJ, Bloch RF, Turpie AGG. Heparin in acute partial stable stroke (abstract). *Annals of Internal Medicine* 1987; 106: 782.

Easton JD, Sherman DG, Hart RG. Heparin in acute partial stable stroke (letter). *Annals of Internal Medicine* 1987; 106: 781.

Loeliger EA. Heparin in acute partial stable stroke (letter). *Annals of Internal Medicine* 1987; 106: 781.

Elias 1990 {published and unpublished data}

**Elias A, Milandre L, Lagrange G, Aillaud MF, Alonzo B, Toulemonde F, Juhan-Vague I, Khalil R, Bayrou B, Serradimigni A. Prevention of deep venous thrombosis of the leg by a very low molecular weight heparin fraction (CY 222) in patients with hemiplegia following cerebral infarction: a randomized pilot study (30 patients). *Review of Medical International* 1990; 11: 95–98.

FISS 1995 {published and unpublished data}

**Kay R, Wong KS, Lu YL, Chan YW, Tsoi TH, Ahuja AT, Chan FL, Fong KY, Law CB, Wong A, Woo J. Low-molecular-weight heparin for the treatment of acute ischemic stroke. *New England Journal of Medicine* 1995; 333: 1588–1593.

Kay R. Fraxiparin in stroke study (abstract). *Stroke* 1994; 25: 253.

FISS-bis 1998 {published data only}

**Hommel M, for the FISS-bis Investigators Group. Fraxiparine in ischaemic stroke study (FISS bis) (abstract). *Cerebrovascular Diseases* 1998; 8 (Suppl 4): 19.

IST 1997 {published data only}

**International Stroke Trial Collaborative Group. The International Stroke Trial (IST): a randomised trial of aspirin, subcutaneous heparin, both, or neither among 19435 patients with acute ischaemic stroke. *Lancet* 1997; 349: 1569–1581.

International Stroke Trial Pilot Study Collaborative Group. Study design of the International Stroke Trial (IST), baseline data, and outcome in 984 randomised patients in the pilot study. *Journal of Neurology Neurosurgery and Psychiatry* 1996; 60: 371–376.

Marshall 1960 {published data only}

**Marshall J, Shaw DA. Anticoagulant therapy in acute cerebrovascular accidents: a controlled trial. *Lancet* 1960; 1: 995–998.

Marshall J, Shaw DA. Anticoagulant therapy in *cerebrovascular disease. Proceedings of the Royal Society of Medicine* 1960: 547–549.

McCarthy 1977 {published and unpublished data}

**McCarthy ST, Turner JJ, Robertson D, Hawkey CJ, Macey DJ. Low dose heparin as a prophylaxis against deep-vein thrombosis after acute stroke. *Lancet* 1977; ii: 800–801.

McCarthy 1986 {published and unpublished data}

**McCarthy ST, Turner J. Low-dose subcutaneous heparin in the prevention of deep-vein thrombosis and pulmonary emboli following acute stroke. *Age and Ageing* 1986; 15: 84–88.

NAT-COOP 1962 {published data only}

**Baker RN, Broward JA, Fang HC, Fisher CM, Groch SN, Heyman A, Karp AR, McDevitt E, Scheinberg P, Schwartz W, Toole JF. Anticoagulant therapy in cerebral infarction. Report on co-operative study. *Neurology* 1962; 12: 823–829.

Miller Fisher C. Anticoagulant therapy in cerebral thrombosis and cerebral embolism. A national cooperative study, interim report. *Neurology* 1961; 11: 119–131.

Pambianco 1995 {published and unpublished data}

**Pambianco G, Orchard T, Landau P. Deep vein thrombosis: prevention in stroke patients during rehabilitation. *Archives of Physical Medicine and Rehabilitation* 1995; 76: 324–330.

Desmukh M, Bisignani M, Landau P, Orchard TJ. Deep vein thrombosis in rehabilitating stroke patients. Incidence, risk factors and prophylaxis. *American Journal of Physical Medicine and Rehabilitation* 1991; 70: 313–316.

Pince 1981 {unpublished data only}

**Pince J. Thromboses veineuses des membres inferieurs et embolies pulmonaires au cours des accidents vasculaires cerebraux. A propos d'un essai comparitif de traitement preventif (These pour le doctorat d'etat en medecine). Toulouse: Universite Paul Sabatier, 1981.

Prins 1989 {published and unpublished data}

**Prins MH, Gelsema R, Sing AK, van Heerde LR, den Ottolander GJ. Prophylaxis of deep venous thrombosis with a low-molecular-weight heparin (Kabi 2165/Fragmin) in stroke patients. *Haemostasis* 1989; 19: 245–250.

Prins MH, den Ottolander GJH, Gelsema R, van Woerkom TCM, Sing AK, Heller I. Deep venous thrombosis prophylaxis with a LMW heparin (KABI 2165) in stroke patients (abstract). *Thrombiosis and Haemostasis* 1987; 58: 117.

Sandset 1990 {published and unpublished data}

**Sandset PM, Dahl T, Stiris M, Rostad B, Scheel B, Abildgaard U. A double-blind and randomized placebo-controlled trial of low molecular weight heparin once daily to prevent deep-vein thrombosis in acute ischemic stroke. *Seminars in Thrombiosis and Hemostasis* 1990; 16 (Suppl): 25–33.

Sandset PM, Dahl T, Abildgaard U. Venous thromboembolic complications in acute thrombotic stroke. Progress report from a randomized trial (abstract). *Acta Neurologica Scandinavica* 1987; 76: 392.

Tazaki 1986 {published data only}

**Tazaki Y, Kobayashi S, Togi H, Ohtomo E, Goto F, Araki G, Kodama R, Ito E, Sawada T, Fujishima M, Nakajima M. Therapeutic effect of thrombin inhibitor MD-805 in acute phase of cerebral thrombosis – Phase II double-blinded clinical trial (English translation). Rinsho to Kenkyu (*Japanese Journal of Clinical and Experimental Medicine*) 1986; 63: 3047–3057.

Tazaki 1992 {published data only}

**Tazaki Y, Kobayashi S, Togi H, Ohtomo E, Goto F, Araki G, Kodama R, Kanda T, Ito E, Sawada T, Fujishima M, Sakuma A, Tsutani K, Kan S. Clinical usefulness of thrombin inhibitor MD-805 in acute phase of cerebral thrombosis – double blinded comparative study using placebo as a control (English translation). Igaku no Ayumi (*Journal of Clinical and Experimental Medicine*) 1992; 161: 887–907.

TOAST 1998 {unpublished data only}

**TOAST Investigators. Low Molecular Weight Heparinoid, ORG 10172 (Danaparoid), and outcome after acute ischaemic stroke. *Journal of the American Medical Association* 1998; 279: 1265–1272.

Adams JHP. Trial of Org 10172 in Acute Stroke Treatment (TOAST) (abstract). *Stroke* 1994; 25: 545.

Turpie 1987 {published and unpublished data}

**Turpie AGG, Levine MN, Hirsh J, Carter CJ, Jay RM, Powers PJ, Andrew M, Magnani HN, Hull RD, Gent M. Double-blind randomised trial of Org 10172 low-molecular-weight heparinoid in prevention of deep-vein thrombosis in thrombotic stroke. *Lancet* 1987; 1: 523–526.

Turpie AGG. Low molecular weight heparins: deep vein thrombosis prophylaxis in elective hip surgery and thrombotic stroke. *Acta Chirurgica Scandinavica* 1988; 543 (Suppl): 85–86.

Turpie AGG, Levine MN, Hirsh J, Carter CJ, Jay RM, Powers PJ, Andrew M, Magnani HN, Hull RD, Gent M. A double-blind randomized trial of Org 10172 Low Molecular Weight Heparinoid in the prevention of deep venous thrombosis in patients with thrombotic stroke (abstract). *Thrombosis and Haemostasis* 1987; 58: 123.

Vissinger 1995 {unpublished data only}

**Vissinger H, Husted S. Trial of tinzaparin vs placebo ischaemic stroke. Unpublished work.

References to studies included in the Cochrane Review by Sandercock *et al.* (2005) of low-molecular-weight heparins or heparinoids versus standard unfractionated heparin for acute ischaemic stroke

Dumas 1994 {published and unpublished data}

Dumas R, Woitinas F, Kutnowski M, Nikolic I, Berberich R, Abedinpour F, Zoeckler S, Gregoire F, Jerkovic M, Egberts JFM, Stiekema JCJ. A multi-centre double blind randomized study to compare the safety and efficacy of once-daily ORG 10172 and twice-daily low-dose heparin in preventing deep-vein thrombosis in patients with acute ischaemic stroke. *Age and Ageing* 1994; 23: 512–516.

Hageluken C, Egberts J, Stiekema J. A multi-centre, assessor-blind, randomised, safety study of Org 10172, administered subcutaneously twice daily, for the prophylaxis of deep vein thrombosis in patients with a non-haemorrhagic stroke of recent onset (protocol 87038). Organon International B.V. (Internal report SDGRR No. 3165), Oss, The Netherlands, 1992.

Hageluken 1992 {unpublished data only}

Hageluken C, Egberts J. A multi-centre, assessor-blind, randomised pilot study of three different doses of Org 10172 (375, 750 and 1250 U), administered subcutaneously once daily, compared with low dose heparin, administered subcutaneously twice daily, in the prophylaxis of deep vein thrombosis (DVT) in patients with a non-haemorrhagic stroke of recent onset (protocol 85144). Organon International B.V. (Internal report SDGRR No. 3158). Oss, The Netherlands, 1992.

Hillbom 1998 {published and unpublished data}

Hillbom M, Erila T, Flosbach C, Sotaniemi K, Tatlisumak T, Sarna S, Kaste M. Enoxaparin, a low-molecular-weight heparin (LWMH) may be superior to standard heparin in the prevention of deep-vein thrombosis (DVT) in stroke patients. *European Journal of Neurology* 1998; 5 (Suppl 3): S110.

Stiekema 1988 {published and unpublished data}

Hossman V, Loettgen J, Auel H, Bewermeyer H, Heiss WD. Prophylaxis of deep vein thrombosis in acute stroke. A prospective, randomised double-blind study. *Haemostasis* 1986; 16 (Suppl 5): 54.

Stiekema JCJ, Egberts JFM, Voerman J. An open, randomised, pilot multi-centre study of Org 10172 versus heparin administered for the purpose of deep vein thrombosis prophylaxis in patients with a non-haemorrhagic stroke of recent onset. Organon International B.V. (Internal report SDGRR No. 2310). Oss, The Netherlands, 1988.

Turpie 1992 {published and unpublished data}

Magnani HN, Egberts JFM. A preliminary report of a multi-centre, assessor-blind, randomised, comparative safety and efficacy study of Org 10172 versus low dose heparin, administered subcutaneously twice daily for the prophylaxis of deep vein thrombosis in patients with acute thrombotic stroke (protocol 004–010). Organon International B.V (Internal report SDGRR No. 3172). Oss, the Netherlands, 1992.

Turpie AGG, Levine MN, Powers PJ, Ginsberg JG, Jay RM, Klimek M, Leclerc J, Cote R, Neemah J, Geerts W, Hirsh J, Gent M. A low-molecular-weight heparinoid compared with unfractionated heparin in the prevention of deep vein thrombosis in patients with acute ischemic stroke. *Annals of Internal Medicine* 1992; 117: 353–357.

Turpie AGG, Levine MN, Powers PJ, Ginsberg JG, Jay RM, Klimek M, Leclerc J, Cote R, Neemeh J, Geerts W, Hirsh J, Gent M. A double blind randomized trial of Org 10172 Low Molecular Weight Heparinoid versus unfractionated heparin in the prevention of deep venous thrombosis in patients.

Long-term prevention in patients with non-cardioembolic ischaemic stroke or TIA

Gorter JW for the SPIRIT and EAFT study groups. Major bleeding during anticoagulation after cerebral ischaemia. Patterns and risk factors. *Neurology* 1999; 53: 1319–1327.

Sandercock P, Mielke O, Liu M, Counsell C. Anticoagulants for preventing recurrence following presumed non-cardioembolic ischaemic stroke or transient ischaemic attack. *The Cochrane Database of Systematic Reviews* 2002, Issue 4. Art. No.: CD000248. DOI: 10.1002/14651858.CD000248.

The Stroke Prevention in Reversible Ischaemia Trial (SPIRIT) Study Group. A randomised trial of anticoagulants versus aspirin after cerebral ischaemia of presumed arterial origin. *Annals of Neurology* 1997; 42: 857–865.

References to studies included in the Cochrane Review of anticoagulants for preventing recurrence following presumed non-cardioembolic ischaemic stroke or transient ischaemic attack by Sandercock *et al.* (2002)

Baker 1964 {published data only}

Baker RN, Schwartz WS, Rose MD. Transient ischemic strokes. A report of a study of anticoagulant therapy. *Neurology* 1966; 16: 841–847.

Bradshaw 1975 {published data only}

Bradshaw P, Brennan S. Trial of long-term anticoagulant therapy in the treament of small stroke associated with a normal carotid angiogram. *Journal of Neurology Neurosurgery and Psychiatry* 1975; 38: 642–647.

Enger 1965 {published data only}

Enger E, Boyesen S. Long-term anticoagulant therapy in patients with cerebral infarction: a controlled clinical study. *Acta Medica Scandinavica* 1965; 178 (Suppl 438): 7–61.

Howard 1963 {published data only}

Howard FA, Cohen P, Hickler RB, Locke S, Newcomb T, Tyler HR. Survival following stroke. *Journal of the American Medical Association* 1963; 183 (11): 921–925.

LHSPS 1999 {published data only}

Fortini A, Bonechi G, Carnovali M, Olivo G, Rinaldi G, Gensini GF. Multi-centric study on ischemic cerebral cerebral re-infarct prevention with low-dose heparin: the informatic system (Sistema informatico dello studio clinico controllato multicentrico sulla prvenzione del reinfarto cerebrale ischemico con eparina a basso dosaggio). AQ35aRivista Di Neurobiologica 1990; 36 (2): 219–221.

*Neri Serneri GG, Gensini GF, Carnovali M, Olivo G, Modesti PA, Inzitari D, Nencini P, Pracucci G. Low-dose heparin stroke prevention study: preliminary efficacy analysis. *Cerebrovascular Diseases* 1999; 9 (Suppl 1): 67.

McDevitt 1959 {published data only}

Groch SN, McDevitt E, Wright IS. A long-term study of cerebral vascular disease. *Annals of Internal Medicine* 1961; 55: 358–367.

McDevitt E, Groch SN, Wright IS. A cooperative study of *cerebrovascular disease. Circulation* 1959; 20: 215–223.

*McDowell F, McDevitt E. Treatment of the completed stroke with long-term anticoagulant: six and one-half years experience. In: Siekert RG, Whisnant JP (eds), *Cerebral Vascular Diseases. Fourth Conference.* New York: Grune & Stratton Inc, 1965: 185–199.

McDowell F, McDevitt E, Wright IS. Anticoagulant therapy: five years experience with the patient with an established cerebrovascular accident. *Archives of Neurology* 1963; 8: 209–214.

Nat-Coop 1962 {published data only}

Baker RN, Broward JA, Fang HC, Fisher CM, Groch SN, Heyman A, Karp HR, McDevitt E, Scheinberg P, Schwartz W, Toole JF. Anticoagulant therapy in cerebral infarction. Report on co-operative study. *Neurology* 1962; 12: 823–829.

Miller Fisher C. Anticoagulant therapy in cerebral thrombosis and cerebral embolism. A national cooperative study interim report. *Neurology* 1961; 11: 119–131.

SWAT 1998 {published data only}

Stewart B, Shuaib F, Veloso F. Stroke Prevention with Warfarin or Aspirin Trial (SWAT). *Stroke* 1998; 29: 304.

Thygesen 1964 {published data only}

Thygesen P, Christensen E, Dyrbye M, Eiken M, Franzen E, Gormsen J, Lademann A, Lennox-Buchthal M, Ronnov-Jessen V, Therkelsen J. Cerebral apoplexy: A clinical, radiological, electroencephalographic and pathological study with special reference to the prognosis of cerebral infarction and the result of long-term anticoagulant therapy. *Danish Medical Bulletin* 1964; 11: 233–257.

VA Study 1961 {published data only}

Baker RN. An evaluation of anticoagulant therapy in the treatment of *cerebrovascular disease*. Report of the Veterans Administration Cooperative Study of Atherosclerosis, Neurology Section. *Neurology* 1961; 11: 132–138.

Wallace 1964 {published data only}

Wallace DC. Cerebral vascular disease in relation to long-term anticoagulant therapy. *Journal of Chronic Diseases* 1964; 17: 527–537.

Chapter 10. Antiplatelet therapy

Acute ischaemic stroke

Antiplatelet vs control

Abciximab Emergent Stroke Treatment Trial (AbESTT) investigators. Emergency administration of abciximab for treatment of patients with acute ischaemic stroke. Results of a randomised phase 2 trial. Stroke 2005; 36: 880–890.

AbESTT investigators. Effects of abciximab for acute ischaemic stroke: final results of Abciximab in Emergent Stroke Treatment Trial (AbESTT) (abstract). *Stroke* 2003; 34: 253.

Adams Jr HP. Abciximab in Emergent Stroke Treatment Trial – II. Ongoing Clinical Trial Abstracts, *29th International Stroke Conference*, 2004, American Stroke Association, CTP32.

Chen ZM, Sandercock P, Pan HC *et al.* Indications for early aspirin use in acute ischaemic stroke. A combined analysis of 40, 000 randomised patients from the Chinese Aspirin Stroke Trial and the International Stroke Trial. *Stroke* 2000; 31: 1240–1249.

Hankey GJ, Eikelboom JW. Adding aspirin to clopidogrel after TIA and ischemic stroke: benefits do not match risks. *Neurology* 2005; 64: 1117–1121.

International Stroke Trial Pilot Study Collaborative Group. Study design of the International Stroke Trial (IST), baseline data and outcome in 984 randomised patients in the pilot study. *Journal of Neurology Neurosurgery and Psychiatry* 1996; 60: 371–376.

Roden-Jullig A, Britton M, Malmkuist K, Leijd B. Aspirin in the prevention of progressing stroke: a randomised controlled study. *J Intern Med* 2003; 254: 584–590.

Sandercock P, Gubitz G, Foley P, Counsell C. Antiplatelet therapy for acute ischaemic stroke. *The Cochrane Database of Systematic Reviews* 2003, Issue 2. Art. No.: CD000029. DOI: 10.1002/14651858.CD00002.

Sarma GR, Roy AK. Nadroparin plus aspirin versus aspirin alone in the treatment of acute ischaemic stroke. *Neurology India* 2003; 51: 208–210.

References to studies included in the Cochrane Review of antiplatelet therapy for acute ischaemic stroke by Sandercock *et al.* (2003)

Abciximab 2000 {published data only}
*The Abciximab in Ischemic Stroke Investigators. Abciximab in acute ischemic stroke. A randomized, double-blind, placebo-controlled, dose escalation study. *Stroke* 2000; 31: 601–609.

CAST 1997 {published and unpublished data}
*CAST (Chinese Acute Stroke Trial) Collaborative Group. A randomised placebo-controlled trial of early aspirin use in 20,000 patients with acute ischaemic stroke. *Lancet* 1997; 349: 1641–1649.

Ciufetti 1990 {published and unpublished data}
*Ciuffetti G, Aisa G, Mercuri M, Lombardini R, Paltriccia R, Neri C, Senin U. Effects of ticlopidine on the neurologic outcome and the hemorheologic pattern in the postacute phase of ischemic stroke: a pilot study. *Angiology* 1990; 41: 505–511.

IST 1997 {published and unpublished data}
*International Stroke Trial Collaborative Group. The International Stroke Trial (IST): a randomised trial of aspirin, subcutaneous heparin, both, or neither among 19435 patients with acute ischaemic stroke. *Lancet* 1997; 349: 1569–1581.

MAST-I 1995 {published and unpublished data}
*Multicentre Acute Stroke Trial-Italy (MAST-I) Group. Randomised controlled trial of streptokinase, aspirin, and combination of both in treatment of acute ischaemic stroke. *Lancet* 1995; 346: 1509–1514.

Ohtomo 1991 {published data only}
*Ohtomo E, Kutsuzawa T, Kogure K, Hirai S, Goto F, Terashi Am Tazaki Y, Araki G, Ito E, Fujishima M, Nakashima M. Clinical usefulness of OKY-046 on the acute stage of cerebral thrombosis – double blind trial in comparison with placebo. Rinsho Iyaku (*Journal of Clinical Therapeutics and Medicine*) 1991; 7 (2): 353–388.

Pince 1981 {unpublished data only}
*Pince J. Thromboses veineuses des membres inferieures et embolies pulmonaires au cours des accidents vasculaires cerebraux. A propos d'un essai comparatif de traitment preventif. (These pour le doctorat d'tat en medicine.) Toulouse: Universite Paul Sabatier, 1981.

Turpie 1983 {unpublished data only}
*Turpie AGG, Dobkin B, McKenna R. A trial of ticlopidine, an antiplatelet agent, for acute cerebral infarction. Guildford: Sanofi Winthrop (*Sanofi Internal Report* 1983.001.6.188) 1983.

Utsumi 1988 {unpublished data only}
*Utsumi H. Evaluation of utility of ticlopidine, an antiplatelet agent, for acute cerebral infarction. Guildford: Sanofi Winthrop (*Sanofi Internal Report* 001.6.128) 1984.

Anticoagulation vs antiplatelet therapy
Berge E, Sandercock P. Anticoagulants versus antiplatelet agents for acute ischaemic stroke. *The Cochrane Database of Systematic Reviews* 2001, Issue 2. Art. No.: CD003242. DOI: 10.1002/14651858.CD003242.

Berge E, Sandercock P. Anticoagulants versus antiplatelet agents for acute ischaemic stroke (Cochrane Corner). *Stroke* 2003; 34: 1571–1572.

Sarma GR, Roy AK. Nadroparin plus aspirin versus aspirin alone in the treatment of acute ischaemic stroke. *Neurology India* 2003; 51: 208–210.

References to studies included in the Cochrane Review of anticoagulants versus antiplatelet agents for acute ischaemic stroke by Berge and Sandercock (2001)

HAEST 2000 {published and unpublished data}

*Berge E, Abdelnoor M, Nakstad PH, Sandset PM. Low molecular-weight heparin versus aspirin in patients with acute ischaemic stroke and atrial fibrillation: a double-blind randomised study. *Lancet* 2000; 355: 1205–1210. 296.

IST 1997 {published and unpublished data}

*International Stroke Trial Collaborative Group. The International Stroke Trial (IST): a randomised trial of aspirin, subcutaneous heparin, both, or neither among 19435 patients with acute ischaemic stroke. *Lancet* 1997; 349 (9065): 1569–1581. 134.

Pince 1981 {published data only}

*Pince J. Thromboses veineuses des membres inferieurs et embolies pulmonaires au cours des accidents vasculaires cerebraux. A propos d'un essai comparatif de traitement preventif (These pour le doctorat d'etat en medecine). Toulouse: Université Paul Sabatier, 1981.

TAIST 2001 {unpublished data only}

*Bath PMW, Lindenstrom E, Boysen G, De Deyn P, Friis P, Leys D, Marttila R, Olsson JE, O'eill D, Orgogozo JM, Ringelstein B, van der Sande JJ, Turpie AGG, for the TAIST Investigators. Tinzaparin in acute ischaemic stroke (TAIST): a randomised aspirin-controlled trial. *Lancet* 2001; 358: 702–710.

Long-term secondary prevention

Antiplatelet therapy vs control or other antiplatelet agents

Akinboboye OO, Idris O, Chou RL, Sciacca RR, Cannon PJ, Bergmann SR. Absolute quantitation of coronary steal induced by intravenous dipyridamole. *Journal of the American College of Cardiology* 2001; 37: 109–116.

Algra A, van Gijn J. Cumulative meta-analysis of aspirin efficacy after cerebral ischemia of arterial origin. *Journal of Neurology Neurosurgery and Psychiatry* 1999; 66: 255.

Algra A, De Schryver ELLM, van Gijn J, Kappelle LJ, Koudstaal PJ. Oral anticoagulants versus antiplatelet therapy for preventing further vascular events after transient ischaemic attack or minor stroke of presumed arterial origin (Cochrane Review). In: *The Cochrane Library*, Issue 2, 2004. Chichester, UK: John Wiley & Sons, Ltd.

Anderson DC, Goldstein LB. Aspirin. It's hard to beat. *Neurology* 2004; 62: 1036–1037.

Antithrombotic Trialists' Collaboration. Collaborative meta-analysis of randomised trials of antiplatelet therapy for prevention of death, myocardial infarction, and stroke in high risk patients. *British Medical Journal* 2002; 324: 71–86.

Benavente O, Hart R. Secondary prevention of small subcortical strokes (SPS3).

Ongoing Clinical Trial Abstracts, *29th International Stroke Conference*, 2004, American Stroke Association, CTP41.

Bennett CL, Weinburg PD, Rozenberg-Ben-Dror K, Yarnold PR, Kwaan HC, Gren D. Thrombotic thrombocytopenic purpura associated with ticlopidine: a review of 60 cases. *Annals of Internal Medicine* 1998a; 128: 541–544.

Bennett CL, Kiss JE, Weinburg PD *et al.* Thrombotic thrombocytopenic purpura after stenting and ticlopidine. *Lancet* 1998b; 352: 1036–1037.

Bennett CL, Davidson CJ, Raisch DW, Weinberg PD, Bennett RH, Feldman MD. Thrombotic thrombocytopenic purpura associated with ticlopidine in the setting of coronary artery stents and stroke prevention. *Archives of Internal Medicine* 1999; 159: 2524–2528.

Bhatt DL, Topol EJ. Scientific and therapeutic advances in antiplatelet therapy. *Nature Review* 2003; 2: 15–28.

Bhatt DL. Aspirin resistance: more than just a laboratory curiosity. *Journal of the American College of Cardiology* 2004; 43: 1–3.

Bhatt DL, Topol E, on behalf of the CHARISMA Executive Committee. Clopidogrel added to aspirin versus aspirin alone in secondary prevention and high-risk primary prevention: rationale and design of the CHARISMA trial. *American Heart Journal* 2004; 148: 263–268.

Caplan LR. Thoughts evoked by MATCH and other trials. *Stroke* 2004; 35: 2604–2605.

CAPRIE Steering Committee. A randomised blinded trial of clopidogrel versus aspirin in patients at risk of ischemic events (CAPRIE). *Lancet* 1996; 348: 1333–1338.

Chew DP, Bhatt DL, Sapp S, Topol EJ. Increased mortality with oral platelet glycoprotein IIb/IIIa antagonists. A meta-analysis of phase III multicenter randomized trials. *Circulation* 2001; 103: 201–206.

The Clopidogrel in Unstable Angina to Prevent Recurrent Events (CURE) Trial Investigators. Effects of clopidogrel in addition to aspirin in patients with acute coronary syndromes without ST-Segment elevation. *New England Journal of Medicine* 2001; 345: 494–502.

Coull AJ, Lovett JK, Rothwell PM, on behalf of the Oxford Vascular Study. Population based study of early risk of stroke after transient ischemic attack or minor stroke: implications for public education and organisation of services. *British Medical Journal* 2004; 328: 326–328.

Culebras A, Rotta-Escalante R, Vila J *et al.* Triflusal versus aspirin for the prevention of cerebral infarction: a randomised stroke study. *Neurology* 2004; 62: 1073–1080.

Derry S, Loke YK. Risk of gastrointestinal hemorrhage with long term use of aspirin: meta-analysis. *British Medical Journal* 2000; 321: 1183–1187.

De Schryver ELLM, on behalf of the European/Australian Stroke Prevention in Reversible Ischemia Trial (ESPRIT) Group. Design of ESPRIT: an international randomised trial for secondary prevention after non-disabling cerebral ischemia of arterial origin. *Cerebrovascular Diseases* 2000; 10: 147–150.

De Schryver ELLM, Algra A, van Gijn J. Dipyridamole for preventing stroke and other vascular events in patients with vascular disease. *The Cochrane Database of Systematic Reviews* 2002, Issue 2. Art. No.: CD001820. DOI: 10.1002/14651858.CD001820.

De Schryver EL, Algra A, van Gijn J. Cochrane Review: Dipyridamole for preventing major vascular events in patients with vascular disease: Dipyridamole in stroke prevention. *Stroke* 2003; 34: 2072–2080.

Diener HC, Cunha L, Forbes C *et al.* European Stroke Prevention Study 2. Dipyridamole and acetylsalicylic acid in the secondary prevention of stroke. *Journal of the Neurological Science* 1996; 143: 1–13.

Diener H-C, Bogousslavsky J, Brass LM *et al.*, on behalf of the MATCH investigators. Aspirin and clopidogrel compared with clopidogrel alone after recent ischemic stroke or transient ischemic attack in high-risk patients (MATCH): randomised, double-blind, placebo-controlled trial. *Lancet* 2004; 364: 331–337.

Dippel DW, Wijnhoud AD, Koudstaal PJ. Prediction of major vascular events after TIA or minor stroke. A comparison of 6 models (abstract). *Cerebrovascular Diseases* 2004; 17 (Suppl 5): 35.

Dusitanond P, Hankey GJ. Ticlopidine. *Journal of Drug Evaluation* 2005 (in press).

Eikelboom JW, Hirsh J, Weitz JI, Johnston M, Yi Q, Yusuf S. Aspirin resistance and the risk of myocardial infarction, stroke, or cardiovascular death in patients at high risk of cardiovascular outcomes. *Circulation* 2002; 105: 1650–1655.

Eikelboom JW, Hankey GJ. Aspirin resistance: a new independent predictor of vascular events? *Journal of the American College of Cardiology* 2003; 41 (6): 966–968.

Gent M, Blakely JA, Easton JD *et al.* The Canadian American Ticlopidine Study (CATS) in thromboembolic stroke. *Lancet* 1989; 1: 1215–1220.

Gorelick PB, Richardson DJ, Kelly M *et al.* for the African American Antiplatelet Stroke Prevention Study (AAAPS) Investigators. Aspirin and ticlopidine for prevention of recurrent stroke in black patients. A randomized trial. *Journal of the American Medical Association* 2003; 289: 2947–2957.

Gotoh F, Toghi H, Hirai S *et al.* The Cilostazol Stroke Prevention Study: a placebo-controlled double-blind trial of secondary prevention of cerebral infarction. *Journal of Stroke and Cerebrovascular Diseases* 2000; 9: 147–157.

Gum PA, Kottke-Marchant K, Welsh PA, White J, Topol EJ. A prospective, blinded determination of the natural history of aspirin resistance among stable patients with cardiovascular disease. *Journal of the American College of Cardiology* 2003; 41: 961–965.

Hankey GJ. Clopidogrel and thrombotic thrombocytopenic purpura. *Lancet* 2000; 356: 269–270.

Hankey GJ. Ongoing and planned trials of antiplatelet therapy in the acute and long-term management of patients with ischaemic brain syndromes: setting a new standard of care. *Cerebrovascular Diseases* 2004; 17 (S3): 11–16.

Hankey GJ, Sudlow CLM, Dunbabin DW. Thienopyridines or aspirin to prevent stroke and other serious vascular events in patients at high risk of vascular disease. *Stroke* 2000; 31: 1779–1784.

Hankey GJ, Eikelboom JW. Aspirin resistance. *British Medical Journal* 2004; 328: 477–479.

Hankey GJ, Eikelboom JW. Adding aspirin to clopidogrel after TIA and ischaemic stroke: benefits do not match risks. *Neurology* 2005; 64: 1117–1121.

Hass WK, Easton JD, Adams Jr HP *et al.* A randomised trial comparing ticlopidine hydrochloride with aspirin for the prevention of stroke in high-risk patients. *New England Journal of Medicine* 1989; 321: 501–507.

He J, Whelton PK, Vu B, Klag MJ. Aspirin and risk of hemorrhagic stroke. A meta-analysis of randomised controlled trials. *Journal of the American Medical Association* 1998; 280: 1930–1935.

Jain A, Suarez J, Mahmarian JJ, Zoghbi WA, Quinones MA, Verani MS. Functional significance of myocardial perfusion defects induced by dipyridamole using thallium-201 single photon emission computed tomography and two-dimensional echocardiography. *American Journal of Cardiology* 1990; 66: 802–806.

Keltz TN, Innerfield M, Gitler B, Copper JA. Dipyridamole-induced myocardial ischemia. *Journal of the American Medical Association* 1987; 257: 1515–1516.

Kennedy J, Eliaasziw M, Buchan A *et al.* The Fast Assessment of Stroke and Transient ischaemic attack (TIA) to prevent Early Recurrence (FASTER) trial – Pilot phase. Ongoing Clinical Trial Abstracts, *29th International Stroke Conference*, 2004, American Stroke Association, CTP31.

Leonard-Bee J, Bath PMW, Bousser M-G *et al.*, on behalf of the Dipyridamole in Stroke Collaboration (DISC). Dipyridamole for preventing recurrent ischaemic stroke and other vascular events. A meta-analysis of individual patient data from randomised controlled trials. *Stroke* 2005; 36: 162–168.

Lovett JK, Coull A, Rothwell PM, on behalf of the Oxford Vascular Study. Early risk of recurrent stroke by etiological subtype: implications for stroke prevention. *Neurology* 2004; 62: 569–574.

Macleod MR, Amarenco P, Davis SM, Donnan GA. Atheroma of the aortic arch: an important and poorly recognised factor in the aetiology of stroke. *Lancet Neurology* 2004; 3: 408–414.

Markus H, Ringlestein EB. The effect of dual antiplatelet therapy compared with aspirin on asymptomatic embolisation in carotid stenosis: the CARESS trial (abstract 4). *Cerebrovascular Diseases* 2004; 17 (Suppl 5): 39.

Markus HS, Droste DW, Kaps M, Larrue V, Lees K, Siebler M, Ringelstein EB. Dual antiplatelet therapy with clopidogrel and aspirin in symptomatic carotid stenosis evaluated using doppler embolic signal detection. The Clopidogrel and Aspirin for Reduction of Emboli in Symptomatic carotid Stenosis (CARESS) trial. Circulation 2005; 111: 2233–2240.

Matiás-Guiu J, Ferro JM, Alvarez-Sabin J *et al.* Comparison of triflusal and aspirin for prevention of vascular events in patients after cerebral infarction: the TACIP Study – a randomised, double-blind, multicentre trial. *Stroke* 2003; 34: 840–848.

Mehta SR, Yusuf S, Peters RJG *et al.*, for the Clopidogrel in Unstable angina to prevent Recurrent Events trial (CURE) Investigators. Effects of pretreatment with clopidogrel and aspirin followed by long-term therapy in patients undergoing percutaneous coronary intervention: the PCI-CURE study. *Lancet* 2001; 358: 527–533.

Nighoghossian N, Hermier M, Adeleine P *et al.* Old microbleeds are a potential risk factor for cerebral bleeding after ischaemic stroke. A gradient-echo T2*-weighted brain MRI study. *Stroke* 2002; 33: 735–742.

Patrono C. Aspirin resistance: definition, mechanisms and clinical read-outs. *Journal of Thrombosis and Haemostasis* 2003; 1: 1710–1713.

Sacco RL, Diener H-C, Yusuf S, PRoFESS Steering Committee and Study Group. Prevention Regimen for Effectively avoiding Second Strokes (PRoFESS). *29th International Stroke Conference*. San Diego: American Stroke Association; 2004: CTP18.

Serebruany VL, Malinin Al, Eisert RM, Sane DC. Risk of bleeding complications with antiplatelet agents: meta-analysis of 338,191 patients enrolled in 50 randomised controlled trials. *American Journal of Hematology* 2004; 75: 40–47.

Steinhubl SR, Tan WA, Foody JM, Topol EJ, for the EPISTENT investigators. Incidence and clinical course of thrombotic thrombocytopenic purpura due to ticlopidine following coronary stenting. *Journal of the American Medical Association* 1999; 281: 806–810.

Steinhubl SR, Berger PB, Mann JT III *et al.*, for the CREDO Investigators. Early and sustained dual oral antiplatelet therapy following percutaneous coronary intervention. A randomized controlled trial. *Journal of the American Medical Association* 2002; 288: 2411–2420.

The Stroke Prevention in Reversible Ischemia Trial (SPIRIT) Study Group. A randomized trial of anticoagulants versus aspirin after cerebral ischemia of presumed arterial origin. *Annals of Neurology* 1997; 42: 857–865.

Topol EJ, Easton JD, Amarenco P *et al*. Design of the blockade of the glycoprotein IIb/IIIa receptor to avoid vascular occlusion (BRAVO) trial. *American Heart Journal* 2000; 139: 927–933.

Tran H, Anand SS. Oral antiplatelet therapy in *cerebrovascular disease*, coronary artery disease, and peripheral arterial disease. *Journal of the American Medical Association* 2004; 292: 1867–1874.

Virtanen KS, Mattila S, Jarvinen A, Frick MH. Angiographic findings in patients exhibiting ischemia after oral dipyridamole. *International Journal of Cardiology* 1989; 23: 33–36.

Oral anticoagulants vs antiplatelet therapy (for non-cardioembolic stroke)

Algra A, De Schryver ELLM, van Gijn J, Kappelle LJ, Koudstaal PJ. Oral anticoagulants versus antiplatelet therapy for preventing further vascular events after transient ischaemic attack or minor stroke of presumed arterial origin (Cochrane Review). In: *The Cochrane Library*, Issue 1, 2002. Oxford: Update Software.

Algra A, De Schryver ELLM, van Gijn J, Kappelle LJ, Koudstaal PJ. Oral anticoagulants versus antiplatelet therapy for preventing further vascular events after transient ischaemic attack or minor stroke of presumed arterial origin (Cochrane Corner). *Stroke* 2003; 34: 234–235.

Chimowitz MI, Lynn MJ, Howlett-Smith H *et al*. Comparison of warfarin and aspirin for sympromatic intracranial arterial stenosis. *New England Journal of Medicine* 2005; 352: 1305–1316.

De Schryver ELLM, on behalf of the European/Australian Stroke Prevention in Reversible Ischaemia Trial (ESPRIT) Group. Design of ESPRIT: an international randomized trial for secondary prevention after non-disabling cerebral ischaemia of arterial origin. *Cerebrovascular Diseases* 2000; 10 (2): 147–150.

De Schryver ELLM. ESPRIT: Protocol change. *Cerebrovascular Diseases* 2001; 11: 286.

The European/Australasian Stroke Prevention in Reversible Ischaemia Trial (ESPRIT) Study Group. Oral anticoagulation in patients after cerebral ischaemia of arterial origin and risk of intracranial haemorrhage. *Stroke* 2003; 34: e45–e47.

Mohr J, Thompson JLP, Lazar RM, Levin B, Sacco RL, Furie KL, Kistler JP, Albers GW, Pettigrew LC, Adams Jr HP, Jackson CM, Pullicino P, for the Warfarin-Aspirin Recurrent Stroke Study Group. A comparison of warfarin and aspirin for the prevention of recurrent ischemic stroke. *New England Journal of Medicine* 2001; 345: 1444–1451.

Torn M, Algra A, Rosendaal FR. Oral anticoagulation for cerebral ischemia of presumed arterial origin. High initial bleeding risk. *Neurology* 2001; 57: 1993–1999.

References to studies included in the Cochrane Review of oral anticoagulants vs antiplatelet therapy by Algra *et al.* (2004)

Garde 1983 {published data only}

Garde A, Samuelsson K, Fahlgren H, Hedberg E, Hjerne L-G, Östman J. Treatment after transient ischemic attacks: a comparison between anticoagulant drug and inhibition of platelet aggregation. *Stroke* 1983; 14 (5): 677–681.

Olsson 1980 {published data only}

Brechter C, Bäcklund H, Krook H, Müller R, Nitelius E, Olsson JE, Olsson O, Thornberg A. Comparison between anticoagulant treatment and anti-platelet therapy in order to prevent cerebral infarction in patients with TIA/RIND (Trombocytehämmande behandling eller antikoagulantia som profylax vid TIA/RIND). Läkartidningen 1980; 77 (52): 4947–4956.

*Olsson JE, Brechter C, Bäcklund H, Krook H, Müller R, Nitelius E, Olsson O, Tornberg A. Anticoagulant vs anti-platelet therapy as prophylactic against cerebral infarction in transient ischemic attacks. *Stroke* 1980; 11 (1): 4–9.

SPIRIT 1997 {published and unpublished data}

The Stroke Prevention In Reversible Ischemia Trial (SPIRIT) Study Group. A randomised trial of anticoagulants versus aspirin after cerebral ischemia of presumed arterial origin. *Annals of Neurology* 1997; 42 (6): 857–865.

SWAT 1998 {published data only}

Stewart B, Shuaib A, Veloso F. Stroke Prevention with Warfarin or Aspirin Trial (SWAT). (Abstract P9) *Stroke* 1998; 29: 304.

WARSS 2001 {published data only}

*Mohr JP *et al.* for the WARSS Group. A comparison of warfarin and aspirin for the prevention of recurrent ischemic stroke. *New England Journal of Medicine* 2001; 345: 1444–1451.

Mohr JP, for the WARSS Group. Design considerations for the Warfarin-Antiplatelet Recurrent Stroke Study. *Cerebrovascular Diseases* 1995; 5: 156–157.

The WARSS, APASS, PICSS, HAS and GENESIS Study Groups. The feasibility of a collaborative double-blind study using an anticoagulant. *Cerebrovascular Diseases* 1997; 7: 100–112.

Chapter 11. Carotid artery revascularisation

Carotid endarterectomy

Ascher E, Markevich N, Hingorani A, Kallakuri S.: Pseudo-occlusions of the internal carotid artery: a rationale for treatment on the basis of a modified duplex scan protocol. *Journal of Vascular Surgery* 2002; 35: 340–350.

Asymptomatic Carotid Atherosclerosis Study Group. Carotid endarterectomy for patients with asymptomatic internal carotid artery stenosis. *Journal of the American Medical Association* 1995; 273: 1421–1428.

Benade M, Warlow CP. Cost of identifying patients for carotid endartectomy. *Stroke* 2002a; 33: 435–439.

Benade M, Warlow CP. Costs and benefits of carotid endartectomy and associated preoperative arterial imaging. A systematic review of health economic literature. *Stroke* 2002b; 33: 629–638.

Bermann SS, Devine JJ, Erdos LS, Hunter GC. Distinguishing carotid artery pseudo-occlusion with colour-flow Doppler. *Stroke* 1995; 26: 434–438.

Bond R, Rerkasem K, Rothwell PM. Routine or selective carotid artery shunting for carotid endarterectomy (and different methods of monitoring in selective shunting). *The Cochrane Database of Systematic Reviews* 2001, Issue 4, Art. No.: CD000190. DOI: 10.1002/14651858. CD000190.

Bond R, Rerkasem K, Rothwell PM. A systematic review of the risks of carotid endarterectomy in relation to the clinical indication and the timing of surgery. *Stroke* 2003a; 34: 2290–2301.

Bond R, Rerkasem K, Rothwell PM. Routine or selective carotid artery shunting for carotid endarterectomy (and different methods of monitoring in selective shunting) (Cochrane Corner). *Stroke* 2003b; 34: 824–825.

Bond R, Rerkasem K, Naylor AR, Rothwell PM. A systematic review of randomised controlled trials of different types of patch materials during carotid endarterectomy. Stroke 2005; 36: 1350–1.

Cina CS, Clase CM, Haynes RB. Carotid endarterectomy for symptomatic carotid stenosis. *The Cochrane Database of Systematic Reviews* 1999, Issue 3. Art. No.: CD001081. DOI: 10.1002/14651858.CD001081.

Coull AJ, Lovett JK, Rothwell PM, on behalf of the Oxford Vascular Study. Population based study of early risk of stroke after transient ischemic attack or minor stroke: implications for public education and organisation of services. *British Medical Journal* 2004; 328: 326–328.

European Carotid Surgery Trialists' Collaborative Group. MRC European Carotid Surgery Trial. Interim results for symptomatic patients with severe (70–99%) or with mild (0–29%) carotid stenosis. *Lancet* 1991; 337: 1235–1243.

European Carotid Surgery Trialists' Collaborative Group. Randomised trial of endarterectomy for recently symptomatic carotid stenosis: Final results of the MRC European Carotid Surgery Trial (ECST). *Lancet* 1998; 351: 1379–1387.

Feasby TE, Quan H, Ghali WA. Hospital and surgeon determinants of carotid endarterectomy outcomes. *Archives of Neurology* 2002; 59: 1877–1881.

Fields WS, Maslenikov V, Meyer JS, Hass WK, Remington RD, MacDonald M. Joint study of extracranial arterial occlusion. V. Progress report on prognosis following surgery or non-surgical treatment for transient cerebral ischaemic attacks and cervical carotid artery lesions. *Journal of the American Medical Association* 1970; 211: 1993–2003.

Goldstein LB, Moore WS, Robertson JT *et al.* Complication rates for carotid endarterectomy: a call for action. *Stroke* 1997; 28: 889–890.

Johnston DC, Goldstein LB: Clinical carotid endarterectomy decision making: non-invasive vascular imaging versus angiography. *Neurology* 2001; 56: 1009–1015.

Lovett J, Dennis M, Sandercock PAG, Bamford J, Warlow CP, Rothwell PM. The very early risk of stroke following a TIA. *Stroke* 2003; 34: e138–e140.

Lovett JK, Coull A, Rothwell PM, on behalf of the Oxford Vascular Study. Early risk of recurrent stroke by aetiological subtype: implications for stroke prevention. *Neurology* 2004; 62: 569–574.

Markus H, Ringlestein EB. The effect of dual antiplatelet therapy compared with aspirin on asymptomatic embolisation in carotid stenosis: the CARESS trial (abstract 4). *Cerebrovascular Diseases* 2004; 17 (Suppl 5): 39.

Mayberg MR, Wilson E, Yatsu F, Weiss DG, Messina L, Hershey LA, Colling C, Eskeridge J, Deykin D, Winn HR. Carotid endarterectomy and prevention of cerebral ischemia in symptomatic carotid stenosis. Veterans Affairs Cooperative Studies Program 309 Trialist Group. *Journal of the American Medical Association* 1991; 266: 3289–3294.

Morgenstern LB, Fox AJ, Sharpe BL, Eliasziw M, Barnett HJ, Grotta JC, for the North American Symptomatic Carotid Endarterectomy Trial (NASCET) Group. The risks and benefits of carotid endarterectomy in patients with near occlusion of the carotid artery. *Neurology* 1997; 48: 911–915.

MRC Asymptomatic Carotid Surgery Trial (ACST) Collaborative Group. Prevention of disabling and fatal strokes by successful carotid endarterectomy in patients without recent neurological symptoms: randomised controlled trial. *Lancet* 2004; 363: 1491–1502.

Norris J, Rothwell PM. Noninvasive carotid imaging to select patients for endarterectomy: Is it really safer than conventional angiography? *Neurology* 2001; 56: 990–991.

North American Symptomatic Carotid Endarterectomy Trial Collaborators. Beneficial effect of carotid endarterectomy in symptomatic patients with high-grade carotid stenosis. *New England Journal of Medicine* 1991; 325: 445–453.

North American Symptomatic Carotid Endarterectomy Trial Collaborators. Benefit of carotid endarterectomy in patients with symptomatic moderate or severe stenosis. *New England Journal of Medicine* 1998; 339: 1415–1425.

Ogata J, Masuda J, Yutani C, Yamaguchi T. Rupture of atheromatous plaque as a cause of thrombotic occlusion of stenotic internal carotid artery. *Stroke* 1990; 21: 1740–1745.

Patel SC, Collie D, Wardlaw JM *et al.* Outcome, observer reliability, and patient preferences if CTA, MRA, or Doppler ultrasound were used, individually or together, instead of digital subtraction angiography before carotid endarterectomy. *Journal of Neurology Neurosurgery and Psychiatry* 2002; 73: 21–28.

Rerkasem K, Bond R, Rothwell P. Local versus general anaesthetic for carotid endarterectomy (Cochrane Corner). *Stroke* 2005; 36: 169–170.

Rerkasem K, Bond R, Rothwell P. Local versus general anaesthetic for carotid endarterectomy (Cochrane Review). In: The Cochrane Library. Issue 1. 2005. Oxford: Update Software. 227 *Cochrane Library*, John Wiley & Sons Ltd.

Rothwell PM, Gibson RJ, Slattery JM *et al.* Equivalence of measurements of carotid stenosis: a comparison of three methods of 1001 angiograms. *Stroke* 1994; 25: 2435–2439.

Rothwell PM, Warlow CP. Is self-audit reliable? *Lancet* 1995; 346: 1623.

Rothwell PM, Slattery J, Warlow CP. A systematic comparison of the risk of stroke and death due to carotid endarterectomy. *Stroke* 1996a; 27: 260–265.

Rothwell PM, Slattery J, Warlow CP. A systematic comparison of the risk of stroke and death due to carotid endarterectomy for symptomatic and asymptomatic carotid stenosis. *Stroke* 1996b; 27: 266–269.

Rothwell P, Slattery J, Warlow C. Clinical and angiographic predictors of stroke and death from carotid endarterectomy: systematic review. *British Medical Journal* 1997; 315: 1571–1577.

Rothwell PM, Warlow CP, on behalf of the European Carotid Surgery Trialists' Collaborative Group. Interpretation of operative risks of individual surgeons. *Lancet* 1999a; 353: 1325.

Rothwell PM, Warlow CP, on behalf of the ECST Collaborators. Prediction of benefit from carotid endarterectomy in individual patients: a risk-modelling study. *Lancet* 1999b; 353: 2105–2110.

Rothwell PM, Warlow CP, for the European Carotid Surgery Trialists' Collaborative Group: low risk of ischaemic stroke in patients with collapse of the internal carotid artery distal to severe carotid stenosis: cerebral protection due to low post-stenotic flow? *Stroke* 2000; 31: 622–630.

Rothwell PM, Gibson R, Warlow CP. Interrelation between plaque surface morphology and degree of stenosis on carotid angiograms and the risk of ischemic stroke in patients with symptomatic carotid stenosis. *Stroke* 2000a; 31: 615–621.

Rothwell PM, Pendlebury ST, Wardlaw J, Warlow CP. Critical appraisal of the design and reporting of studies of imaging and measurement of carotid stenosis. *Stroke* 2000b; 31: 1444–1450.

Rothwell PM, Gutnikov SA, Warlow CP, for the ECST. Re-analysis of the final results of the European Carotid Surgery Trial. *Stroke* 2003a; 34: 514–523.

Rothwell PM, Eliasziw M, Gutnikov SA, Fox AJ, Taylor W, Mayberg MR, Warlow CP, Barnett HJ, for the Carotid Endarterectomy Trialists' Collaboration. Pooled analysis of individual patient data from randomised controlled trials of endarterectomy for symptomatic carotid stenosis. *Lancet* 2003b; 361: 107–116.

Rothwell PM. ACST: Which subgroups will benefit most from carotid endarterectomy? *Lancet* 2004; 364: 1122–1123.

Rothwell PM, Eliasziw M, Gutnikov SA, Warlow CP, Barnett HJ, for the Carotid Endarterectomy Trialists' Collaboration. Endarterectomy for symptomatic carotid stenosis in relation to clinical subgroups and the timing of surgery. *Lancet* 2004; 363: 915–924.

Rothwell PM. With what to treat which patient with recently symptomatic carotid stenosis? *Practical Neurology* 2005; 5: 68–83.

Rothwell PM, Mehta Z, Howard SC, Gutnikov SA, CP Warlow. From subgroups to individuals: general principles and the example of carotid endarterectomy. *Lancet* 2005; 365: 256–265.

Sandercock PA, Warlow CP, Jones LN, Starkey IR. Predisposing factors for cerebral infarction: the Oxfordshire community stroke project. *British Medical Journal* 1989; 298: 75–80.

Shaw DA, Venables GS, Cartlidge NE, Bates D, Dickinson PH. Carotid endarterectomy in patients with transient cerebral ischaemia. *Journal of the Neurological Sciences* 1984; 64: 45–53.

Torvik A, Svindland A, Lindboe CF. Pathogenesis of carotid thrombosis. *Stroke* 1989; 20: 1477–1483.

Local versus general anaesthesia for carotid endarterectomy

McCleary AJ, Maritati G, Gough MJ. Carotid endarterectomy: local or general anaesthesia? *European Journal of Vascular and Endovascular Surgery* 2001; 22: 1–12.

Rerkasem K, Bond R, Rothwell PM. Local versus general anaesthesia for carotid endarterectomy. *The Cochrane Database of Systematic Reviews* 2004, Issue 2. Art. No.: CD000126. DOI: 10.1002/14651858.CD000126.pub2.

Rerkasem K, Bond R, Rothwell PM. Local versus general anaesthesia for carotid endarterectomy (Cochrane Corner). *Stroke* 2005; 36: 169–170.

References to trials included in the Cochrane Review by Rerkasem *et al.* (2004) entitled Local versus general anaesthesia for carotid endarterectomy

Binder 1999 {published and unpublished data}

Binder M, Fitzgerald R, Fried H, Schwarz S. Carotid endarterectomy surgery in cervical block: an economic alternative to general anaesthesia? (Karotisdesobliteration in cervicalisblockade: eine okonomische alternative zur vollnarkose?). Gesundheitsökonomie & Qualitätsmanagement 1999; 4: 19–24.

Forssell C, Takolander R, Bergqvist D, Johansson A, Persson NH. Local versus general anaesthesia in carotid surgery. A prospective, randomised study. *European Journal of Vascular Surgery* 1989; 3: 503–509.

Kasprzak P, Topel I, Mann S, Altmeppen J, Mackh J, Angerer M. General versus regional anesthesia and perioperative cardiopulmonary complications in carotid surgery: a prospective randomized study. *European Journal of Vascular and Endovascular Surgery* (submitted).

McCarthy 2001b {published data only}

*McCarthy RJ, Walker R, McAteer P, Budd JS, Horrocks M. Patient and hospital benefits of local anaesthesia for carotid endarterectomy. *European Journal of Vascular and Endovascular Surgery* 2001; 22: 13–18.

Pluskwa 1989 {published data only}

Pluskwa F, Bonnet F, Abhay K, Touboul C, Rey B, Marcandoro J *et al.* Blood pressure profiles during carotid endarterectomy. Comparing flunitrazepam/fentanyl/nitrous oxide with epidural anaesthesia (author's translation). *Annales Françaises D'anesthèsie et De Rèanimation* 1989; 8: 26–32.

Prough 1989 {published data only}

Prough DS, Scuderi PE, McWhorter JM, Balestrieri FJ, Davis CH, Stullken EH. Hemodynamic status following regional and general anesthesia for carotid endarterectomy. *Journal of Neurosurgical Anesthesiology* 1989; 1: 35–40.

Sbarigia 1999 {published and unpublished data}

Sbarigia E, DarioVizza C, Antonini M, Speziale F, Maritti M, Fiorani B *et al.* Locoregional versus general anesthesia in carotid surgery in carotid surgery: Is there an impact on perioperative myocardial ischemia? Results of a prospective monocentric randomized trial. *Journal of Vascular Surgery* 1999; 30: 131–138.

Eversion versus conventional carotid endarterectomy

Cao PG, De Rango P, Zannetti S, Giordano G, Ricci S, Celani MG. Eversion versus conventional carotid endarterectomy for preventing stroke. *The Cochrane Database of Systematic Reviews* 2000, Issue 4, Art. No.: CD001921. DOI: 10.1002/14651858.CD001921.

References to studies included in the Cochrane Review of Eversion versus conventional carotid endarterectomy by Cao *et al.* (2000)

Ballotta E, Da Giau G, Saladini M, Abbruzzese E, Renon L. Toniato A. Carotid endarterectomy with patch closure versus carotid eversion endarterectomy and reimplantation: a prospective randomized study. *Surgery* 1999; 125: 271–279.

Ballotta E, Renon L, Da Giau G, Toniato A, Baracchini C, Abbruzzese E. A prospective randomized study on bilateral carotid endarterectomy: patching versus eversion. Clinical outcome and restenosis. *Annals of Surgery* 2000; 232: 119–125.

Balzer K. Eversion versus conventional carotid endarterectomy. In: Horsch S, Ktenidis K (eds), Perioperative monitoring in carotid surgery. *Darmstadt Steinkopff Springer* 1998; 159–165: 2836.

Cao P, Giordano G, De Rango P, Zannetti S, Chiesa R, Coppi G, Palombo D, Spartera C, Stancanelli V, Vecchiati E, and collaborators of the EVEREST Study Group. A randomized study on eversion versus standard carotid endarterectomy: study design and preliminary results: the EVEREST trial. *Journal of Vascular Surgery* 1998; 27: 595–605: 2720.

Vanmaele RG. The technique of division-endarterectomy-anastomosis for the surgical treatment of extracranial carotid artery atheromatosis. Antwerp: Antwerp University UIA, 1992.

Vanmaele RG, Van Schil PE, DeMaeseneer MG, Lehert P, Van Look RF. Endarterectomy and reimplantation for carotid stenosis. In: Chang JB (ed.), *Modern Vascular Surgery*. New York: Springer-Verlag, 1994; 85–96: 2680.

Vanmaele RG, Van Schil PE, DeMaeseneer MG, Meese G, Lehert PH, Van Look RF. Division-endarterectomy-anastomosis of the internal carotid artery: a prospective randomized comparative study. *Cardiovascular Surgery* 1994; 2 (5): 573–581: 1814.

Routine or selective carotid artery shunting for carotid endarterectomy (and different methods of monitoring in selective shunting)

Bond R, Rerkasem K, Rothwell PM. Routine or selective carotid artery shunting for carotid endarterectomy (and different methods of monitoring in selective shunting). *The Cochrane Database of Systematic Reviews* 2001, Issue 4, Art. No.: CD000190. DOI: 10.1002/14651858. CD000190.

References to studies included in the Cochrane review by Bond *et al.* (2001) on routine or selective carotid artery shunting for carotid endarterectomy (and different methods of monitoring in selective shunting)

Fletcher JP, Morris JGL, Little JM, Kershaw LZ. EEG monitoring during carotid endarterectomy. *Australia and NewZealand Journal of Surgery* 1988; 58: 285–288.

Gumerlock MK, Neuwelt EA. Carotid endarterectomy: to shunt or not to shunt. *Stroke* 1988; 19: 1485–1490.

Sandmann W, Kolvenbach R, Willeke F. Risks and benefits of shunting in carotid endarterectomy (letter). *Stroke* 1993; 24: 1098.

Sandmann W, Willeke F, Kovenbach R, Benecke R, Godehardt E. To shunt or not to shunt: the definite answer with a randomized study. In: Veith FJ (ed.), *Current Critical Problems in Vascular Surgery*. Vol. 5. St Louis, Missouri: Quality Medical Publishing Inc, 1993: 434–440.

Patches of different types for carotid patch angioplasty

Bond R, Rerkasem K, Naylor R, Rothwell PM. Patches of different types for carotid patch angioplasty. *The Cochrane Database of Systematic Reviews* 2003, Issue 3. Art. No.: CD000071. DOI: 10.1002/14651858.CD000071.pub2.

References to studies included in this review of patches of different types for carotid patch angioplasty by Bond *et al.* (2003d)

AbuRahma AF, Khan JH, Robinson PA, Saiedy S, Short YS, Boland JP *et al.* Prospective randomized trial of carotid endarterectomy with primary closure and patch angioplasty with saphenous vein, jugular vein, and polytetrafluoroethylene: perioperative (30 day) results. *Journal of Vascular Surgery* 1996; 24: 998–1007.

AbuRahma AF, Robinson PA, Saiedy S, Kahn JH, Boland JP. Prospective randomized trial of carotid endarterectomy with primary closure and patch angioplasty with saphenous vein, jugular vein, and polytetrafluoroethylene: long-term follow-up. *Journal of Vascular Surgery* 1998; 27 (2): 222–232.

AbuRahma A, Hannay S, Khan JH, Robinson PA, Hudson JK, Davis EA. Prospective randomised study of carotid endarterectomy with polytetrafluoroethylene versus collagen-impregnated Dacron (Hemashield) patching: perioperative (30-day) results. *Journal of Vascular Surgery* 2002; 35: 125–130.

Gonzalez-Fajardo JA, Perez JL, Mateo AM. Saphenous vein patch versus polytetrafluoroethylene patch after carotid endarterectomy. *Journal of Cardiovascular Surgery* 1994; 35: 523–528.

Perez-Burckhardt JL, Gonzalez-Fajardo JA, Mateo AH. Saphenous vein patch versus politetra-fluoroethylene patch after carotid endarterectomy. *International Angiology* 1995; 14 (Suppl 1): 346.

Hayes PD, Allroggen H, Steel S, Thompson MM, London NJ, Bell PR *et al.* Randomized trial of vein versus Dacron patching during carotid endarterectomy: influence of patch type on post-operative embolization. *Journal of Vascular Surgery* 2001; 33 (5): 994–1000.

Katz SG, Kohl RD. Does the choice of material influence early morbidity in patients undergoing carotid patch angioplasty? *Surgery* 1996; 119: 297–301.

Lord RSA, Raj TB, Stary DL, Nash PA, Graham AR, Goh KH. Comparison of saphenous vein patch, polytetrafluoroethylene patch, and direct arteriotomy closure after carotid endarterec-tomy. Part I: Perioperative results. *Journal of Vascular Surgery* 1989; 9: 521–529.

O'Hara PJ, Hertzer NR, Mascha EJ, Krajewski LP, Clair DG, Ouriel K. A prospective, randomized study of saphenous vein patching versus synthetic patching during carotid endarterectomy. *Journal of Vascular Surgery* 2002; 35(2): 324–330.

Ricco J-B, Demarque C, Bouin-Pineau M-H, Camiade C. Vein patch versus PTFE patch for carotid endarterectomy. A randomized trial in a selected group of patients. *European Journal of Vascular Surgery* 1996 (submitted).

Ricco JB, Gauthier J-B, Bodin-Pineau M-H. Enlargement patch after carotid endarterectomy. Polytetrafluoroethylene (PTFE) or saphenous patch? Results of a randomized study after 3 years (abstract). Paper presented at *The French-Language Society of Vascular Surgery Annual Congress of Reims* 19–20 June 1992.

Patch angioplasty versus primary closure for carotid endarterectomy

Bond R, Rerkasem K, AbuRahma AF, Naylor AR, Rothwell PM. Patch angioplasty versus primary closure for carotid endarterectomy. *The Cochrane Database of Systematic Reviews* 2003, Issue 3. Art. No.: CD000160. DOI: 10.1002/14651858.CD000160.pub2.

References to studies included in the review by Bond *et al.* (2003c), entitled: Patch angioplasty versus primary closure for carotid endarterectomy.

AbuRahma AF, Khan JH, Robinson PA, Saiedy S, Short YS, Boland JP *et al.* Prospective random-ized trial of carotid endarterectomy with primary closure and patch angioplasty with saphe-nous vein, jugular vein, and polytetrafluoroethylene: perioperative (30 day) results. *Journal of Vascular Surgery* 1996; 24: 998–1007.

AbuRahma AF, Robinson PA, Saiedy S, Kahn JH, Boland JP. Prospective randomized trial of carotid endarterectomy with primary closure and patch angioplasty with saphenous vein, jugular vein, and polytetrafluoroethylene: long-term follow-up. *Journal of Vascular Surgery* 1998; 27 (2): 222–232.

Eikelboom BC, Ackerstaff RGA, Hoeneveld H, Ludwig JW, Teeuwen C, Vermeulen FEE et al. Benefits of carotid patching: a randomized study. *Journal of Vascular Surgery* 1988; 7: 240–247.

de Letter JAM, Moll FL, Welten RJT, Eikelboom BC, Ackerstaff RGA, Vermeulen FEE et al. Benefits of carotid patching: a prospective randomized study with long-term follow-up. *Annals of Vascular Surgery* 1994; 8: 54–58.

Katz D, Snyder SO, Gandhi RH, Wheeler JR, Gregory RT, Gayle RG et al. Long-term follow up for recurrent stenosis: a prospective randomized study of expanded polytetrafluoroethylene patch angioplasty versus primary closure after carotid endarterectomy. *Journal of Vascular Surgery* 1994; 19: 198–205.

Lord RSA, Raj TB, Stary DL, Nash PA, Graham AR, Goh KH. Comparison of saphenous vein patch, polytetrafluoroethylene patch, and direct arteriotomy closure after carotid endarterectomy. Part 1: Perioperative results. *Journal of Vascular Surgery* 1989; 9: 521–529.

Clagett GP, Patterson CB, Fisher Jr DF, Fry RE, Eidt JF, Humble TH et al. Vein patch versus primary closure for carotid endarterectomy. A randomized prospective study in a selected group of patients. *Journal of Vascular Surgery* 1989; 9: 213–223.

Myers SI, Valentine RJ, Chervu A, Bowers BL, Clagett GP. Saphenous vein patch versus primary closure for carotid endarterectomy: long term assessment of a randomized prospective study. *Journal of Vascular Surgery* 1994; 19: 15–22.

Ranaboldo CJ, Barros D'Sa ABB, Bell PRF, Chant ADB, Perry PM, for the Joint Vascular Research Group. Randomized controlled trial of patch angioplasty for carotid endarterectomy. *British Journal of Surgery* 1993; 80: 1528–1530.

De Vleeschauwer P, Wirthle W, Holler L, Krause E, Horsch S. Is venous patch grafting after carotid endarterectomy able to reduce the rate of restenosis? Prospective randomized pilot study with stratification. *Acta Chirurgica Belgica* 1987; 87: 242–246.

Adjunct medical therapies

Antiplatelet therapy

Antithrombotic Trialists' Collaboration: Collaborative meta-analysis of randomized trials of antiplatelet therapy for prevention of death, myocardial infarction, and stroke in high risk patients. *British Medical Journal* 2002; 324: 71–86.

CAPRIE Steering Committee. A randomised, blinded, trial of clopidogrel versus aspirin in patients at risk of ischaemic events (CAPRIE). CAPRIE Steering Committee. *Lancet* 1996; 348: 1329–1339.

Diener HC, Bogousslavsky J, Brass LM, Cimminiello C, Csiba L, Kaste M, Leys D, Matias-Guiu J, Rupprecht HJ, MATCH Investigators. Aspirin and clopidogrel compared with clopidogrel alone after recent ischaemic stroke or transient ischaemic attack in high-risk patients (MATCH): randomised, double-blind, placebo-controlled trial. *Lancet* 2004; 364: 331–337.

Engelter S, Lyrer P. Antiplatelet therapy for preventing stroke and other vascular events after carotid endarterectomy. *The Cochrane Database of Systematic Reviews* 2003, Issue 2. Art. No.: CD001458. DOI: 10.1002/14651858.CD001458.

Engelter S, Lyrer P. Antiplatelet therapy for preventing stroke and other vascular events after carotid endarterectomy (Cochrane Corner). *Stroke* 2004; 35: 1227–1228.

Hankey GJ. Ongoing and planned trials of antiplatelet therapy in the acute and long-term management of patients with ischaemic brain syndromes: setting a new standard of care. *Cerebrovascular Diseases* 2004; 17 (Suppl 3): 11–16.

Markus HS, Ringelstein EB. The effect of dual antiplatelet therapy compared with aspirin on asymptomatic embolisation in carotid stenosis: the CARESS Trial. *Cerebrovascular Diseases* 2004; 17 (Suppl 5): 39.

Markus HS, Droste DW, Kaps M, Larrue V, Lees K, Siebler M, Ringelstein EB. Dual antiplatelet therapy with clopidogrel and aspirin in symptomatic carotid stenosis evaluated using doppler embolic signal detection. The Clopidogrel and Aspirin for Reduction of Emboli in Symptomatic carotid Stenosis (CARESS) trial. Circulation 2005; 111: 2233–40.

Molloy J, Markus HS. Asymptomatic embolization predicts stroke and TIA risk in patients with carotid artery stenosis. *Stroke* 1999; 30: 1440–1443.

Payne DA, Jones CI, Hayes PD, Thompson MM, London NJ, Bell PR, Goodall AH, Naylor AR. Beneficial effects of clopidogrel combined with aspirin in reducing cerebral emboli in patients undergoing carotid endarterectomy. *Circulation* 2004; 109: 1476–1481.

Sivenius J, Riekkinen PJ, Smets P, Laakso M, Lowenthal A: The European Stroke Prevention Study (ESPS). Results by arterial distribution. *Annals of Neurology* 1991; 29: 596–600.

Valton L, Larrue V, Pavy la Traon A *et al*. Microembolic signals and risk of early recurrence in patients with stroke or transient ischemic attack. *Stroke* 1998; 29: 2125–2128.

References to studies included in the Cochrane Review by Engelter and Lyrer (2003) entitled: Anti-platelet therapy for preventing stroke and other vascular events after carotid endarterectomy

Antithrombotic Trialists' Collaboration. Collaborative meta-analysis of randomised trials of antiplatelet therapy for prevention of death, myocardial infarction, and stroke in high risk patients. *British Medical Journal* 2002; 324: 71–86.

Bischoff G, Pratschner T, Kail M *et al*. Anticoagulants, antiaggregants or nothing following carotid endarterectomy? *European Journal of Vascular Surgery* 1993; 7: 364–369.

Boysen G. Danish very-low dose aspirin after carotid endarterectomy trial. *Personal Communication* August 2001.

Boysen G, Sorensen PS, Juhler M, Andersen AR, Boas J, Olsen JS, Joensen P. Danish very-low dose aspirin after carotid endarterectomy trial. *Stroke* 1988; 19 (10): 1211–1215.

Boysen G, Sorensen PS, Juhler M, Andersen AR, Boas J, Olsen JS, Joensen P. Low-dose aspirin after carotid surgery. *Stroke* 1988; 19: 148 (abstract).

Fields WS, Lemak NA. Controlled trial of Aspirin in cerebral ischemia; study design, surveillance, and results. In: Breddin K, Dorndorf W, Loew D, Marx R (eds), Acetylsalicylic Acid in Cerebral Ischemia and Coronary Heart Disease, 1st edition. Stuttgartt, New York: Schattauer, 1978: 85–91.

Fields WS, Lemak NA, Frankowski RF, Hardy RJ. Controlled trial of aspirin in cerebral ischemia. Part II: surgical group. *Stroke* 1978; 9 (4): 309–319.

Harker LA, Bernstein EF, Dilley RB, Scala TE, Sise MJ, Hye RJ, Otis SM, Roberts RS, Gent M. Failure of aspirin plus dipyridamole to prevent restenosis after carotid endarterectomy. *Annals of Internal Medicine* 1992; 116 (9): 731–736.

Hansen F, Lindblad B, Persson NH, Bergquist D. Can recurrent stenosis after carotid endarterectomy be prevented by low-dose acetylsalicylic acid? A double-blind, randomised and placebo-controlled study. *European Journal of Vascular Surgery* 1993; 7 (4): 380–385.

Kretschmer G, Pratschner T, Prager M *et al.* Antiplatelet treatment prolongs survival after carotid endarterectomy. Analysis of the clinical series followed by a controlled trial. *Annals of Surgery* 1990; 211: 317–322.

Lemak NA, Fields WS, Gary Jr HE. Controlled trial of aspirin in cerebral ischemia: an addendum. *Neurology* 1986; 36: 705–710.

Lindblad B, Persson NH, Takolander R, Bergquist D. Does low-dose acetylsalicylic acid prevent stroke after carotid surgery? A double-blind, placebo-controlled randomized trial. *Stroke* 1993; 24 (8): 1125–1128.

Pratesi C, Pulli R, Milanesi G, Lavezzari M, Pamparana F, Bertini D. Indobufen versus placebo in the prevention of restenosis after carotid endarterectomy: a double-blind pilot study. *Journal of International Medical Research* 1991; 19 (3): 202–209.

Pratschner T, Kretschmer P, Prager M *et al.* Antiplatelet therapy following carotid bifurcation endarterectomy. Evaluation of a controlled clinical trial. Prognostic significance of histologic plaque examination on behalf of survival. *European Journal of Vascular Surgery* 1990; 4: 285–289.

Taylor DW, Barnett HJ, Haynes RB, Ferguson GG, Sackett DL, Thorpe KE, Simard D, Silver FL, Hachinski V, Clagett GP, Barnes R, Spence JD. Low-dose and high dose acetylsalicylic acid for patients undergoing carotid endarterectomy: a randomised controlled trial. ASA and Carotid Endarterectomy (ACE) Trial Collaborators. *Lancet* 1999; 353 (9171): 2179–2184.

Anticoagulants

Algra A, Francke CL, Koehler PJ. A randomized trial of anticoagulants versus aspirin after cerebral ischaemia of presumed arterial origin. *Annals of Neurology* 1997; 42: 857–865.

European Atrial Fibrillation Trial (EAFT) Study Group. Secondary prevention in non-rheumatic atrial fibrillation after transient ischaemic attack or minor stroke. *Lancet* 1993; 342: 1255–1262.

Kanter MC, Tegeler CH, Pearce LA *et al.* Carotid stenosis in patients with atrial fibrillation. Prevalence, risk factors, and relationship to stroke in the Stroke Prevention in Atrial Fibrillation Study. *Archives of Internal Medicine* 1994; 154: 1372–1377.

The Stroke Prevention in Reversible Ischaemia Trial (SPIRIT) Study Group. A randomised trial of anticoagulants versus aspirin after cerebral ischaemia of presumed arterial origin. *Annals of Neurology* 1997; 42: 857–865.

Warfarin Aspirin Recurrent Stroke Study Group. A comparison of warfarin and aspirin for the prevention of recurrent ischemic stroke. *New England Journal of Medicine* 2001; 345: 1444–1451.

Lowering blood pressure

Gorelick PB. Distribution of atherosclerotic cerebrovascular lesions. Effects of age, race, and sex. *Stroke* 1993; 24: 116–119.

Grubb Jr RL, Derdeyn CP, Fritsch SM, Carpenter DA, Yundt KD, Videen TO, Spitznagel EL, Powers WJ. Importance of hemodynamic factors in the prognosis of symptomatic carotid occlusion. *Journal of the American Medical Association* 1998; 280: 1055–1060.

PROGRESS Collaborative Group: Randomised trial of a perindopril-based blood-pressure-lowering regimen among 6,105 individuals with previous stroke or transient ischaemic attack. *Lancet* 2001; 358: 1033–1041.

Rothwell PM, Howard SC, Spence D. Relationship between blood pressure and stroke risk in patients with symptomatic carotid occlusive disease. *Stroke* 2003; 34: 2583–2590.

Spence JD. Management of resistant hypertension in patients with carotid stenosis: High prevalence of renovascular hypertension. *Cerebrovascular Diseases* 2000; 10: 249–254.

Thiele BL, Young JV, Chikos PM, Hirsch JH, Strandness DE. Correlation of arteriographic findings and symptoms in cerebrovascular disease. *Neurology* 1980; 30: 1041–1046.

Van der Grond J, Balm R, Kappelle J, Eikelboom BC, Mali WP: Cerebral metabolism of patients with stenosis or occlusion of the internal carotid artery. *Stroke* 1995; 26: 822–828.

Lowering blood cholesterol

Cannon CP, Braunwald E, McCabe CH *et al.* Intensive versus moderate lipid lowering with statins after acute coronary syndromes. *New England Journal of Medicine* 2004; 350: 1495–1504.

Heart Protection Study Collaborative Group: MRC/BHF Heart Protection Study of cholesterol lowering with simvastatin in 20,536 high-risk individuals: a randomised placebo-controlled trial. *Lancet* 2002; 360: 7–22.

Heart Protection Study Collaborative Group. Effects of cholesterol-lowering with simvastatin on stroke and other major vascular events in 20,536 people with cerebrovascular disease or other high-risk conditions. *Lancet* 2004; 363: 757–767.

Mercuri M, Bond MG, Sirtori CR, Veglia F, Crepaldi G, Feruglio FS, Descovich G, Ricci G, Rubba P, Mancini M, Gallus G, Bianchi G, D'Alo G, Ventura Al. Pravastatin reduces carotid intima-media thickness progression in an asymptomatic hypercholesterolemic Mediterranean population: the Carotid Atherosclerosis Italian Ultrasound Study. *American Journal of Medicine* 1996; 101: 627–634.

Waters DD, Schwartz GG, Olsson AG, Zeiher A, Oliver MF, Ganz P, Ezekowitz M, Chaitman BR, Leslie SJ, Stern T, MIRACL Study Investigators. Effects of atorvastatin on stroke in patients with unstable angina or non-Q-wave myocardial infarction: a myocardial ischemia reduction with aggressive cholesterol lowering (MIRACL) substudy. *Circulation* 2002; 106: 1690–1695.

Carotid stenting

Alberts MJ, for the Publications Committee of the WALLSTENT. Results of a multicentre prospective randomised trial of carotid artery stenting vs. carotid endarterectomy (abstract). *Stroke* 2001; 32: 325d.

Brooks WH, McClure RR, Jones MR *et al.* Carotid angioplasty and stenting versus carotid endarterectomy: randomized trial in a community hospital. *Journal of the American College of Cardiology* 2001; 38: 1589–1595.

Brooks WH, McClure RR, Jones MR, Coleman TC, Breathitt L. Carotid angioplasty and stenting versus carotid endarterectomy for treatment of asymptomatic carotid stenosis: a randomised trial in a community hospital. Neurosurgery 2004; 54: 318–325.

CAVATAS Investigators. Endovascular versus surgical treatment in patients with carotid stenosis in the Carotid and Vertebral Transluminal Angioplasty Study (CAVATAS): a randomised trial. *Lancet* 2001; 357: 1729–1737.

Connors JJ, Sacks D, Furlan AJ *et al.* Training, competency, and credentialing standards for diagnostic cervicocerebral angiography, carotid stenting and cerebrovascular intervention. *Neurology* 2005; 64: 190–198.

Coward LJ, Featherstone RL, Brown MM. Percutaneous transluminal angioplasty and stenting for carotid artery stenosis. The Cochrane database of systematic reviews 2004, Issue 1. Art. No.: CD 000515. DOI: 10.1002/14651858.CD000515.pub2.

Coward LJ, Featherstone RL, Brown MM. Safety and efficacy of endovascular treatment of carotid artery stenosis compared with carotid endarterectomy. A Cochrane Systematic Review of the Randomised Evidence. *Stroke* 2005; 36: 905–911.

Dotter CT, Judkins MP, Rosch J. Nonoperative treatment of arterial occlusive disease: a radiologically facilitated technique. *Radiologic Clinics of North America* 1967; 5: 531–542.

Featherstone R, Coward LC, Brown MM. International Carotid Stenting Study (ICSS). Ongoing Clinical Trial Abstracts, *29th International Stroke Conference*, 2004, American Stroke Association, CTP9.

Higashida RT, Meyers PM, Phatouros CC *et al.* Reporting standards for carotid artery angioplasty and stent placement. *Stroke* 2004; 35: e112–e133.

Howard VJ, Sheffet AJ, Brott TG *et al.* Progress report of the Carotid Revascularisation Endarterectomy vs Stenting Trial (CREST). Ongoing Clinical Trial Abstracts, *29th International Stroke Conference*, 2004, American Stroke Association, CTP21.

Naylor AR, London NJ, Bell PR. Carotid and Vertebral Artery Transluminal Angioplasty Study. *Lancet* 1997; 349: 1324–1325.

Reimers B, Corvaja N, Moshiri S, Sacca S, Albiero R, Di Mario C, Pascotto P, Colombo A. Cerebral protection with filter devices during carotid artery stenting. *Circulation* 2001; 104: 12–15.

Ringleb PA, Kunze A. Stent-supported Percutaneous Angioplasty of the Carotid artery versus Endartectomy. An update of the German and Austrian randomised multicentre study. Ongoing Clinical Trial Abstracts, *29th International Stroke Conference*, 2004, American Stroke Association, CTP20.

Yadav JS, Wholey MH, Kuntz RE *et al.*, for the Stenting and Angioplasty with Protection in Patients at High Risk for Endarterectomy Investigators. Protected carotid-artery stenting versus endarterectomy in high-risk patients. *New England Journal of Medicine* 2004; 351: 1493–1501.

Chapter 12. Lowering blood pressure

Bath PM. Major ongoing stroke trials: Efficacy of Nitric Oxide in Stroke (ENOS) Trial (abstract). *Stroke* 2001; 32: 2450–2451.

Bath P, Chalmers J, Powers W, Beilin L, Davis S, Lenfant C, Mancia G, Neal B, Whitworth J, Zanchetti A. International Society of Hypertension Writing Group. International Society of Hypertension (ISH): statement on the management of blood pressure in acute stroke. *Journal of Hypertension* 2003; 21: 665–672.

Barer DH, Cruickshank JM, Ebrahim SB, Mitchell JR. Low dose beta blockade in acute stroke ('BEST' trial): an evaluation. *British Medical Journal* 1988; 296: 737–741.

Blood Pressure in Acute Stroke Collaboration (BASC). Interventions for deliberately altering blood pressure in acute stroke. *The Cochrane Database of Systematic Reviews* 2001, Issue 2, Art. No.: CD000039. DOI: 10.1002/14651858.CD000039.

Blood Pressure Lowering Treatment Trialists' Collaboration. Effect of ACE inhibitors, calcium antagonists, and other blood-pressure-lowering drugs: results of prospectively designed overviews of randomised trials. *Lancet* 2000; 355: 1955–1964.

Blood Pressure Lowering Treatment Trialists' Collaboration. Effect of different blood-pressure-lowering regimens on major cardiovascular events: results of prospectively designed overviews of randomised trials. *Lancet* 2003; 362: 1527–1535.

Bosch J, Yusuf S, Pogue J, Sleight P, Lonn E, Rangoonwala B, Davies R, Ostergren J, Probstfield J, on behalf of the HOPE Investigators. Use of ramipril in preventing stroke: double-blind randomised trial. *British Medical Journal* 2002; 324: 1–5.

Carter A. Hypotensive therapy in stroke survivors. *Lancet* 1970; 1: 485–489.

Chapman N, Huxley R, Anderson C *et al.* effects of a perindopril-based blood pressure-lowering regimen on the risk of recurrent stroke according to stroke subtype and medical history. The PROGRESS Trial. *Stroke* 2004; 35: 116–121.

Collins R, Peto R, MacMahon S. Blood pressure, stroke and coronary heart disease. Part 2: Short-term reductions in blood pressure: overview of randomised drug trials in their epidemiological context. *Lancet* 1990; 335: 827–838.

The Dutch TIA Study Group. Trial of secondary prevention with atenolol after transient ischemic attack or nondisabling ischemic stroke. *Stroke* 1993; 24: 543–548.

Eriksson S, Olofsson B-O, Wester P-O. Atenolol in secondary prevention after stroke. *Cerebrovascular Diseases* 1995; 5: 21–25.

Gueyffier F, Boutitie F, Boissel J, Coope J, Cutler J, Ekbom T, Fagard R, Friedman L, Perry HM, Pocock S *et al.* INDANA: a meta-analysis on individual patient data in hypertension: protocol and preliminary results. *Therapie* 1995; 50: 353–362.

Gueyffier F, Boissel J-P, Boutitie F, Pocock S, Coope J, Cutler J, Ekbom T, Fagard R, Friedman L, Kerlikowske K *et al.*, for the INDANA (Individual Data Analysis of Antihypertensive Intervention Trial) Project Collaborators. Effect of antihypertensive treatment in patients having already suffered from stroke: gathering the evidence. *Stroke.* 1997; 28: 2557–2562.

The Heart Outcomes Prevention Evaluation Study Investigators. Effects of an angiotensin-converting-enzyme inhibitor, ramipril, on cardiovascular events in high-risk patients. *New England Journal of Medicine* 2000; 342: 145–153.

Hypertension-Stroke Cooperative Study Group. Effect of antihypertensive treatment on stroke recurrence. *Journal of the American Medical Association*, 1974; 229: 409–418.

Lawes CMM, Bennett DA, Feigin VL, Rodgers A. Blood pressure and stroke. An overview of published reviews. *Stroke* 2004; 35: 1024–1033.

MacMahon S, Peto R, Cutler J, Collins R, Sorlie P, Neaton J. Blood pressure, stroke and coronary heart disease. Part I: Effects of prolonged differences in blood pressure: evidence from nine prospective observational studies corrected for the regression dilution bias. *Lancet* 1990; 335: 765–774.

PATS Collaborating Group. Post-Stroke Antihypertensive Treatment Study: a preliminary result. *Chinese Medical Journal* 1995; 108: 710–717.

PROGRESS Collaborative Group. Randomised trial of a perindopril-based blood-pressure-lowering regimen among 6105 individuals with previous stroke or transient ischaemic attack. *Lancet* 2001; 358: 1033–1041.

Rashid P, Leonardi-Bee J, Bath P. Blood pressure reduction and secondary prevention of stroke and other vascular events a systematic review. *Stroke* 2003; 34: 2741–2749.

Rodgers A, MacMahon S, Gamble G, Slattery J, Sandercock P, Warlow C, for the United Kingdom Transient Ischaemic Attack Collaborative Group. Blood pressure and risk of stroke in patients with *cerebrovascular disease. British Medical Journal* 1996; 313: 147.

Schrader J, Lüders S, Kulschewski A *et al.* Morbidity and mortality after stroke, eprosartan compared with nitrendipine for secondary prevention. Principal results of a prospective, randomised controlled study (MOSES). *Stroke* 2005; 36: 1218–1226.

Sleight P, Yusuf S, Pogue J, Tsuyuki R, Diaz R, Probstfield J, for the Heart Outcomes Prevention Evaluation (HOPE) Study Investigators. Blood-pressure reduction and cardiovascular risk in HOPE study. *Lancet* 2001; 358: 2130–2131.

Staessen JA, Fagard R, Thijs L *et al.* Randomised double-blind comparison of placebo and active treatment for older patients with isolated systolic hypertension. The systolic hypertension in Europe (SYST-EUR) Trial Investigators. *Lancet* 1997; 350: 757–764.

Svensson P, de Faire U, Sleight P, Yusuf S, Östergren J. Comparative effects of ramipril on ambulatory and office blood pressures. A HOPE substudy. *Hypertension*, 2001; 38: e28–e32.

Chapter 13. Lowering blood cholesterol concentration

Acheson J, Hutchinson EC. Controlled trial of clofibrate in cerebral vascular disease. *Atherosclerosis* 1972; 15: 177–183.

AFCAPS/TexCAPS Research Group, Downs JR, Clearfield M, Weis S *et al.* Primary prevention of acute coronary events with lovastatin in men and women with average cholesterol levels. Results of AFCAPS/TexCAPS. *Journal of the American Medical Association* 1998; 279: 1615–1622.

Amarenco P, Tonkin AM. Statins for stroke prevention. Disappointment and hope. *Circulation* 2004; 109 (Suppl III): III-44–III-49.

Arntz H-R, Agrawal R, Wunderlich W *et al.* Beneficial effects of pravastatin (+cholestyramine/niacin) initiated immediately after a coronary event: the randomised Lipid-Coronary Artery Disease (L-CAD) study. *American Journal of Cardiology* 2000; 86: 1293–1298.

Asia Pacific Cohort Studies Collaboration. Cholesterol, coronary heart disease, and stroke in the Asia Pacific region. *International Journal of Epidemiology* 2003; 32: 563–572.

Bhatia M, Howard SC, Clarke TG, Murphy MFG, Rothwell PM. Apolipoproteins predict ischaemic stroke in patients with a previous transient ischaemic attack. Presented at the *World Stroke Congress*, Vancouver, Canada, June 23, 2004.

BIP Study Group. Secondary prevention by raising HDL cholesterol and reducing triglycerides in patients with coronary artery disease. *Circulation* 2000; 102: 21–27.

Byington RP, Davis BR, Plehn J *et al.* Reduction of stroke events with pravastatin: the Prospective Pravastatin Pooling (PPP) Project. *Circulation* 2001; 103: 387–392.

Cannon CP, Braunwald E, McCabe CH *et al.* Intensive versus moderate lipid lowering with statins after acute coronary syndromes. *New England Journal of Medicine* 2004; 350: 1495–1504.

Cholesterol Treatment Trialists' (CTT) Collaboration. Protocol for a prospective collaborative overview of all current and planned randomised trials of cholesterol treatment regimens. *American Journal of Cardiology* 1995; 75: 1130–1134.

Colhoun HM, Betteridge DJ, Durrington PN, on behalf of the CARDS investigators. Primary prevention of cardiovascular disease with atorvastatin in type 2 diabetes in the Colloborative Atorvastatin Diabetes Study (CARDS): multicentre randomised placebo-controlled trial. *Lancet* 2004; 364: 685–696.

Corvol J-C, Bousamondo A, Sirol M *et al.* Differential effects of lipid-lowering therapies on stroke prevention. A meta-analysis of randomised trials. *Archives of Internal Medicine* 2003; 163: 669–676.

Di Mascio R, Marchioli R, Tognoni G. Cholesterol reduction and stroke occurrence: an overview of randomised clinical trials. *Cerebrovascular Diseases* 2000; 10: 85–92.

Eastern Stroke and Coronary Heart Disease Collaborative Research Group. Blood pressure, cholesterol and stroke in Eastern Asia. *Lancet* 1998; 352: 1801–1807.

Heart Protection Study Collaborative Group. MRC/BHF Heart Protection Study of cholesterol lowering with simvastatin in 20, 536 high-risk individuals: a randomised placebo-controlled trial. *Lancet* 2002; 360: 7–22.

Heart Protection Study Collaborative Group. Effects of cholesterol-lowering with simvastatin on stroke and other major vascular events in 20,536 people with cerebrovascular disease or other high-risk conditions. *Lancet* 2004; 363: 757–767.

Horenstein RB, Smith DE, Mosca L, for the Women's Pooling Project Investigators. Cholesterol predicts stroke mortality in the Women's Pooling Project. *Stroke* 2002; 33: 1863–1868.

Iso H, Jacobs DR, Wentworth D, Neaton JD, Cohen JD, for the MRFIT Research Group. Serum cholesterol levels and six-year mortality from stroke in 350,977 men screened for the Multiple Risk Factor Intervention Trial. *New England Journal of Medicine* 1989; 320: 904–910.

Koren-Morag N, Tanne D, Graff E, Goldbourt U, for the Bezafibrate Infarction Prevention Study Group. Low- and high-density lipoprotein cholesterol and ischemic *cerebrovascular disease*. The Bezafibrate Infarction Prevention Registry. *Archives of Internal Medicine* 2002; 162: 993–999.

Law MR, Wald NJ, Rudnicka AR. Quantifying effect of statins on low density lipoprotein cholesterol, ischaemic heart disease and stroke: systematic review and meta-analysis. *British Medical Journal* 2003; 326: 1423–1429.

Leppala JM, Virtamo J, Fogelholm R, Albanes D, Heinonen OP. Different risk factors for different stroke subtypes. *Stroke* 1999; 30: 2535–2540.

Liem A, van Boven AJ, Withagen AP *et al.* Fluvastatin in acute myocardial infarction: effects of early and late ischaemia and events – the FLORIDA trial. *Circulation* 2000; 102: 2672-d (abstract).

Manktelow B, Gillies C, Potter JF. Interventions in the management of serum lipids for preventing stroke recurrence. *The Cochrane Database of Systematic Reviews* 2002, Issue 3. Art. No.: CD002091. DOI: 10.1002/14651858.CD002091.

Plehn JF, Davis BR, Sacks FM, Rouleau JL, Pfeffer MA, Bernstein V, Cuddy TE, Moyé LA, Piller LB, Rutherford JD, Simpson LM, Braunwald E. Reduction of stroke incidence after myocardial infarction with pravastatin: the Cholesterol and Recurrent Events (CARE) study. The CARE Investigators. *Circulation* 1999; 99: 216–223.

Prospective Studies Collaboration. Cholesterol, diastolic blood pressure, and stroke: 13,000 strokes in 450,000 people in 45 prospective cohorts. *Lancet* 1995; 346: 1647–1653.

Rubins HB, Robins SJ, Collins D *et al.* Gemfibrozil for the secondary prevention of coronary heart disease in men with low levels of high-density lipoprotein cholesterol. *New England Journal of Medicine* 1999; 341: 410–417.

Scandinavian Simvastatin Survival Study Group. Randomised trial of cholesterol lowering in 4444 patients with coronary disease: the Scandinavian Simvastatin Survival Study (4S). *Lancet* 1994; 344: 1383–1389.

Schwartz GG, Olsson AG, Ezekowitz MD, Ganz P, Oliver MF, Waters D *et al.*, for the Myocardial Ischemia Reduction with Aggressive Cholesterol Lowering (MIRACL) Study Investigators. Effects of atrovastatin on early recurrent ischaemic events in acute coronary syndromes. The MIRACL Study: A randomised controlled trial. *Journal of the American Medical Association* 2001; 285: 1711–1718.

Simons LA, McCallum J, Friedlander Y, Simons J. Risk factors for ischaemic stroke. *Stroke* 1998; 29: 1341–1346.

Simons LA, Simons J, Friedlander Y, McCallum J. Cholesterol and other lipids predict CHD and ischaemic stroke in the elderly, but only in those below 70 years. *Atherosclerosis* 2001; 159: 201–208.

The SPARCL Investigators. Design and baseline characteristics of the Stroke Prevention by Aggressive Reduction in Cholesterol Levels (SPARCL) Study. *Cerebrovascular Diseases* 2003; 16: 389–395.

Tanne D, Yaari S, Goldbourt U. High-density lipoprotein cholesterol and risk of ischaemic stroke mortality. *Stroke* 1997; 28: 83–87.

White HD, Simes RJ, Anderson NE, Hankey GJ, Watson JDG, Hunt D, Colquhoun DM, Glasziou P, MacMahon SR, Kirby AC, West MJ, Tonkin AM. Pravastatin therapy and the risk of stroke. *New England Journal of Medicine* 2000; 343: 317–326.

The Veterans Administration Cooperative Study Group. The treatment of cerebrovascular disease with Clofibrate. Final report of the Veterans Administration Cooperative Study of Atherosclerosis, Neurology Section. *Stroke* 1973; 4: 684–693.

Chapter 14. Control of lifestyle and other vascular risk factors

Alam S, Johnson AG. A meta-analysis of randomised controlled trials (RCT) among healthy normotensive and essential hypertensive elderly patients to determine the effect of high salt (NaCl) diet on blood pressure. *Journal of Human Hypertension* 1999; 13: 367–374.

American Diabetes Association. Standards of medical care for patients with diabetes mellitus. *Diabetes Care* 2003; 26: (Suppl 1): S33–S50.

Antithrombotic Trialists' Collaboration. Collaborative meta-analysis of randomised trials of antiplatelet therapy for prevention of death, myocardial infarction, and stroke in high risk patients. *British Medical Journal* 2002; 324: 71–86.

Appel LJ, Moore TJ, Obarzanek E *et al.* A clinical trial of the effects of dietary patterns on blood pressure. *New England Journal of Medicine* 1997; 336: 1117–1123.

Appel LJ, Champagne CM, Harsha DW *et al.* Effects of comprehensive lifestyle modification on blood pressure control. Mains results of the PREMIER clinical trial. *Journal of the American Medical Association* 2003; 289: 2083–2093.

Asia Pacific Cohort Studies Collaboration. Blood glucose and risk of cardiovascular disease in the Asia Pacific region. *Diabetes Care* 2004; 27: 2836–2842.

B-Vitamin Treatment Trialists' Collaboration. Homocysteine-lowering trials for prevention of cardiovascular events: a review of the design and power of the large randomised trials. *American Heart Journal* 2005 (in press).

Bath PMW, Gray LJ. Association between hormone replacement therapy and subsequent stroke. *British Medical Journal* 2005; 330: 342–345.

Beral V, Banks E, Reeves G. Evidence from randomised trials on the long-term effects of hormone replacement therapy. *Lancet* 2002; 360: 942–944.

Bonita R, Duncan J, Truelson T, Jackson R, Beaglehole R. Passive smoking as well as active smoking increases the risk of stroke. Tobacco Control 8, 1999; 156–160.

Chan WS, Ray J, Wai EK *et al.* Risk of stroke in women exposed to low-dose oral contraceptives. *Archives of Internal Medicine* 2004; 164: 741–747.

Chiasson J-L, Josse RG, Gomis R *et al.* for the STOP-NIDDM Trial Research Group. Acarbose for prevention of type 2 diabetes mellitus: the STOP-NIDDM randomised trial. *Lancet* 2002; 359: 2072–2077.

Chiasson J-L, Joss RG, Gomis R *et al.* Acarbose treatment and the risk of cardiovascular disease and hypertension in patients with impaired glucose tolerance. The STOP-NIDDM trial. *Journal of the American Medical Association* 2003; 290: 486–494.

Colhoun HM, Betteridge DJ, Durrington PN, on behalf of the CARDS investigators. Primary prevention of cardiovascular disease with atorvastatin in type 2 diabetes in the Collaborative Atorvastatin Diabetes Study (CARDS): multicentre randomised placebo-controlled trial. *Lancet* 2004; 364: 685–696.

Collins R, MacMahon S. Blood pressure, antihypertensive drug treatment and the risks of stroke and of coronary heart disease. *British Medical Bulletin* 1994; 50 (2): 272–298.

Cook NR, Cohen J, Hebert PR, Tayloer JO, Hennekens CH. Implications of small reductions in diastolic blood pressure for primary prevention. *Archives of Internal Medicine* 1995; 155: 701–709.

Crawford F, Langhorne P. Time to review all the evidence for hormone replacement therapy. *British Medical Journal* 2005; 330: 345.

Cutler JA, Follmann D, Allender PS. Randomised trials of sodium restriction: an overview. *American Journal of Clinical Nutrition* 1997; 65 (Suppl 2): 643–651S.

Davey Smith G. Effect of passive smoking on health. *British Medical Journal* 2003; 326: 1048–1049.

Daviglus ML, Orencia AJ, Dyer AR *et al.* Dietary vitamin C, beta-carotene and 30-year risk of stroke: results from the Western Electric Study. *Neuroepidemiology* 1997; 16: 69–77.

The Diabetes Control and Complications Trial/Epidemiology of Diabetes Interventions and Complications Research Group. Intensive diabetes therapy and carotid intima-media thickness in type 1 diabetes mellitus. *New England Journal of Medicine* 2003; 348: 2294–2303.

Diabetes Prevention Program Research Group. Reduction in the incidence of type 2 diabetes with lifestyle intervention or metformin. *New England Journal of Medicine* 2002; 346: 393–403.

Donnan GA, You R, Thrift A, Mcneil JJ Smoking as a risk factor for stroke. *Cerebrovascular Diseases* 1993; 3: 129–138.

Faraci FM, Lentz SR. Hyperhomocysteinemia, oxidative stress, and cerebral vascular dysfunction. *Stroke* 2004; 35: 345–347.

Foster C, Murphy M, Nicholas JJ, Pignone M, and Bazian Ltd. Cardiovascular disorders. Primary Prevention. In: *Clinical Evidence* F. Godlee (ed.), BMJ Publishing Group Ltd, London, 2004.

Fung T, Stampfer M, Manson J *et al.* Prospective study of major dietary patterns and stroke risk in women. *Stroke* 2004; 35: 2014–2019.

Gaede P, Vedel P, Larsen N *et al.* Multifactorial intervention and cardiovascular disease in patients with type 2 diabetes. *New England Journal of Medicine* 2003; 348: 383–393.

Gillum LA, Mamidipudi SK, Johnston SC. Ischaemic stroke risk with oral contraceptives. A meta-analysis. *Journal of the American Medical Association* 2000; 284: 72–78.

GISSI-Prevenzione Investigators. Dietary supplementation with n-3 polyunsaturated fatty acids and vitamin E after myocardial infarction: results of the GISSI-Prevenzione trial. *Lancet* 1999; 354: 447–455.

Grady D, Yaffe K, Kristof M *et al.* Effect of postmenopausal hormone replacement therapy on cognitive function: the Heart and Estrogen/progestin Replacement Study. *American Journal of Medicine* 2002; 113: 543–548.

Graudal NA, Galloe AM, Garred P. Effects of sodium restriction on blood pressure, renin, aldosterone, catecholamines, cholesterols, and triglyceride: a meta-analysis. *Journal of the American Medical Association* 1998; 279: 1383–1391.

Green DM, Ropper AH, Kronmal RA *et al.* Serum potassium level and dietary potassium intake as risk factors for stroke. *Neurology* 2002; 59: 314–320.

Hankey GJ. Smoking and risk of stroke. *Journal of Cardiovascular Risk* 1999; 6: 207–211.

Hankey GJ, Eikelboom JW. Folic acid-based multivitamin therapy to prevent stroke – the jury is still out. *Stroke* 2004; 35: 1995–1998.

Hankey GJ, Eikelboom JW. Homocysteine and stroke. *Lancet* 2005; 365: 194–196.

Hart RG, Pearce LA. Serum potassium level and dietary potassium intake as risk factors for stroke. *Neurology* 2003; 60: 1869–1870.

He FJ, MacGregor GA. Effect of longer-term modest salt reduction on blood pressure. *The Cochrane Database of Systematic Reviews* 2004, Issue 1. Art. No.: CD004937. DOI: 10.1002/14651858. CD004937.

He K, Rimm EB, Merchant A *et al.* Fish consumption and risk of stroke in men. *Journal of the American Medical Association* 2002; 288: 3130–3136.

He K, Merchant A, Rimm EB *et al.* Dietary fat intake and risk of stroke in male US healthcare professionals: 14 year prospective cohort study. *British Medical Journal* 2003; 327: 777–781.

He K, Merchant A, Rimm EB *et al.* Folate, vitamin B6, and B12 intakes in relation to risk of stroke among men. *Stroke* 2004; 35: 169–174.

Heart Protection Study Collaborative Group. MRC/BHF Heart Protection Study of antioxidant vitamin supplementation in 20,536 high-risk individuals: a randomised placebo-controlled trial. *Lancet* 2002; 360: 23–33.

Heart Protection Study Collaborative Group. MRC/BHF Heart Protection Study of cholesterol-lowering with simvastatin in 5963 people with diabetes: a randomised placebo-controlled trial. *Lancet* 2003; 361: 2005–2016.

Heart Outcomes Prevention Evaluation (HOPE) Study Investigators. Effects of ramipril on cardiovascular and microvascular outcomes in people with diabetes mellitus: results of the HOPE study and MICRO-HOPE substudy. *Lancet* 2000a; 355: 253–259.

Heart Outcomes Prevention Evaluation Study Investigators Vitamin E supplementation and cardiovascular events in high-risk patients. *New England Journal of Medicine* 2000b; 342: 154–160.

Heart Outcomes Prevention Evaluation Study Investigators Effects of an agiotensin-converting enzyme inhibitor, ramipiril, on cardiovascular events in high-risk patients. *New England Journal of Medicine* 2000c; 342: 145–153.

Hillbom M, Juvela S, Numminen H. Alcohol intake and risk of stroke. *Journal of Cardiovascular Risk* 1999; 6: 223–228.

Hommel M, Jaillard A. Alcohol and stroke prevention. *New England Journal of Medicine* 1999; 341: 1605–1606.

Homocysteine Lowering Trialists' Collaboration. Lowering blood homocysteine with folic acid based supplements: meta-analysis of randomised trials. *British Medical Journal* 1998; 316: 894–898.

The Homocysteine Studies Collaboration. Homocysteine and risk of ischemic heart disease and stroke. A meta-analysis. *Journal of the American Medical Association* 2002; 288: 2015–2022.

Hooper L, Bartlett C, Davey Smith G, Ebrahim S. Systematic review of long term effects of advice to reduce dietary salt in adults. *British Medical Journal* 2002; 325: 628–637.

Hooper L, Bartlett C, Davey Smith G, Ebrahim S. Advice to reduce dietary salt for prevention of cardiovascular disease. *The Cochrane Database of Systematic Reviews* 2004, Issue 1. Art. No.: CD003656.pub2. DOI: 10.1002/14651858.CD003656.pub2.

Jamrozik K, Anderson CA, Stewart-Wynne EG. The role of lifestyle factors in the etiology of stroke. A population- based case–control study in Perth, Western Australia. *Stroke* 1994; 25: 51–59.

Jacques PF, Selhub J, Bostom AG, Wilson PW, Rosenberg IH: The effect of folic acid fortification on plasma folate and total homocysteine concentrations. *New England Journal of Medicine* 1999; 340: 1449–1454.

John JJ, Ziebland S, Yudkin P, Roe LS, Neil HAW, for the Oxford Fruit and Vegetable Study Group. Effects of fruit and vegetable consumption on plasma antioxidant concentrations and blood pressure: a randomised controlled trial. *Lancet* 2002; 359: 1969–1974.

Kawachi I, Colditz GA, Stampfer MJ *et al.* Smoking cessation and decreased risk of stroke in women. *Journal of the American Medical Association* 1993; 269: 232–236.

Keli SO, Hertog MGL, Feskens EJM, Kromhout D. Dietary flavonoids, antioxidant vitamins, and incidence of stroke. *Archives of Internal Medicine* 1996; 156: 637–642.

Kris-Etherton PM, Harris WS, Appel LJ, for the Nutrition Committee. Fish consumption, fish oil, omega-3 fatty acids, and cardiovascular disease. *Circulation* 2002; 106: 2747–2757.

Kurth T, Gaziano JM, Berger K *et al.* Body mass index and the risk of stroke in men. *Archives of Internal Medicine* 2002; 162: 2557–2562.

Lancaster T, Stead LF. Physician advice for smoking cessation. *The Cochrane Database of Systematic Reviews* 2004, Issue 4. Art. No.: CD000165.pub2. DOI: 10.1002/14651858. CD000165.pub2.

Law MR, Frost CD, Wald NJ. By how much does dietary salt reduction lower blood pressure? III-Analysis of data from trials of salt reduction. *British Medical Journal* 1991a; 302: 819–824.

Law MR, Frost CD, Wald NJ I. By how much does dietary salt reduction lower blood pressure? I Analysis of observational data among populations. *British Medical Journal* 1991b; 302: 811–815.

Lawlor DA, Davey Smith G, Kundu D, Bruckdorfer KR, Ebrahim S. Those confounded vitamins: What can we learn from the differences between observational versus randomised trial evidence? *Lancet* 2004; 363: 1724–27.

Lee CD, Folsom AR, Blair SN. Physical activity and stroke risk. A meta-analysis. *Stroke* 2003; 34: 2475–2482.

Legge SD, Spence JD, Tamayo A, Hachinski V. Serum potassium level and dietary potassium intake as risk factors for stroke. *Neurology* 2003; 60: 1869–1870.

Liu S, Manson JE, Stampfer MJ *et al.* Whole grain consumption and risk of ischaemic stroke in women. A prospective study. *Journal of the American Medical Association* 2000; 284: 1534–1540.

MacMahon S, Rodgers A. The epidemiological association between blood pressure and stroke: implications for primary and secondary prevention. *Hypertension Research* 1994a; 17 (Suppl I): S23–S32.

MacMahon S, Rodgers A. Blood pressure, antihypertensive treatment and stroke risk. *Journal of Hypertension* 1994b; 12 (Suppl 10): S5–S14.

MacMahon S, Peto R, Cutler J *et al.* Blood pressure, stroke and coronary heart disease. Part 1 – prolonged differences in blood pressure: prospective observational studies corrected for the regression dilution bias. *Lancet* 1990; 335: 765–774.

Manson JE, Stampfer MJ, Willett WC, Colditz GA, Speitzer FE, Hennekens CH. Antioxidant vitamin consumption and incidence of stroke in women (abstract). *Circulation* 1993; 87: 678.

Midgley JP, Matthew AG, Greenwood CM, Logan AG. Effect of reduced dietary sodium on blood pressure: a meta-analysis of randomised controlled trials. *Journal of the American Medical Association* 1996; 275: 1590–1597.

Morris CD, Carson S. Routine vitamin supplementation to prevent cardiovascular disease: a summary of the evidence for the US Preventive Services Task Force. *Annals of Internal Medicine* 2003; 139: 56–70.

Nelson HD, Humphrey LL, Nygren P *et al.* Postmenopausal hormone replacement therapy: scientific review. *Journal of the American Medical Association* 2002; 288: 872–881.

Ness A, Powles J. The role of diet, fruit and vegetables and antioxidants in the aetiology of stroke. *Journal of Cardiovascular Risk* 1999; 6: 229–234.

Peters MJ, Morgan LC. The pharmacotherapy of smoking cessation. *Medical Journal of Australia* 2002; 176: 486–490.

Peto, R. Smoking and death: the past 40 years and the next 40. *British Medical Journal* 1994; 309: 937–939.

Quinlivan EP, McPartlin J, McNulty H, Ward M, Strain JJ, Weir DG *et al.* Importance of both folic acid and vitamin B12 in reduction of risk of vascular disease. *Lancet* 2002; 359: 227–228.

Quist-Paulsen P, Gallefoss, F. Randomised controlled trial of smoking cessation intervention after admission for coronary heart disease. *British Medical Journal* 2003; 327: 1254–1257.

Rajan S, Wallace JI, Brodkin KI, Beresford SA, Allen RH, Stabler SP. Response of elevated methylmalonic acid to three dose levels of oral cobalamin in older adults. *Journal of the American Geriatrics Society* 2002; 50: 1789–1795.

Reynolds K, Lewis LB, Nolen JDL *et al.* Alcohol consumption and risk of stroke. A meta-analysis. *Journal of the American Medical Association* 2003; 289: 579–588.

Rothwell PM, Eliasziw M, Gutnikov SA, Fox AJ, Taylor W, Mayberg MR, Warlow CP, Barnett HJ, for the Carotid Endarterectomy Trialists' Collaboration. Pooled analysis of individual patient data from randomised controlled trials of endarterectomy for symptomatic carotid stenosis. *Lancet* 2003; 361: 107–116.

Sacco M, Pellegrini F, Roncaglioni MC *et al.* Primary prevention of cardiovascular events with low-dose aspirin and vitamin E in type 2 diabetic patients. Results of the Primary Prevention Project (PPP) trial. *Diabetes Care* 2003; 26: 3264–3272.

Saunders DH, Greig CA, Young A, Mead GE. Physical fitness training for stroke patients (Cochrane Corner). *Stroke* 2004; 35: 2235.

Sauvaget C, Nagano J, Allen N, Kodama K. Vegetable and fruit intake and stroke mortality in the Hiroshima/Nagasaki Life Span Study. *Stroke* 2003; 34: 2355–2360.

Seibert C, Barbouche E, Fagan J *et al.* Prescribing oral contraceptives for women older than 35 years of age. *Annals of Internal Medicine* 2003; 138: 54–64.

Shinton R, Beevers G. Meta-analysis of relation between cigarette smoking and stroke. *British Medical Journal* 1989; 298: 789–794.

Silagy C, Lancaster T, Stead L, Mant D, Fowler G. Nicotine replacement therapy for smoking cessation. The Cochrane Database of Systematic Reviews 2004, Issue 3. Art. No.: CD000146. pub2. DOI: 10.1002/14651858.CD000146.pub2.

Singh RB, Dubnov G, Niaz MA *et al.* Effect of an Indo-Mediterranean diet on progression of coronary artery disease in high risk patients (Indo-Mediterranean Diet Heart Study): a randomised single-blind trial. *Lancet* 2002; 360: 1455–1461.

Solomon CG. Reducing cardiovascular risk in type 2 diabetes. *New England Journal of Medicine* 2003; 348: 457–458.

Toole JF, Malinow R, Chambless L, Spence JD, Pettigrew LC, Howard VJ, Sides EG, Wang C-H, Stampfer M. Lowering homocysteine in patients with ischemic stroke to prevent recurrent stroke, myocardial infarction and death. The Vitamin Intervention for Stroke Prevention (VISP) randomised controlled trial. *Journal of the American Medical Association* 2004; 291: 565–575.

Trichopoulou A, Costacou T, Barnia C, Trichopoulos D. Adherence to a Mediterranean diet and survival in a Greek population. *New England Journal of Medicine* 2003; 348: 2599–2608.

Tuomilehto J, Rastenye D. Diabetes and glucose intolerance as risk factors for stroke. *Journal of Cardiovascular Risk* 1999; 6: 241–249.

UK Prospective Diabetes Study (UKPDS) Group. Intensive blood-glucose control with sulphonylureas or insulin compared with conventional treatment and risk of complications in patients with type 2 diabetes (UKPDS 33). *Lancet* 1998a; 352: 837–853. (Erratum, *Lancet* 1999; 354: 602).

UK Prospective Diabetes Study (UKPDS) Group. Effect of intensive blood-glucose control with metformin on complications in overweight patients with type 2 diabetes (UKPDS 34). *Lancet* 1998b; 352: 854–865. (Erratum, *Lancet* 1998; 352: 1557).

US Preventive Services Taks Force. Routine vitamin supplementation to prevent cancer and cardiovascular disease: recommendations and rationale. *Annals of Internal Medicine* 2003; 139: 51–55.

Vandenbroucke JP. When are observational studies as credible as randomised trials? *Lancet* 2004; 363: 1728–1731.

Vessey M, Painter R, Yeates. Mortality in relation to oral contraceptive use and cigarette smoking. *Lancet* 2003; 362: 185–191.

The VITATOPS Trial Study Group. The VITATOPS (Vitamins To Prevent Stroke) trial: Rationale and design of an international, large, simple, randomised trial of homocysteine-lowering multivitamin therapy in patients with recent transient ischaemic attack or stroke. *Cerebrovascular Diseases* 2002; 13: 120–126.

Vivekananthan DP, Penn MS, Sapp SK, Hsu A, Topol EJ. Use of antioxidant vitamins for the prevention of cardiovascular disease: meta-analysis of randomised trials. *Lancet* 2003; 361: 2017–2023.

Vokó Z, Hollander M, Hofman A, Koudstaal PJ, Breteler M. Dietary antioxidants and the risk of ischemic stroke. The Rotterdam Study. *Neurology* 2003; 61: 1273–1275.

Wald DS, Law M, Morris JK. Homocysteine and cardiovascular disease: evidence on causality from a meta-analysis. *British Medical Journal* 2002; 325: 1202–1206.

Wald DS, Law M, Morris JK. The dose–response relation between serum homocysteine and cardiovascular disease: implications for treatment and screening. *Eur J Cardiovasc Prevention Rehab* 2004; 11: 250–253.

Wassertheil-Smoller S, Hendrix SL, Limacher M *et al.*, for the WHI Investigators. Effect of oestrogen plus progestin on stroke in postmenopausal women. The Women's Health Initiative: a randomised trial. *Journal of the American Medical Association* 2003; 289: 2673–2684.

Whelton PK, He J, Cutler JA, Brancati FL, Appel LJ, Follmann D, Klag MJ. Effects of oral potassium on blood pressure: meta-analysis of randomized controlled clinical trials. *Journal of the American Medical Association* 1997; 277: 1624–1632.

Whelton PK, Appel LJ, Espeland MA, Applegate WB, Ettinger Jr WH, Kostis JB. Sodium reduction and weight loss in the treatment of hypertension in older persons: a randomized controlled trial of nonpharmacologic interventions in the elderly (TONE). *Journal of the American Medical Association* 1998; 279: 839–846.

Whincup PH, Gilg JA, Emberson JR *et al.* Passive smoking an risk of coronary heart disease and stroke: prospective study with cotinine measurement. *British Medical Journal* 2004; 329: 200–204.

WHO Collaborative Study of Cardiovascular Disease and Steroid Hormone Contraception. Haemorrhagic stroke, overall stroke risk, and combined oral contraceptives: results of an international, multicentre, case–control study. *Lancet* 1996; 348: 505–510.

Witzum JL. The oxidation hypothesis of atherosclerosis. *Lancet* 1994; 344: 793–795.

Chapter 15. Antithrombotic therapy for preventing recurrent cardiogenic embolism

Atrial fibrillation

Atrial Fibrillation Investigators. Risk factors for stroke and efficacy of antithrombotic therapy in atrial fibrillation. Analysis of pooled data from five randomised controlled trials. *Archives of Internal Medicine* 1994; 154: 1449–1457.

Berge E, Abdelnoor M, Nakstad PH, Sandset PM, on behalf of the HAEST Study Group. Low molecular-weight heparin versus aspirin in patients with acute ischaemic stroke and atrial fibrillation: a double-blind randomised study. *Lancet* 2000; 355: 1205–1210.

Bo S, Ciccone G, Scaglione L *et al.* Warfarin for non-valvular atrial fibrillation: still underused in the 21st century? *Heart* 2003; 89: 553–554.

Eikelboom J, Hankey G. Ximelagatran or warfarin in atrial fibrillation? *Lancet* 2004; 363: 734.

Executive Steering Committee, on behalf of the SPORTIF III Investigators. Stroke prevention with the oral direct thrombin inhibitor ximelagatran compared with warfarin in patients with non-valvular atrial fibrillation (SPORTIF III): randomised controlled trial. *Lancet* 2003; 362: 1691–1698.

Furuya H, Fernandez-Salguero P, Gregory W *et al.* Genetic polymorphism of CYP2C9 and its effect on warfarin maintenance dose requirement in patients undergoing anticoagulant therapy. *Pharmacogenetics* 1995; 5: 389–392.

Gage BF, Van Walraven C, Pearce L *et al.* Selecting patients with atrial fibrillation for anticoagulation. Stroke risk stratification in patients taking aspirin. *Circulation* 2004; 110: 2287–2292.

Gallus AS, Baker RI, Chong BH, Ockleford PA, Street AM, on behalf of the Australasian Society of Thrombosis and Haemostasis. Consensus guidelines for warfarin therapy. Recommendations from the Australasian Society of Thrombosis and Haemostasis. *Medical Journal of Australia* 2000; 172: 600–605.

Hankey GJ, Klijn CJM, Eikelboom JW. Ximelagatran or warfarin for stroke prevention in patients with atrial fibrillation? *Stroke* 2004; 35: 389–391.

Hart RG, Boop BS, Anderson DC. Oral anticoagulants and intracranial haemorrhage. Facts and hypotheses. *Stroke* 1995; 26: 1471–1477.

Hart RG, Benavente O, McBride R, Pearce LA. Antithrombotic therapy to prevent stroke in patients with atrial fibrillation: A meta-analysis. *Annals of Internal Medicine* 1999; 131: 492–501.

Hart RG, Halperin JL. Atrial fibrillation and stroke: concepts and controversies. *Stroke* 2001; 32: 803–808.

Hart RG, Palacio S, Pearce LA. Atrial fibrillation, stroke and acute antithrombotic therapy. Analysis of randomised clinical trials. *Stroke* 2002; 33: 2722–2727.

Heppell RM, Berkin KE, McLenachan JM, Davies JA. Haemostatic and haemodynamic abnormalities associated with left atrial thrombosis in non-rheumatic atrial fibrillation. *Heart* 1997; 77: 407–411.

Hirsh J, Dalen JE, Anderson DR *et al.* Oral anticoagulants. Mechanism of action, clinical effectiveness, and optimal therapeutic range. *Chest* 2001; 119: 8S–21S.

Kannel WB, Wolf PA, Benjamin EJ, Levy D. Prevalence, incidence, prognosis, and predisposing conditions for atrial fibrillation: population-based estimates. *American Journal of Cardiology* 1998; 82: 2N.

Lee WM, Larrey D, Olsson R *et al.* Hepatic findings in long-term clinical trials of ximelagatran. *Drug Safety* 2005; 28: 351–370.

Lip GY, Lip PL, Zarifis J *et al.* Fibrin D-dimer and beta-thromboglobulin as markers of thrombogenesis and platelet activation in atrial fibrillation: effects of introducing ultra-low-dosee warfarin and aspirin. *Circulation* 1996; 94 (3): 425–431.

McNamara RL, Tamariz LJ, Segal JB, Bass EB. Management of atrial fibrillation: review of the evidence for the role of pharmacologic therapy, electrical cardioversion, and echocardiography. *Annals of Internal Medicine* 2003; 139: 1018–1033.

Oldenburg J, Quenzel EM, Harbrecht U *et al.* Missense mutations at ALA-10 in the factor IX propeptide: an insignificant variant in normal life but a decisive cause of bleeding during oral anticoagulant therapy. *British Journal of Haematology* 1997; 98: 240–244.

Pérez-Gómez F, Alegría E, Brejón J *et al.* Comparative effects of antiplatelet, anticoagulant, or combined threapy in patients with valvular and nonvalvular atrial fibrillation. *Journal of the American College of Cardiology* 2004, 44: 1557–1566.

Peters NS, Schilling RJ, Kanagaratnam P, Markides V. Atrial fibrillation: strategies to control, combat, and cure. *Lancet* 2002; 359: 593–603.

Peterson GM, Boom K, Jackson L, Vial JH. Doctor's beliefs on the use of antithrombotic therapy in atrial fibrillation: identifying barriers to stroke prevention. *Internal Medicine Journal* 2002; 32: 15–23.

Sandercock PAG, Warlow CP, Jones LN, Starkey IR. Predisposing factors for cerebral infraction: the Oxfordshire Community Stroke Project. *British Medical Journal* 1989; 298: 75–80.

Sandercock P, Bamford J, Dennis M, Burn J, Slattery J, Jones L, Boonyakarnkul S, Warlow C. Atrial fibrillation and stroke: prevalence in different types of stroke and influence on early and long term prognosis (Oxfordshire Community Stroke Project). *British Medical Journal* 1992; 305: 1460–1465.

Saxena R, Lewis S, Berge E, Sandercock PAG, Koudstaal PJ, for the International Stroke Trial Collaborative Group. Risk of early death and recurrent stroke and effect of heparin in 3169 patients with acute ischaemic stroke and atrial fibrillation in the International Stroke Trial. *Stroke* 2001; 32: 2333–2337.

Shirani J, Alaeddini J. Structural remodeling of the left atrial appendage in patients with chronic non-valvular atrial fibrillation: implications for thrombus formation, systemic embolism, and assessment by transesophageal echocardiography. *Cardiovascular Pathology* 2000; 9: 95–101.

SPORTIF Executive Steering Committee for the SPORTIF V investigators. Ximelagatran vs warfarin for stroke prevention in patients with nonvalvular atrial fibrillation. A randomised Trial. *Journal of the American Medical Association* 2005; 293: 690–698.

Van Walraven C, Hart RG, Singer DE, Laupacis A, Connolly S, Petersen P, Koudstaal PJ, Chang Y, Hellemons B. Oral anticoagulants vs aspirin in nonvalvular atrial fibrillation: an individual patient meta-analysis. *Journal of the American Medical Association* 2002; 288: 2441–2448.

Longer-term prevention of recurrent cardiogenic ischaemic stroke
Anticoagulation vs control

Hart RG, Palacio S, Pearce LA. Atrial fibrillation, stroke and acute antithrombotic therapy. Analysis of randomised clinical trials. *Stroke* 2002; 33: 2722–2727.

Saxena R, Koudstaal PJ. Anticoagulants for preventing stroke in patients with nonrheumatic atrial fibrillation and a history of stroke or transient ischaemic attack. *The Cochrane Database of Systematic Reviews* 2004, Issue 1. Art. No.: CD000185. DOI: 10.1002/14651858.CD000185.pub2.

Saxena R, Koudstaal PJ. Anticoagulants for preventing stroke in patients with nonrheumatic atrial fibrillation and a history of stroke or transient ischaemic attack (Cochrane Corner). *Stroke* 2004b; 35: 1782–1783.

References to studies included in the Cochrane Review of oral anticoagulants vs control by Saxena and Koudstaal (2004)

EAFT 1993 {published data only}

EAFT (European Atrial Fibrillation Trial) Study Group. Secondary prevention in non-rheumatic atrial fibrillation after transient ischaemic attack or minor stroke. *Lancet* 1993; 342: 1255–1262.

VA-SPINAF 1992 {published data only}

Ezekowitz MD, Bridgers SL, James KE *et al.*, for the Veterans Affairs Stroke Prevention in Nonrheumatic Atrial Fibrillation Investigators. Warfarin in the prevention of stroke associated with nonrheumatic atrial fibrillation. *New England Journal of Medicine* 1992; 327: 1406–1412.

Additional references

AFASAK 1989

Petersen P, Boysen G, Godtfredsen J, Andersen ED, Andersen B. Placebo-controlled, randomised trial of warfarin and aspirin for prevention of thromboembolic complications in chronic atrial fibrillation. The Copenhagen AFASAK Study. *Lancet* 1989; i: 175–179.

AFI 1994

Atrial Fibrillation Investigators. Risk factors for stroke and efficacy of antithrombotic therapy in atrial fibrillation. *Archives of Internal Medicine* 1994; 154: 1449–1457.

BAATAF 1990

The Boston Area Anticoagulation Trial for Atrial Fibrillation Investigators. The effect of low-dose warfarin on the risk of stroke in patients with non-rheumatic atrial fibrillation. *New England Journal of Medicine* 1990; 323: 1505–1511.

Berge 2000

Berge E, Abdelnoor M, Nakstad PH, Sandset PM. Low molecular-weight heparin versus aspirin in patients with acute ischaemic stroke and atrial fibrillation: a double-blind randomised study. HAEST Study Group. *Lancet* 2000; 355: 1205–1210.

Bogousslavsky 1986

Bogousslavsky J, Hachinski VC, Boughner DR *et al.* Cardiac lesions and arterial lesions in carotid transient ischaemic attacks. *Archives of Neurology* 1986; 43: 223–228.

CAFA 1991

Connolly SJ, Laupacis A, Gent M, Roberts RS, Cairns JA, Joyner C, for the CAFA Study Coinvestigators. Canadian Atrial Fibrillation Anticoagulation (CAFA) Study. *Journal of the American College of Cardiology* 1991; 18: 349–355.

CETF 1986

Cerebral Embolism Task Force. Cardiogenic brain embolism. *Archives of Neurology* 1986; 43: 71–84.

EAFT 1995

EAFT Study Group. Optimal oral anticoagulant therapy in patients with nonrheumatic atrial fibrillation and recent cerebral ischemia. *New England Journal of Medicine* 1995; 333: 5–10.

Fisher 1979

Fisher CM. Reducing risks of cerebral embolism. *Geriatrics* 1979; 34: 59–66.

Flegel 1987

Flegel KM, Shipley MJ, Rose G. Risk of stroke in non-rheumatic atrial fibrillation. *Lancet* 1987; i: 526–529.

Harrison 1984

Harrison MJG, Marshall J. Atrial fibrillation, TIAs and completed stroke. *Stroke* 1984; 15: 441–442.

Hylek 1996

Hylek EM, Skates SJ, Sheehan MA, Singer DE. An analysis of the lowest effective intensity of prophylactic anticoagulation for patients with nonrheumatic atrial fibrillation. *New England Journal of Medicine* 1996; 335: 540–546.

Hylek 2003

Hylek EM, Go A, Chang Y, Jensvold M, Henault L, Selby J, Singer DE. Effect of intensity of oral anticoagulation on stroke severity and mortality in atrial fibrillation. *New England Journal of Medicine* 2003; 349: 1019–1026.

Kannel 1982

Kannel WB, Abbott RD, Savage DD, McNamara PM. Epidemiologic features of chronic atrial fibrillation: The Framingham study. *New England Journal of Medicine* 1982; 306: 1018–1022.

Kopecky 1987

Kopecky Sl, Gersh BJ, McGoon MD *et al*. The natural history of lone atrial fibrillation. *New England Journal of Medicine* 1987; 317: 669–674.

Koudstaal 1986

Koudstaal PJ, van Gijn J, Klootwijk APJ *et al*. Holter monitoring in patients with transient and focal ischaemic attacks of the brain. *Stroke* 1986; 17: 192–195.

Larrue 1997

Larrue V, von Kummer R, del Zoppo G, Bluhmki E. Hemorrhagic transformation in acute ischemic stroke. Potential contributing factors in the European Cooperative Acute Stroke Study. *Stroke* 1997; 28: 957–960.

Martin 1977

Martin A. Atrial fibrillation in the elderly. *British Medical Journal* 1977; 1: 712.

Olsson 1980

Olsson SB. Atrial fibrillation – some current problems. *Acta Medica Scandinavica* 1980; 207: 1–4.

Sandercock 1992

Sandercock P, Bamford J, Dennis M, Burn J, Slattery J, Burns L, Boonyakarnkul S, Warlow C. Atrial fibrillation and stroke: prevalence in different types of stroke and influence on early and long term prognosis (Oxfordshire community stroke project). *British Medical Journal* 1992; 305: 1460–1465.

Saxena 2001

Saxena R, Lewis S, Berge E, Sandercock PA, Koudstaal PJ. Risk of early death and recurrent stroke and effect of heparin in 3169 patients with acute ischemic stroke and atrial fibrillation in the International Stroke Trial. *Stroke* 2001; 32: 2333–2337.

Sherman 1986

Sherman DG, Goldman L, Whiting RB *et al*. Risk of thrombo-embolism in patients with atrial fibrillation. *Archives of Neurology* 1986; 43: 68–70.

SPAF 1991

The Stroke Prevention in Atrial Fibrillation Investigators. Stroke prevention in atrial fibrillation. Final results. *Circulation* 1991; 84: 527–539.

Whisnant 1999

Whisnant JP, Brown RD, Petty GW, O'Fallon WM, Sicks JD, Wiebers DO. Comparison of population-based models of risk factors for TIA and ischemic stroke. *Neurology* 1999; 53: 532–536.

Wolf 1983

Wolf PA, Dawber TR, Thomas HE. Epidemiologic assessment of chronic atrial fibrillation and risk of stroke: The Framingham study. *Neurology* 1983; 28: 973–977.

Wolf 1991

Wolf PA, Abbott RD, Kannel WB. Atrial fibrillation as an independent risk factor for stroke: the Framingham Study. *Stroke* 1991; 22: 983–988.

Antiplatelet therapy vs control

Antithrombotic Trialists' Collaboration. Collaborative meta-analysis of randomised trials of antiplatelet therapy for prevention of death, myocardial infarction, and stroke in high risk patients. *British Medical Journal* 2002; 324: 71–86.

Koudstaal PJ. Antiplatelet therapy for preventing stroke in patients with nonrheumatic atrial fibrillation and a history of stroke or transient ischemic attacks. *The Cochrane Database of Systematic Reviews* 1996, Issue 1. Art. No.: CD000186. DOI: 10.1002/14651858.CD000186.

References to studies included in the Cochrane Review of antiplatelet therapy vs control by Koudstaal (1996)

EAFT 1993 {published data only}

EAFT (European Atrial Fibrillation Trial) Study Group. Secondary prevention in nonrheumatic atrial fibrillation after transient ischaemic attack or minor stroke. *Lancet* 1993; 342: 1255–1262.

Anticoagulation vs antiplatelet therapy

Saxena R, Koudstaal PJ. Anticoagulants versus antiplatelet therapy for preventing stroke in patients with nonrheumatic atrial fibrillation and a history of stroke or transient ischemic attack. The Cochrane Database of Systematic Reviews 2003, Issue 4. Art. No.: CD000187.pub2. DOI: 10.1002/14651858.CD000187.pub2.

Saxena R, Koudstaal PJ. Anticoagulants versus antiplatelet therapy for preventing stroke in patients with nonrheumatic atrial fibrillation and a history of stroke or transient ischaemic attack. *Stroke* 2005; 36: 914–915.

Van Walraven C, Hart RG, Singer DE, Laupacis A, Connolly S, Petersen P, Koudstaal PJ, Chang Y, Hellemons B. Oral anticoagulants vs aspirin in nonvalvular atrial fibrillation: an individual patient meta-analysis. *Journal of the American Medical Association* 2002; 288: 2441–2448.

References to studies included in the Cochrane Review of anticoagulation versus antiplatelet therapy by Saxena and Koudstaal (2003)

EAFT 1993 {published data only}

EAFT (European Atrial Fibrillation Trial) Study Group. Secondary prevention in nonrheumatic atrial fibrillation after transient ischaemic attack or minor stroke. *Lancet* 1993; 342: 1255–1262.

SIFA 1997

Morocutti C, Amabile G, Fattapposta F, Nicolosi A, Matteoli S, Trappolini M *et al.* for the SIFA (Studio Italiano Fibrillazione Atriale) Investigators. Indobufen versus warfarin in the secondary prevention of major vascular events in nonrheumatic atrial fibrillation. *Stroke* 1997; 28: 1015–1021.

Patent Foramen Ovale

Braun MU, Fassbender D, Schoen SP *et al.* Transcatheter closure of patent foramen ovale in patients with cerebral ischaemia. *Journal of the American College of Cardiology* 2002; 39: 2019–2025.

Devuyst G, Bogousslavsky J, Ruchat P *et al.* Prognosis after stroke followed by surgical closure of patent foramen ovale: a prospective follow-up study with brain MRI and simultaneous trans-oesophageal and transcranial Doppler ultrasound. *Neurology* 1996; 47: 1162–1166.

Donnan GA, Davis SM. Patent foramen ovale and stroke: closure by further randomised trial is required! *Stroke* 2004; 35: 806.

Homma S, Di Tullio MR, Sacco RL, Sciacca RR, Smith C, Mohr JP. Surgical closure of patent foramen ovale in cyptogenic stroke patients. *Stroke* 1997; 28: 2376–2381.

Homma S, Di Tullio MR, Sacco RL, Sciacca RR, Smith C, Mohr JP, PFO in Cryptogenic Stroke Study (PICSS) Investigators. Effect of medical treatment in stroke patients with patent foramen ovale: patent foramen ovale in Cryptogenic Stroke Study. *Circulation* 2002; 105: 2625–2631.

Horton SC, Bunch TJ. Patent foramen ovale and stroke. *Mayo Clinic Proceedings* 2004; 79: 79–88.

Hung J, Landzberger MJ, Jenkins KJ *et al.* Closure of patent foramen ovale for paradoxical emboli: intermediate-term risk of recurrent neurological events following transcatheter device placement. *Journal of American College of Cardiology* 2000; 35: 1311–1316.

Jones EG, Calafiore P, Donnan GA, Tonkin AM. Evidence that patent foramen ovale is not a risk factor for cerebral ischaemic in the elderly. *American Journal of Cardiology* 1994; 74: 596–599.

Khairy P, O'Donnell CP, Landzberg MJ. Transcatheter closure versus medical therapy of patent foramen ovale and presumed paradoxical thromboemboli. *Annals of Internal Medicine* 2003; 139: 753–760.

Martin F, Sanchez PL, Doherty E *et al.* Percutaneous transcatheter closure of patients foramen ovale in patients with paradoxical embolism. *Circulation* 2002; 106: 1121–1126.

Mas JL, Arquizan C, Lamy C *et al.* Patent Foramen Ovale and Atrial Septal Aneurysm Study Group. Recurrent cerebrovascular events associated with patients foramen ovale, atrial septal aneurysm, or both. *New England Journal of Medicine* 2001; 345. 1740–1746.

Mattle HP, Meier B, Windecker S. PC trial Patent foramen ovale and Cryptogenic embolism. Ongoing Clinical Trial Abstracts, *International Stroke Conference, 2005*, New Orleans, Louisiana, CTP55.

Mohr JP, Thompson JL, Lazar RM *et al.* A comparison of warfarin and aspirin for the prevention of recurrent ischaemic stroke. *New England Journal of Medicine* 2001; 345: 1444–1451.

Mohr JP. Patent cardiac foramen ovale: stroke risk and closure. *Annals of Internal Medicine* 2003; 139: 787–788.

Petty GW, Khanderia BK, Meissner I *et al.* A population-based study of the relationship between patent foramen ovale and cerebrovascular ischaemic events (abstract). *Neurology* 2003; 60: A256.

Saver JL, Carroll JD, Hijazi ZM *et al.* Randomised evaluation of Recurrent Stroke comparing PFO closure to Established Current standard of care Treatment (RESPECT). Ongoing Clinical Trial Abstracts, *International Stroke Conference*, 2005, American Stroke Association, CTP42.

Tong DC, Becker KJ. Patent foramen ovale and recurrent stroke: closure is the best option: No. *Stroke* 2004; 35: 804–805.

US Food and Drug Administration. Humanitarian Device Exemption. HDE #H990011 February 2000.

Windecker S, Wahl A, Chatterjee T *et al.* Percutaneous closure of patent foramen ovale in patients with paradoxical embolism: long-term risk of recurrent thromboembolic events. *Circulation* 2000; 101: 893–898.

Infective endocarditis

Hart RG, Foster JW, Luther MF, Kanter MC. Stroke in infective endocarditis. *Stroke* 1990; 21: 695–700.

Hart RG, Boop BS, Anderson DC. Oral anticoagulants and intracranial haemorrhage. Facts and hypotheses. *Stroke* 1995; 26: 1471–1477.

Jones HR, Siekert RG. Neurological manifestations of infective endocarditis: review of clinical and therapeutic challenges. *Brain* 1989; 112: 1295–1315.

Kanter MC, Hart RG. Neurologic complications of infective endocarditis. *Neurology* 1991; 41: 1015–1020.

Krapf H, Skalej M, Voigt K. Subarachnoid hemorrhage due to septic embolic infarction in infective endocarditis. *Cerebrovascular Diseases* 1999; 9: 182–184.

Masuda J, Yutani C, Waki R, Ogata J, Kuriyama Y, Yamaguchi T. Histopathological analysis of the mechanisms of intracranial haemorrhage complicating infective endocarditis. *Stroke* 1992; 23: 843–850.

Moreillon P, Que Y-A. Infective endocarditis. *Lancet* 2004; 363: 139–149.

van der Meulen JHP, Weststrate W, van Gijn J, Habbema JDF. Is cerebral angiography indicated in infective endocarditis? *Stroke* 1992; 23: 1662–1667.

Salgado AV. Central nervous system complications of infective endocarditis. *Stroke* 1991; 22: 1461–1463.

Chapter 16. Arterial dissection and arteritis

Arterial dissection

Bassetti C, Carruzzo A, Sturzenegger M, Tuncdogan E. Recurrence of cervical artery dissection: a prospective study of 81 patients. *Stroke* 1996; 27: 1804–1807.

Brandt T, Grond-Ginsbach C. Spontaneous cervical artery dissection. From risk factors toward pathogenesis. *Stroke* 2002; 33: 657–658.

Gallai V, Caso V, Paciaroni M *et al.* Mild hyperhomocyst(e)inaemia: a possible risk factor for cervical artery dissection. *Stroke* 2001; 32: 714–718.

Grau AJ, Brandt T, Buggle F *et al.* Association of cervical artery dissection with recent infection. *Archives of Neurology* 1999; 56, 851–856.

Guillon B, Brunereau L, Biousse V, Djouhri H, Levy C, Bousser M-G. Long-term follow-up of aneurysms developed during extracranial internal carotid artery dissection. *Neurology* 1999; 53, 117–122.

Leys D, Moulin Th, Stojkovic *et al.* Follow-up of patients with history of cervical artery dissection. *Cerebrovascular Diseases* 1995; 5: 43–49.

Lyrer P, Engelter S. Antithrombotic drugs for carotid artery dissection. *The Cochrane Database of Systematic Reviews* 2003, Issue 1. Art. No.: CD000255. DOI: 10.1002/14651858.CD000255.

Lyrer P, Engelter S.(b) Antithrombotic drugs for carotid artery dissection (Cochrane Corner). *Stroke* 2004; 35: 613–614.

Mokri B, Sundt TM, Houser W, Piepgras DG. Spontaneous dissection of the cervical internal carotid artery. *Annals of Neurology* 1986; 19: 126–138.

O'Connell BK, Towfighi J, Brennan RW *et al.* Dissecting aneurysms of head and neck. *Neurology* 1985; 35: 993–997.

Pepin M, Schwarze U, Superti-Furga A, Byers PH. Clinical and genetic features of Ehlers-Danlos syndrome type IV, the vascular type. *New England Journal of Medicine* 2000; 342: 673–680.

Peters M, Bohl J, Thomke F *et al.* Dissection of the internal carotid artery after chiropractic manipulation of the neck. *Neurology* 1995; 45: 2284–2286.

Pezzini A, Del Zotto E, Archetti S *et al.* Plasma homocysteine concentration, C677T *MTHFR* genotype, and 844ins68bp *CBS* genotype in young adults with spontaneous cervical artery dissection and atherothrombotic stroke. *Stroke* 2002; 33: 664–669.

Rothwell DM, Bondy SJ, Williams JI. Chiropractic manipulation and stroke: a population-based case–control study. *Stroke* 2001; 32: 1054–1060.

Schievink WI, Mokri B, Piepgras DG, Kuiper JD. Recurrent spontaneous arterial dissections: risk in familial versus non-familial disease. *Stroke* 1996; 27, 622–624.

Schievink WI, Wijdicks EFM, Michels VV, Vockley J, Godfrey M. Heritable connective tissue disorders in cervical artery dissections: a prospective study. *Neurology* 1998; 50: 1166–1169.

Schievink W. Spontaneous dissection of the carotid and vertebral arteries. *New England Journal of Medicine* 2001; 344: 898–906.

Sturzenegger M, Mattle HP, Rivoir A, Baumgartner RW. Ultrasound findings in carotid artery dissection. Analysis of 43 patients. *Neurology* 1995; 45: 691–698.

Arteritis

Calvo-Romero JM. Giant cell arteritis. *Postgraduate Medical Journal* 2003; 79: 511–515.

Caselli RJ, Hunder GG, Whisnant JP. Neurologic disease in biopsy-proven giant cell (temporal) arteritis. *Neurology* 1988; 38: 685–689.

Hankey GJ: Isolated angiitis/angiopathy of the central nervous system. *Cerebrovascular Diseases* 1991; 1: 2–15.

Hayreh SS, Steroid therapy for visual loss in patients with giant-cell arteritis. *Lancet* 2000; 355: 1572–1574.

Moore PM, Richardson B. Neurology of the vasculitides and connective tissue diseases. *Journal of Neurology Neurosurgery and Psychiatry* 1998; 65: 10–22.

Moore PM. Central nervous system vasculitis. *Current Opinion on Neurology* 1998; 11: 241–246.

Salvarani C, Cantini F, Boiardi L, Hunder GG. Polymyalgia rheumatic and giant-cell arteritis. *New England Journal of Medicine* 2002; 347: 261–271.

Scolding NJ, Wilson H, Hohlfeld *et al.*, for the EFNS Cerebral Vasculitis Taks Force. The recognition, diagnosis and management of cerebral vasculitis: a European survey. *European Journal of Neurology* 2002; 9: 343–347.

Swannell AJ. Polymyalgia rheumatica and temporal arteritis: diagnosis and management. *British Medical Journal* 1997; 314: 1329–1332.

Woolfenden AR, Tong DC, Marks MP, Ali AO, Albers GW. Angiographically defined primary angiitis of the CNS: is it really benign? *Neurology* 1998; 51, 183–188.

Chapter 17. Treatment of intracerebral haemorrhage

Adams RE, Diringer MN. Response to external ventricular drainage in spontaneous intracerebral hemorrhage with hydrocephalus. *Neurology* 1998; 50: 519–523.

Arkin S, Cooper HA, Hutter JJ, Miller S, Schmidt ML, Seibel NL, Shapiro A, Warrier I. Activated recombinant human coagulation factor VII therapy for intracranial hemorrhage in patients with hemophilia A or B with inhibitors. Results of the NovoSeven emergency-use program. *Haemostasis* 1998; 28: 93–98.

Auer LM, Deinsberger W, Neiderkorn K, Gell G, Kleinert R, Schneider G, Holzer P, Bone G, Mokry M, Korner E, Kleinert G, Hanusch S. Endoscopic surgery versus medical treatment for spontaneous intracerebral haematoma: a randomised study. *Journal of Neurosurgery* 1989; 70: 530–535.

Batjer HH, Reisch JS, Allen BC, Plaizier LJ, Jen Su C. Failure of surgery to improve outcome in hypertensive putaminal hemorrhage: a prospective randomised trial. *Archives of Neurology* 1990; 47: 1103–1106.

Beatty RM, Zervas NT. Stereotactic aspiration of a brain stem hematoma. *Neurosurgery* 1973; 13: 204–207.

Becker KJ, Baxter AB, Bybee HM, Tirschwell DL, Abouelsaad T. Extravasation of radiographic contrast is an independent predictor of death in primary intracerebral hemorrhage. *Stroke* 1999: 30: 2025–2032.

Bell BA, Smith MA, Kean DM, McGhee CN *et al.* Brain water measured by magnetic resonance imaging: correlation with direct estimation and changes after mannitol and dexamethasone. *Lancet* 1987; 1: 66–69.

Bosch DA, Beute GN. Successful stereotaxic evacuation of an acute pontomedullary hematoma: case report. *Journal of Neurosurgery* 1985; 62: 153–156.

Broderick JP, Brott T, Tomsick T, Tew J, Duldner J, Huster G. Management of intracerebral hemorrhage in a large metropolitan population. *Neurosurgery* 1994; 34: 882–887.

Broderick JP, Adams Jr HP, Barsan W *et al.* Guidelines for the management of spontaneous intracerebral hemorrhage: a statement for healthcare professionals from a special writing group of the Stroke Council, American Heart Association. *Stroke* 1999; 30: 905–915.

Brott T, Broderick J, Kothari R, Barsan W, Tomsick T, Sauerbeck L, Spilker J, Duldner J, Khoury J. Early hemorrhage growth in patients with intracerebral hemorrhage. *Stroke* 1997; 28: 1–5.

Brown DL, Morgenstern LB. Stopping the bleeding in intracerebral haemorrhage. *New England Journal of Medicine* 2005; 352: 828–830.

Butler AC, Tait RC. Management of oral anticoagulant-induced intracranial haemorrhage. *Blood Reviews* 1998; 12: 35–44.

Collins R, Scrimgeour A, Yusuf S, Peto R Reduction in fatal pulmonary embolism and venous thrombosis by perioperative administration of subcutaneous heparin: overview of results of randomized trials in general, orthopedic, and urologic surgery. *New England Journal of Medicine* 1988; 318: 1162–1173.

Darby JM, Yonas H, Marion DW, Latchaw RE Local 'inverse steal' induced by hyperventilation in head injury. *Neurosurgery* 1988; 23: 84–88.

Daverat P, Castel JP, Dartigues JF, Orgogozo JM. Death and functional outcome after spontaneous intracerebral hemorrhage: a prospective study of 166 cases using multivariate analysis. *Stroke* 1991; 22: 1–6.

Dickmann U, Voth E, Schicha H, Henze T, Prange H, Emrich D. Heparin therapy, deep-vein thrombosis and pulmonary embolism after intracerebral hemorrhage. *Klinische Wochenschrift* 1988; 66: 1182–1183.

Dunne JW, Chakera T, Kermode S. Cerebellar haemorrhage: diagnosis and treatment: a study of 75 consecutive cases. *Quarterly Journal of Medicine* 1987; 64: 739–754.

Eleff SM, Borel C, Bell WR, Long DM. Acute management of intracranial hemorrhage in patients receiving thrombolytic therapy: case reports. *Neurosurgery* 1990; 26, 867–869.

Fernandes H, Mendelow A. Spontaneous intracerebral hemorrhage: a surgical dilemma. *British Journal of Neurosurgery* 1999; 13: 389–394.

Fernandes HM, Gregson B, Siddique S, Mendelow AD. Surgery in intracerebral hemorrhage. The uncertainty continues. *Stroke* 2000; 31: 2511–2516.

Fewel ME, Park P. The emerging role of recombinant-activated factor VII in neurocritical care. *Neurocritical Care* 2004; 1: 19–30.

Fisher CM, Picard EH, Polak A, Dalal P. Ojemann R. Acute hypertensive cerebellar hemorrhage. *Journal of Nervous and Mental Disease* 1965; 140: 38–57.

Fogelholm R, Avikainen S, Murros K. Prognostic value and determinants of first-day mean arterial pressure in spontaneous supratentorial intracerebral hemorrhage. *Stroke* 1997; 28: 1396–1400.

Franke CL, van Swieten JC, Algra A, van Gijn J. Prognostic factors in patients with intracerebral haematoma. *Journal of Neurology Neurosurgery and Psychiatry* 1992; 55: 653–657.

Fredriksson K, Norrving B, Stromblad LG. Emergency reversal of anticoagulation after intracerebral hemorrhage. *Stroke* 1992; 23: 972–977.

Grandi FC, Sandercock P, Miccio M, Salvi RM. Physical methods for preventing deep vein thrombosis in stroke. *Stroke* 2005; 36: 1102–1103 (Cochrane Corner).

Hemphill JC, Bonovich DC, Besmertis L *et al.* The ICH Score: a simple, reliable grading scale for intracerebral haemorrhage. *Stroke* 2001; 32: 891–897.

Hosseini H, Leguerinel C, Hariz M *et al.* Stereotactic aspiration of deep intracerebral haematomas under computed tomographic control. A multicenter prospective randomised trial. *12th European Stroke Conference 2003*, Valencia, Spain, 57.

Juvela S, Heiskanen O, Poranen A, Valtonen S, Kuurne T, Kaste M, Troupp H. The treatment of spontaneous intracerebral hemorrhage: a prospective randomised trial of surgical and conservative treatment. *Journal of Neurosurgery* 1989; 70: 755–758.

Kase CS, Robinson RK, Stein RW *et al.* Anticoagulant-related intracerebral hemorrhage. *Neurology* 1985; 35: 943–948.

Kazui S, Naritomi H, Yamamoto H, Sawada T, Yamaguchi T. Enlargement of spontaneous intracerebral hemorrhage. Incidence and time course. *Stroke* 1996; 27: 1783–1787.

Keir SL, Lewis SC, Wardlaw JM, Sandercock PA, on behalf of IST and CAST Collaborative Groups Effect of aspirin or heparin given to patients with hemorrhagic stroke (abstract). *Stroke* 2000; 31: 314.

Kobayashi S, Sato A, Kageyama Y, Nakamura H, Watanabe Y, Yamaura A. Treatment of hypertensive cerebellar hemorrhage: surgical or conservative management? *Neurosurgery* 1994; 34: 246–250.

Kushner MJ, Bressman SB. The clinical manifestations of pontine hemorrhage. *Neurology* 1985; 35: 637–643.

Lapointe M, Haines S. Fibrinolytic therapy for intraventricular hemorrhage in adults. *The Cochrane Database of Systematic Reviews* 2002, Issue 2. Art. No.: CD003692. DOI: 10.1002/14651858.CD003692.

Leker RR, Abramsky O. Early anticoagulation in patients with prosthetic heart valves and intracerebral hematoma. *Neurology* 1998; 50: 1489–1491.

Lisk DR, Pasteur W, Rhoades H, Putnam RD, Grotta JC. Early presentation of hemispheric intracerebral hemorrhage: prediction of outcome and guidelines for treatment allocation. *Neurology* 1994; 44: 133–139.

Lui TN, Fairholm DJ, Shu TF, Chang CN, Lee ST, Chen HR. Surgical treatment of spontaneous cerebellar hemorrhage. *Surgical Neurology* 1985; 23: 555–558.

McKissock W, Richardson A, Taylor J. Primary intracerebral haemorrhage: a controlled trial of surgical and conservative treatment in 180 unselected cases. *Lancet* 1961; ii: 221–226.

Mahaffey KW, Granger CB, Sloan MA *et al.* Neurosurgical evacuation of intracranial hemorrhage after thrombolytic therapy for acute myocardial infarction: experience from the GUSTO-I Trial. *American Heart Journal* 1999; 138: 493–499.

Masiyama S, Niizuma H, Suzuki J. Pontine haemorrhage: a clinical analysis of 26 cases. *Journal of Neurology Neurosurgery and Psychiatry* 1985; 48: 658–662.

Mathew P, Teasdale G, Bannan A, Oluoch-Olunya D. Neurosurgical management of cerebellar haematoma and infarct. *Journal of Neurology Neurosurgery and Psychiatry* 1995; 59: 287–292.

Mayer SA, Brun N, Davis S, Broderick J, Diringer MN, Steiner T, for the US NovoSeven ICH Trial Investigators. Safety and preliminary efficacy of recombinant coagulation factor VIIa in acute intracerebral hemorrhage: US Phase 2A Study (abstract). *Stroke* 2004; 35: 332.

Mayer SA, Brun NC, Broderick J *et al.*, for the Europe/Australasia NovoSeven ICH Trial Investigators. Safety and feasibility of recombinant factor VIIa for acute intracerebral hemorrhage. *Stroke* 2005a; 36: 74–79.

Mayer SA, Brun NC, Begtrup K *et al.* Recombinant activated factor VII for acute intracerebral haemorrhage. *New England Journal of Medicine* 2005b; 352: 777–785.

Mendelow AD Mechanisms of ischemic brain damage with intracerebral hemorrhage. *Stroke* 1993; 24 (Suppl I): 115–117.

Mendelow AD, Gregson BA, Fernandes HM, Murray GD, Teasdale GM, Hope DT, Karimi A, Shaw MDM, Barer DH, for the STICH Investigators. Early surgery versus initial conservative treatment in patients with spontaneous supratentorial intracerebral haematomas in the International Surgical Trial in Intracerebral Haemorrhage (STICH): a randomised trial. *Lancet* 2005; 365: 387–397.

Monroe DM, Hoffman M, Oliver JA, Roberts HR. Platelet activity of high-dose factor VIIa is independent of tissue factor. *British Journal of Haematology* 1997; 99: 542–547.

Morgenstern LB, Frankowski RF, Shedden P, Pasteur W, Grotta JC. Surgical treatment for intracerebral hemorrhage (STICH): a single-center, randomised clinical trial. *Neurology* 1998; 51: 1359–1363.

Muizelaar JP, Lutz HA, Becker DP. Effect of mannitol on ICP and CBF and correlation with pressure autoregulation in severely head-injured patients. *Journal of Neurosurgery* 1984; 61: 700–706.

Muizelaar JP, Marmarou A, Ward JD *et al.* Adverse effects of prolonged hyperventilation in patients with severe head injury: a randomized clinical trial. *Journal of Neurosurgery* 1991; 75, 731–739.

Nieuwkamp DJ, de Gans K, Rinkel GJE, Algra A. Treatment and outcome of severe intraventricular extension in patients with subarachnoid or intracerebral hemorrhage: a systematic review of the literature. *Journal of Neurology* 2000; 247: 117–121.

Niizuma H, Suzuki J. Computed tomography-guided stereotactic aspiration of posterior fossa hematomas: a supine lateral retromastoid approach. *Neurosurgery* 1987; 21: 422–427.

NINDS ICH Workshop participants. Priorities for clinical research in intracerebral haemorrhage. *Stroke* 2005; 36: e23–e41.

Park P, Fewel ME, Garton HJ, Thompson BG, Hoff JT. Recombinant activated factor VII for the rapid correction of coagulopathy in nonhemophilic neurosurgical patients. *Neurosurgery* 2003; 53: 34–39.

Patrono C, Ciabattoni G, Patrignani P *et al.* Clinical pharmacology of platelet cyclooxygenase inhibition. *Circulation* 1985; 72: 1177–1184.

Portenoy RK, Lipton RB, Berger AR, Lesser ML, Lantos G. Intracerebral haemorrhage: a model for the prediction of outcome. *Journal of Neurology Neurosurgery and Psychiatry* 1987; 50: 976–979.

Poungvarin N, Bhoopat W, Viriyavejakul A *et al.* Effects of dexamethasone in primary supratentorial intracerebral hemorrhage. *New England Journal of Medicine* 1987; 316: 1229–1233.

Prasad K, Shrivastava A. Surgery for primary supratentorial intracerebral haemorrhage. *The Cochrane Database of Systematic Reviews* 1999, Issue 2. Art. No.: CD000200. DOI: 10.1002/14651858.CD000200.

Ramas R, Salem BI, De Pawlikowski MP, Goordes C, Eisenberg S, Leidenfrost R. The efficacy of pneumatic compression stockings in the prevention of pulmonary embolism after cardiac surgery. *Chest* 1996; 109: 82–85.

Roberts HR, Monroe III DM, Hoffman M. Safety profile of recombinant factor VIIa. *Seminars in Hematology* 2004; 41 (Suppl 1): 101–108.

Ropper AH. Lateral displacement of the brain and level of consciousness in patients with an acute hemispheral mass. *New England Journal of Medicine* 1986; 314: 953–958.

Ropper AH. Treatment of intracranial hypertension. In: *Neurological and Neurosurgical Intensive Care* 3rd edition, Ropper AH (ed.), New York: Raven Press, 1993: 29–52.

Sandercock P, Collins R, Counsell C *et al.* The International Stroke Trial (IST): a randomised trial of aspirin, subcutaneous heparin, both, or neither among 19,435 patients with acute ischaemic stroke. *Lancet* 1997; 349: 1569–1581.

St Louis EK, Wijdicks EFM, Li HZ. Predicting neurologic deterioration in patients with cerebellar hematomas. *Neurology* 1998; 51: 1364–1369.

Taneda M, Hayakawa T, Mogami H. Primary cerebellar hemorrhage: quadrigeminal cistern obliteration on CT scans as a predictor of outcome. *Journal of Neurosurgery* 1987; 67: 545–552.

Teernstra O, Evers S, Lodder J, Leffers P, Franke C, Blaauw G. Stereotactic treatment of intracerebral haematoma by means of plasminogen activator. A multicenter randomised controlled trial (SICHPA). *Stroke* 2003; 34: 968–974.

Tellez H, Bauer RB. Dexamethasone as treatment in cerebrovascular disease, 1: a controlled study in intracerebral hemorrhage. *Stroke* 1973; 4: 541–546.

Tuhrim S, Dambrosia JM, Price TR *et al.* Intracerebral hemorrhage: external validation and extension of a model for prediction of 30-day survival. *Annals of Neurology* 1991; 29: 658–663.

Wells PS, Lensing AWA, Hirsh J. Graduated compression stockings in the prevention of postoperative venous thromboembolism: a meta-analysis. *Archives of Internal Medicine* 1994; 154: 67–72.

Wijdicks EFM, Schievink WI, Brown RD, Mullany CJ. The dilemma of discontinuation of anticoagulation therapy for patients with intracranial hemorrhage and mechanical heart valves. *Neurosurgery* 1998; 42, 769–773.

Young WB, Lee KP, Pessin MS, Kwan ES, Rand WM, Caplan LR. Prognostic significance of ventricular blood in supratentorial hemorrhage: a volumetric study. *Neurology* 1990; 40: 616–619.

Yu YL, Kumana CR, Lauder IJ *et al.* Treatment of acute cerebral hemorrhage with intravenous glycerol: a double-blind, placebo-controlled, randomized trial. *Stroke* 1992; 23: 967–971.

Zuccarello M, Brott T, Derex L, Kothari R, Sauerbeck L, Tew J, Van Loveren H, Yeh HS, Tomsick T, Pancioli A, Khoury J, Broderick J. Early surgical treatment for supratentorial intracerebral hemorrhage: a randomised feasibility study. *Stroke* 1999; 30: 1833–1839.

Chapter 18. Treatment of subarachnoid haemorrhage

Agnelli G, Piovella F, Buoncristiani P *et al.* Enoxaparin plus compression stockings compared with compression stockings alone in the prevention of venous thromboembolism after elective neurosurgery. *New England Journal of Medicine* 1998; 339: 80–85.

Amin-Hanjani S, Schwartz RB, Sathi S, Stieg PE. Hypertensive encephalopathy as a complication of hyperdynamic therapy for vasospasm: report of two cases. *Neurosurgery* 1999; 44: 1113–1116.

Anon. Protease inhibitors for delayed cerebral ischemia after subarachnoid haemorrhage? *Lancet* 1992; 339: 1199–1200.

Asano T, Takakura K, Sano K *et al.* Effects of a hydroxyl radical scavenger on delayed ischemic neurological deficits following aneurysmal subarachnoid hemorrhage: results of a multicenter, placebo-controlled double-blind trial. *Journal of Neurosurgery* 1996; 84: 792–803.

Awad IA, Carter LP, Spetzler RF, Medina M, Williams Jr FC. Clinical vasospasm after subarachnoid hemorrhage: response to hypervolemic hemodilution and arterial hypertension. *Stroke* 1987; 18: 365–372.

Ayus JC, Krothapalli RK, Arieff AI. Treatment of symptomatic hyponatremia and its relation to brain damage: a prospective study. *New England Journal of Medicine* 1987; 317: 1190–1195.

Bauer LA. Interference of oral phenytoin absorption by continuous nasogastric feedings. *Neurology* 1982; 32: 570–572.

Bavinzski G, Talazoglu V, Killer M *et al.* Gross and microscopic histopathological findings in aneurysms of the human brain treated with Guglielmi detachable coils. *Journal of Neurosurgery* 1999a; 91: 284–293.

Bejjani GK, Bank WO, Olan WJ, Sekhar LN. The efficacy and safety of angioplasty for cerebral vasospasm after subarachnoid hemorrhage. *Neurosurgery* 1998; 42: 979–986.

van den Bergh WM, on behalf of the MASH Study Group. Magnesium Sulphate in aneurysmal subarachnoid haemorrhage. A randomised, controlled trial. Stroke 2005; 36: 1011–1015.

Biller J, Godersky JC, Adams Jr HP. Management of aneurysmal subarachnoid hemorrhage. *Stroke* 1988; 19: 1300–1305.

Black PM, Crowell RM, Abbott WM. External pneumatic calf compression reduces deep venous thrombosis in patients with ruptured intracranial aneurysms. *Neurosurgery* 1986; 18: 25–28.

Brilstra EH, Rinkel GJE, van der Graaf Y, van Rooij WJJ, Algra A. Treatment of intracranial aneurysms by embolization with coils: a systematic review. *Stroke* 1999; 30: 470–476.

Broderick JP, Brott TG, Duldner JE, Tomsick T, Leach A. Initial and recurrent bleeding are the major causes of death following subarachnoid hemorrhage. *Stroke* 1994; 25: 1342–1347.

Brouwers PJAM, Wijdicks EFM, Hasan D *et al.* Serial electrocardiographic recording in aneurysmal subarachnoid hemorrhage. *Stroke* 1989; 20: 1162–1167.

Brouwers PJAM, Wijdicks EFM, van Gijn J. Infarction after aneurysm rupture does not depend on distribution or clearance rate of blood. *Stroke* 1992; 23: 374–379.

Calhoun DA, Oparil S. Treatment of hypertensive crisis. *New England Journal of Medicine* 1990; 323: 1177–1183.

Candia GL, Heros RC, Lavine MH *et al.* Effect of intravenous sodium nitroprusside on cerebral blood flow and intracranial pressure. *Neurosurgery* 1978; 3: 50–53.

Crawford MD, Sarner M. Ruptured intracranial aneurysm: a community study. *Lancet* 1965; ii: 1254–1257.

Eskridge JM, McAuliffe W, Song JK *et al.* Balloon angioplasty for the treatment of vasospasm: results of first 50 cases. *Neurosurgery* 1998; 42: 510–516.

Farhat SM, Schneider RC Observations on the effect of systemic blood pressure on intracranial circulation in patients with cerebrovascular insufficiency. *Journal of Neurosurgery* 1967; 27: 441–445.

Findlay JM, Kassell NF, Weir BKA *et al.* A randomized trial of intraoperative, intracisternal tissue plasminogen activator for the prevention of vasospasm. *Neurosurgery* 1995; 37: 168–178.

Fodstad H, Pilbrant A, Schannong M, Strömberg S. Determination of tranexamic acid and fibrin/fibrinogen degradation products in cerebrospinal fluid after aneurysmal subarachnoid haemorrhage. *Acta Neurochirurgica* (Wien) 1981; 58: 1–13.

Foy PM, Chadwick DW, Rajgopalan N, Johnson AL, Shaw MD. Do prophylactic anticonvulsant drugs alter the pattern of seizures after craniotomy? *Journal of Neurology Neurosurgery and Psychiatry* 1992; 55: 753–757.

Fujii Y, Takeuchi S, Sasaki O, Minakawa T, Koike T, Tanaka R. Ultra-early rebleeding in spontaneous subarachnoid hemorrhage. *Journal of Neurosurgery* 1996; 84: 35–42.

Gifford RW Jr. Management of hypertensive crises. *Journal of the American Medical Association* 1991; 266: 829–835.

van Gijn J, van Dongen KJ. The time course of aneurysmal haemorrhage on computed tomograms. *Neuroradiology* 1982; 23: 153–156.

van Gijn J, Hijdra A, Wijdicks EFM, Vermeulen M, van Crevel H. Acute hydrocephalus after aneurysmal subarachnoid hemorrhage. *Journal of Neurosurgery* 1985; 63: 355–362.

Greenberg DA. Calcium channels and calcium channel antagonists. *Annals of Neurology* 1987; 21: 317–330.

Gruber A, Ungersböck K, Reinprecht A *et al.* Evaluation of cerebral vasospasm after early surgical and endovascular treatment of ruptured intracranial aneurysms. *Neurosurgery* 1998a; 42: 258–267.

Guglielmi G, Vinuela F, Duckwiler G *et al.* Endovascular treatment of posterior circulation aneurysms by electrothrombosis using electrically detachable coils. *Journal of Neurosurgery* 1992; 77: 515–524.

Haley Jr EC, Kassell NF, Apperson-Hansen C, Maile MH, Alves WM. A randomized, double-blind, vehicle-controlled trial of tirilazad mesylate in patients with aneurysmal subarachnoid hemorrhage: a cooperative study in North America. *Journal of Neurosurgery* 1997; 86: 467–474.

Harrier HD. Use of labetalol in trauma. *Critical Care Medicine* 1988; 16: 1159–1160.

Harrigan MR. Cerebral salt wasting syndrome: a review. *Neurosurgery* 1996; 38: 152–160.

Hart RG, Byer JA, Slaughter JR, Hewett JE, Easton JD. Occurrence and implications of seizures in subarachnoid hemorrhage due to ruptured intracranial aneurysms. *Neurosurgery* 1981; 8: 417–421.

Hasan D, Vermeulen M, Wijdicks EFM, Hijdra A, van Gijn J. Effect of fluid intake and antihypertensive treatment on cerebral ischemia after subarachnoid hemorrhage. *Stroke* 1989a; 20: 1511–1515.

Hasan D, Lindsay KW, Wijdicks EFM *et al.* Effect of fludrocortisone acetate in patients with subarachnoid hemorrhage. *Stroke* 1989b; 20: 1156–1161.

Hasan D, Vermeulen M, Wijdicks EFM, Hijdra A, van Gijn J. Management problems in acute hydrocephalus after subarachnoid hemorrhage. *Stroke* 1989c; 20: 747–753.

Hasan D, Wijdicks EFM, Vermeulen M. Hyponatremia is associated with cerebral ischemia in patients with aneurysmal subarachnoid hemorrhage. *Annals of Neurology* 1990; 27: 106–108.

Hasan D, Lindsay KW, Vermeulen M. Treatment of acute hydrocephalus after subarachnoid hemorrhage with serial lumbar puncture. *Stroke* 1991; 22: 190–194.

Hasan D, Schonck RS, Avezaat CJ, Tanghe HL, van Gijn J, van der Lugt PJ. Epileptic seizures after subarachnoid hemorrhage. *Annals of Neurology* 1993; 33: 286–291.

Hauerberg J, Eskesen V, Rosenorn J. The prognostic significance of intracerebral haematoma as shown on CT scanning after aneurysmal subarachnoid haemorrhage. *British Journal of Neurosurgery* 1994; 8: 333–339.

Heiskanen O, Poranen A, Kuurne T, Valtonen S, Kaste M. Acute surgery for intracerebral haematomas caused by rupture of an intracranial arterial aneurysm: a prospective randomized study. *Acta Neurochirurgica* (Wien) 1988; 90: 81–83.

Higashida RT, Halbach VV, Cahan LD *et al.* Transluminal angioplasty for treatment of intracranial arterial vasospasm. *Journal of Neurosurgery* 1989; 71: 648–653.

Hijdra A, van Gijn J. Early death from rupture of an intracranial aneurysm. *Journal of Neurosurgery* 1982; 57: 765–768.

Hijdra A, Vermeulen M, van Gijn J, van Crevel H. Respiratory arrest in subarachnoid hemorrhage. *Neurology* 1984; 34: 1501–1503.

Hijdra A, van Gijn J, Stefanko S *et al.* Delayed cerebral ischemia after aneurysmal subarachnoid hemorrhage: clinicoanatomic correlations. *Neurology* 1986; 36: 329–333.

Hijdra A, Braakman R, van Gijn J, Vermeulen M, van Crevel H. Aneurysmal subarachnoid hemorrhage: complications and outcome in a hospital population. *Stroke* 1987a; 18: 1061–1067.

Hijdra A, Vermeulen M, van Gijn J, van Crevel H. Rerupture of intracranial aneurysms: a clinicoanatomic study. *Journal of Neurosurgery* 1987b; 67: 29–33.

Honma Y, Fujiwara T, Irie K, Ohkawa M, Nagao S. Morphological changes in human cerebral arteries after percutaneous transluminal angioplasty for vasospasm caused by subarachnoid hemorrhage. *Neurosurgery* 1995; 36: 1073–1081.

Hop JW, Rinkel GJE, Algra A, van Gijn J. Case-fatality rates and functional outcome after subarachnoid hemorrhage: a systematic review. *Stroke* 1997; 28: 660–664.

Hop JW, Rinkel GJE, Algra A, van Gijn J. Quality of life in patients and partners after aneurysmal subarachnoid hemorrhage. *Stroke* 1998; 29: 798–804.

Hop JW, Rinkel GJE, Algra A, van Gijn J. Initial loss of consciousness and risk of delayed cerebral ischemia after aneurysmal subarachnoid hemorrhage. *Stroke* 1999; 30: 2268–2271.

Inagawa T, Kamiya K, Ogasawara H, Yano T. Rebleeding of ruptured intracranial aneurysms in the acute stage. *Surgical Neurology* 1987; 28: 93–99.

Inagawa T, Tokuda Y, Ohbayashi N, Takaya M, Moritake K. Study of aneurysmal subarachnoid hemorrhage in Izumo City, Japan. *Stroke* 1995; 26: 761–766.

International Subarachnoid Aneurysm Trial (ISAT) Collaborative Group. International Subarachnoid Aneurysm Trial (ISAT) of neurosurgical clipping versus endovascular coiling in 2143 patients with ruptured intracranial aneurysms: a randomised trial. *Lancet* 2002; 360: 1267–1274.

Kaneko T, Sawada T, Niimi T Lower limit of blood pressure in treatment of acute hypertensive intracranial hemorrhage (AHCH). *Journal of Cerebral Blood Flow and Metabolism* 1983; 3 (Suppl 1): S51–S52.

Kassell NF, Torner JC. Aneurysmal rebleeding: a preliminary report from the Cooperative Aneurysm Study. *Neurosurgery* 1983; 13: 479–481.

Kassell NF, Peerless SJ, Durward QJ, Beck DW, Drake CG, Adams Jr HP. Treatment of ischemic deficits from vasospasm with intravascular volume expansion and induced arterial hypertension. *Neurosurgery* 1982; 11: 337–343.

Kassell NF, Torner JC, Haley Jr EC, Janc JA, Adams Jr HP, Kongable GL. The International Cooperative Study on the Timing of Aneurysm Surgery. 1: Overall management results. *Journal of Neurosurgery* 1990; 73: 18–36.

Kassell NF, Haley Jr EC, Apperson-Hansen C *et al*. Randomized, double-blind, vehicle-controlled trial of tirilazad mesylate in patients with aneurysmal subarachnoid hemorrhage: a cooperative study in Europe, Australia, and New Zealand. *Journal of Neurosurgery* 1996; 84: 221–228.

Kawai K, Nagashima H, Narita K *et al*. Efficacy and risk of ventricular drainage in cases of grade V subarachnoid hemorrhage. *Neurological Research* 1997; 19: 649–653.

Koivisto T, Vanninen R, Hurskainen H, Saari T, Hernesniemi J, Vapalahti M. Outcomes of early endovascular versus surgical treatment of ruptured cerebral aneurysms: a prospective randomized study. *Stroke* 2000; 31: 2369–2377.

Kosnik EJ, Hunt WE. Postoperative hypertension in the management of patients with intracranial arterial aneurysms. *Journal of Neurosurgery* 1976; 45: 148–154.

Lanzino G, Kassell NF. Double-blind, randomized, vehicle-controlled study of high-dose tirilazad mesylate in women with aneurysmal subarachnoid hemorrhage. 2: A cooperative study in North America. *Journal of Neurosurgery* 1999; 90: 1018–1024.

Lanzino G, Kassell NF, Dorsch NWC *et al*. Double-blind, randomized, vehicle-controlled study of high dose tirilazad mesylate in women with aneurysmal subarachnoid hemorrhage. 1: A cooperative study in Europe, Australia, New Zealand, and South Africa. *Journal of Neurosurgery* 1999b; 90: 1011–1017.

Lennihan L, Mayer SA, Fink ME *et al*. Effect of hypervolemic therapy on cerebral blood flow after subarachnoid hemorrhage: a randomized controlled trial. *Stroke* 2000; 31: 383–391.

Linskey ME, Horton JA, Rao GR, Yonas H. Fatal rupture of the intracranial carotid artery during transluminal angioplasty for vasospasm induced by subarachnoid hemorrhage: case report. *Journal of Neurosurgery* 1991; 74: 985–990.

Ljunggren B, Saveland H, Brandt L, Zygmunt S. Early operation and overall outcome in aneurysmal subarachnoid hemorrhage. *Journal of Neurosurgery* 1985; 62: 547–551.

Locksley HB. Report of the Cooperative Study on intracranial aneurÿysms and subarachnoid hemorrhage: Section V, part II. Natural history of subarachnoid hemorrhage, intracranial aneurysms, and arteriovenous malformations. *Journal of Neurosurgery* 1996; 25: 321–368.

McDougall CG, Halbach VV, Dowd CF, Higashida RT, Larsen DW, Hieshima GB. Causes and management of aneurysmal hemorrhage occurring during embolization with Guglielmi detachable coils. *Journal of Neurosurgery* 1998; 89: 87–92.

McKissock W, Richardson A, Walsh L. 'Posterior-communicating aneurysms': a controlled trial of conservative and surgical treatment of ruptured aneurysms of the internal carotid artery at or near the point of origin of the posterior communicating artery. *Lancet* 1960; I: 1203–1206.

McKissock W, Richardson A, Walsh L. Anterior communicating aneurysms: a trial of conservative and surgical treatment. *Lancet* 1965; I: 873–876.

Malek AM, Higashida RT, Phatouros CC, Dowd CF, Halbach VV. Treatment of an intracranial aneurysm using a new three-dimensional-shape Guglielmi detachable coil: technical case report. *Neurosurgery* 1999; 44: 1142–1144.

Manninen PH, Ayra B, Gelb AW, Pelz D. Association between electrocardiographic abnormalities and intracranial blood in patients following acute subarachnoid hemorrhage. *Journal of Neurosurgical Anesthesiology* 1995; 7: 12–16.

Mayer SA, Solomon RA, Fink ME *et al.* Effect of 5% albumin solution on sodium balance and blood volume after subarachnoid hemorrhage. *Neurosurgery* 1998; 42: 759–767.

Mendelow AD, Stockdill G, Steers AJ, Hayes J, Gillingham FJ. Double-blind trial of aspirin in patient receiving tranexamic acid for subarachnoid hemorrhage. *Acta Neurochirurgica* (Wien) 1982; 62: 195–202.

Miller JA, Dacey Jr RG, Diringer MN. Safety of hypertensive hypervolemic therapy with phenylephrine in the treatment of delayed ischemic deficits after subarachnoid hemorrhage. *Stroke* 1995; 26: 2260–2266.

Mizukami M, Kawase T, Usami T, Tazawa T. Prevention of vasospasm by early operation with removal of subarachnoid blood. *Neurosurgery* 1982; 10: 301–307.

Molyneux AJ, Ellison DW, Morris J, Byrne JV. Histological findings in giant aneurysms treated with Guglielmi detachable coils: report of two cases with autopsy correlation. *Journal of Neurosurgery* 1995; 83, 129–132.

Mori T, Katayama Y, Kawamata T, Hirayama T. Improved efficiency of hypervolemic therapy with inhibition of natriuresis by fludrocortisone in patients with aneurysmal subarachnoid hemorrhage. *Journal of Neurosurgery* 1999; 91: 947–952.

Newell DW, Eskridge JM, Mayberg MR, Grady MS, Winn HR. Angioplasty for the treatment of symptomatic vasospasm following subarachnoid hemorrhage. *Journal of Neurosurgery* 1989; 71: 654–660.

Nibbelink DW, Torner JC, Henderson WG. Randomised treatment study: drug-induced hypotension. In: Aneurysmal Subarachnoid Haemorrhage. Report of the Cooperative Study (eds Sahs AL, Nibbelink DW & Torner JC), Baltimore: Urban & Schwarzenberg, 1981: 77–106.

Nurmohamed MT, van Riel AM, Henkens CM *et al.* Low molecular weight heparin and compression stockings in the prevention of venous thromboembolism in neurosurgery. *Thrombosis and Haemostasis* 1996; 75: 233–238.

Öhman J, Heiskanen O. Timing of operation for ruptured supratentorial aneurysms: a prospective randomized study. *Journal of Neurosurgery* 1989; 70: 55–60.

Öhman J, Servo A, Heiskanen O. Risks factors for cerebral infarction in good-grade patients after aneurysmal subarachnoid hemorrhage and surgery: a prospective study. *Journal of Neurosurgery* 1991; 74, 14–20.

Olafsson E, Hauser WA, Gudmundsson G. A population-based study of prognosis of ruptured cerebral aneurysm: mortality and recurrence of subarachnoid hemorrhage. *Neurology* 1997; 48, 1191–1195.

O'Sullivan MG, Doward N, Whittle IR *et al.* Management and long-term outcome following subarachnoid haemorrhage and intracranial aneurysm surgery in elderly patients: an audit of 199 consecutive cases. *British Journal of Neurosurgery* 1994; 8: 23–30.

Paré L, Delfino R, Leblanc R. The relationship of ventricular drainage to aneurysmal rebleeding. *Journal of Neurosurgery* 1992; 76: 422–427.

Pickard JD, Murray GD, Illingworth R *et al.* Effect of oral nimodipine on cerebral infarction and outcome after subarachnoid haemorrhage: British aneurysm nimodipine trial. *British Medical Journal* 1989; 298: 636–642.

Pinto AN, Canhao P, Ferro JM. Seizures at the onset of subarachnoid haemorrhage. *Journal of Neurology* 1996; 243: 161–164.

Rinkel GJE, Wijdicks EFM, Ramos LMP, van Gijn J. Progression of acute hydrocephalus in subarachnoid haemorrhage: a case report documented by serial CT scanning. *Journal of Neurology Neurosurgery and Psychiatry* 1990; 53: 354–355.

Rinkel GJE, Feigin VL, Algra A, Vermeulen M, van Gijn J. Calcium antagonists for aneurysmal subarachnoid haemorrhage. *The Cochrane Database of Systematic Reviews* 2005, Issue 2. Art. No.: CD000277. DOI: 10.1002/14651858.CD000277.pub2.

Rinkel GJE, Feigin VL, Algra A, van Gijn J. Circulatory volume expansion therapy for aneurysmal subarachnoid haemorrhage. *The Cochrane Database of Systematic Reviews* 2004, Issue 1. Art. No.: CD000483. DOI: 10.1002/14651858.CD000483.pub2.

Rinkel GJE, Feigin VL, Algra A, van Gijn J. Hypervolaemia in aneurysmal subarachnoid haemorrhage. *Stroke* 2005; 36: 1104–1105 (Cochrane Corner).

Roos YBWEM, Beenen LF, Groen RJ, Albrecht KW, Vermeulen M. Timing of surgery in patients with aneurysmal subarachnoid haemorrhage: rebleeding is still the major cause of poor outcome in neurosurgical units that aim at early surgery. *Journal of Neurology Neurosurgery and Psychiatry* 1997; 63: 490–493.

Roos YBWEM, for the STAR Study Group. Antifibrinolytic treatment in subarachnoid hemorrhage: a randomized placebo-controlled trial. *Neurology* 2000; 54: 77–82.

Roos YBWEM, Rinkel GJE, Vermeulen M, Algra A, van Gijn J. Antifibrinolytic therapy for aneurysmal subarachnoid haemorrhage. *The Cochrane Database of Systematic Reviews* 2003, Issue 2. Art. No.: CD001245. DOI: 10.1002/14651858.CD001245.

Roos Y, Rinkel G, Vermeulen M, Algra A, van Gijn J. Antifibrinolytic therapy for aneurysmal subarachnoid haemorrhage. A major update of a Cochrane Review (Cochrane Corner). *Stroke* 2003; 34: 2308–2309.

Rose FC, Sarner M. Epilepsy after ruptured intracranial aneurysm. *British Medical Journal* 1965; 1: 18–21.

Rosenwasser RH, Delgado TE, Buchheit WA, Freed MH. Control of hypertension and prophylaxis against vasospasm in cases of subarachnoid hemorrhage: a preliminary report. *Neurosurgery* 1983; 12: 658–661.

Rosenwasser RH, Jallo JI, Getch CC, Liebman KE. Complications of Swan-Ganz catheterisation for haemodynamic monitoring in patients with subarachnoid haemorrhage. *Neurosurgery* 1995; 37: 872–875.

Rousseaux P, Scherpereel R, Bernard MH, Graftieaux JP, Guyot JF. Fever and cerebral vasospasm in intracranial aneurysms. *Surgical Neurology* 1980; 14: 459–465.

Saito I, Asano T, Ochiai C, Takakura K, Tamura A, Sano K. A. double-blind clinical evaluation of the effect of nizofenone (Y-9179) on delayed ischemic neurological deficits following aneurysmal rupture. *Neurological Research* 1983; 5: 29–47.

Saito I, Asano T, Sano K *et al.* Neuroprotective effect of an antioxidant, ebselen, in patients with delayed neurological deficits after aneurysmal subarachnoid hemorrhage. *Neurosurgery* 1998; 42: 269–277.

Schievink WI, Wijdicks EFM, Parisi JE, Piepgras DG, Whisnant JP. Sudden death from aneurysmal subarachnoid hemorrhage. *Neurology* 1995; 45: 871–874.

Schoser BG, Heesen C, Eckert B, Thie A. Cerebral hyperperfusion injury after percutaneous transluminal angioplasty of extracranial arteries. *Journal of Neurology* 1997; 244: 101–104.

Shaw MD, Foy PM, Conway M *et al.* Dipyridamole and postoperative ischemic deficits in aneurysmal subarachnoid hemorrhage. *Journal of Neurosurgery* 1985; 63: 699–703.

Shimoda M, Oda S, Shibata M, Tominaga J, Kittaka M, Tsugane R. Results of early surgical evacuation of packed intraventricular hemorrhage from aneurysm rupture in patients with poor-grade subarachnoid hemorrhage. *Journal of Neurosurgery* 1999; 91: 408–414.

Spetzger U, Reul J, Thron A, Warnke JP, Gilsbach JM. Microsurgical embolectomy and removal of a migrated coil from the middle cerebral artery. –*Cerebrovascular Diseases* 1997; 7: 226–231.

Sterns RH, Riggs JE, Schochet Jr SS. Osmotic demyelination syndrome following correction of hyponatremia. *New England Journal of Medicine* 1986; 314: 1535–1542.

Stiver SI, Porter PJ, Willinsky RA, Wallace C. Acute human histopathology of an intracranial aneurysm treated using Guglielmi detachable coils: case report and review of the literature. *Neurosurgery* 1998; 43: 1203–1207.

Suzuki S, Sano K, Handa H *et al.* Clinical study of OKY-046, a thromboxane synthetase inhibitor, in prevention of cerebral vasospasms and delayed cerebral ischaemic symptoms after subarachnoid haemorrhage due to aneurysmal rupture: a randomized double-blind study. *Neurological Research* 1989; 11: 79–88.

Theodore J, Robin ED. Speculations on neurogenic pulmonary oedema. *American Review of Respiratory Disease* 1976; 113: 405–411.

Tokiyoshi K, Ohnishi T, Nii Y. Efficacy and toxicity of thromboxane synthetase inhibitor for cerebral vasospasm after subarachnoid hemorrhage. *Surgical Neurology* 1991; 36: 112–118.

Torner JC, Nibbelink DW, Burmeister LF. Statistical comparisons of end results of a randomised treatment study. In: Sahs, AL, Nibbelink, DW, Torner, JC (eds), *Aneurysmal Subarachnoid Hemorrhage. Report of the Cooperative Study.* Baltimore: Urban & Schwarzenberg, 1981b: 249–275.

Vanninen R, Koivisto T, Saari T, Hernesniemi J, Vapalahti M. Ruptured intracranial aneurysms — acute endovascular treatment with electrolytically detachable coils: a prospective randomized study. *Radiology* 1999; 211: 325–336.

Vermeij FH, Hasan D, Bijvoet HWC, Avezaat CJJ. Impact of medical treatment on the outcome of patients after aneurysmal subarachnoid hemorrhage. *Stroke* 1998; 29: 924–930.

Vermeulen M, Lindsay KW, Murray GD *et al.* Antifibrinolytic treatment in subarachnoid hemorrhage. *New England Journal of Medicine* 1984a; 311: 432–437.

Vora YY, Suarez-Almazor M, Steinke DE, Martin ML, Findlay JM. Role of transcranial Doppler monitoring in the diagnosis of cerebral vasospasm after subarachnoid hemorrhage. *Neurosurgery* 1999; 44: 1237–1247.

Weir B, Grace M, Hansen J, Rothberg C. Time course of vasospasm in man. *Journal of Neurosurgery* 1978; 48: 173–178.

Wells PS, Lensing AWA, Hirsh J. Graduated compression stockings in the prevention of postoperative venous thromboembolism: a meta-analysis. *Archives of Internal Medicine* 1994; 154: 67–72.

Whitfield PC, Moss H, O'Hare D, Smielewski P, Pickard JD, Kirkpatrick PJ. An audit of aneurysmal subarachnoid haemor/rhage: earlier resuscitation and surgery reduces inpatient stay and deaths from rebleeding. *Journal of Neurology Neurosurgery and Psychiatry* 1996; 60: 301–306.

Whitfield PC, Kirkpatrick PJ. Timing of surgery for aneurysmal subarachnoid haemorrhage. *The Cochrane Database of Systematic Reviews* 2001, Issue 1. Art. No.: CD001697. DOI: 10.1002/14651858.CD001697.

Wijdicks EFM, Vermeulen M, ten Haaf JA, Hijdra A, Bakker WH, van Gijn J. Volume depletion and natriuresis in patients with a ruptured intracranial aneurysm. *Annals of Neurology* 1985a; 18: 211–216.

Wijdicks EFM, Vermeulen M, Hijdra A, van Gijn J. Hyponatremia and cerebral infarction in patients with ruptured intracranial aneurysms: is fluid restriction harmful? *Annals of Neurology* 1985b; 17: 137–140.

Wijdicks EFM, Vermeulen, M, van Brummelen P, van Gijn J. The effect of fludrocortisone acetate on plasma Volume and natriuresis in patients with aneurysmal subarachnoid hemorrhage. *Clinical Neurology and Neurosurgery* 1988a; 90: 209–214.

Wijdicks EFM, Vermeulen M, Murray GD, Hijdra A, van Gijn J. The effects of treating hypertension following aneurysmal subarachnoid hemorrhage. *Clinical Neurology and Neurosurgery* 1990; 92: 111–117.

Wijdicks EFM, Kokmen E, O'Brien, PC. Measurement of impaired consciousness in the neurological intensive care unit: a new test. *Journal of Neurology Neurosurgery and Psychiatry* 1998; 64: 117–119.

Wohns RN, Tamas L, Pierce KR, Howe JF. Chlorpromazine treatment for neurogenic pulmonary edema. *Critical Care Medicine* 1985; 13: 210–211.

References to studies included in the Cochrane Review by Roos *et al.* (2003) of antifibrinoytic treatment for SAH

Chandra 1978 {published data only}

Chandra B. Treatment of subarachnoid hemorrhage from ruptured intracranial aneurysm with tranexamic acid: a double-blind clinical trial. *Annals of Neurology* 1978; 3: 502–504.

Fodstad 1981 {published data only}

Fodstad H, Forssell A, Liliequist B, Schannong M. Antifibrinolysis with tranexamic acid in aneurysmal subarachnoid hemorrhage: a consecutive controlled clinical trial. *Neurosurgery* 1981; 8: 158–165.

Girvin 1973 {published and unpublished data}

Girvin JP. The use of antifibrinolytic agents in the preoperative treatment of ruptured intracranial aneurysms. *Transactions of the American Neurological Association* 1973; 98: 150–152.

Kaste 1979 {published data only}

Kaste M, Ramsay M. Tranexamic acid in subarachnoid hemorrhage. A double-blind study. *Stroke* 1979; 10: 519–522.

Maurice 1978 {published data only}

Maurice-Williams RS. Prolonged antifibrinolysis: an effective non-surgical treatment for ruptured intracranial aneurysms? *British Medical Journal* 1978; 1: 945–947.

Roos 2000 {published data only}

Roos Y, for the STAR-Study Group. Antifibrinolytic treatment in aneurysmal subarachnoid haemorrhage: A randomized placebo-controlled trial. *Neurology* 2000; 54: 77–82.

Tsementzis 1990 {published data only}

Tsementzis SA, Hitchcock ER, Meyer CH. Benefits and risks of antifibrinolytic therapy in the management of ruptured intracranial aneurysms. A double-blind placebo-controlled study. *Acta Neurochirurgica* 1990; 102: 1–10.

Tsementzis SA, Honan WP, Nightingale S, Hitchcock ER, Meyer CH. Fibrinolytic activity after subarachnoid haemorrhage and the effect of tranexamic acid. *Acta Neurochirurgica* 1990; 103: 116–121.

v. Rossum 1977 {published data only}

Van Rossum J, Wintzen AR, Endtz LJ, Schoen JHR, de Jonge H. Effect of tranexamic acid on rebleeding after subarachnoid hemorrhage: a double-blind controlled clinical trial. *Annals of Neurology* 1977; 2: 238–242.

Vermeulen 1984 {published data only}

Vermeulen M, Lindsay KW, Murray GD *et al.* Antifibrinolytic treatment in subarachnoid hemorrhage. *New England Journal of Medicine* 1984; 311: 432–437.

References to studies included in the Cochrane Review of calcium antagonists after SAH by Rinkel *et al.* (2001)

Allen 1983 {published data only}

Allen GS, Ahn HS, Preziosi TJ, Battye R, Boone SC, Chou SN, Kelly DL, Weir BK, Crabbe RA, Lavik PL, Rosenbloom SB, Dorsey FC, Ingram CR, Mellits DE, Bertsch LA, Boisvert DP, Hundley MB, Johnson RK, Strom JA, Transou CR. Cerebral arterial spasm – a controlled trial of Nimodipine in patients with subarachnoid hemorrhage. *New England Journal of Medicine* 1983; 308: 619–624.

Ferro 1990 {unpublished data only}

Ferro JM, Melo TP, Oliveira V, Trindade AM, Lobo-Antunes J, Campos JC. Prevention of vasospasm in subarachnoid hemorrhage with oral nicardipine. Unpublished study (personal communication) 1990.

Haley 1993 {published data only}

Haley EC, Kassell NF, Torner JC. A randomised controlled trial of high-dose intravenous nicardipine in aneurysmal subarachnoid hemorrhage. *Journal of Neurosurgery* 1993; 78: 537–547.

Haley EC, Kassell NF, Torner JC. A randomized trial of nicardipine in subarachnoid hemorrhage: angiographic and transcranial Doppler ultrasound results. *Journal of Neurosurgery* 1993; 78: 548–553.

Haley EC, Kassell NF, Torner JC, Kongable G. Nicardipine ameliorates angiographic vasospasm following subarachnoid hemorrhage (SAH) (abstract). *Neurology* 1991; 41 (Suppl 1): 346.

Han 1993 {published and unpublished data}

Han DH, Lee SH, Lee SH. Effect of nimodipine treatment on outcome in surgical cases of aneurysmal SAH. *Journal of Neurosurgery* 1993; 78: 346A.

Messeter 1987 {published data only}

Messeter K, Brandt L, Ljunggren B, Svendgaard NA, Algotsson L, Romner B, Ryding E. Prediction and prevention of delayed ischemic dysfunction after aneurysmal subarachnoid hemorrhage and early operation. *Neurosurgery* 1987; 20: 548–553.

Neil-Dwyer 1987 {published data only}

Mee E, Dorrance D, Lowe D, Neil-Dwyer G. Controlled study of nimodipine in aneurysm patients treated early after subarachnoid hemorrhage. *Neurosurgery* 1988; 22: 484–491.

Mee EW, Dorrance DE, Low D, Neil-Dwyer G. Cerebral blood flow and neurological outcome: a controlled study of nimodipine in patients with subarachnoid haemorrhage (abstract). *Journal of Neurology Neurosurgery and Psychiatry* 1986; 49: 469.

Neil-Dwyer G, Mee E, Dorrance D, Lowe D. Early intervention with nimodipine in subarachnoid haemorrhage. *European Heart Journal* 1987; 8: 41–47.

Ohman 1991 {published data only}

Juvela S, Kaste M, Hillbom M. Effect of nimodipine on platelet function in patients with subarachnoid hemorrhage. *Stroke* 1990; 21: 1283–1288.

Ohman J. Surgery for ruptured intracranial aneurysms: defining the present optimal conditions Dissertation. Finland: Helsingin Yliopisto, 1991.

Ohman J, Heiskanen O. Effect of nimodipine on the outcome of patients after aneurysmal subarachnoid hemorrhage and surgery. *Journal of Neurosurgery* 1988; 69(5): 683–686.

Ohman J, Servo A, Heiskanen O. Long-term effects of nimodipine on cerebral infarcts and outcome after aneurysmal subarachnoid hemorrhage and surgery. *Journal of Neurosurgery* 1991; 74: 8–13.

Petruk 1988 {published data only}

Disney LB. Cerebral vasospasm following subarachnoid hemorrhage: clinical investigation of oral nimodipine and factors influencing outcome (hemorrhage) Dissertation. *Dissertation Abstracts International* 1990; 52/11-B: 221.

Petruk KC, West M, Mohr G, Weir BKA, Benoit BG, Gentili F, Disney LB, Khan MI, Grace M, Holness RO, Karwon MS, Ford RM, Cameron GS, Tucker WS, Purves GB, Miller JDR, Hunter KM, Richard MT, Durity FA, Chan R, Clein LJ, Maroun FB, Godon A. Nimodipine treatment in poor-grade aneurysm patients. Results of a multicentre double-blind placebo-controlled trial. *Journal of Neurosurgery* 1988; 68: 505–517.

Philippon 1986 {published data only}

Philippon J, Grob R, Dagreou F, Guggiari M, Rivierez M, Viars P. Prevention of vasospasm in subarachnoid haemorrhage. A controlled study with Nimodipine. *Acta Neurochirurgica* 1986; 82: 110–114.

Pickard 1989 {published data only}

Pickard JD, Murray GD, Illingworth R, Shaw MDM, Teasdale GM, Foy PM, Humphrey PRD, Lang DA, Nelson R, Richards P, Sinar J, Bailey S, Skene A. Effect of oral nimodipine on cerebral infarction and outcome after subarachnoid haemorrhage: British aneurysm nimodipine trial. *British Medical Journal* 1989; 298: 636–642.

Shibuya 1992 {published data only}

Shibuya M, Suzuki Y. [Treatment of cerebral vasospasm by a protein kinase inhibitor AT877] [Japanese]. No to Shinkei – *Brain and Nerve* 1993; 45: 819–824.

Shibuya M, Suzuki Y, Sugita K, Saito I, Sasaki T, Takakura K, Nagata I, Kikuchi H, Takemae T, Hidaka H. Effect of AT877 on cerebral vasospasm after aneurysmal subarachnoid hemorrhage. Results of a prospective placebo controlled double blind trial. *Journal of Neurosurgery* 1992; 76: 571–577.

References to studies included in the Cochrane Review of circulatory volume expansion after SAH by Rinkel *et al.* (2004)

CPMC {published data only}

Klebanoff L, Fink ME, Lennihan L, Solomon RA, Mayer SA, Beckford AR *et al.* Management of cerebral vasospasm in the 1990s. *Clinical Neuropharmacology* 1995; 18 (2): 127–137.

Lennihan L, Mayer SA, Fink ME, Beckford A, Paik MC, Zhang H *et al.* Effect of hypervolemic therapy on cerebral blood flow after subarachnoid hemorrhage: a randomized controlled trial. *Stroke* 2000; 31: 383–391.

Lennihan L, Solomon RA, Beckford AR, Fink ME, Paik M *et al.* Comparison of effects of hypervolemia and normovolemia on cerebral blood flow after subarachnoid hemorrhage. *Stroke* 1997; 28: 249.

Lennihan L, Solomon RA, Fink ME, Paik M, Klebanoff L, Beckford AR *et al.* Comparison of effects of hypervolemia and normovolemia on clinical outcome and medical complications after subarachnoid hemorrhage. *Neurology* 1997; 3: 365.

Lennihan L, Solomon RA, Mayer SA, Prohovnik I, Fink ME, Klebanoff L *et al.* Effect of volume therapy on cerebral blood flow after subarachnoid hemorrhage. *Neurology* 1994; 44 (Suppl 2): 862S.

Mayer SA, Solomon RA, Fink ME, Lennihan L, Stern L, Beckford AR *et al.* Effect of 5% albumin solution on sodium balance and blood volume after subarachnoid hemorrhage. *Neurosurgery* 1998; 42: 759–768.

Index